Pediatric Cataract Surgery

Techniques, Complications, and Management

Pediatric Cataract Surgery
Techniques, Complications, and Management

EDITORS

M. Edward Wilson, Jr., M.D.

Director, Storm Eye Institute, Department of Ophthalmology
Medical University of South Carolina, Charleston, South Carolina

Rupal H. Trivedi, M.D.

Assistant Professor, Storm Eye Institute, Department of Ophthalmology
Medical University of South Carolina, Charleston, South Carolina

Suresh K. Pandey, M.D.

Assistant Professor, Department of Ophthalmology & Visual Sciences
John A. Moran Eye Center, University of Utah, Salt Lake City, Utah

Intraocular Implant Unit, Sydney Hospital & Sydney Eye Hospital
Scholar to the University of Sydney, Save Sight Institute and
Discipline of Ophthalmology, Sydney, NSW, Australia

Formerly Post-Doctoral Fellow, Storm Eye Institute
Department of Ophthalmology, Medical University of South Carolina
Charleston, South Carolina

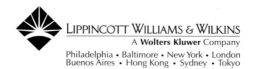

LIPPINCOTT WILLIAMS & WILKINS
A **Wolters Kluwer** Company
Philadelphia • Baltimore • New York • London
Buenos Aires • Hong Kong • Sydney • Tokyo

Acquisitions Editor: Jonathan Pine
Managing Editor: Lisa Kairis
Project Manager: Nicole Walz
Senior Manufacturing Manager: Ben Rivera
Senior Marketing Manager: Adam Glazer
Design Coordinator: Teresa Mallon
Cover Designer: Joseph DePinho
Production Service: TechBooks
Printer: Quebecor World–Kingsport

© 2005 by LIPPINCOTT WILLIAMS & WILKINS
530 Walnut Street
Philadelphia, PA 19106 USA
LWW.com

Printed in USA

Library of Congress Cataloging-in-Publication Data

Pediatric cataract surgery : techniques, complications, and management / edited by M. Edward Wilson Jr., Rupal H. Trivedi, Suresh K. Pandey.
    p. ; cm.
    Includes bibliographical references and index.
    ISBN 0-7817-4307-9 (casebound)
    1. Cataract in children—Surgery. I. Wilson, M. Edward. II. Trivedi, Rupal H. III. Pandey, Suresh K.
  [DNLM: 1. Cataract Extraction—Child. WW 260 P371 2005]
RE451.P42 2005
617.7′42059—dc22

2005000396

10 9 8 7 6 5 4 3 2 1

PREFACE

Pediatric cataracts are common and represent one of the most treatable causes of lifelong visual impairment in this population. The global estimate of 1.5 million severely visually impaired and blind children is relatively low compared to the 17 million adults who are blind owing to cataracts. However, the burden of disability in terms of "blind-years" is approximately 75 million (1.5 million children × 50 years of age) because of the child's life expectancy after developing the visual disability.

Presently, the only known treatment for a cataract is the surgical removal of the opaque lens. This is often followed by implantation of an intraocular lens (IOL), even in early childhood. Management of congenital and childhood cataracts is more challenging than cataract management in adults. Increased intraoperative difficulties, a propensity for increased postoperative inflammation, the changing refractive state of the eye, more common postoperative complications, such as capsule opacification, secondary membranes, and postoperative glaucoma, and the tendency to develop amblyopia all add to the difficulty of achieving a good outcome. Development of techniques for cataract surgery specific to children is necessary because of the low scleral rigidity, increased elasticity of the anterior capsule, and high vitreous pressure. Also, microphthalmia and pupillary miosis often add to the surgical complexity. Finally, surgical timing and adequate visual rehabilitation are paramount to avoiding irreversible visual damage secondary to amblyopia.

Dr. Edward Epstein and Professor D. Peter Choyce (UK) performed the first IOL implantations in children in the late 1950s. However, ophthalmologists continued to be hesitant to implant IOLs in the pediatric population because of the unknown long-term effect of synthetic material, the changing refractive status of the developing eye, and the increased inflammatory response that occurs in pediatric eyes. As time passed and technology improved, publications appeared supporting the safety and effectiveness of IOLs in children of nearly all ages. Advances in microsurgical techniques and the availability of better viscoelastic materials and appropriately sized and styled implants, suitable for small eyes, have greatly increased the success of pediatric cataract–IOL surgery worldwide. Many significant surgical advances for cataract management in children have occurred in the last two decades.

In light of these advances, we were surprised that there existed no single reference textbook on pediatric cataract surgery. Cataract surgeons worldwide face the unique challenges posed by children's eyes, often without knowing how to alter the familiar adult approach to maximize the chance for a successful outcome. This book is directed to both the pediatric ophthalmologist and the adult cataract surgeon. Childhood cataracts will be seen in nearly all ophthalmic practices, but not often enough for most surgeons to feel maximally comfortable with the treatment options.

This textbook on pediatric cataract surgery is our effort to provide an overview of state-of-the-art cataract management for children. We hope that it is both practical and scholarly, both easy to read and comprehensive. In its 57 chapters, grouped into nine sections, we have tried to cover all the necessary details on the detection, analysis, and management of pediatric cataracts. We hope that this book will be useful for ophthalmic surgeons at all levels, from novice or occasional pediatric surgeons to leaders in the field.

Note: Supported in part by an unrestricted grant to SEI from Research to Prevent Blindness, New York, NY; and the Grady Lyman Fund, MUSC Health Science Foundation, Charleston, SC.

CONTENTS

Hamid Ahmadieh, M.D.
Professor, Department of Ophthalmology, Shahid Beheshti University; Chief, Vitreoretinal Service, Labbafinejad Medical Center, Tehran, Iran
20. Postoperative Medications and Follow-up; 43. Opacification of the Ocular Media

Irene Anteby, M.D.
Ophthalmic Surgeon, Department of Ophthalmology, Hadassah University Hospital, Jerusalem, Israel
31. Persistent Fetal Vasculature

Luanna R. Bartholomew, Ph.D
Medical Editor, Storm Eye Institute, Medical University of South Carolina, Charleston, South Carolina
55. Pediatric Cataract Surgery and Intraocular Lens Implantation: Practice Styles and Preferences of the 2001 ASCRS and AAPOS Membership

Linda S. Dancy, CRNA
Department of Anesthesia and Perioperative Medicine, Medical University of South Carolina, Charleston, South Carolina
10. Anesthetic Management of the Pediatric Patient with Cataracts

John M. Facciani, M.D.
Vistar Eye Center, Roanoke, Virginia
44. Postoperative Glaucoma

Elizabeth M. Hofmeister, M.D.
Staff, Department of Ophthalmology, Naval Medical Center, San Diego, California
7. Intraocular Lens Power Calculation for Children

M.R. Ja'farinasab, M.D.
Department of Ophthalmology, Shahid Beheshti University; Vitreoretinal Service, Labbafinejad Medical Center, Tehran, Iran
20. Postoperative Medications and Follow-up

Mohammad Ali Javadi, M.D.
Professor, Department of Ophthalmology, Shahid Beheshti University; Chief, Department of Ophthalmology, Labbafinejad Medical Center, Tehran, Iran
43. Opacification of the Ocular Media

Stacey J. Kruger, M.D.
Faculty, Miami Children's Hospital; Voluntary Associate Professor, Department of Ophthalmology, Bascom Palmer Eye Institute/University of Miami, Miami, Florida
37. Lowe Syndrome

Vanita Kumar, Ph.D
Senior Scientific Officer, Center for Genetic Disorders, Guru Nanak Dev University, Amritsar, Punjab, India
3. Genetics of Congenital Cataracts

Scott K. McClatchey, M.D.
Assistant Professor, Department of Surgery, Uniformed Services, University of the Health Sciences, Bethesda, Maryland; Chairman, Department of Ophthalmology, Naval Medical Center, San Diego, California
7. Intraocular Lens Power Calculation for Children

Bharti Nihalani, M.S.
Junior Consultant, Iladevi Cataract and IOL Research Center, Memnagar, Ahmedabad, India
14. Multiquadrant Hydrodissection

Randall J. Olson, M.D.
Presidential Professor and Director, Department of Ophthalmology and Visual Sciences, John A. Moran Eye Center, University of Utah, Salt Lake City, Utah
21. Posterior Chamber Lens Implants: Currently Available Lens Designs and Future Application

Suresh K. Pandey, M.D.
Assistant Professor, Department of Ophthalmology and Visual Sciences, John A. Moran Eye Center, University of Utah, Salt Lake City, Utah; Intraocular Implant Unit, Sydney Hospital & Sydney Eye Hospital; Scholar to the University of Sydney, Save Sight Institute and Discipline of Ophthalmology, Sydney, NSW, Australia; Formerly Post-Doctoral Fellow, Storm Eye Institute, Department of Ophthalmology, Medical University of South Carolina, Charleston, South Carolina
1. Embryology and Anatomy of the Human Crystalline Lens; 2. Etiology and Morphology of Pediatric Cataracts; 5. Evaluation of Visually Significant Cataracts; 8. Historical Overview; 13. Anterior Capsule Management; 17. Dye-Enhanced Pediatric Cataract Surgery; 19. Lensectomy and Anterior Vitrectomy When an Intraocular Lens Is Not Being Implanted; 21. Posterior Chamber Lens Implants: Currently Available Lens Designs and Future Application; 22. Intraocular Lens Types and Sizes for Pediatric Cataract Surgery; 28. Transscleral Suture Fixation of Posterior Chamber Intraocular Lenses; 39. Pediatric Cataract Surgery in Eyes with Uveitis; 40. Intraoperative Complications of Pediatric Cataract–Intraocular Lens Surgery and Their Management; 47. Retinal Detachment; 48. Management of Residual Refractive Error After Intraocular Lens Implantation; 50. Assessment of Visual Functions (Acuity, Contrast Sensitivity) and Amblyopia Management; 53. Traumatic Cataracts in Children; 56. Step-by-Step Approach for Management of Pediatric Cataracts

Srinivas K. Rao, M.D.
Senior Consultant, Cornea Service, Director, International Relationships Sankara Nethralaya, Chennai, Tamil Nadu, India
46. Cystoid Macular Edema

Daljit Singh, M.S., D.Sc.
Professor Emeritus, Department of Human Genetics, Guru Nanak Dev University; Director, Daljit Singh Eye Hospital, Amritsar, Punjab, India
3. Genetics of Congenital Cataracts; 18. Applications of the Fugo Blade; 25. The Iris-Claw Lens (Artisan); 34. Preexisting Posterior Capsule Defects; 38. Dislocated Crystalline Lenses; 51. Phakic Intraocular Lenses in Children

Indu R. Singh, M.S.
Consultant Ophthalmologist, Dr. Daljit Singh Eye Hospital, Amritsar, Punjab, India
38. Dislocated Crystalline Lenses

Jai Rup Singh, Ph.D.
Professor and Coordinator, Center for Genetic Disorders, Guru Nanak Dev University, Amritsar, Punjab, India
3. Genetics of Congenital Cataracts

Kiranjit Singh, M.S.
Consultant Ophthalmologist, Dr. Daljit Singh Eye Hospital, Amritsar, Punjab, India
25. The Iris-Claw Lens (Artisan); 34. Preexisting Posterior Capsule Defects; 38. Dislocated Crystalline Lenses

Ravijit Singh, M.S.
Consultant Ophthalmologist, Dr. Daljit Singh Eye Hospital, Amritsar, Punjab, India
38. Dislocated Crystalline Lenses; 51. Phakic Intraocular Lenses in Children

Ravi Shankar Jit Singh, MBBS, M.S.
Postdoctoral Fellow, Department of Ophthalmology, Penn State M.S. Hershey Medical Center, Hershey, Pennsylvania; Clinical Fellow, Department of Ophthalmology, Dr. Daljit Singh Eye Hospital, Amritsar, Punjab, India
18. Applications of the Fugo Blade; 25. The Iris-Claw Lens (Artisan)

Seema K. Singh, M.S.
Consultant Ophthalmologist, Dr. Daljit Singh Eye Hospital, Amritsar, India
34. Preexisting Posterior Capsule Defects

Catherine M. Suttle, B.Sc, Ph.D., MCOptom
Lecturer, School of Optometry, University of New South Wales, Sydney, New South Wales, Australia
50. Assessment of Visual Functions (Acuity, Contrast Sensitivity) and Amblyopia Management

Rupal H. Trivedi, M.D.
Assistant Professor, Storm Eye Institute, Department of Ophthalmology, Medical University of South Carolina, Charleston, South Carolina
4. Epidemiology of Pediatric Cataracts and Associated Blindness; 6. Informed Consent; 9. Planning Pediatric Cataract Surgery: Diverse Issues; 11. Principles of Incision Construction in Pediatric Cataract Surgery; 12. Ophthalmic Viscosurgical Devices; 14. Multiquadrant Hydrodissection; 15. Lens Substance Aspiration; 16. Posterior Capsulotomy and Anterior Vitrectomy for the Management of Pediatric Cataracts; 23. Primary Intraocular Lens Implantation in Infantile Cataract Surgery; 24. AcrySof Intraocular Lens Implantation in Eyes with Pediatric Cataracts; 26. Role of Optic Capture in Pediatric Cataract–Intraocular Lens Surgery; 27. Polypseudophakia; 29. Secondary Intraocular Lens Implantation; 30. Cataracts Associated with Type I Diabetes Mellitus; 32. Cataract Surgery in Eyes with Retinopathy of Prematurity; 33. Cataract Surgery in Eyes Treated for Retinoblastoma; 35. Anterior Lenticonus in Alport Syndrome; 36. Aniridia and Cataracts; 37. Lowe Syndrome; 39. Pediatric Cataract Surgery in Eyes with Uveitis; 42. Growth of Aphakic and Pseudophakic Eyes; 44. Postoperative Glaucoma; 45. Strabismus in Pediatric Aphakia and Pseudophakia; 49. Aphakia; 52. Pediatric Refractive Surgery; 53. Traumatic Cataracts in Children; 54. Pediatric Cataracts in Developing-World Settings; 55. Pediatric Cataract Surgery and Intraocular Lens Implantation: Practice Styles and Preferences of the 2001 ASCRS and AAPOS Membership; 56. Step-by-Step Approach for Management of Pediatric Cataracts; 57. My Preferred Approach

Abhay R. Vasavada, M.S., FRCS
Director, Iladevi Cataract and IOL Research Center, Memnagar, Ahmedabad, India
14. Multiquadrant Hydrodissection; 26. Role of Optic Capture in Pediatric Cataract–Intraocular Lens Surgery

Arun Verma, M.S.
Consultant Ophthalmologist, Dr. Daljit Singh Eye Hospital, Amritsar, India
25. The Iris-Claw Lens (Artisan)

Charles T. Wallace, M.D.
Professor of Anesthesiology, Department of Anesthesiology, Anesthesia, and Perioperative Medicine, Children's Hospital, Charleston, South Carolina
10. Anesthetic Management of the Pediatric Patient with Cataracts

M. Edward Wilson, M.D.
Director, Storm Eye Institute, Department of Ophthalmology, Medical University of South Carolina, Charleston, South Carolina
2. Etiology and Morphology of Pediatric Cataracts; 4. Epidemiology of Pediatric Cataracts and Associated Blindness; 6. Informed Consent; 8. Historical Overview; 9. Planning Pediatric Cataract Surgery: Diverse Issues; 11. Principles of Incision Construction in Pediatric Cataract Surgery; 12. Ophthalmic Viscosurgical Devices; 13. Anterior Capsule Management; 15. Lens Substance Aspiration; 16. Posterior Capsulotomy and Anterior Vitrectomy for the Management of Pediatric Cataracts; 19. Lensectomy and Anterior Vitrectomy When an Intraocular Lens Is Not Being

Implanted; **22.** *Intraocular Lens Types and Sizes for Pediatric Cataract Surgery;* **23.** *Primary Intraocular Lens Implantation in Infantile Cataract Surgery;* **24.** *AcrySof Intraocular Lens Implantation in Eyes with Pediatric Cataracts;* **27.** *Polypseudophakia;* **28.** *Transscleral Suture Fixation of Posterior Chamber Intraocular Lenses;* **29.** *Secondary Intraocular Lens Implantation;* **30.** *Cataracts Associated with Type I Diabetes Mellitus;* **31.** *Persistent Fetal Vasculature;* **32.** *Cataract Surgery in Eyes with Retinopathy of Prematurity;* **34.** *Preexisting Posterior Capsule Defects; 35. Anterior Lenticonus in Alport Syndrome;* **36.** *Aniridia and Cataracts;* **37.** *Lowe Syndrome;* **39.** *Pediatric Cataract Surgery in Eyes with Uveitis;* **40.** *Intraoperative Complications of Pediatric Cataract–Intraocular Lens Surgery and Their Management;* **41.** *Postoperative Complications of Pediatric Cataract–Intraocular Lens Surgery and Their Management;* **42.** *Growth of Aphakic and Pseudophakic Eyes;* **44.** *Postoperative Glaucoma;* **45.** *Strabismus in Pediatric Aphakia and Pseudophakia;* **48.** *Management of Residual Refractive Error After Intraocular Lens Implantation;* **49.** *Aphakia;* **52.** *Pediatric Refractive Surgery;* **53.** *Traumatic Cataracts in Children;* **54.** *Pediatric Cataracts in Developing-World Settings;* **55.** *Pediatric Cataract Surgery and Intraocular Lens Implantation: Practice Styles and Preferences of the 2001 ASCRS and AAPOS Membership;* **56.** *Step-by-Step Approach for Management of Pediatric Cataracts;* **57.** *My Preferred Approach*

Invited Physicians

David BenEzra, M.D., Ph.D., Israel; Al Biglan, M.D., Pittsburgh, Pennsylvania; Earl Crouch, M.D., Norfolk, Virginia; Elie Dahan, M.D., South Africa; Scott Lambert, M.D., Atlanta, Georgia; Sam Masket, M.D., Los Angeles, California; Michael O'Keefe, M.D., Ireland; David Plager, M.D., Indianapolis, Indiana; Abhay Vasavada, M.S., FRCS, India; David Yorston, M.D., Kenya; Charlota Zetterstom, M.D., Sweden

57. *My Preferred Approach*

Characteristics of Cataracts in Children

Chapter 1

Embryology and Anatomy of the Human Crystalline Lens

Suresh K. Pandey

EMBRYOLOGY OF THE CRYSTALLINE LENS

The crystalline lens is derived from the embryonic surface ectoderm after contact and interaction of the anterior wall of the neuroectodermal optical vesicle with the epithelial lining of the embryo. The first trace of the crystalline lens plate appears at 25 days of gestation in the form of thickening of the surface ectoderm at the site of previous contact with the optical vesicle.[1-3] As the optical vesicle enlarges, it becomes closely opposed to the surface ectoderm, which is a single layer of cuboidal cells. Figure 1-1 illustrates stages of lens development.

Lens Plate

The cells of the surface ectoderm that overlie the optic vesicles become columnar at about 27 days of gestation in the form of thickening of the surface ectoderm. This area of thickened cells is called the lens plate or the lens placode. A chemical mediator from the neuroectoderm is believed to stimulate formation of the lens plate.

Lens Pit

At approximately 22 to 23 days of gestation, the cells of the lens plate arch posteriorly, forming a concave depression, the lens pit. The lens pit deepens by a process of cellular multiplication and invaginates.

Lens Vesicle

As the lens pit continues to invaginate, the stalk of cells that connects it to the surface ectoderm constricts and eventually disappears. The resultant sphere is a single layer of cuboidal cells encased within a periodic acid/Schiff–positive basement membrane (lens capsule). The remaining overlying surface ectoderm re-forms to create an uninterrupted layer anteriorly; this layer becomes the corneal epithelium.

Lens Fibers

Soon after the lens vesicle forms, the anterior and posterior walls of the lens vesicle differentiate into dissimilar structures. The anterior wall remains a single layer of cuboidal epithelium, but the cells on the posterior wall increase in length and form elongated fibers that project into the lumen of the vesicle. Their nuclei migrate forward from the posterior pole toward the middle of the vesicle. The vesicle remains spherical, but the lumen of the vesicle becomes much smaller and is eventually obliterated by these fibers. This process results in the solid embryonic lens nucleus, which is completely developed by the end of the fourth week.

The formation of all subsequent fibers occurs around the embryonic region at the lens bow. The anterior lens epithelial cells migrate equatorially, undergo mitotic division, and form new elongated lens fibers concentrically at the equator around the older central fibers. This growth of new fibers continues throughout life so that the lens increases in weight and size, although at a much slower rate in later years. As new fibers are formed, the nuclei of the cells gradually disappear, resulting in a lens center normally devoid of cellular nuclei.

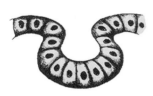

1. Lens plate

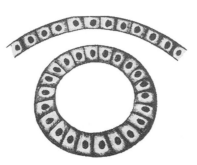

4. Lens vesicle (early)

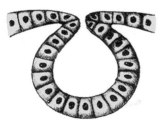

2. Lens pit (early)

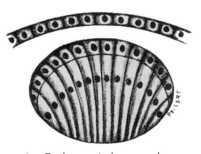

5. Lens vesicle (late)

3. Lens pit (late)

6. Embryonic lens nucleus

FIGURE 1-1. Stages of growth and development of the embryonic lens. (Reprinted with permission from Apple DJ, Rabb MF. *Ocular Pathology, Clinical Applications and Self-Assessment,* Mosby-Yearbook Inc., St. Louis, Missouri, Chapter 4, Lens and Pathology of Intraocular Lenses, Page 118, Figure 4-1.

Lens Nuclei

As development progresses, the earlier-formed deep fibers become more homogeneous than younger superficial ones, resulting in a definite stratification. Chronologically, one can identify the following stages of differentiation.

The embryonic nucleus. Situated in the central part of the lens, the embryonic nucleus constitutes the primitive lens fibers formed by elongation of the posterior epithelial cells. It is devoid of sutures.

The fetal nucleus. The fetal nucleus contains "Y" sutures that develop during the third month. Growth of this nucleus may continue until the eighth month.

The adult nucleus. From birth onwards, lens fibers continue to be added, forming the adult nucleus. The successive concentric layers of lens fibers become very tightly opposed.

Lens Sutures

The succeeding generations of lens fibers extend anteriorly and posteriorly from the equator beneath the capsule. The lens fibers are shorter in the deeper plane than in the superficial plane. Moreover, the fibers in any plane are not long enough to reach from the anterior to the posterior pole. When the lens fibers extend more anteriorly, they fall short posteriorly, and vice versa. The lens sutures began to appear in the second month, immediately after formation of the primary lens nucleus from the lens vesicle. The purpose of the sutures is to ensure that the lens becomes a flattened biconvex sphere rather than retaining its initial spherical shape.

Initially two Y-shaped sutures are present: the upright anterior Y suture and the inverted posterior suture. During later gestation and after birth, growth of the lens sutures is much more irregular. Instead of simple Y sutures, more complicated dendritic patterns caused by asymmetric fiber growth are observed.

GROWTH OF THE HUMAN CRYSTALLINE LENS

Pediatric ocular structures, including the crystalline lens, are significantly smaller than those in the adult, especially in the first 1 to 3 years of life. The human crystalline lens grows throughout life by the deposition of new fibers. At birth the human lens weighs approximately 90 mg, and it increases in mass at a rate of 2 mg per year as new fibers form. The most rapid lens growth occurs from birth to 2 years of age.[4] The mean diameter of the capsular bag is about 7.0 to 7.5 mm at birth, increasing to about 9.0 to 9.5 mm by the age of 2 years. Figure 1-2 illustrates gross features of pediatric and adult crystalline lenses.

Human crystalline lens growth is slower after the second decade. The lens does not increase much in size thereafter because of the relative loss of hydration and shrinkage of the lens nucleus, which offsets some of the growth

from new fiber deposition. Also, the lens capsule thickens with age and loses some of its inherent elasticity, which further decreases its capacity for accommodation and helps lead to presbyopia.

ANATOMY OF THE HUMAN CRYSTALLINE LENS

The adult crystalline lens measures approximately 9.6 ± 0.4 mm in diameter, with an approximate anterior–posterior diameter of 4.2 ± 0.5 mm.[5] The anterior and posterior poles form the optical and geometrical axis of the lens. Although the normal lens is transparent and clear in vivo, it is seldom completely colorless; even in childhood a slight yellowish tint is present, which tends to intensify with age.

The crystalline lens is a unique, transparent, biconvex intraocular structure that lies in the anterior segment of the eye, suspended radially at its equator by the zonular fibers and the ciliary body, between the iris and the vitreous body. Enclosed in an elastic capsule, the lens has no innervation or blood supply after fetal development. Its nourishment must be obtained from the surrounding aqueous and vitreous humors, and the same media must also remove metabolic waste products. Therefore, disturbances in circulation of these fluids, or inflammatory processes in these chambers, play a large role in the pathogenesis of lens abnormalities. The aqueous humor continuously flows from the ciliary body to the anterior chamber, bathing the anterior surface of the lens.

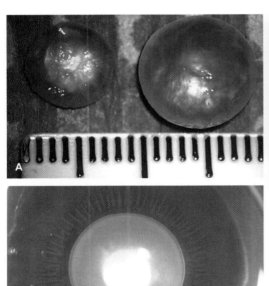

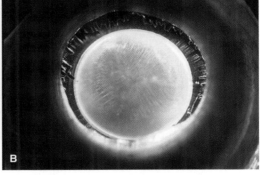

FIGURE 1-2. Human pediatric and adult crystalline lenses. (**A**) Gross photograph of human crystalline lenses from a child aged 4 months (left) and from an adult aged 70 years. (**B**) Gross photograph of a 20-month human lens obtained postmortem, showing the crystalline lens zonules and ciliary body (anterior or surgeon's view). Diameter of the lens, 8.5 mm. (**C**) Gross photograph of a 20-month human lens obtained postmortem, showing the crystalline lens zonules and ciliary body (Miyake–Apple posterior view).

Disturbances in permeability of the lens capsule and epithelium can occur, leading to the formation of cataracts. Posteriorly, the crystalline lens is supported by the vitreous (hyaloid) face and lies in a small depression called the *patellar fossa*. In younger eyes, the vitreous comes in contact with the posterior capsule in a circular area of thickened vitreous, the ligamentum hyaloideocapsulare. The potential space between the capsule and the circle of condensed vitreous is called Berger's space. The lateral border of the lens is the equator, formed by the joining of the anterior and posterior capsules, and is the site of insertion of the zonular fibers.

The lens consists of three components: capsule, epithelium, and lens substance. The lens substance is a product of the continuous growth of the epithelium and consists of the cortex and nucleus. The transition between the cortex and the nucleus is gradual. It does not reveal a concise line of demarcation in histological sections. The lines of demarcation are often better visualized by slit-lamp microscopy.

Lens Capsule

The lens capsule is a basement membrane elaborated by the lens epithelium anteriorly and by superficial fibers posteriorly. On light microscopy the lens capsule appears as a structureless, elastic membrane that completely surrounds the lens. It is a true periodic acid/Schiff–positive basement membrane, a secretory product of the lens epithelium. The capsule functions as a metabolic barrier and may play a role in shaping the lens during accommodation. The lens capsule varies in thickness in different zones. At its thickest

the lens capsule represents the thickest basement membrane in the body. The relative thickness of the anterior capsule compared with the much thinner posterior capsule may result from the fact that the former lies directly adjacent to, and is actively secreted by, the epithelium, whereas the lens epithelium is not present on the posterior surface. Local differences in capsular thickness are important surgically, particularly because of the danger of tears or rupture of the thin posterior capsule during cataract surgery. Remnants of the tunica vasculosa lentis are common and appear as light-gray opacities (Mittendorf dots) at or near the posterior pole. These opacities are rarely responsible for significant visual loss.

Lens Epithelial Cells

Some details about the lens epithelial cells and their behavior after pediatric cataract surgery are pertinent. Postoperative proliferation of these cells may lead to opacification of the visual axis, which in turn may contribute to decreased vision after cataract surgery.[6] The lens epithelium is confined to the anterior surface and the equatorial lens bow (Fig.1-3). It consists of a single row of cuboidal–cylindrical cells, which can be divided biologically into two zones with two different types of cells.

A Cells

The A cells are located in the anterior–central zone (corresponding to the central zone of the anterior lens capsule). They consist of relatively quiescent epithelial cells with minimal mitotic activity. When disturbed, they

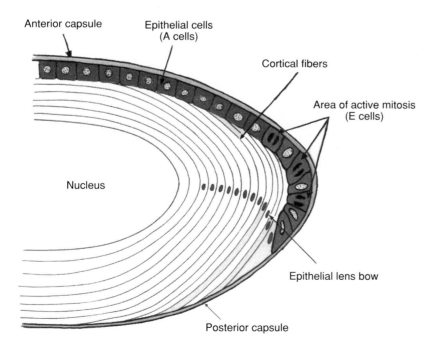

FIGURE 1-3. Schematic illustration of the microscopic anatomy of the lens, showing the A cells of the anterior epithelium and the E cells, the important germinal epithelial cells of the equatorial lens bow. These lens epithelial cells play a prominent role in the pathogenesis of various complications such as postoperative opacification of the anterior and posterior capsules.

tend to remain in place and not migrate. However, in a variety of disorders (e.g., inflammation, trauma), an anterior subcapsular epithelial plaque may form. The primary response of the anterior epithelial cells is to proliferate and form fibrous tissue by undergoing fibrous metaplasia.

Recently a new potential complication caused by A-cell proliferation has emerged in the field of cataract-refractive surgery. The anterior subcapsular opacities that have been described with various phakic posterior chamber intraocular lenses are based on A-cell proliferation. The fibrotic response of the anterior lens epithelium is what determines the degree of anterior capsular thickening following implantation of a phakic posterior chamber intraocular lens in close proximity to (or on) the anterior surface of the crystalline lens.

E Cells

E cells are located in the second zone, as a continuation of the anterior lens epithelial cells around the equator, forming the equatorial lens bow, with the germinal cells. These cells normally show mitotic capability, and new lens fibers are continuously produced at this site. Because cell production in this region is relatively active, the cells are rich in enzymes and have extensive protein metabolism. E cells are responsible for the continuous formation of all cortical fibers, and they account for the continuous growth in size and weight of the lens throughout life. During lens enlargement the location of older fibers becomes more central as new fibers are formed at the periphery.

In pathologic states, the E cells tend to migrate posteriorly along the posterior capsule; instead of undergoing a fibrotic transformation, they tend to form large, balloonlike bladder cells (i.e., Wedl cells), which are visible clinically as "pearls." These equatorial cells are the primary source of classic secondary cataracts, especially the pearl form of posterior capsule opacification. E cells are responsible for the formation of a Soemmering's ring, which is a donut-shaped lesion composed of retained/regenerated lens cortex and cells that may form following any disruption of the anterior lens capsule. This lesion was initially described in connection with ocular trauma. It is the basic precursor of classic posterior capsule opacification. E cells have also been implicated in the pathogenesis of opacification between piggyback intraocular lenses, also termed interlenticular opacification.

Lens Substance (Cortex and Nucleus)

The lens substance consists of the lens fibers themselves, which are derived from the equatorial lens epithelium. On cross section these cells are hexagonal and are bound together by ground substance. After formation, the cellular nuclei of the lens fibers are present only temporarily. Subsequently they disappear, leaving the lens center devoid of cell nuclei except in certain pathologic situations (e.g., maternal rubella syndrome).

The original lens vesicle represents the primary embryonic nucleus; in later stages of gestation the fetal nucleus encircles the embryonic nucleus. The various layers surrounding the fetal nucleus are designated according to stages of growth. The most peripherally located fibers, which underlie the lens capsule, form the lens cortex. The designation cortex is actually an arbitrary term signifying a peripheral location within the lens, rather than specific fibers.

In summary, the crystalline lens is a unique, transparent, biconvex intraocular structure that consists of three components: capsule, epithelium, and lens substance. The lens is formed from the optic vesicle. The human crystalline lens grows throughout life by the deposition of new fibers, with the most rapid lens-growth occuring in the first 2 years after birth.

ACKNOWLEDGMENT

The author gratefully acknowledges the partial support of an unrestricted grant from Research to Prevent Blindness, Inc., New York.

REFERENCES

1. Duke-Elder S, Cook C. Normal and abnormal development. Part 1. Embryology. In: Duke-Elder S, ed. *System of Ophthalmology.* Vol III. St. Louis: Mosby, 1963:127–138.
2. Kuszak JR, Brown HG. Embryology and anatomy of the lens. In: Albert DM, Jacobeic FA, eds. *Principles and Practice of Ophthalmology.* Philadelphia: Saunders, 1994:82–96.
3. Apple DJ, Rabb MF. Lens and Pathology of Intraocular Lenses. In: Apple DJ, Rabb MF. *Ocular Pathology, Clinical Applications and Self-Assessment.* St. Louis: Mosby, 1998;117–204.
4. Bluestein EC, Wilson ME, Wang XH, et al. Dimensions of the pediatric crystalline lens: implications for intraocular lenses in children. *J Pediatr Ophthalmol Strabismus* 1996;33:18–20.
5. Assia EI, Castaneda VE, Legler UFC, et al. Studies on cataract surgery and intraocular lenses at the Center for Intraocular Lens Research. *Ophthalmol Clin North Am* 1991;4:251–266.
6. Apple DJ, Solomon DK, Tetz MR, et al. Posterior capsule opacification. *Surv Ophthalmol* 1992;37:73–116.

Etiology and Morphology of Pediatric Cataracts

Suresh K. Pandey and M. Edward Wilson, Jr.

Childhood cataracts can be classified as congenital, infantile, or juvenile, depending on the age at onset. Congenital cataracts are present at birth but may go unnoticed until an effect on the child's visual function is noticed or a white pupil reflex develops. Infantile cataracts develop in the first 2 years of life, and juvenile cataracts have an onset within the first decade of life.[1,2] The term *presenile* cataract is sometimes seen in the literature. This term refers to cataracts with an onset prior to 45 years of age. *Age-related* or so-called "senile" cataracts occur at or after age 45 years. Congenital and infantile cataracts are responsible for about 10% of all blindness worldwide.[3]

Childhood cataracts can also be classified according to etiology (e.g., traumatic cataract, autosomal dominant cataract) or morphology.[4–8] Both of these classifications are discussed in this chapter.

ETIOLOGY OF PEDIATRIC CATARACTS

It is important to consider the origin of a cataract. The common teaching for many years has been that roughly one-third of childhood cataracts are inherited, one-third are associated with other diseases or syndromes, and the remaining one-third are idiopathic. The etiology of pediatric cataracts has been reviewed by several authors and several classifications have been proposed.[1,3,8] Table 2-1 presents an etiological classification of congenital cataracts.[3] The etiology of pediatric cataracts can be broadly classified and summarized in the following seven subgroups.

Hereditary Cataracts

Hereditary cataracts are passed from one generation to the next. Autosomal dominant transmission is responsible for 75% of congenital hereditary cataracts. Affected individuals are usually otherwise perfectly well and have no as-

sociated systemic illness. Less commonly, the inheritance may be autosomal recessive. These cataracts are bilateral but may be asymmetric. Also, marked variability can be seen between affected family members. Some cataracts are so mild that family members do not know they have them.

There are also a number of rare hereditary syndromes in which the affected individual not only has cataracts but also has an associated systemic illness. Less commonly, the inheritance may be autosomal recessive. Cataracts may be associated with renal and cerebral disease in Lowe's oculocerebrorenal syndrome, which is X linked recessive. It is therefore important that all children with bilateral congenital cataracts are examined by a pediatrician to exclude a systemic disorder.

Metabolic Cataracts

Congenital, infantile, or juvenile lens opacities may have an underlying metabolic cause. Galactosemia, for example, is a metabolic disorder in which the child's body cannot metabolize galactose, a major component of milk and milk products. The baby will have vomiting and diarrhea and may develop "oil droplet" cataracts. It is thought that 10% to 30% of newborns with classic galactosemia develop cataracts in the first few days or weeks of life. Once a newborn is put on a galactose-restricted diet, cataracts usually clear. Surgery is sometimes necessary when dietary treatment is delayed. Many galactosemia patients have eye examinations to check for the presence of cataracts on a regular basis. These examinations are required more frequently during the first year of life (e.g., every 3–4 months) but less often (e.g., one or two times a year) in older children. It is a good idea to have an eye exam if galactose-1-phosphate levels are observed to rise above a "target" range.

Glucose 6-phosphatase dehydrogenase deficiency is an X-linked disorder and therefore affects mainly males.

▶ **TABLE 2-1** **Etiological Classification of Congenital Cataracts**

Isolated Findings
Hereditary
  Autosomal dominant
  Autosomal recessive
  X Linked
  Sporadic (one-third of all congenital cataracts)

Part of Syndrome or Systemic Disease
Hereditary
  With renal disease
    Lowe's oculocerbrorenal syndrome
    Alport syndrome (autosomal dominant)
  With central nervous system disease
    Marinesco Sjögren's syndrome (autonomic recessive)
    Sjögren's syndrome (autosomal recessive)
    Smith–Lemli–Opitz syndrome
    Laurence–Moon–Bardet–Biedel syndrome
  With skeletal disease
    Conradi's syndrome (presence of cataract indicates worse prognosis)
    Marfan's syndrome
    Stippled epiphysis
  With abnormalities of head and face
    Hallermann–Streiff syndrome
    Francois dyscephalic syndrome
    Pierre Robin syndrome
    Oxycephaly
    Crouzon's disease
    Acrocephalosyndactyly (Apert's syndrome)
  With polydactyly
    Rubinstein–Taybi syndrome
  With skin disease
    Bloch–Sulzberger syndrome
    Congenital ectodermal dysplasia of the anhidrotic type
    Rothmund Thomson syndrome
    Schafer's syndrome
    Siemen's syndrome
    Incontinential pigmenti
    Atopic dermatitis
    Cockayne's syndrome
    Marshall syndrome
  With chromosomal disorders
    Trisomy 13 (usually die within 1 year)
    Trisomy 18: Edward's syndrome
    Trisomy 21: Down's syndrome (often cataract formation delayed until approximately age 10)
    Turner's syndrome
    Patau's syndrome
  With metabolic disease
    Galactosemia (autosomal recessive)
    Galactokinase deficiency
    Congenital hemolytic jaundice
    Fabry's disease
    Refsum's disease
    Mannosidosis
  With miscellaneous hereditary syndromes
    Norrie's disease

▶ **TABLE 2-1** **(Continued)**

    Hereditary spherocytosis
    Myotonic dystrophy
Nonhereditary
  Prenatal causes
    Rubella syndrome
    Toxoplasmosis
    Varicella
    Cytomegalovirus
    Herpes simplex virus
    Measles
    Mumps
    Vaccinia
    Intrauterine hypoxia or malnutrition
  Postnatal causes
    Retinopathy of prematurity
    Hypoglycemia
    Hypocalcemia
    Radiation
    Trauma
    Chronic uveitis
    Diabetes mellitus
    Wilson's disease
    Renal insufficiency
    Drug induced
    High-voltage electric shock
  Associated with another ocular abnormality
    PFV (persistence of fetal vasculature)
    Microphthalmos
    Aniridia
    Retinitis pigmentosa
    Norrie's disease
    Colobomas
    Lenticonus

Modified with permission from Arkin M, Azar D, Fraioli A. Infantile cataracts. *Int Ophthalmol Clin* 1992;32(1):110–111.

These babies present with jaundice and hemolytic anemia and may also develop infantile cataracts. Infection, acute illness, and ingestion of fava beans will precipitate an attack of hemolysis in these children. Death may result unless the condition is diagnosed and treated with an urgent blood transfusion.

Hypoglycemia of whatever cause may give rise to lens opacities in children. The majority of babies with profound hypoglycemia also have convulsions and may have permanent brain damage. Hypocalcemia may results in cataracts, although these are usually functionally less significant than cataracts resulting from hypoglycemia.

Traumatic Cataracts

Traumatic cataracts are a common cause of unilateral loss of vision in children (Fig. 2-1). Penetrating injuries are usually more common than blunt injuries. Most of the injuries that result in a traumatic cataract occur in children while

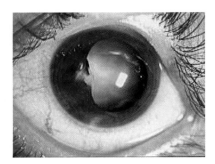

FIGURE 2-1. Pediatric uniocular cataract following trauma. Photograph of the eye of a 6-year-old male child showing a traumatic cataract after blunt trauma (firecracker injury). Note the iris tear and synechia along with the diffuse cortical cataract. (Courtesy of Jagat Ram, MD, Chandigarh, India.)

they are playing or involved in a sport-related activity. Injuries are also caused by thorns, firecrackers, sticks, arrows, darts, BB pellets, and automobile airbags. Cataracts caused by blunt trauma classically form stellate- or rosette-shaped posterior axial opacities that may be stable or progressive, whereas penetrating trauma with disruption of the lens the capsule forms cortical changes that may remain focal if small or may progress rapidly to total cortical opacification.

Secondary Cataracts

The most common type of secondary cataract is a result of uveitis occurring in conjunction with arthritis (juvenile chronic arthritis) or as a result of intermediate or posterior uveitis of any cause. The cataract may be a direct result of inflammation within the eye or can result from the steroids used to treat the condition. Cataracts caused by steroid ingestion are usually posterior subcapsular.

Less frequently, a cataract may be seen secondary to an intraocular tumor, a foreign body, or a chronic retinal detachment. Cataracts have also been reported after laser treatment for threshold retinopathy of prematurity.

Cataracts Secondary to Maternal Infection During Pregnancy

The most common maternal infection leading to congenital cataracts in children is rubella, also known as German measles. Maternal infection with the rubella virus, an RNA toga virus, can cause fetal damage, especially if the infection occurs during the first trimester of pregnancy. Systemic manifestations of congenital rubella infection include cardiac defects, deafness, and mental retardation.

Cataracts resulting from congenital rubella syndrome are characterized by pearly white nuclear opacity. Sometimes the entire lens is opacified (complete cataract) and the cortex may liquefy. Histologically, lens fiber nuclei are retained deep within the lens substance. Cataract removal may be complicated by excessive postoperative inflammation caused by release of these virus particles. Congenital rubella syndrome, which occurred in epidemic proportions in the United States in the early 1960s, is manifest in its complete form by several systemic findings. These include failure to thrive, deafness, cardiac anomalies, patent ductus arteriosus, and thrombocytopenic rash. While congenital rubella remains common in some parts of the developing world, it is practically nonexistent in the United States because of widespread rubella vaccination of the population.

Other infectious diseases that may have affected the mother during pregnancy, such as toxoplasmosis, toxocariasis, and cytomegalovirus, can also cause congenital cataracts along with systemic illness in the newborn baby.

Iatrogenic Cataracts

Iatrogenic cataracts are most commonly seen in children who have had total-body irradiation for leukemia and in children who have had organ transplants and are on long-term systemic steroid therapy. These are usually older children who do very well after cataract surgery. As stated above, cataracts have been reported after laser treatment for threshold retinopathy of prematurity.[9] Also, cataracts may develop after vitrectomy to remove a vitreous hemorrhage from birth trauma or to treat retinal detachment.

Syndromes and Congenital Cataracts

There is a large variety of chromosomal and dysmorphic syndromes in which the child will have a high risk of having congenital cataracts. It is important to notice any abnormal features in children presenting with cataracts, such as unusual facial features, extra digits, unusual skin, short stature, developmental delay, and microcephaly or hydrocephaly, as it is essential that a diagnosis is made such that the child receives any necessary treatment and the parents receive genetic counseling about the possible risks of producing other offspring with similar problems.

Cataracts of Unknown Etiology (Idiopathic or Sporadic)

The vast majority of nontraumatic unilateral cataracts fall into this category. Many surgeons would say that this is the most common single category. It is, of course, a diagnosis of exclusion. Unilateral cataracts will not be metabolic or hereditary. A search for signs of trauma or eye inflammation is warranted. Bilateral cataracts may also be of unknown etiology. However, the hereditary nature of some cataracts will not be evident from the history alone. A careful examination of the parents may reveal visually insignificant cataracts that a parent did not know were present. In the context of the overall medical and developmental history and the age at onset of the cataract, a metabolic and genetic workup may be indicated before an idiopathic etiology can be declared. These workups should be customized with the assistance of a developmental pediatrician so that every test ordered is done so with a real suspicion for a positive finding. Shotgun workups directed by the ophthalmologist should be discouraged.

MORPHOLOGY OF PEDIATRIC CATARACTS

Congenital, developmental, and traumatic cataracts can have different morphological characteristics. For surgeons, a classification based on morphological type is most useful. The classification recommended below is in common clinical use and emphasizes those cataract types most likely to be visually significant. It is a modified (added-to) form of a clinical descriptive classification published in 1982[10] and affirmed in a follow-up article in 1993.[11] These simple labels lend themselves to easy stratification of a pediatric surgical case series but do not include some of the myriad rare visually insignificant variations and patterns that have been described by genetic researchers. Terms such as punctate, pulverulent, coraliform, coronary, floriform, retrodot, sunflower, blue-dot, and sutural, while possibly important to etiology, are not included here since they are used to describe lens changes that are nearly always static and visually insignificant. The "oil droplet" type of cataract is also excluded here even though it has a classic appearance, since it either resolves when the galactosemia is treated or becomes a "lamellar" cataract. At the time of surgery, this cataract would be grouped with other lamellar opacities, rather than carrying a label based on its earlier appearance.

In this section, we have chosen to emphasize childhood cataract types based on their anatomical location within the lens and their characteristic natural history (Figs. 2-2 to 2-9). They are all surgical or potentially surgical cataract types. Visual outcome and complications, too, can sometimes be predicted based on these lens types. This can help guide the follow-up as well as the informed consent leading to surgery.

Morphological Classification and Characteristics of Pediatric Cataracts

The categories below are each discussed separately.

1. Diffuse/total
2. Anterior polar
3. Lamellar
4. Nuclear
5. Posterior polar
6. Posterior lentiglobus
7. Posterior (and anterior) subcapsular
8. Persistent hyperplastic primary vitreous
9. Traumatic

Diffuse/Total Cataracts

Diffuse or "total" cataracts are seen most commonly after trauma. However, since trauma is a separate category, only nontraumatic total cataracts are discussed here. In the United States, nontraumatic total cataracts are not common. In a previous pediatric cataract series from the United States, only 4 of 199 eyes were classified as total. However, in the developing world, total cataracts are commonly seen in children (Fig. 2-2). This difference probably relates to the timing of detection of the cataracts in the developing world. Many cataract types, if left untreated, will slowly become diffuse, total cataracts. This is especially true of lamellar cataracts, posterior lentiglobus, and posterior polar opacities. Some total cataracts represent spontaneously ruptured posterior lentiglobus, neglected lamellar opacities, or occult trauma. A B-scan ultrasound is indicated whenever the retina cannot be visualized using an ophthalmoscope. Surgery on total cataracts may reveal watery or partially absorbed lens material within the capsular bag. Occasionally, the total cataract will be little more than a white membrane representing a fused and fibrotic anterior and posterior lens capsule.

Anterior Polar Cataracts

Anterior polar cataracts are often bilateral, hereditary, and visually insignificant. However, notable exceptions occur. If neither parent has anterior polar cataracts, the child may have a sporadic (nonhereditary) form or may have a new mutation and thus pass on some risk of recurrence to the next generation. The most common type of

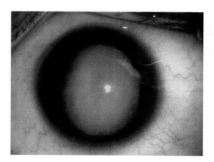

FIGURE 2-2. Diffuse/total infantile cataract. Total cataracts are commonly seen in children in the developing world, which probably relates to the delay in detection of the cataracts. Even in the developed world, nuclear and cortical cataracts may eventually because diffuse/total opacities.

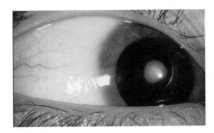

FIGURE 2-3. Anterior polar cataract. A pyramidal shape is seen in more severe anterior polar cataracts, as shown here. The chances of the cataract's becoming visually significant are higher with the pyramidal shape compared to the isolated white dot variety.

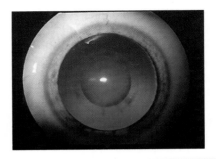

FIGURE 2-4. Lamellar cataract. A layer of semi-opaque cortex is shown surrounding a clear nucleus. These cataracts are usually bilateral and slowly become more dense over time.

anterior polar cataract presents as a tiny white dot in the center of the anterior capsule. These cataracts are usually bilateral but may be unilateral and probably represent a mild abnormality of lens vesicle detachment. They are usually 1 mm or less in diameter and almost never progress. Corneal astigmatism may be present, however, and can cause amblyopia.[12]

Pyramidal cataracts are a distinct and more severe form of anterior polar opacity, named because the shape of the anterior opacity resembles a pyramid (Fig. 2-3). A more accurate and modern description is a likeness to the shape of the chocolate candy called the Hershey's Kiss. The tips of these opacities extend into the anterior chamber and rarely have even been known to be fused with the cornea.[13] They are fibrous and may be associated with an anterior subcapsular cataract that, when present, often progresses to become visually significant. At surgery, the fibrous "Hershey's Kiss" is not easily removed with the vitreous cutter. After it is detached from the anterior capsule, it usually spins around the anterior chamber and has to be delivered through the incision using forceps. These pyramidal cataracts are almost always bilaterally symmetric and may be dominantly inherited.

Anterior lenticonus is less common than the posterior variety and is usually associated with Alport's syndrome. Cataracts are a late finding in anterior lenticonus. However, the secondary refractive error may cause enough visual symptoms to require clear lens extraction and intraocular lens placement. Rarely, the lens will spontaneously rupture, causing lens hydration and total cataract. See Chapter 35 for more on Alport's syndrome and anterior lenticonus.

Lamellar Cataracts

Lamellar cataracts are usually acquired (rather than congenital) and involve a layer (lamellae) of cortex surrounding the fetal nucleus, peripheral to the "Y" sutures. They are almost always bilateral but are commonly asym-

metric (Fig. 2-4). Microphthalmia is not usually associated with this cataract type and the risk of secondary aphakic/pseudophakic glaucoma is much lower than with fetal nuclear opacities. Lamellar cataracts are often hereditary, following an autosomal dominant transmission pattern. The visual prognosis is usually better with lamellar cataracts (even when surgery is delayed) than with cataract types that are densely opaque at birth such as fetal nuclear opacities (discussed below). This improved prognosis is related to the later development of the cataract such that during the critical period of visual development, the cataract did not preclude normal visual development. Lamellar cataracts are characteristically mild initially and slowly worsen with time. Nystagmus does not often develop as a result of these cataracts. Remarkably, children can sometimes function quite well visually even when the lamellar opacity blackens the retinoscopic reflection completely. These cataracts are usually about 5 to 6 mm in diameter and characteristically have a thin layer of clear cortex external to the opacity. The nucleus, internal to the cataract, is also characteristically clear. At surgery, the lamellar opacity will sometimes pop out of the capsular bag as soon as the anterior capsule is opened and the cortex is hydrated. Care must be taken to avoid an extension of the anterior capsulotomy edge when this happens. Despite this tendency to pop out of the bag, lamellar cataracts are soft and can be aspirated easily.

Nuclear Cataracts

The most common congenital cataract is the fetal nuclear cataract. This classic form of cataract usually presents with a white central opacity (unilateral or bilateral) about 3.5 mm in diameter (between the "Y" sutures) surrounded by mostly clear cortex (Fig. 2-5). As time passes from birth, the surrounding cortex may become more opaque diffusely or in radial extensions called "riders." Microphthalmia and microcornea are usually present. The iris often dilates poorly and appears immature, with few crypts,

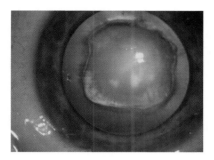

FIGURE 2-5. Fetal nuclear cataract. A dense white fetal nuclear cataract is shown, which is 3.5 mm wide initially and spreads into the surrounding cortical layers.

a poorly formed papillary ruff, and no collarette. These cataracts can be unilateral or bilateral (Fig. 2-6) and can lead to deprivation amblyopia if not removed early in life (before 6 weeks of age if unilateral or before nystagmus appears if bilateral). Sometimes a hyaloid artery remnant is also present, but unlike classic forms of severe persistence of fetal vasculature (PFV), the cataract is predominantly nuclear and no ciliary process traction is seen. Less common nuclear opacities include the varieties of pulverulent (pulverized tiny dots) cataract. These, as stated above, are usually static and do not often need surgery.

Posterior Polar Cataracts

Posterior polar cataracts are usually sporadic cortical opacities with a propensity for spontaneous posterior capsule rupture. These cataracts can be unilateral or bilateral, mild or severe. Caution is in order when doing surgery for posterior polar opacities since the posterior capsule may already be ruptured or honeycombed into a weakened meshwork. Aggressive hydrodissection is discouraged when any posterior polar opacity is seen since it may result in a large uncontrolled posterior capsular tear, with cortical lens material pushed back into the vitreous gel.

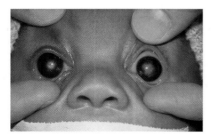

FIGURE 2-6. Fetal nuclear cataracts bilaterally. These cataracts are located predominantly in the fetal nucleus of the lens and are, therefore, truly congenital.

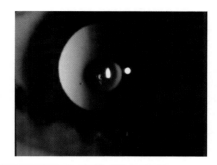

FIGURE 2-7. Posterior lentiglobus. Slit-lamp photograph showing bowing of the posterior capsule, termed *posterior lenticonus*. The term *lentiglobus* better reflects the globular shape of the bowing of the capsule. Cataract formation and even spontaneous rupture can follow the progressive nature of the posterior capsule changes.

Posterior Lentiglobus

Posterior lentiglobus is mostly unilateral and not associated with microphthalmia. It represents the most common type of developmental cataract in a normal-sized eye. Most forms are sporadic, but occasionally an autosomal dominant inherited bilateral form will be encountered. The lens changes begin in the posterior capsule, possibly secondary to a weakness in the area of prior contact with the hyaloid artery. The bulge in the posterior capsule is usually not present at birth but becomes more exaggerated as the intralenticular pressure increases with age. Although some publications refer to this lens capsule bulge as a posterior "lenticonus" (Fig. 2-7), the term *lentiglobus* better reflects the globular, not conical, bowing of the capsule. The disorder is progressive and usually requires surgery. Cataractous changes occur in the posterior cortical layers as the lentiglobus bulge worsens. Spontaneous rupture may occur, leading to a total white cortical cataract. In these cases, the true nature of the lentiglobus may not be discovered until after the lens is entered during surgery. However, posterior capsule rupture can be diagnosed preoperatively even in a total white cataract by careful emmersion A-scan ultrasound. The visual prognosis, on average, is good since the condition tends to progress slowly over time and is not as likely as fetal nuclear opacities to cause a severe deprivation amblyopia.

Posterior (and Anterior) Subcapsular Cataracts

Anterior subcapsular cataracts are often associated with trauma, radiation, or acquired diseases such as uveitis, Alport's syndrome (cataracts associated with anterior lenticonus), and atopic skin disease (shieldlike anterior subcapsular cataracts are classic). Anterior subcapsular opacities may also be part of a more widespread multilayer cataract.

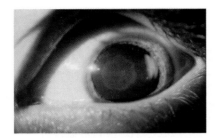

FIGURE 2-8. Posterior subcapsular cataract. Slit-lamp photographs showing an example of a posterior subcapsular cataract in a child secondary to radiotherapy treatment.

Posterior subcapsular cataracts are often "crystalline" in appearance, resembling, at times, the look of frosted glass. This type of cataract is seen in association with inflammatory conditions, especially after steroid use or after radiation (Fig. 2-8). It can also be idiopathic. Unlike posterior cortical or posterior polar opacities, posterior subcapsular cataracts are not associated with defects in the posterior capsule. Most are progressive and reduce visual acuity early in the course of progression, especially in bright light.

Persistent Hyperplastic Primary Vitreous (Now Called Persistence of Fetal Vasculature)

An important and varied type of capsular opacity is associated with PFV (Fig. 2-9). This new term, suggested by Goldberg[14] in 1997, has replaced the older term, persistent hyperplastic primary vitreous. The cardinal features of this spectrum include a membrane behind, but inseparable from, the posterior lens capsule with blood vessels coursing through it. The membrane is often attached to the ciliary processes, pulling them in toward the center of the papillary space. A persistent hyaloid artery is present that can, in rare cases, have enough persistent blood flow to cause hemorrhage when cut by the vitrector handpiece at surgery. Posterior retinal involvement portends a poor prognosis for visual outcome. Surgical aggressiveness is usually reserved for those cases with little or no posterior involvement. Mild cases of PFV are also seen, with only a few, less visually significant, findings. Readers should refer to Chapter 31 for more information on PFV.

Traumatic Cataracts

Since trauma is an etiology rather than a morphology, this type of cataract is discussed above in the section on etiology. However, it is also included here since it does not fit into any one anatomical category. A postsurgical database of patients classified morphologically or anatomically would still need a separate trauma category. Penetrating trauma most often causes a total cataract since the lens is usually ruptured. Blunt traumas cause cataracts that are variable in severity but often appear plaquelike and fibrotic, with anterior and posterior subcapsular opacity as well. Zonular disruption is common, as is anterior chamber angle recession. Chapter 53 covers traumatic cataracts in more detail.

In summary, congenital, infantile, and juvenile onset cataracts represent important causes of visual impairment in childhood. A thorough ocular and systemic examination will often be needed to uncover valuable information needed to assign the appropriate etiology and develop the best treatment plan for the child. The morphological features of childhood cataracts are varied. A classification system based on categories commonly used by surgeons and in clinics is presented and recommended. Segregating childhood cataracts in this way may also help predict the prognosis and the risk for later complications.

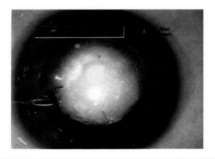

FIGURE 2-9. Persistence and hyperplasia of the primary vitreous. This entity is now called persistent fetal vasculature (PFV) because it represents a spectrum, from the severe variety shown here to much less significant fetal remnants. Note the presence of multiple vessels between the fibrous plaque, the crystalline lens, and the iris. (Courtesy of Abhay R. Vasavada, MD, FRCS, Ahmedabad, India)

REFERENCES

1. Lambert SR, Drack AV. Infantile cataracts. *Surv Ophthalmol* 1996;40:427–458.
2. Bardelli AM, Lasorella G, Vanni M. Congenital and developmental cataracts and multimalformation syndromes. *Ophthalmic Pediatr Genet* 1989;10:93–298.
3. Arkin M, Azar D, Fraioli A. Infantile cataracts. *Int Ophthalmol Clin* 1992;32:110–111.
4. Jain IS, Pillai P, Gangwar DN, Gopal L, Dhir SP. Congenital cataract: management and results. *J Pediatr Ophthalmol Strabismus* 1983;20:243–246.
5. Moore DB. Pediatric cataracts—Diagnosis and treatment. *Optom Vis Sci* 1994;71:168–173.
6. Eckstein M, Vijayalakshmi P, Killedar M, Gilbert C, Foster A. Aetiology of childhood cataract in south India. *Br J Ophthalmol* 1996;80:628–632.
7. Jaafar MS, Robb RM. Congenital anterior polar cataract: a review of 63 cases. *Ophthalmology* 1984;91:249.
8. Amaya L, Taylor D, Russell-Eggitt I, Nischal KK, Lengyel D. The morphology and natural history of childhood cataracts. *Surv Ophthalmol* 2003;48:125–144.

9. O'Neil JW, Hutchinson AK, Saunders RA, Wilson ME. Acquired cataracts after argon laser photocoagulation for retinopathy of prematurity. *J AAPOS* 1998;2:48–51.
10. Parks MM. Visual results in aphakic children. *Am J Ophthalmol* 1982;94:441–449.
11. Parks MM, Johnson DA, Reed GW. Long-term visual results and complications in children with aphakia: a function of cataract type. *Ophthalmology* 1993;100:826–841.
12. Jaafar MS, Robb RM. Congenital anterior polar cataract: a review of 63 cases. *Ophthalmology* 1984;91:249–254.
13. Hiles DA, Carter BT. Classification of cataracts in children. *Int Ophthalmol Clin* 1977;17:15–29.
14. Goldberg MF. Persistent fetal vasculature (PFV): an integrated interpretation of signs and symptoms associated with persistent hyperplastic primary vitreous (PHPV). LIV Edward Jackson Memorial Lecture. *Am J Ophthalmol* 1997;124:587–626.

Genetics of Congenital Cataracts

Vanita Kumar, Jai Rup Singh, and Daljit Singh

Congenital cataract is highly heterogeneous clinically, as various types and subtypes have been documented. It also exhibits wide inter- and intrafamilial heterogeneity.[1,2] Genetically, also, it is heterogeneous, as all three Mendelian modes of inheritance have been reported for it.[3] In nonconsanguineous populations, most inherited nonsyndromic cataracts show an autosomal dominant mode of inheritance, but X-linked and autosomal recessive forms are also common. Nearly one-third of congenital cataract patients have a positive family history.[4]

Eighteen independent genetic loci on many different chromosomes have been identified to date for nonsyndromic autosomal dominant congenital cataract (ADCC). Mutations in 11 genes, including 6 genes for crystallins (αA, αB, βA3/A1, βB2, γC, γD), 2 for gap junctional proteins (GJA-3 and GJA-8), 1 for beaded filament chain protein (BFSP-2), 1 for major intrinsic protein (MIP), and 1 for heat shock factor (HSF-4), have been identified for its different phenotypes (Table 3-1).

Of 18 loci mapped for ADCC, 3 were mapped by Vanita and coworkers, in three large ADCC families of Indian origin, having unique phenotypes.[5,6,10] In one of these families, in seven generations, 74 members were identified as being affected by congenital cataract. The phenotype of this cataract is unique, as it differs completely from the previously reported phenotypes and is described as a "central pouch-like cataract with sutural opacities."[5] It appears as a six-sided pouch with anterior and posterior Y-sutural opacities with prominences at their ends. The anterior and posterior Y sutures end in dumbbell- and knob-shaped opacities. To identify the disease locus in this family, initially we performed a linkage analysis using highly polymorphic microsatellite markers from known candidate regions and excluded all the known loci. In a genomewide scan using 360 markers, linkage to a novel locus on chromosome 15 was detected.[5] A maximum positive 2-point lod score of 5.98 at $\theta = 0.000$ was obtained with marker D15S117. Two-point linkage data were further supported by haplotype and multipoint linkage analysis with chromosome 15 markers with a maximum multipoint lod score of 5.98 with marker D15S117.

In another family, 33 members spread over five generations were diagnosed as being affected by a unique form of "sutural cataract with punctate and cerulean opacities" (Fig. 3-1). Slit-lamp examination showed prominent, dense white opacification around the anterior and posterior Y sutures, and the posterior sutures were more severely affected. Also, grayish, bluish, sharply defined, elongated, spindle-shaped, oval, punctate, and cerulean opacities of various sizes, arranged in a lamellar form, were observed. Linkage analysis to identify the disease locus was carried out for the known candidate regions, and on excluding the loci on chromosomes 1, 2, 12–14, 16, 17, and 19, we obtained positive lod scores on chromosome 22. A maximum positive 2-point lod score of 8.50 at $\theta = 0.050$ was obtained with marker D22S315 at 22q11.2-12.1.[6] Of four β-crystalline genes, *CRYBA4*, *CRYBB1*, *CRYBB2*, and *CRYBB3*, and a pseudogene, *CRYBP1*, localized close to the mapped locus, the investigators screened *CRYBB2*, which is highly expressed in adult human lenses, to identify the molecular defect for this phenotype. A C → T mutation was identified at nucleotide position 475 (Q155X) in the *CRYBB2* gene in all affected subjects in this family. Apart from this mutation, a variant 483C → T was identified in the sixth exon of the *CRYBB2* gene, segregating only in the affected individuals, and not in the unaffected individuals, in this family. These two sequence alterations are identical to the sequence of the *CRYBP1* pseudogene, which is placed very close to the *CRYBB2* gene. Also ≤104 bp *CRYBP1*-like fragment flanked by chromosomal junction sequences, is observed in *CRYBB2* gene sequence. Therefore, gene conversion between the *CRYBB2* gene and its pseudogene *CRYBP1* is the most likely mechanism for this unique phenotype.[7] As the same mutation, Q155X, has been reported for two different phenotypes of ADCC in two different families, of different origins,[8,9] it can be concluded that the mutant *CRYBB2* causes cataract formation but other

▶ **TABLE 3-1** **Mapped Loci for Nonsyndromic Autosomal Dominant Congenital Cataracts**

Locus	Type of Cataract	Mutated Gene	Reference
1pter-p36.13	i. Posterior polar	Unknown	Ionides et al. 1997 [14]
	ii. Volkmann		Eiberg et al. 1995 [15]
1q12-25	Zonular pulverulent	Connexin-50 (GJA-8)	Renwick and Lawler 1963 [16]
			Shiels et al. 1998 [17]
2p12	Nuclear cataract	Unknown	Khaliq et al. 2002 [18]
2q33-35	i. Coppock-like	Gamma C	Lubsen et al. 1987 [19]
	ii. Polymorphic	Unknown	Rogaev et al. 1996 [20]
	iii. Aculeiform	Gamma D	Héon et al. 1999 [21]
3q21-22	ADCC-3	BFSP-2/phakinin	Jakobs et al. 2000 [22]
11q22-22.3	Posterior polar	Crystalline αB	Berry et al. 2001 [23]
12q13	i. Polymorphic lamellar	MIP	Berry et al. 2000 [24]
	ii. ADCC-2	MIP	Bateman et al. 2000 [25]
13q11-12	Zonular pulverulent	Connexin-46 (GJA-3)	Mackay et al. 1997 [26]
15q21-22	Central pouchlike with sutural opacities[a]	Unknown	Vanita et al. 2001 [5]
16q22.1	i. Posterior polar	Unknown	Richards et al. 1984 [27]
	ii. Marner	HSF-4	Eiberg et al. 1988 [28]
	iii. Lamellar	HSF-4	Bu et al. 2002 [29]
16q23.1	Cerulean[b]	Unknown	Kumar et al. 2002 [10]
17p13	Anterior polar	Unknown	Berry et al. 1996 [13]
17q11.2-12	Zonular sutural	Crystalline βA3/A1	Padma et al. 1995 [30]
			Kannabiran et al. 1999 [31]
17q23.1-23.2	Zonular pulverulent	Crystalline βA3/A1	Bateman et al. 2000 [25]
17q24	Cerulean	Unknown	Armitage et al. 1995 [32]
20p12-q12	Posterior polar	Unknown	Yamada et al. 2000 [33]
21q22.3	Zonular	Crystalline αA	Litt et al. 1998 [34]
22q11.2-12.1	i. Cerulean	Crystalline βB2	Kramer et al. 1996 [35]
	ii. Coppock-like	Crystalline βB2	Gill et al. 2000 [9]
	iii. Sutural cataract with punctate & cerulean opacities[a]	Crystalline βB2 & crystalline βB2P	Vanita et al. 2001 [7]

[a] Novel phenotype documented and mapped by authors.
[b] Novel locus mapped by authors.

modifying factors determine the exact phenotype of the cataract.

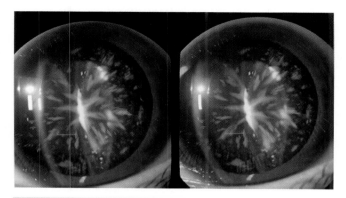

FIGURE 3-1. "Sutural cataract with punctate and cerulean opacities" mapped to a locus at 22q11.2-12.1.

In another ADCC family, 12 members of three generations were diagnosed to be affected by "cerulean cataract." Initially linkage analysis was performed for known cerulean cataract loci at 17q24 and 22q11.2-12.1 and excluded these as candidates for our cerulean cataract family. The other candidate loci, on chromosomes 1–3, 9–17, 19, and 21 were also excluded by analyzing more than 100 markers (nearly one-third of the genome), and positive 2-point lod scores >3 were obtained with three markers on chromosome 16 at a novel locus at 16q23.1.[10] Two-point linkage data at this region were further supported by haplotype and multipoint analysis, and a multipoint lod score of 3.612 was obtained between marker D16S518 and marker D16S511.

On the basis of mapping data also, the genetic heterogeneity of congenital cataract is evident. The same phenotype has been mapped on different chromosomes. For example, zonular pulverulent cataract has been mapped to chromosome 1 in one family and to chromosome 13 in another, and cerulean cataract in three families has been mapped to three different chromosomes: 16, 17, and 22. Similarly for posterior polar cataract, four different loci have been identified, on chromosomes 1, 11, 16, and 20. Also, for anterior polar cataract, Moross et al.[11] reported a balanced translocation between chromosome 2 and chromosome 14 in a three-generation ADCC family, Rubin et al.[12] reported an unbalanced translocation between chromosome 3 and chromosome 18 in two affected sisters, and Berry et al.[13] identified a locus for anterior polar cataract at 17p13 in an ADCC family. On the other hand, an identical mutation, a 475C → T transition in the sixth exon of the *CRYBB2* gene, has been identified for totally different phenotypes, i.e., cerulean cataract and Coppock-like cataract.[8,9]

The α-, β-, and γ-crystallines are the major structural proteins of the lens, constituting more than 90% of the soluble lens proteins. Their highly ordered arrangement in the lens is responsible for the consistent refractive index and transparency. Most of the mutations reported in crystallins are predicted to disrupt the tertiary structure, resulting in an increased tendency of these crystallins to aggregate and precipitate. Apart from crystallins, the mutations identified in cytoskeletal components, membrane proteins, gap junctional channels, and heat shock factors indicate their role in maintaining and regulating transparency and homeostasis in the eye lens. Also, the mechanism of cataract formation is not as simple as one gene mutation resulting in one phenotype. Rather, genetic as well as environmental factors may also modify the expression and hence the phenotype. Therefore, these factors also need to be identified. Identification of the exact molecular defects underlying the different phenotypes of congenital cataracts will improve our understanding, not only of the pathogenesis of childhood cataracts and the developmental biology of the lens, but also of age-related cataracts.

REFERENCES

1. Francois J. Genetics of cataract. *Ophthalmologica* 1982;184:61–71.
2. Luis A, David T, Isabelle RE, Ken KN, Dora L. The morphology and natural history of childhood cataracts. *Surv Ophthalmol* 2003;48:125–144.
3. McKusick VA. *Mendelian Inheritance in Man: Catalogs of Autosomal Dominant, Autosomal Recessive, and X-Linked Phenotypes.* 10th Ed. Baltimore, MD: The Johns Hopkins University Press, 1992.
4. Vanita, Singh JR, Singh D. Genetic and segregation analysis of congenital cataract in the Indian population. *Clin Genet* 56:389–393.
5. Vanita, Singh JR, Sarhadi VK, et al. A novel form of central pouch-like cataract with sutural opacities maps to chromosome 15q21-22. *Am J Hum Genet* 2001;68:509–514.
6. Vanita. *Genetical Investigations in Congenital Cataract Cases* [PhD thesis]. Amritsar, India: Guru Nanak Dev University.
7. Vanita, Sarhadi VK, Andre R, et al. A unique form of autosomal dominant cataract explained by gene conversion between β-crystalline B2 and its pseudogene. *J Med Genet* 2001;38:392–396.
8. Litt M, Valenzuela RC, LaMorticella DM, et al. Autosomal dominant cerulean cataract is associated with a chain termination mutation in the human crystallin gene CRYβB2. *Hum Mol Genet* 1997;6:665–668.
9. Gill D, Klose R, Munier FL, et al. Genetic heterogeneity of the Coppock-like cataract: a mutation in CRYBB2 on chromosome 22q11.2. *Invest Ophthalmol Vis Sci* 2000;41:159–165.
10. Kumar V, Singh JR, Singh D, Sperling K. A new locus for cerulean cataract on chromosome 16. *Am J Hum Genet* 2002;71:2107.
11. Moross T, Vaithilingam SS, Styles S, Gardner HA. Autosomal dominant anterior polar cataracts associated with a familial 2;14 translocation. *J Med Genet* 1984;21;52–53.
12. Rubin SE, Nelson LB, Pletcher BA. Anterior polar cataract in two sisters with an unbalanced 3;18 translocation. *Am J Ophthalmol* 1994;117:512–515.
13. Berry V, Ionides ACW, Moore AT, Plant C, Bhattacharya SS, Shiels A. A locus for autosomal dominant anterior polar cataract on chromosome 17p. *Hum Mol Genet* 1996;5:415–419.
14. Ionides ACW, Berry V, Mackay DS, et al. A locus for autosomal dominant posterior polar cataract on chromosome 1p. *Hum Mol Genet* 1997;6:47–51.
15. Eiberg H, Lund AM, Warburg M, Rosenberg T. Assignment of congenital cataract Volkmann type (CCV) to chromosome 1p36. *Hum Genet* 1995;96:33–38.
16. Renwick JK, Lawler SD. Probable linkage between a congenital cataract locus and the Duffy blood group locus. *Ann Hum Genet* 1963;27:67–84.
17. Shiels A, Mackay D, Ionides A, Berry V, Moore A, Bhattacharya SS. A missense mutation in the human connexin50 gene (GJA8) underlies autosomal dominant zonular pulverulent cataract on chromosome 1q. *Am J Hum Genet* 1998;62:526–532.
18. Khaliq S, Hameed A, Ismail M, Anwar K, Mehdi SQ. A novel locus for autosomal dominant nuclear cataract mapped to chromosome 2p12 in a Pakistani family. *Invest Ophthal Vis Sci* 2002;43:2083–2087.
19. Lubsen N, Renwick J, Tsui LC, Breitman M, Schoenmackers J. A locus of a human hereditary cataract is closely linked to the gamma-crystalline gene family. *Proc Natl Acad Sci USA* 1987;84:489–492.
20. Rogaev EI, Rogaeva EA, Korovaitseva GI, et al. Linkage of polymorphic congenital cataract to the γ-crystalline gene locus on human chromosome 2q33-35. *Hum Mol Genet* 1996;5:699–703.
21. Héon E, Priston M, Schorderet DF, et al. The γ-crystallines and human cataracts: a puzzle made clearer. *Am J Hum Genet* 1999;65:1261–1267.
22. Jakobs PM, Hess JF, FitzGerald PG, Kramer P, Weleber RG, Litt M. Autosomal dominant congenital cataract associated with a deletion mutation in the human beaded filament protein gene BFSP2. *Am J Hum Genet* 2000;66:1432–1436.
23. Berry V, Francis P, Reddy MA, et al. Alpha-B crystalline gene (CRYAB) mutation causes dominant congenital posterior polar cataract in humans. *Am J Hum Genet* 2001;69:1141–1145.
24. Berry V, Francis P, Kaushal S, Moore A, Bhattacharya SS. Missense mutation in MIP underlie autosomal dominant polymorphic and lamellar cataracts linked to 12q. *Nature Genet* 2000;25:15–17.
25. Bateman JB, Geyer DD, Flodman P, et al. A new betaA1-crystalline splice junction mutation in autosomal dominant cataract. *Invest Ophthalmol Vis Sci* 2000;41:3278–3285.
26. Mackay D, Ionides A, Berry V, Moore A, Bhattacharya SS, Shiels A. Autosomal dominant congenital cataract linked to chromosome 13. *Am J Hum Genet* 1997;60:1474–1478.
27. Richards J, Maumenee IH, Rowe S, Lovrien EW. Congenital cataract possibly linked to haptoglobin. *Cytogenet Cell Genet* 1984;37:570.
28. Eiberg H, Marner E, Rosenberg T, Mohr J. Marner's cataract (CAM) assigned to chromosome 16: linkage to haptoglobin. *Clin Genet* 1988;34:272–275.
29. Bu L, Jin Y, Shi Y, et al. Mutant DNA binding domain of HSF4 is associated with autosomal dominant lamellar and Marner cataract. *Nature Genet* 2002;31:276–278.
30. Padma T, Ayyagari R, Murty JS, et al. Autosomal dominant zonular cataract with sutural opacities localized to chromosome 17q11-12. *Am J Hum Genet* 1995;57:840–845.

31. Kannabiran C, Wawrousek E, Sergeev Y, Rao GN, Kaiser-Kupfer M, Hejtmancik JF. Mutation of beta A3/A1 crystalline gene in autosomal dominant zonular cataract with sutural opacities results in a protein with single globular domain. *Invest Ophthal Vis Sci* 1999;40:S786 (abstract).

32. Armitage MM, Kivlin JD, Ferell RE. A progressive early onset cataract gene maps to human chromosome 17q24. *Nature Genet* 1995;9:37–40.

33. Yamada K, Tomita H, Yoshiura K, et al. An autosomal dominant posterior polar cataract locus maps to human chromosome 20p12-q12. *Eur J Hum Genet* 2000;8:535–539.

34. Litt M, Kramer P, LaMorticella DM, Murphey W, Lovrien EW, Weleber RG. Autosomal dominant congenital cataract associated with a missense mutation in the human alpha crystalline gene CRYAA. *Hum Mol Genet* 1998;7:471–474.

35. Kramer P, Yount J, Mitchell T, et al. A second locus for cerulean cataract maps to the β crystalline region on chromosome 22. *Genomics* 1996;35:539–542.

Epidemiology of Pediatric Cataracts and Associated Blindness

Rupal H. Trivedi and M. Edward Wilson, Jr.

According to the World Health Organization (WHO), every minute one child goes blind somewhere in the world.[1] In 1992 WHO estimated that there are 1.5 million children with severe visual impairment (SVI) or blindness (BL) in the world.[2] The incidence of SVI in children is not precisely known. The WHO report[1] gave an estimated figure of 500,000 new cases a year, of which at least 50% of the children are believed eventually to die because of associated illness.

Children who are born blind or who become blind after birth have a lifetime of BL ahead of them that includes all the associated socioeconomic impacts to the child, the family, and the society. Indeed, the number of "blind years" because of all causes of BL in children is almost equal to the number of "blind years" because of cataracts in adults.[3] Because of the impact of BL in children, several programs are seeking to fight this problem, including a 5-year program launched in June 2002 by WHO to reduce the burden of avoidable BL in children in 30 developing countries.[4] The Lions Club's International Foundation is contributing $3.75 million toward this goal.

One of the leading etiologies of BL in children, especially in the developing world, is cataracts. Using a standardized classification and coding system, Gilbert and colleagues[5] evaluated 9,293 children in 40 countries and reported that the lens is responsible for 12% (range, 7 to 20%) of anatomical abnormalities in children. Because of the high incidence and treatable nature of the condition, it is reasonable to think that an improved approach to the management of childhood cataracts would have a large impact on childhood BL as a whole.

In this chapter we describe the epidemiology of childhood cataracts and the BL associated with them.

DIFFICULTIES IN DATA COLLECTION

Several articles have been published that attempt to quantitate BL from childhood cataracts. The reliability of these studies and their usefulness for comparison are uncertain for various reasons, which include the following.

1. *Noncataractous reasons for BL.* Most of the studies define BL as being caused by pediatric cataracts. However, besides cataracts, there are many conditions that can prevent the achievement of normal visual acuity (e.g., amblyopia, secondary opacification of the visual axis, residual refractive error). It should also be noted that lesser degrees of visual loss, visual field defects, or unilateral BL can also result in significant visual disability in children, which has not been accounted for in most studies.

2. *Varying standards between studies.* Standards for "visual impairment" and "age at childhood cataract" vary between studies. This makes comparison of data difficult. WHO defines the visually impaired (VI) child as having a corrected visual acuity of <20/60 in the better eye, SVI as having a corrected visual acuity of <20/200, and BL as having a corrected visual acuity of <20/400. Gilbert and coworkers[5] tried to improve the overall collection of data by publishing standardized SVI forms for childhood data collection. Widespread use of these standardized forms will hopefully lead to more meaningful data collection that will allow comparison between studies.

3. *Different methods for collecting data.* Registration data, population surveys, and studies of children in schools for the blind have been found to vary widely in the methods used for data collection. Differences may underestimate or overestimate the severity of disease. Comparisons between these studies are therefore unreliable.

4. *Difficulty in assessing childhood visual function.* Visual function can be difficult to assess accurately in children even under ideal conditions. This can lead to variations between examinations of the same children and unreliable visual function reporting.

PREVALENCE AND INCIDENCE

Prevalence

Prevalence can be defined as the total number of cases of a disease in a given population at a specific time.

Childhood Cataracts

The prevalence of childhood cataracts has been reported as 1 to15 per 10,000 children.[6] The wide range is because of the variety of methods, different age groups, and varying case definitions used in the studies, as well as true differences between populations.[6] Foster and colleagues[6] also noted that available information suggests that the birth prevalence of congenital bilateral cataracts in industrialized countries is 1 to 3 per 10,000 children.

They have calculated that approximately 4 children/ million total population per year will be born with bilateral cataracts in industrialized countries, and the figure for developing countries is likely to be 10 children/million total population per year. They have estimated that currently 200,000 children globally are blind owing to bilateral cataracts.

The birth defect monitoring program (BDMP) in the United States reported the prevalence of congenital cataracts as 0.8/10,000 births for 1970–1987.[7] A cluster of areas with a significantly high prevalence was found in Michigan in a geographic band from the southwestern to the east–central section of the state. Edmonds and James,[8] examining the BDMP data, have shown that from 1979/1980 to 1988/1989 there was a 6.8% rate increase (range, 0.7 to 1.3 per 10,000 births). James[7] reported the 1988/1989 BDMP/Commission on Professional and Hospital Activities prevalence of 1.2/10,000 births, with the highest rates found in the Northeast (1.7/10,000). The Metropolitan Atlanta Congenital Defects Program surveillance reported a congenital cataract prevalence of 2.1/10,000 live births from 1988 to 1991.[9] Kocur and Resnikoff[10] have reported that cataracts are the leading cause of BL in the middle-income countries of Europe.

▶ **TABLE 4-1** **Worldwide Regional Distribution of Cataract as a Cause of Visual Impairment and Blindness in Children**

Region	Reference [No.], Year(s) of Study	Number of Patients Examined	Percentage Visual Impairment (%)	Cause of Visual Impairment	Population Studied
Canada	Pearce [16], 1970–1973	1,046	13	Cataract	School for blind
Jamaica	Moriarty [17], 1986	108	39	Cataract	School for blind
Bolivia	Foster [18], 1988	78	21	Cataract	School for blind
Thailand, Philippines	Gilbert & Foster [19], 1993	65, 113	16.9, 16.8	Cataract	School for blind
West Africa, South India, Chile	Gilbert et al. [20], NA	284, 305, 217	15.5, 7.4, 9.2	Cataract	School for blind
Argentina	Gilbert et al. [21], 1993	573	8	Cataract	School for blind
Sri Lanka	Eckstein et al. [22], 1995	226	17	Cataract	School for blind
East Africa	Gilbert et al. [23], 1995	244	13.5	Cataract	School for blind
USA	Decarlo & Nowakowski [24], 1996–1997	123	13	Cataract, aphakia	School for blind
China	Hornby et al. [25], 1998	1,245	18.8	Lens	School for blind
India	Rahi et al. [26], 1995	1,318	12.3	Cataract, uncorrected aphakia, amblyopia	School for blind
Brazil	de Carvalho et al. [27], 1982–1992	395	10.4	Cataract	Low-vision service
Uganda	Waddell [28], 1984–1998	443; 692	21.7 (school); 36.4 (community)	Cataract, aphakia	School for blind; community
India	Hornby et al. [29], NA	291	7.9	Lens	School for blind
Poland	Seroczynska et al. [30], 1979–1999	3,000	14.1	Cataract	School for blind
Malaysia	Reddy & Tan [31], 2001	358	22.3	Lens	School for blind
Mongolia	Bulgan & Gilbert [32], 2002	64	34	Lens	School for blind + community

Screening of 2,447 4-year-olds yielded a rate of 7.7 cataracts/10,000 live births,[11] while two other cohort birth studies suggested a prevalence of 5.3[12] and 4.4[13] cataracts/10,000 live births. A prospective collaborative perinatal project conducted by 12 U.S. universities reported the prevalence of infantile cataract as 13.6/10,000 infants.[14] The report further noted that isolated infantile cataracts occurred 3.8 times as often among infants born weighting ≤2,500 g than among those born at >2,500 g. In 2003 Holmes et al.[15] reported, in a retrospective population-based medical record retrieval in the U.S. population, that the birth prevalence of visually significant cataracts was 3.0/10,000 (infantile cataract) to 4.5/10,000 (possible infantile cataract, defined as a cataract diagnosed after the first year for which there is no evidence of an acquired etiology). The authors estimated a total of 1,774 cases a year, with a prevalence rate of 4.5/10,000 live births.

Blindness Associated with Childhood Cataracts

The prevalence of BL from cataracts in children in developing countries is probably 1 to 4/10,000, compared with approximately 0.1 to 0.4/10,000 children in the industrialized world.[6] Table 4-1 reports the regional distributions of cataracts as a cause of VI and BL in children around the world.[16-32]

Incidence

The incidence is the number of new cases that develop in a population during a specified time interval. Although the incidence of pediatric cataracts is difficult to ascertain, Wirth and coworkers[33] have indirectly calculated it for Australia during their 25-year study (1975–2000). Over these 25 years, 421 index cases with congenital and pediatric cataracts were identified (16.8% a year), giving an incidence of pediatric cataracts in Australia of 2.2/10,000 (i.e., 1 in 4,500).

CONTROL OF CATARACT BLINDNESS IN CHILDREN

Pediatric cataract–associated BL can be avoided or treated using a combination of preventive services at the community level, specialized surgical services in pediatric ophthalmic units, and low-vision devices and services. This discussion is mostly applicable to the developing world. Most developing nations provide health delivery services through a tiered system, with central hospitals supporting smaller and rural hospitals and health delivery centers. In Africa and Asia, for example, many countries have established a three-tiered system, consisting of primary, secondary, and tertiary levels.

Primary Level of Care

Primary eye care includes services provided by trained community health workers. Their main responsibility is to prevent BL from occurring. Personnel trained in primary eye care are essential for the control of BL in children. Primary care providers should

- provide ophthalmoscopic screening of neonates and identify patients who need referrals;
- refer such patients for ophthalmologic assessment and treatment;
- encourage and motivate parents and/or children regarding patching, when suggested by secondary and/or tertiary eye care providers;
- provide services for immunization;
- encourage long-term ocular follow-up;
- provide counseling to avoid consensual marriages between families with histories of childhood cataracts; and
- educate people to use preventive measures to avoid sports-related and other ocular trauma.

Secondary Level of Care

At the secondary level the main responsibility is to maintain or improve functional visual outcome. The eye surgeon should

- be able to carry out a full eye examination and assessment and make a provisional diagnosis;
- arrange surgery for the affected eye at the tertiary center;
- follow up postoperative eyes to detect secondary opacities;
- work as a joining link between primary-level care and tertiary centers;
- help patients to follow patching instructions;
- effectively communicate with parents to ensure their involvement; and
- arrange screening for children in their schools.

Tertiary Level of Care

Tertiary care services should include facilities for the trained ophthalmologist, optometrist, anesthetist, pediatrician, and neonatologist. Their main responsibility is to restore vision to patients blinded by anatomical and/or functional causes. The central hospital, usually attached to a medical school, is the tertiary resource. There may be several tertiary hospitals in larger countries serving large geographic regions. This facility usually is a large general hospital and offers a wide range of specialty services. Although it consumes a high proportion of the health budget, it often is overwhelmed by the demand for services. The tertiary eye center provides more sophisticated eye care than that available at the provincial hospital, and ophthalmic subspecialists, if available, are likely to be assigned there.

Tertiary care centers should

- be able to provide surgical services within well-equipped centers containing vitrectomy instruments, high-viscosity viscoelastic agents, and high-quality intraocular lens material;
- organize and provide low-vision services;
- responsibly participate in research;
- train the faculty of primary- and secondary-level programs;
- support, supervise, motivate, and provide feedback to staff at secondary-level centers;
- correct residual refractive error when needed;
- provide long-term regular follow-up with assessment and treatment of posterior capsule opacification, glaucoma, refractive error, and amblyopia, to achieve a good visual outcome; and
- provide guidance to improve the infrastructure and technology that will ensure the development of low-cost, high-quality, low-vision devices, which should be widely available, even in low-income countries.

Globally, an estimated 200,000 children are bilaterally blind from cataract. Many more suffer from partial cataracts that progress and cause increasing visual difficulty as the child ages. Exact epidemiological data for children of all ages are difficult to gather. However, because of the number of blind years presented, treatment of partial cataracts is among the most cost-effective intervention in all of ophthalmology. Management of pediatric cataracts is often difficult and tedious, and it requires a dedicated team effort by the parents, pediatrician, surgeon, anesthesiologist, orthoptist, and community health worker. We should concentrate on not only improving, but also maintaining both anatomical and functional outcomes in eyes with pediatric cataracts and prepare for lifelong follow-up.

REFERENCES

1. WHO. Press release. Geneva: World Health Organization, 2002.
2. WHO. *Prevention of Childhood Blindness.* Geneva: World Health Organization, 1992.
3. Gilbert C, Foster A. Childhood blindness in the context of VISION 2020—The right to sight. *Bull WHO* 2001;79:227–232.
4. Ahmad K. WHO launches international program to combat childhood blindness. *Lancet* 2002;359:2258.
5. Gilbert C, Foster A, Negrel AD, Thylefors B. Childhood blindness: a new form for recording causes of visual loss in children. *Bull WHO* 1993;71:485–489.
6. Foster A, Gilbert C, Rahi J. Epidemiology of cataract in childhood: a global perspective. *J Cataract Refract Surg* 1997;23:601–604.
7. James LM. Maps of birth defects occurrence in the U.S., Birth Defects Monitoring Program (BDMP)/CPHA, 1970–1987. *Teratology* 1993;48:551–646.
8. Edmonds LD, James LM. Temporal trends in the prevalence of congenital malformations at birth based on the birth defects monitoring program, United States, 1979–1987. *MMWR CDC Surveill Summ* 1990;39:19–23.
9. MACDP. Metropolitan Atlanta congenital defects program (MACDP) surveillance data, 1988–1991. *Teratology* 1993;48:695–709.
10. Kocur I, Resnikoff S. Visual impairment and blindness in Europe and their prevention. *Br J Ophthalmol* 2002;86:716–722.
11. Kohler L, Stigmar G. Vision screening of four-year-old children. *Acta Physiol Scand* 1973;62:17–27.
12. Stewart-Brown SL, Haslum MN. Partial sight and blindness in children of the 1970 birth cohort at 10 years of age. *J Epidemiol Commun Health* 1988;42:17–23.
13. Stayte M, Reeves B, Wortham C. Ocular and vision defects in preschool children. *Br J Ophthalmol* 1993;77:228–232.
14. SanGiovanni JP, Chew EY, Reed GF, et al. Infantile cataract in the collaborative perinatal project: prevalence and risk factors. *Arch Ophthalmol* 2002;120:1559–1565.
15. Holmes JM, Leske DA, Burke JP, Hodge DO. Birth prevalence of visually significant infantile cataract in a defined U.S. population. *Ophthal Epidemiol* 2003;10:67–74.
16. Pearce WG. Causes of blindness in children. 1046 cases registered with the Canadian National Institute for the Blind 1970–1973. *Can J Ophthalmol* 1975;10:469–472.
17. Moriarty BJ. Childhood blindness in Jamaica. *Br J Ophthalmol* 1988;72:65–67.
18. Foster A. Childhood blindness. *Eye* 1988;2:S27–S36.
19. Gilbert C, Foster A. Causes of blindness in children attending four schools for the blind in Thailand and the Philippines. A comparison between urban and rural blind school populations. *Int Ophthalmol* 1993;17:229–234.
20. Gilbert CE, Canovas R, Hagan M, et al. Causes of childhood blindness: results from West Africa, South India and Chile. *Eye* 1993;7:184–188.
21. Gilbert CE, Canovas R, Kocksch de Canovas R, Foster A. Causes of blindness and severe visual impairment in children in Chile. *Dev Med Child Neurol* 1994;36:326–333.
22. Eckstein MB, Foster A, Gilbert CE. Causes of childhood blindness in Sri Lanka: results from children attending six schools for the blind. *Br J Ophthalmol* 1995;79:633–636.
23. Gilbert CE, Wood M, Waddel K, Foster A. Causes of childhood blindness in East Africa: results in 491 pupils attending 17 schools for the blind in Malawi, Kenya and Uganda. *Ophthal Epidemiol* 1995;2:77–84.
24. DeCarlo DK, Nowakowski R. Causes of visual impairment among students at the Alabama School for the Blind. *J Am Optom Assoc* 1999;70:647–652.
25. Hornby SJ, Xiao Y, Gilbert CE, et al. Causes of childhood blindness in the People's Republic of China: results from 1131 blind school students in 18 provinces. *Br J Ophthalmol* 1999;83:929–932.
26. Rahi JS, Sripathi S, Gilbert CE, Foster A. Childhood blindness in India: causes in 1318 blind school students in nine states. *Eye* 1995;9:545–550.
27. de Carvalho KM, Minguini N, Moreira Filho DC, Kara-Jose N. Characteristics of a pediatric low-vision population. *J Pediatr Ophthalmol Strabismus* 1998;35:162–165.
28. Waddell KM. Childhood blindness and low vision in Uganda. *Eye* 1998;12:184–192.
29. Hornby SJ, Adolph S, Gothwal VK, et al. Evaluation of children in six blind schools of Andhra Pradesh. *Ind J Ophthalmol* 2000;48:195–200.
30. Seroczynska M, Prost ME, Medrun J, et al. The causes of childhood blindness and visual impairment in Poland. *Klin Oczna* 2001;103:117–120.
31. Reddy SC, Tan BC. Causes of childhood blindness in Malaysia: results from a national study of blind school students. *Int Ophthalmol* 2001;24:53–59.
32. Bulgan T, Gilbert C. Prevalence and causes of severe visual impairment and blindness in children in Mongolia. *Ophthal Epidemiol* 2002;9:271–281.
33. Wirth MG, Russell-Eggitt IM, Craig JE, et al. Aetiology of congenital and paediatric cataract in an Australian population. *Br J Ophthalmol* 2002;86:782–786.

Preoperative Workup

Chapter 5

Evaluation of Visually Significant Cataracts

Suresh K. Pandey

Cataracts remain one of the most important surgically treated causes of blindness in children and represents the major preventable cause of lifelong visual handicap. The importance of careful evaluation of visually significant cataracts cannot be overemphasized. Only a small minority of childhood cataracts present clinically with subjective complaints relating to vision. Therefore all newborns deserve a screening eye examination, which should include an evaluation of the red fundus reflexes and ophthalmoscopy. Often the first sign of the lenticular opacity is a white or partially white pupil noted by the parents or caretaker. Increasingly, congenital cataracts are detected by pediatricians, who in recent years have been well trained to inspect the red fundus reflex in every newborn. Examination of the red reflex can reveal even minute lenticular opacities. Detailed evaluation of the normally symmetrical red fundus reflexes is easily accomplished in a darkened room by shining a bright direct ophthalmoscope into both eyes simultaneously. This test, called the illumination test, red reflex test, or Bruckner test, can be easily used for routine ocular screening by nurses, pediatricians, neonatologist and family physicians. Retinoscopy through the child's undilated pupil is helpful for estimating potential vision in an eye harboring a cataract. Any central opacity or surrounding cortical distortion >3 mm can be assumed to be visually significant.[1-4]

In addition to the white pupillary reflex, strabismus may be the initial manifestation, especially in unilateral cataract cases. Nystagmus or poor visual fixation may herald the presence of bilateral lens opacities in infancy.[5]

A significant fraction of childhood cataracts is detected in the course of routine school or preschool vision screening.

EVALUATION OF VISUAL ACUITY

Accurate and reliable assessment of visual function in infants and young children is important for ensuring optimal management of those at risk of abnormal visual development. It is important to quantify the visual acuity of children with cataracts as precisely as possible. Visual function can be assessed by history, observation of the ocular fixation and following reflex, behavioral testing, and electrophysiologic examination.

Infants with complete bilateral congenital cataracts usually demonstrate decreased visual interest and experience delayed milestones of development. Ocular fixation and following movements may be decreased or absent. Nystagmus results from early visual deprivation and signals that vision may be poor even after treatment. Various methods have been used for evaluation of visual function in infants and children. In general, most developmentally normal children older than 3 years of age can be tested reliably using Snellen's equivalents. Interested readers should refer to Chapter 50 to become famaliar with details on visual function in children.

HISTORY

A detailed history concerning the age at onset of visual signs and symptoms and the ocular status at previous eye examinations can be helpful in assessing the visual prognosis after treatment.

The etiology and morphology of the lens opacity may help elucidate their origin.[3-8] Interested readers should refer to Chapter 2 to learn details on etiology and morphology of pediatric cataracts. In brief, the common causes of cataracts in children include intrauterine infections, metabolic disorders, and genetically transmitted syndromes. Approximately one third of cataracts in children are sporadic; they are not associated with any systemic or ocular diseases. However, they may be spontaneous mutations and may lead to cataract formation in the patient's offspring. About one third of congenital cataracts are familial. The most frequent mode of transmission is autosomal dominant with complete penetrance. This type of cataract may appear as a total cataract, polar cataract, lamellar cataract, or nuclear opacity. All close family members should be examined. Infectious causes of cataracts include rubella (the most common), chicken pox, cytomegalovirus, herpes simplex, herpes zoster, poliomyelitis, influenza, Epstein–Barr virus, syphilis, and toxoplasmosis.

Unilateral cataracts occupying primarily the posterior cortex (with or without extension forward to involve the nucleus) are usually the result of isolated, idiopathic, sporadic malformation involving the posterior capsule, either posterior bulging of abnormally thin capsular membrane (posterior lenticonus or lentiglobus) or fibrous thickening of the capsule resulting from persistent fetal vasculature.[9] Bilateral posterior polar cataracts (with or without associated lenticonus) are typically familial.

Bilateral or unilateral anterior polar opacities are usually idiopathic, while unilateral or bilateral anterior lenticonus is most often associated with Alport's syndrome. Anterior subcapsular localization may be associated with atopic dermatitis. Nuclear, lamellar, and diffuse multipunctate cataracts may result from a wide variety of causes including chromosomal abnormalities (Down syndrome), metabolic disturbances (primarily hypocalcemia and hypoglycemia), and hereditary transmission, but very often no etiology can be determined.

In contrast to posterior cortical cataracts associated with lenticonus or persistent fetal vasculature, and in marked contrast to the adult situation, isolated posterior subcapsular (PSC) opacification is seldom seen as a sporadic idiopathic occurrence in childhood. Unilateral occurrence should prompt a careful search for evidence of trauma. Reported causes of bilateral PSC cataracts include chronic uveitis, metabolic disorders, prolonged corticosteroid treatment for chronic disease, radiation treatment for malignancy, nonaccidental injury. Posterior subcapsular cataract is also seen in older children and young adults with atopic dermatitis and type 2 (central) neurofibromatosis, and are known complications of systemic steroid therapy. Previous studies have not clearly identified the asthmatic children at risk for development of PSC cataracts. However, recent studies concluded that asthmatic children receiving steroids for 2 years or longer and having a markedly delayed bone age are at a greater risk for development of PSC.[10]

Traumatic cataract in children is a common cause of unilateral visual loss, after penetrating injuries. Eighty percent of traumatic cataracts occur during play or sport-related activities. Injuries caused by BB guns, firecrackers, sticks, and bows and arrows are common causes of traumatic cataracts in children as reported in some studies.[11,12] A history of physical and/or ocular injury is not always available either because there was no adult witness or because the injury resulted from physical abuse that was denied by the caretaker responsible. Crystalline lens dislocation, angle recession, or iridodialysis, and viteous, retinal hemorrhages are associated findings that should immediately suggest traumatic origin.

At the time of first presentation after trauma to the eye, primary repair of the corneal or scleral wound is usually preferred. Cataract surgery with intraocular lens implantation is performed 1–4 weeks after a complete evaluation of damage to intraocular structures (e.g., posterior capsule rupture, vitreous hemorrhage, and retinal detachment) with ancillary methods such as B-scan ultrasonography.

ANTERIOR SEGMENT EVALUATION

Congenital, developmental, and traumatic cataracts can have different morphological characteristics. Slit-lamp examination clarifies the morphology of the cataract and may help determine, along with associated findings, the cause and prognosis. Associated abnormalities of the cornea, iris, and pupil should be noted. A portable handheld slit lamp is especially helpful for examining infants and young children. Glaucoma should be ruled out because cataracts and glaucoma are associated with congenital rubella and Lowe syndrome.[13]

FUNDOSCOPIC EXAMINATION

An attempt should be made to visualize the retina, fovea, and optic disc to estimate the visual potential for the eye. When the cataract completely obstructs the visual axis, B-scan ultrasonography may be used to rule out potential retinal and vitreous pathology.

The anterior segment and fundus examination may need to be done under sedation or examination under anesthesia in young children. The surgeon may elect to prepare for surgery but delay the final decision on surgery until the time of the examination under anesthesia.

PREOPERATIVE PREPARATION AND WORKUP

In some cases, the cause of the cataract is obvious and costly laboratory tests are not warranted. A positive family history of childhood cataract or evidence of a minor opacity of the same type in one parent confirms a diagnosis of hereditary congenital cataract. Unilateral cataracts usually are isolated sporadic incidents. Bilateral cataracts often are inherited but can be associated with other diseases. A metabolic, infectious, systemic, and genetic workup should be considered. The common causes are hypoglycemia, trisomy (Down, Edward, and Patau syndromes), myotonic dystrophy, infectious diseases (toxoplasmosis, rubella, cytomegalovirus, and herpes simplex [TORCH]), posterior lenticonus, persistent hyperplastic primary vitreous, and prematurity. Other ocular abnormalities associated with cataract often provide diagnostic clues or require attention as problems in their own right. Elevated intraocular pressure may accompany congenital cataract associated with congenital rubella syndrome or Lowe syndrome.[13] Posterior segment malformation can be detected by B scan ultrasonography in some cases of persistent fetal vasculature. Rhegmatogenous retinal detachment occurs in a significant number of patients with cataracts caused by atopic dermatitis. Pigmentary retinopathy (salt and pepper fundus) may be visible in eyes afflicted with rubella or other congenital infection. Signs of uveitis indicate the presence of an underlying disorder such as juvenile rheumatoid arthritis, Fuchs' heterochromic iridocylclitis, or pars planitis (intermediate uveitis).[14] Interested readers should refer to Chapter 39 to learn details of pediatric cataract surgery in uveitis.

Serologic screening for congenital infection (TORCH) titers, including testing for rubella and syphilis, is indicated for any infant with bilateral cataracts of uncertain origin. It is particularly important to identify the baby with rubella prior to surgery, because exposure of operating room personnel to lens material containing the virus may cause harm. TORCH testing in older children often gives misleading results and should be reserved for cases in which there is specific clinical evidence for one of those conditions.

INDICATIONS FOR TREATMENT

To avoid the development of deprivational amblyopia, prompt diagnosis and treatment are necessary for visually significant cataracts in neonates, infants, or toddlers. A study by Birch and Stager[15] suggested that intervention before 6 weeks of age may minimize the effects of congenital unilateral deprivation on the developing visual system and provide for optimal rehabilitation of visual acuity. Indications for cataract surgery with or without intraocular lens implantation as reported in the literature include central cataracts >3 mm in diameter (visually significant); dense nuclear cataracts; cataracts obstructing the examiner's view of the fundus or preventing refraction of the patient, if the contralateral cataract has been removed; and cataracts associated with strabismus and/or nystagmus.[16–24]

When children beyond infancy present with dense, central opacities of uncertain duration and Snellen visual acuity cannot be accurately measured, surgery within a few weeks of detection is indicated. Nonsurgical methods such as patching and pharmacological pupillary dilation can be useful to manage partial cataracts.

The threshold for surgical removal of a partial cataract in a child capable of Snellen visual acuity has often been stated to be 20/50 or worse. However, each child must be approached individually. The loss of accommodation after the cataract is removed may negatively affect visual functioning more than the partial cataract did. Vision charts such as Lea Hyvarinen symbol charts and HOTV matching charts are very useful in assessment of visual status in a young child unable to read. However, individual judgments need to be made (especially in children too young for Snellen visual acuity testing) based on documented progression of the partial cataract and on the child's visual functioning, visual needs, and expected best visual outcome. When possible, low-contrast sensitivity testing may provide a helpful guideline for deciding the need for either cataract surgery or treatment for posterior capsule opacification.

In summary, a thorough ocular and systemic examination is mandatory in every child for accurate diagnosis of the type and severity of the cataract. Ocular examination should include assessment of visual acuity, retinoscopy for red fundus reflex, ocular motility, and pupillary response and posterior segment evaluation. When feasible, biomicroscopic examination of the anterior segment should be performed to evaluate the size, density, and location of the cataract so as to plan the surgical procedure and to determine the anticipated visual outcome. Fundus examination should be carried out after pupillary dilatation. "A"-scan ultrasound helps to measure the axial length for calculating the intraocular lens power and monitoring the globe elongation postoperatively. For an eye with a total cataract, a B-scan ultrasound evaluation is useful for detection of vitreoretinal pathology. A history from the parents is useful to determine whether the cataract is congenital, developmental, or traumatic in origin. One must ascertain if there is any history of maternal drug use, infection, or exposure to radiation during pregnancy. Each child should be thoroughly examined by a pediatrician to rule out systemic associations, anomalies, or congenital rubella syndrome.

REFERENCES

1. Lambert SR, Drack AV. Infantile cataracts. *Surv Ophthalmol* 1996;40:427–428.
2. Hamill MB, Koch DD. Pediatric cataracts. *Curr Opin Ophthalmol* 1999;10:4–9.
3. Amaya L, Taylor D, Russell-Eggitt I, et al. The morphology and natural history of childhood cataracts. *Surv Ophthalmol* 2003;48:125–144.

4. Nelson LB, Wagner RS. Pediatric cataract surgery. *Int Ophthalmol Clin* 1994;34:165–169.

5. Hiles DA, Sheridan SJ. Strabismus associated with infantile cataracts. *Int Ophthalmol Clin* 1977;17:193–202.

6. Jain IS, Pillai P, Gangwar DN, et al. Congenital cataract: etiology and morphology. *J Pediatr Ophthalmol Strabismus* 1983;20:238–242.

7. Potter WS. Pediatric cataracts. *Pediatr Clin North Am* 1993;40:841–853.

8. Wilson ME. Clinician's corner. In: Ruttum MS, ed. *Childhood Cataracts*. American Academy of Ophthalmology, Focal Points, Clinical Modules for Ophthalmologists. March 1996;14(1):10.

9. Morita S, Kora Y, Takahasi K, Fukai H, Hayashi H. Intraocular lens implantation in a child with monocular cataract and anterior persistent hyperplastic primary vitreous. *J Cataract Refract Surg* 2001;27:477–480.

10. Bhagat RG, Chai H. Development of posterior subcapsular cataracts in asthmatic children. *Pediatrics* 1984;73:626–630.

11. Churchill AJ, Noble BA, Etchells DE, George NJ. Factors affecting visual outcome in children following uniocular traumatic cataract. *Eye* 1995;9:285–291.

12. Pandey SK, Ram J, Werner L, et al. Visual results and postoperative complications of capsular bag versus sulcus fixation of posterior chamber intraocular lenses for traumatic cataract in children. *J Cataract Refract Surg* 1999;25:1576–1584.

13. Kruger SJ, Wilson ME Jr, Hutchinson AK, et al. Cataracts and glaucoma in patients with oculocerebrorenal syndrome. *Arch Ophthalmol* 2003;121:1234–1237.

14. Foster CS, Barrett F. Cataract development and cataract surgery in patients with juvenile rheumatoid arthritis-associated iridocyclitis. *Ophthalmology* 1993;100:809–817.

15. Birch EE, Stager DR. The critical period for surgical treatment of dense, congenital, unilateral cataracts. *Invest Ophthalmol Vis Sci* 1996;37:1532–1538.

16. Helveston EM. Infantile cataract surgery. *Int Ophthalmol Clin* 1977;17:75–82.

17. Pandey SK, Wilson ME, Trivedi RH, et al. Pediatric cataract surgery and intraocular lens implantation: current techniques, complications and management. *Int Ophthalmol Clin* 2001;41:175–196.

18. Basti S, Greenwald MJ. Principles and paradigms of pediatric cataract management. *Indian J Ophthalmol* 1995;43:159–176.

19. Nelson LB. Diagnosis and management of cataracts in infancy and childhood. *Ophthalm Surg* 1984;15:688–697.

20. Hiles DA. Implant surgery in children. *Int Ophthalmol Clin* 1979;19:95–123.

21. Sinskey RM, Karel F, Dal Ri E. Management of cataracts in children. *J Cataract Refract Surg* 1979;15:196–200.

22. Morgan KS. Pediatric cataract and lens implantation. *Curr Opin Ophthalmol* 1995;6:9–13.

23. Hiles DA, Biglan AW. Indications for infantile cataract surgery. *Int Ophthalmol Clin* 1977;17:39–45.

24. Dahan E. Pediatric cataract surgery. In: Yanoff M, Ducker JS, eds. *Ophthalmology*. St. Louis: Mosby-Yearbook, 1998;30:1–30.

Informed Consent

M. Edward Wilson, Jr. and Rupal H. Trivedi

As soon as surgery is proposed for a cataract in a child, the informed consent process begins. As with many other aspects of medicine, this process is both a *science* and an *art*. The ophthalmologist must be able to explain to the patient's parents or legal guardian (and to the child as well, if appropriate) the nature of the problem and why surgery is being recommended to alleviate it. Appropriate available options for managing the cataract should be explained in terms that the family can understand. In this electronic age, with nearly everyone having access to Internet information, families often arrive in the office with much more knowledge about their child's condition than would have been true only a few years ago. While not all of the information available on the Internet is scientifically based, overall the availability of information has led to a more knowledgeable and inquisitive patient population. Surgeons who perform pediatric cataract surgery should be prepared for sometimes quite lengthy discussions with this new breed of patient. The extra time is not wasted, however, because a better-informed family is much more likely to comply with the frequent follow-ups, medications, patching, glasses wear, etc., that are so essential to an eventual visual acuity outcome from the surgery.

Spaeth has written that *"informed consent is, in many ways, at the heart of the American system of medical and surgical practice."*[1] When informed consent is done properly, the parents and the physician become partners with the common goal of doing what is best for the patient's health and well-being. Time spent establishing this partnership prior to surgery will help assure compliance with the often difficult aftercare and follow-up. Parents have a right to understand the treatment that is being recommended for their child. The surgeon must use language that best accomplishes that goal. While the signing of the surgical consent form can sometimes be delegated to an assistant, the surgeon should be the one who informs parents about the treatment details, alternatives, and meaningful risks of the proposed surgery. A request for a second opinion during the informed consent decision usually indicates that the surgeon has not communicated well and in a manner that the parents can understand. Surgeons should be prepared for the common question, *"What would you do if this were your child?"*

Some surgeons view the informed consent process as primarily a method to help prevent malpractice lawsuits. However, the signed consent document does little more than prevent accusations of battery. The family may state at a later time that they did not understand the nature or the risks of the surgery and that they signed the form because they were told to sign it. An informed consent form in itself will not effectively prevent the filing of malpractice lawsuits. On the other hand, a meaningful exchange of information that leads to the partnership mentioned earlier will significantly decrease the risk of a lawsuit even if the surgery has a poor outcome. A family that agrees wholeheartedly on the decision to pursue a particular surgical option is much less likely to file a lawsuit when a complication occurs, even if that particular complication was not specifically discussed preoperatively. Lack of adequate information about a particular complication is not often the basis for a malpractice claim. In one study, only 2.5% of malpractice claims were based on the failure to obtain adequate informed consent.[2]

Negligence is a more common claim by a prosecuting attorney. When families feel that the surgical procedure adopted was not indicated, they are much less understanding when a complication occurs. Plaintiffs' lawyers plead lack of informed consent only as a last resort, and not usually as the primary charge against a negligent surgeon.

In addition to the commonsense considerations discussed above, specific professional responsibilities also govern the discussion of risks, benefits, and alternatives when medical or surgical treatments are proposed. The following advisory opinion, based on the American Academy of Ophthalmology (AAO)'s Code of Ethics, is reprinted from the AAO Web site (http://www.aao.org/aao/member/ethics/informed_consent.cfm):

When medical and surgical procedures are proposed, both ethical principle and the law require discussion of significant associated risk. Although legal requirements are a minimum standard that may be routinely exceeded by practice of good professional ethics, they are an important benchmark on which to build. Clearly an ophthalmologist must understand and conform to the minimum required by applicable law. In some states, a community standard is used by which a physician must disclose any information about risks and other factors that the average prudent physician in the community would disclose. Most other states set a higher standard, requiring disclosure of all information possessed by a doctor that a reasonable patient would find significant in deciding whether or not to undergo a procedure. In no case does the law require the physician to give each patient a comprehensive seminar of their condition.

In general, any risks or potential complications that are sufficiently common or significant that they might reasonably influence the patient's judgment must be disclosed. Exclusions may include very minor, rare, or inconsequential risks. Similarly, if a risk is readily apparent to people of common sense, then discussion can reasonably be excluded unless the physician has reason to believe that such a disclosure is necessary or appropriate to obtain truly informed consent. Essentially, the physician must explain the nature of the treatment, significant risks, and reasonable alternatives to the treatment proposed in language that the patient can understand. When a patient is too young to legally consent to care, or when a patient lacks the capacity to decide independently, the informed consent must be obtained from a surrogate acting on the patient's behalf. The same procedure for explaining the risks, benefits and alternatives should be followed with a guardian or surrogate.

In the specific instance of pediatric cataract surgery, the informed consent discussion should include the criteria used by the surgeon to decide that the cataract is visually significant, the details of the surgical procedure being proposed (i.e., whether a posterior capsulectomy and anterior vitrectomy will be used and whether an intraocular lens [IOL] will be placed), whether the surgery will result in the postoperative need for glasses, contacts, and/or patching for amblyopia, and the importance of postoperative follow-up and postoperative medications as well as the importance of avoiding postoperative trauma to the recently operated eye. A general discussion of operative and postoperative risks should include a discussion of visual axis opacification, IOL malposition, abnormalities of the size and shape of the pupil, and variability in the postoperative residual refractive error. Endophthalmitis and retinal detachment are rare after pediatric cataract surgery but are of such significance to vision that they should be mentioned as part of the informed consent. Complicating conditions that may occur unrelated to the surgical event itself are nonetheless very important as part of the informed consent process. The partnership being developed with the parents is meant to help assure appropriate follow-up and appropriate attention to complicating conditions that may not appear for years after the surgery. Aphakic/pseudophakic glaucoma, deprivation amblyopia, strabismus, and changing refractive error are conditions in this category and are ideally discussed as part of the preoperative knowledge exchange.

The lion's share of the informed consent discussion with regard to pediatric cataract surgery will concern issues related to the placement of an IOL. While IOL implantation has become the most common method used to correct aphakia in children overall, it is still considered "off label." This designation means that the IOLs implanted in children were tested as part of their FDA market approval process only in adults. It does not mean that the FDA has disallowed their use in children. It implies only that the device is being used for a purpose or in a patient population that is different from the one for which it was tested as part of the market approval process. The following paragraph is taken directly from the FDA Web site and serves to give surgeons some guidance on the legality of IOL use in children and whether institutional review board oversight is indicated when these devices are implanted in children.[3]

Good medical practice in the best interests of the patient requires that physicians use legally available drugs, biologics and devices according to their best knowledge and judgment. If physicians use a product for an indication not in the approved labeling, they have the responsibility to be well informed about the product, to base its use on a firm scientific rationale and on sound medical evidence, and to maintain records of the products use and effects. Use of a marketed product in this manner when the intent is the "practice of medicine" does not require the submission of an investigational new drug application (IND), investigational device exemption (IDE) or review by an institutional review board (IRB). However, the institution at which the product will be used may, under its own authority, require IRB review or other institutional oversight.

Parents should be made aware that IOL implantation in children is considered off label. However, they should also be made aware that IOL implantation at the time of cataract surgery has become the treatment of choice for a large majority of surgeons when the recipient is beyond infancy. As Levin[4] has stated, patients and their families come to us "with a trust that we cannot betray." The foundation of that trust is that we will act in their best interests and that we will tell them the truth at all times. We must openly and honestly discuss with our patients the innovative nature of proposed treatments, such as IOL implantation and its variations, including the degree of newness, the past experience of others and ourselves, and even the disclosure that "I have never done this before." Conversations are also needed about potential conflicts of interest, academic, financial, or otherwise.

There is no doubt that the informed consent process surrounding pediatric cataract surgery is more time-consuming and in many ways more complex than for most other ophthalmic procedures. Truth telling and the artful transfer of knowledge in terms appropriate for the family will help assure that a physician–patient relationship built on trust will develop.

In summary, informed consent is an essential part of a surgical practice. It is the physician's ethical responsibility to be honest with the patient. It is the parents' right to make decisions regarding the destiny of their children. These guardians are not in a position to do this without appropriate knowledge. The process of obtaining informed consent is based on both science and art but it is one of the most important practical ways of assuring high standards and ongoing improvement of quality medical care. Finally, the physician is legally obligated to obtain such consent.

REFERENCES

1. Spaeth GL, ed. *Ophthalmic Surgery, Principles and Practices.* 3rd Ed. Philadelphia: WB Saunders, 2003:12.
2. Fasanella RM, ed. *Eye Surgery: Innovations and Trends, Pitfalls, Complications.* Springfield, IL: Charles C Thomas, 1977.
3. Wilson ME. Intraocular lenses for children in the year 2000: when is oversight by the institutional review board or food and drug administration required? *J AAPOS* 2000;4(6):325.
4. Levin AV. IOLs, innovation, and ethics in pediatric ophthalmology: let's be honest. *J AAPOS* 2002;6(3):133–135.

Intraocular Lens Power Calculation for Children

Scott K. McClatchey and Elizabeth M. Hofmeister

The eyes of children are constantly growing. Just as the body grows fastest in infancy and early childhood, most ocular growth occurs in the first few years of life. This growth has significant optical implications. In adult cataract surgery, calculation of the desired intraocular lens (IOL) power is relatively simple, requiring only knowledge of the axial length (AL), cornea power, and IOL parameters. The constant size of the adult eye ensures that the refraction of an adult pseudophakic eye is stable. The optics of a child's eye are also simple at any given point in time. However, ocular growth has profound effects on refraction, potentially causing a large myopic shift.

Ideally, we would like for a child who has cataract surgery to grow up to have good visual acuity and emmetropia in adulthood. Achieving this goal requires consideration of many factors, including IOL power, patient age and cooperation, family concerns, and clinical management issues. Family issues and the maturity of the child may determine the effectiveness of amblyopia management, and this in turn can impact the surgeon's choice of IOL power. The development of good vision is dependent on complex interactions between the binocular visual input and the brain's development: differences in image quality between the eyes rapidly lead to amblyopia and strabismus in young children. Therefore, whether the cataract is unilateral or bilateral must be factored into the choice of optical management.

In this chapter, we discuss biometry, IOL formula use, growth of the eye, and practical and research considerations that come from the refractive growth of the eye.

BIOMETRY

Two ocular measurements are critical to IOL calculation: axial length (AL) and cornea power (K). In addition, several other measurements are useful in the management of the pseudophakic child, including cornea diameter, intraocular pressure (IOP), and cornea thickness. These can be done while the child is awake in patients as young as 3 years, using gentle reassurance.

Office measurement of AL and cornea curvature can be challenging or impossible in very young children. Fortunately, these measurements can be done quite easily in the operating room while the child is asleep. A-Scan ultrasound can be done using either contact or immersion methods. Care must be taken that the scan is directed toward the macula and that the tip does not indent the relatively soft cornea. We have found handheld keratometry (e.g., using the Retinomax [Keeler, Windsor, Berkshire, UK] or others by Alcon and Marco) to be useful in anesthetized children, both for IOL calculations and for rigid contact lens fitting. Harvey et al. showed that the Alcon portable autokeratometer (PAK) produces accurate measurements of surface curvature under a variety of suboptimal conditions in infants and children.[1]

For secondary IOLs, the correct power can be calculated without AL or K simply by using the aphakic refraction. For a given aphakic refraction, the relative proportions of AL and K can vary: as AL increases, K must decrease. It turns out optically that these relative proportions of AL and K make very little difference in the refraction after an IOL is implanted.[2] We are not aware of a program that does these calculations directly. However, the Pediatric IOL Calculator,[3] a free computer program for Windows, can be used to do this indirectly. To use this program for a secondary IOL, put in the child's age, the A-constant of the IOL, and an approximate K and AL (a guess will do for K and for AL). Put in a power of "0" for "IOL power," and the program will tell you the predicted "resulting refraction." Next, adjust the value of AL until the "resulting refraction" equals the measured refraction for that eye. Finally, put in your "goal refraction"; the resulting "IOL to use" output should be accurate.

Glaucoma is a frequent occurrence in aphakic and pseudophakic children's eyes, and we think that IOP should also be measured at the initiation of anesthesia whenever a child has cataract-related surgery and at subsequent examinations under anesthesia. Because applanation tonometry can be significantly affected by cornea thickness, we also recommend pachymetry at least once during the initial cataract surgery and occasionally at older ages in the clinic if glaucoma is suspected.

IOL FORMULAS

The optics of an aphakic eye is simple. For all practical purposes, the refraction depends on AL and cornea power alone. A pseudophakic eye has two additional factors to consider: the IOL power and its position in the eye. Any of a number of IOL formulas can be used to calculate the refraction of an aphakic or pseudophakic eye, given these parameters. The child's eye is no different in this respect, although differences in children's anterior segment anatomy may affect the position of the IOL immediately after surgery, thus slightly changing the initial postoperative refraction. As we discuss later in the chapter, inaccuracies in formula predictions tend to be overwhelmed by the optical effects of the growth of the eye and by the variance in the rate of refractive growth.

The formulas used for calculation of IOL powers are designed to account for the final position of the IOL in the eye. Variances in IOL design, surgical technique, and anterior segment anatomy result in variances in the position of the IOL in the pseudophakic eye. An IOL that is relatively anterior in the eye will have a greater refractive effect than one that is relatively posterior. The effect of IOL design is accounted for by the various constants used in formulas, such as the A-constant (SRK formulas) and pACD (Hoffer Q). Variance in surgical technique can be accounted for by empiric surgeon factors in modern computer-based formulas.

One of the first IOL calculation formulas was the SRK formula, an empiric, linear formula that made calculations by hand quite simple. This formula worked well for most eyes but gave incorrect calculations for eyes that were short or long or had an unusual anterior segment anatomy. The effects of variance in anterior segment anatomy on IOL calculation have been accounted for by newer generations of IOL formulas. Modern theoretic formulas, such as the SRK-T, Holladay I and II, Hoffer Q, and Haigis, take these factors into account. In adults, the theoretic formulas are more accurate than the SRK I or SRK II formulas, and in published series they show a mean absolute error of $< \pm 0.6$ D (diopter).[4]

Several studies of children have shown larger errors in IOL formula predictions than are found in adults.

Andreo et al. studied 47 consecutive pseudophakic pediatric patients, age 3 months to 16 years.[5] They compared the actual initial postoperative pseudophakic refractions to those predicted by four formulas (SRK-II, SRK-T, Holladay, and Hoffer Q). They found no significant difference in accuracy between the formulas: the average initial postoperative refractive error was between 1.2 and 1.4 D in all formulas. Another study found that the mean difference between the predicted and the actual postoperative refractions was slightly more accurate using theoretic formulas (1.06 D, vs. 1.22 D with regression formulas).[6]

Which IOL formula should be used for children? Because of the relatively large IOL formula errors demonstrated in pediatric studies, it is not clear that any formula can be considered accurate for all children. Although no formula has been proven to have an advantage, we prefer to use the theoretic formulas because they are generally more accurate for small eyes, and may be more accurate in general.

The newest formulas such as Holladay II take anterior segment measurements into account, resulting in more accurate calculations in very short eyes. This type of formula might be useful for initial refraction calculations. However, it is unclear whether the growth of the anterior segment might ultimately negate these advantages in pediatric eyes: the very anatomy that makes a difference in Holladay II may change substantially as the eye grows.

One of the critical steps in the IOL calculation process is recognizing potential measurement errors. In "A Three-Part System for Refining Intraocular Lens Power Calculations," Holladay et al. described techniques for reducing errors in IOL calculation.[18] They stated that mismeasurement of K or AL is the most significant factor leading to large refractive surprises. One part of this system was to consider remeasurement if the biometry measurements (AL and K) were outside the average range, if the IOL power was outside the expected range, or if there was significant asymmetry between the eyes. Children have naturally small eyes that vary in size with age. Fortunately, Gordon and Donzis published the normative data on AL and K, based on a cross-sectional series of children of all ages.[7] These data were used to theoretically extend Holladay and coworkers' remeasurement criteria to children in the Pediatric IOL Calculator computer program. Because of the frequent ocular size asymmetry found in unilateral congenital cataracts, this computer program warns of possible errors in AL and K only if they are unexpectedly large or small for a given age. In addition, the surgeon should be aware that some types of cataract, such as persistent fetal vasculature (PFV; formerly known as PHPV) and congenital nuclear cataract, are known to be associated with eyes smaller than expected for age.

THE GROWTH OF THE EYE

The growth of the eye follows a logarithmic curve. The greatest change is in early childhood, but there is no sharp cutoff: the refractive growth continues up to age 20 years. This growth has profound effects on the refraction of aphakic and pseudophakic eyes.

In normal children, the growth of the eye affects both the AL and the cornea curvature. Most of the growth occurs in the first 2 years of life, but there is a smoothly changing curve, with some growth until adulthood. The AL increases from an average of 16.8 mm at birth to 23.6 mm in adulthood, while K decreases from an average power of 51.2 to 43.5 D.[7]

Aphakic children's eyes become less hyperopic with time: they have an average myopic shift of 10 D from infancy to adulthood.[8] In contrast, the refraction of normal eyes changes much less, approximately −0.9 D. Why is this? Gordon and Donzis performed a biometric study of normal children of various ages and found that the natural lens power decreases dramatically as the eye grows.[7] Indeed, this must be true for the optical system of the eye to focus on the retina at all ages: as long as all parts of the eye grow proportionally from infancy, the focus will remain unchanged. As the natural lens is scaled up in size with the growth of the eye, the surfaces of the lens have greater radii of curvature. This causes the lens to have a longer focal length (lower power) and thus focus well onto the more distant retina. If a child has a lens removed, the eye is left hyperopic in relation to the power of the lens that was removed. Thus, the quantity of hyperopia of a child's aphakic growing eye decreases with time, just as the power of the natural lens decreases with time.

The "aphakic refractions" of normal eyes can be calculated from Gordon and Donzis's biometric data. The refractions of aphakic eyes and the calculated aphakic refractions of normal eyes follow the same smooth curve from infancy to 20 years (Fig. 7-1). Thus the refractive growth of aphakic eyes is very close to that of normal eyes. This "refractive growth" is due to a combination of changes in AL and cornea power.

THE LOGARITHMIC REFRACTIVE GROWTH OF THE APHAKIC EYE

Inspection of the graph of aphakic refraction versus age (Fig. 7-1) shows a curve with a slope that decreases with age. Curve-fitting analysis shows that it closely follows a logarithmic curve. A plot of mean refraction versus log of age for aphakic eyes is a straight line from age 3 months to age 20 years (Fig. 7-2).[8] This fit of the data points is extraordinarily good, with $R^2 = 0.97$ (indicating that the logarithmic curve can account for 97% of the variance in the mean aphakic refractions with age).

The slope of the line in the semilog plot is a measurement of the rate of refractive growth of the eye. This slope can be calculated for any aphakic eye with at least two measurements of refraction separated by sufficient time. The slope of any straight line drawn between any two points (x_1, y_1) and (x_2, y_2) is given by the equation

$$\text{slope} = [y_2 - y_1]/[x_2 - x_1] \qquad (7.1)$$

In the semilog plot of mean refraction versus log of age,

$$\text{slope} = [\text{refraction}_2 - \text{refraction}_1]/ \\ [\log(\text{age}_2) - \log(\text{age}_1)] \qquad (7.2)$$

where age_1 and refraction_1 are from the younger age, and age_2 and refraction_2 are from the older age. Because of the

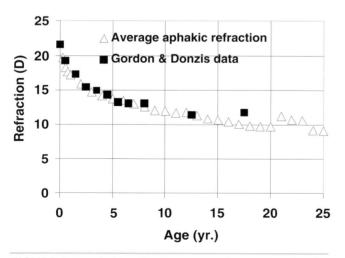

FIGURE 7-1. Aphakic refraction vs. age for a series of aphakic children and for the calculated "aphakic refractions" of the eyes of normal children. (Adapted from McClatchey SK, Parks MM. Myopic shift after cataract removal in childhood. *J Pediatr Ophthalmol Strabismus* 1997;34:88–95.)

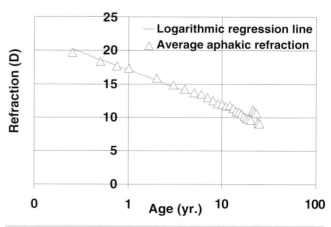

FIGURE 7-2. Semilogarithmic plot of aphakic refraction vs. age for aphakic children.

properties of logarithms, the denominator of this equation can be expressed as the log of a fraction:

$$\log(\text{age}_2) - \log(\text{age}_1) = \log(\text{age}_2/\text{age}_1) \qquad (7.3)$$

In the fraction $\text{age}_2/\text{age}_1$, the unit of time drops out, so the slope in Eq. (7.2) has units of diopters. The slope is therefore independent of the unit of time: it will be the same whether the age is measured in days, months, or years. The slope of this line was originally given the name "rate of myopic shift" when it applied only to aphakic children.[8] In all published descriptions of the logarithmic model, refractions were measured at the spectacle plane, and the logarithm was base 10.[2,3,8–10]

The slope in the logarithmic model can be calculated for pseudophakic eyes by mathematically removing the optical effect of the IOL.[2] The slope in this case is not a direct measure of myopic shift, so it was renamed "rate of refractive growth" (RRG), because it is analogous to other rates and is a measure of the refractive change due to the growth of the eye.

For this model to be extended to pseudophakic eyes, we must know the effect of IOL implantation on the growth of the eye. The largest long-term studies of refractive growth in aphakic and pseudophakic children show that the eyes of aphakic and pseudophakic children have a similar growth curve, with a slightly lower rate of refractive growth in pseudophakic eyes. Most of the refractive change occurs in the first few years of life, with a gradually decreasing rate of myopic shift (reduction in hyperopia).[10]

RRG is lower in children <6 months of age at surgery. However, in children ≥6 months old at surgery, RRG is not affected by age at surgery, type of cataract, initial postoperative refraction, or controlled glaucoma. No other factor studied has been found to consistently and substantially influence RRG. Calculation of RRG eliminates the confounding factors of nonlinear growth of children's eyes and the variables of age at surgery, length of follow-up, and variations in IOL power.[2,3,8–10]

The equivalent aphakic refractions from Gordon and Donzis[7] data (Fig. 7-1) can be used to calculate the mean RRG for these normal children: −5.3 D, versus −6.1 D in aphakic and −5.0 D in pseudophakic children (all ≥6 months old at surgery). Recent data,[11] combined with the previous pseudophakic data in a meta-analysis, gives an RRG of −5.4 D for pseudophakic children. The mean RRG is therefore not very different in aphakic, pseudophakic, and normal children. Cataract surgery after 6 months of age has little effect on the growth of the eye, with or without IOL implantation.

When the ratio of final to initial ages $\text{age}_2/\text{age}_1 = 10$, then the denominator in Eq. (7.2) is $\log(10) = 1.0$. One way to understand the logarithmic model is to consider that when an aphakic child's age increases 10-fold, his or her refraction will change by the quantity given by the RRG value. Since the mean RRG for pseudophakic children was −5.4 D, these eyes had a mean decline in hyperopia of

5.4 D when the ages compared were 10-fold different, for example, from age 0.5 year to age 5 years or from age 2 years to age 20 years.

Based on analysis of the pseudophakic eyes with the highest ratios of final to initial age, we think that the true standard deviation in RRG is 2.4 D. A simple way of understanding the variability in RRG is to acknowledge that some eyes grow faster than others.

EXTENDING THE REFRACTIVE GROWTH MODEL TO EARLY INFANCY

The discussion to this point has concerned children >6 months of age at surgery. There is evidence in the literature that early cataract surgery may slow the growth of both monkey and human eyes. Lambert[12] showed that lens removal at 2 weeks in neonatal monkeys retarded axial elongation. Because monkeys mature four times faster than humans, a 2-week-old monkey is equivalent to a 2-month-old human. Another study showed that in neonatal monkeys, pseudophakic eyes had a slightly lower rate of growth than aphakic eyes, although this was not statistically significant.[13]

The RRG model can be extended to younger ages, based on data. It turns out that children who have surgery at between 3 and 6 months of age have a lower RRG. A study of children who had surgery at between 3 and 6 months of age found an RRG lower than that seen in older children. Pseudophakic eyes had an RRG = −3.3 D, and aphakic eyes had an RRG = −4.6 D ($P = .09$ for the difference between the RRG values).[10]

Logarithmic plots become asymptotic near zero, thus the logarithmic model is not valid in early infancy. The cutoff age is not inherently obvious, but by inspection of the refraction graphs, the age of 3 months was chosen. Therefore, a different model must be used for ages <3 months. Using computer programming, it is a simple matter to take the biometric data from Gordon and Donzis[7] for ages <3 months and prefix them to the logarithmic model. This grafted model can then be used to predict refractions of pseudophakic infants, in theory. We used this grafted model to develop the predictions in Table 7-1. Please note that the predictions for such young pseudophakic children are entirely theoretical and await confirmation.

IOLs *INCREASE* MYOPIC SHIFT OWING TO AN OPTICAL EFFECT

As the pseudophakic eye grows, the distance from the IOL to the retina increases. This effectively moves the focal point of the IOL anterior in the eye. This refractive change is analogous to the refractive difference between contacts and spectacles: the optical effect of vertex distance for a

▶ **TABLE 7-1** Predictions for *Typical* [a] Pseudophakic Eyes

Age at Surgery (yr) [b]	IOL Power [c]	Initial Postop [c]	Predicted Refraction (D) at a Given Age (yr) [a]				
			1	2	4	8	20
−0.15	30.0	+12.00	2.31	0.79	−0.73	−2.24	−4.23
−0.06	29.3	+9.00	2.53	1.03	−0.47	−1.96	−3.92
0.00	28.2	+8.00	2.78	1.31	−0.15	−1.61	−3.53
0.25	26.9	+7.00	3.68	2.24	0.81	−0.61	−2.49
0.5	26.0	+6.50	4.02	1.71	−0.59	−2.86	−5.81
1	24.5	+5.00	5.00	2.61	0.37	−1.84	−4.71
2	22.3	+4.00		4.00	1.85	−0.28	−3.04
3	22.3	+3.00			2.10	−0.04	−2.82
4	22.0	+2.25			2.25	0.12	−2.64
6	21.0	+1.50				0.63	−2.08
8	20.4	+1.00				1.00	−1.69

[a]The rate of refractive growth (RRG) for children with surgery at age ≥0.5 year is assumed to be −5.4 D; for children with surgery at age <0.5 years it is assumed to be −3.3 D after age 0.25 year. The predictions for infants with surgery at age <0.25 year are theoretical. Variations in RRG and initial ocular measurements will significantly affect these predictions: the large variance in RRG will lead to a large range of ultimate refractions; these are the expected means.
[b]The age groups in the first two rows are premature babies (e.g., −0.06 year is equivalent to 37 weeks corrected gestational age, 3 weeks before due date).
[c]IOL power and initial refractions are for example only and are not our recommendations. Assumed A-constant = 118.0. All IOL powers and refractions are given as diopters.

high-power correction is significant. For example, an aphakic patient who is corrected with a +12.00-D spectacle lens at a vertex distance of 12 mm would require a contact lens power of +14.0 D. The need for increased power in the contact lens is caused by the optical effect of vertex distance. The higher the power of the lens, the greater the effect. For example, a patient who required a +20.00-D spectacle lens would require a contact lens power of +26.3 D.

Just as in the contact lens analogy, where vertex distance has a greater effect at high refractive powers, high-power IOLs result in a greater myopic shift for the same increase in AL. As an example, we took a hypothetical patient who had cataract surgery at age 9 months and a typical eye. We calculated what the myopic shift would be if the child was left aphakic or given one of three IOL powers, assuming that ocular growth was unchanged by any of these things. The results (Table 7-2) show that using a high-power IOL

can result in a substantially greater myopic shift than using a low-power IOL, owing to optics alone.

PRACTICAL CONSIDERATIONS IN IOL POWER CHOICE

We think it is useful to start with the goal in mind. Ideally, we would like the child to grow up to have good visual acuity and emmetropia in adulthood. The IOL power choice is only one step in the path to this goal, which also includes amblyopia management and refractive correction with glasses or contact lenses. Ultimately a refractive surgery such as photorefractive keratectomy can eliminate any significant refractive error in adulthood. Of course, not all young children with cataracts will end up with this ideal, because of coexisting ocular abnormalities,

▶ **TABLE 7-2** Calculated Refractive Outcomes for Various IOLs, for a Hypothetical Child with Cataract Surgery at Age 9 Months and a Final Refraction at Age 20 Years [a]

	IOL Power (D)	Initial Refraction (D)	Final Refraction (D)	Myopic Shift (D)
Aphakia	0.0	+17.53	+9.84	7.69
Low-power IOL	17.5	+9.31	−0.05	9.36
Medium-power IOL	32.0	−0.02	−11.82	11.80
High-power IOL	36.0	−3.17	−15.93	12.76

[a]The refraction predictions assume that IOL power has no effect on the physical growth of the eye (axial length and cornea curvature). RRG is assumed to be −5.4 D in all eyes. High-power intraocular lenses increase the quantity of myopic shift that comes with growth.

complications such as glaucoma, or difficulties in amblyopia management. We think the surgeon should choose an IOL power that will help achieve the ideal to the greatest extent possible.

Surgeons have taken four approaches to IOL power choice. At first, when biometry was difficult, some surgeons chose to use an IOL with a typical adult power.[14] With biometry readily available, surgeons can now choose an initial postoperative refractive goal. Some choose hyperopia, with the expectation of myopic shift with time; others choose emmetropia or myopia to help with amblyopia management.[15] Each of these approaches has advantages and disadvantages (Table 7-3). There is no study showing a visual advantage of one approach over the other. We prefer to leave the eye moderately hyperopic, using a logical approach based on knowledge of how the refraction is likely to change with age. We also customize the choice of initial postoperative refraction based on the child, accounting for the refraction of the opposite eye and whether the surgery is unilateral or bilateral, among other factors.

In infants and in very small eyes, refractive correction may require more than a single IOL. The surgeon may choose to leave the pseudophakic eye strongly hyperopic and to correct the hyperopia with a contact lens or spectacles. Another option is to place piggyback IOLs, with a high-power IOL in the bag and a second, lower-power IOL in the sulcus.[16] Piggyback IOLs offer unique advantages and challenges in this situation, and long-term studies in children have not yet been published. As the eye grows, the refraction may become dramatically less hyperopic; in this case the piggyback IOL can be easily removed. On the other hand, some eyes have little refractive growth with age, and the two lenses could be left in place indefinitely. If piggyback IOLs are placed, we think that care should be taken to remove as many of the lens epithelial cells as possible. The space between the two IOLs can provide a scaffold for the rapidly growing lens cells, resulting in obscuration of the visual pathway.

Calculation of predicted refractions of pseudophakic children as they grow can be done in several ways, including spreadsheets and commercial IOL programs. To date, the authors are not aware of a commercial program that uses the logarithmic model. Perhaps the simplest and easiest option is to use the Pediatric IOL Calculator program. This program takes the biometric data, IOL parameters, and age for input and produces a graphical representation of the future refractions, with upper and lower lines representing standard deviations. The program was written in 1997, so the values for RRG and standard deviation need to be modified to match the updated ones listed in this chapter.

Another method for choosing an IOL power is to use a look-up table (such as Table 7-1) and decide on a goal postoperative refraction based on age. This can work well for typical eyes in patients without extraordinary circumstances. However, because of the optics involved, eyes that are unusually long or short for the age of the child will have different quantities of myopic shift, even with the same RRG. In addition, the surgeon should keep in mind that the goal postoperative refraction may be different for children with bilateral cataracts than for those with unilateral cataracts, and account may need to be taken for difficult social circumstances or other factors.

▶ **TABLE 7-3** **Advantages and Disadvantages of Various IOL Power Choice Approaches**

IOL Choice Approach	*Advantage(s)*	*Disadvantage(s)*	*Adult Refraction*
Initial hyperopia	Hyperopia will improve as the eye grows. Less myopic shift	Initial spectacle or contact lens correction is required	Low myopia or emmetropia, with a possibility of hyperopia
Initial emmetropia	No spectacle or contact lens needed initially	Large myopic shift may occur with growth of the eye	Myopia, moderate to high
Initial myopia	At first, may not require contact lens or spectacle correction to prevent amblyopia	Large myopic shift can be expected with growth of the eye	Myopia, possibly very high
Standard adult-power IOL	No need to measure the eye	Unpredictable initial refraction, which can make clinical management much more difficult	High myopia to hyperopia

Because of variability in RRG, a child who is left with initial hyperopia may end up in adult life with either myopia, emmetropia, or hyperopia. Low myopia is useful for near work without correction, but hyperopia and moderate to high myopia require correction with contacts, glasses, or surgery. Because hyperopia greater than about 3 D is difficult to treat well with current refractive surgery techniques, we suggest that this be considered in choosing the IOL power for young children. We suggest that the ideal IOL power should give a low chance (given the variability in RRG) of leaving the child with more than 3 D of hyperopia in adult life.

Because no study has shown a definite advantage of one refractive strategy over another, we think that in equivocal cases, parents should be given an informed choice. They may be in a good position to understand how compliant the child will be with glasses and patching. Some may choose emmetropia in childhood; others may choose emmetropia in adulthood (without further refractive surgery).

RESEARCH CONSIDERATIONS

We are concerned that most research to date on refractive changes in aphakic and pseudophakic children does not use the logarithmic model of refractive growth as a basis for analysis. Many studies attempt to assess the refractive effect of cataract surgery by calculating the absolute myopic shift or by calculating the rate of myopic shift per year. Thus, many published statements are made erroneously, based on large confounding effects owing to age at surgery, age at refraction measurements, length of follow-up, and optical effects of an IOL. These confounding effects can be completely eliminated by using the logarithmic model of refractive growth (RRG) for analysis. The logarithmic model is therefore very useful in comparing refractive growth between eyes in studies of these patients. Indeed, the authors are not aware of another analytic method for studying refractive growth that is not confounded by these factors.

For research that does make proper use of the logarithmic model, two factors should be strongly considered in study design: measurement error and the inherent variability in RRG. The length of time needed to accurately calculate RRG is determined primarily by the uncertainty in measurements of refraction and age. Because age can be identified precisely, the uncertainty in refraction measurement limits the accuracy of RRG calculations for any given patient. In a study of the repeatability of refractions in normal adults, the standard deviation for cycloplegic retinoscopy was found to be 0.48 D.[17] We think this value is close to the real measurement error in refractions of pseudophakic children.

This refraction measurement uncertainty overwhelms the RRG if the refractions are measured too close together in time. Measurements of refractions at two points in time (ages) are required to calculate RRG for any given eye. These measurements must be separated by a time long enough to allow the resulting change in refraction to overcome the effects of measurement error. If the measurements are taken too closely together, there is not enough time for the growth of the eye to show up as a measurable change in refraction. Thus to accurately calculate RRG for a given eye, a large amount of time must separate the initial and final measurements, and the time required must be greater at older ages.

An approximation of the measurement error in RRG can be calculated using the following method. First, assume that the true ages are age_1 and age_2 and that the true refractions are $refraction_{1\_true}$ and $refraction_{2\_true}$. From these numbers, the true RRG (RRG_{true}) can be calculated. Second, assume that the first refraction ($refraction_1$) is actually *measured* in error too high and the second ($refraction_2$) is in error too low by the known uncertainty in refraction measurement. Third, use the two data points thus derived in the semilog plot ([$\log(age_1)$, $refraction_1$] and [$\log(age_2)$, $refraction_2$]) to calculate the RRG: this gives an RRG that is *too high due to measurement error alone*. The difference between this hypothetical measured RRG (with its measurement errors) and RRG_{true} is an estimate of the uncertainty in RRG owing to errors in the measurement of refractions.

If the uncertainty in refraction measurement of pseudophakic children is assumed to be 0.4 D, and data points for a given child are taken at ages 3.0 and 6.0 years, then the uncertainty in RRG would be ±1.3 D (22%). If the data points had instead been taken at ages 5.0 and 6.0 years, the uncertainty in RRG would have been ±5.1 D (83%).

To reduce the error in calculation of RRG for each patient, the length of follow-up should be maximized. Because of the logarithmic nature of refractive growth, the ratio of final to initial age should be at least 2.0 to reduce the uncertainty to 22% or less for each RRG. Thus, the required follow-up time must be much greater in older children. This is why a minimum follow-up time greater than or equal to the age at surgery was required in the multicenter study of pseudophakic children.[10] All studies of refractive change in children should account for this: including eyes with insufficient follow-up time in such studies may cause the measurement error itself to overwhelm the effects of ocular growth, leading to erroneous conclusions.

CONCLUSION

The growth of a child's eye causes a myopic shift that is substantial and predictable. This refractive growth is one of the factors to consider in achieving the ultimate goal: a child who grows up to have good visual acuity and emmetropia in adulthood.

The empiric, logarithmic model of refractive growth has been found to be useful in clinical practice and research. This simple model can be used to predict future refractions of any patient and at any age. In research, it eliminates the confounding effects of many factors that can wrongly bias conclusions.

In 1992, one of the authors (S.K.M.) found that his 1-year-old son had a unilateral posterior lenticonus cataract. At that time the optics of growing eyes were little understood, and there was no model of refractive growth or way to predict the ultimate refraction after lens implantation. At the age of 3 years, this child had cataract removal with IOL implantation, resulting in an initial refraction of +1.50 D, versus +1.00 D in his normal eye. His refraction at age 13 years is now −6.50 D (spherical equivalent), versus +0.50 D in his normal eye. He currently wears a contact lens; when he reaches adulthood, he may have refractive surgery to reach emmetropia. It is our hope that the logarithmic model and other considerations discussed in this chapter will help to guide those surgeons who place IOLs in children's eyes. We also hope that future studies will identify and refine refractive and clinical management strategies that will improve the ultimate vision of these children.

REFERENCES

1. Harvey EM, Miller JM, Dobson V. Reproducibility of corneal astigmatism measurements with a hand held keratometer in preschool children. *Br J Ophthalmol* 1995;79:983–990.
2. McClatchey SK, Parks MM. Theoretic refractive changes after lens implantation in childhood. *Ophthalmology* 1997;104:1744–1751.
3. McClatchey SK. An IOL calculator for childhood cataracts. *J Cataract Refract Surg* 1998;24:1125–1129.
4. Hoffer KJ. The Hoffer Q formula: a comparison of theoretic and regression formulas. *J Cataract Refract Surg* 1993;19:700–712.
5. Andreo LK, Wilson ME, Saunders RA. Predictive value of regression and theoretical IOL formulas in pediatric intraocular lens implantation. *J Pediatr Ophthalmol Strabismus* 1997;34:240–243.
6. Mezer E, Rootman DS, Abdolell M, et al. Early postoperative refractive outcomes of pediatric intraocular lens implantation. *J Cataract Refract Surg* 2004;30:603–610.
7. Gordon RA, Donzis PB. Refractive development of the human eye. *Arch Ophthalmol* 1985;103:785–789.
8. McClatchey SK, Parks MM. Myopic shift after cataract removal in childhood. *J Pediatr Ophthalmol Strabismus* 1997;34:88–95.
9. McClatchey SK. Refractive changes after lens implantation in childhood [letter]. *Ophthalmology* 1998;105:1572–1573.
10. McClatchey SK, Dahan E, Maselli E, et al. A comparison of the rate of refractive growth in pediatric aphakic and pseudophakic eyes. *Ophthalmology* 2000;107:118–122.
11. Plager DA, Kipfer H, Sprunger DT, et al. Refractive change in pediatric pseudophakia: 6-year follow-up. *J Cataract Refract Surg* 2002;28:810–815.
12. Lambert SR. The effect of age on the retardation of axial elongation following a lensectomy in infant monkeys. *Arch Ophthalmol* 1998;116:781–784.
13. Lambert SR, Fernandes A, Drews-Botsch C, Tigges M. Pseudophakia retards axial elongation in neonatal monkey eyes. *Invest Ophthalmol Vis Sci* 1996;37:451–458.
14. Hiles DA. Intraocular lens implantation in children. *Ann Ophthalmol* 1977;9:789–797.
15. Masket S, ed. Consultation Section. *J Cataract Refract Surg* 1991;17:512–518.
16. Wilson ME, Peterseim MW, Englert JA, Lall-Trail JK, Elliott LA. Pseudophakia and polypseudophakia in the first year of life. *J AAPOS* 2001;5:238–245.
17. Zadnik K, Mutti DO, Adams AJ. The repeatability of measurement of the ocular components. *Invest Ophthalmol Vis Sci* 1992;33:2325–2333.
18. Holladay JT, Prager TC, Chandler TY, et al. A three-part system for refining intraocular lens power calculations. *J Cataract Refract Surg,* 1998;14:17–24.

Cataract Surgery in Children

Chapter 8

Historical Overview

Rupal H. Trivedi, M. Edward Wilson, Jr., and Suresh K. Pandey

This chapter highlights the historical aspects of cataract management in children. We also take an opportunity to give credit to the innovators whose efforts have helped us reach the current level of success in the surgical management of pediatric cataracts. In the past, poor outcomes from pediatric cataract surgery prompted many surgeons to use a *conservative approach* (described in Chapter 9). Since then, many surgical strategies have come and gone. They have, however, led us to where we are today. Our current "modern" techniques will also, someday, be included in the historical approach category. Surgeons need to study the past so the lessons learned do not have to be learned again. Also, one must not forget the giants of thought and skill on whose shoulders we now stand. They led the way to our current understanding and our current technology.

OPTICAL IRIDECTOMY

In the 1950s, thick secondary membranes, glaucoma, and corneal decompensation occurred so frequently after pediatric cataract surgery that surgical aggressiveness seemed pointless to many surgeons. In fact, in 1957, Costenbader and Albert[1] stated that they had not seen a single child benefited from surgery for congenital cataracts.

For visually significant congenital cataracts, some surgeons resorted to an optical iridectomy to avoid the inflammatory response and membranes that developed when the

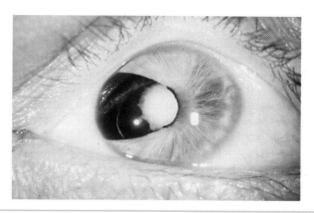

FIGURE 8-1. Optical iridectomy in an eye with congenital nuclear cataract.

lens was entered (Figure 8.1). This technique preserved accommodation and avoided secondary membranes.[1] In multi-handicapped children with bilateral central cataracts, this technique was advocated also to avoid contact lens and spectacle problems. However, the visual results were not satisfactory. Unilateral treatment was rarely advocated. Despite bilateral surgery, nystagmus nearly always developed and vision was rarely better than 20/200 even when a clear zone existed peripheral to the fetal nuclear opacity.[2] Optical iridectomy was useless when total cataracts were present.

DISCISSION/NEEDLING

Needling/discission is probably the oldest of all surgeries for removal of congenital cataracts. Aurelius Cornelius, a Roman physician who lived 2000 years ago (quoted in Ref. 3), first described discission of soft cataracts. The technique used by the ancients was credited to Potts in 1775 (quoted in Ref. 2). Because of its simplicity, discission remained the method of choice until the middle of the twentieth century.

The discission was developed because of surgeons' experiences with the couching operation. It is based on the observation that the lens material of small children is comprised of soluble protein, which is absorbed over weeks or months following an incision of the anterior lens capsule. The discission involves lacerating the anterior capsule of the lens (in one of several shapes and sizes) and allowing the lens material to be absorbed by the aqueous. Most practitioners used an anterior approach but Saunders advocated a posterior approach, because he considered the dispersion of the lens material into the vitreous to be more effective (cited in Ref. 4).

Chandler[5,6] reported the outcome of discission surgery without iridectomy in 33 eyes. Nearly one fifth of the eyes were eventually lost owing to complications related to pupillary block. A thick capsular membrane developed in nearly all eyes undergoing this procedure and secondary glaucoma also occurred frequently. Derby, in 1885, stressed the importance of a widely dilated pupil (quoted in Ref. 2). He felt that the degree of pupillary dilation should be determined before deciding on the type of surgery to be performed. If the pupil failed to dilate, he advised preliminary iridectomy 3 or 4 weeks before doing a discission. Scheie[2] noted, in 1960, that this rule is equally valid for all types of operations for congenital cataract.

Through-and-Through Discission

This variation of the discission procedure was described by Ziegler.[7] He incised the lens through both its anterior and its posterior capsule so as to disperse the lens proteins into both the aqueous and the vitreous humor in hopes of promoting complete absorption. The procedure did not find widespread acceptance, although a Ziegler knife is still included on some surgical trays.

LINEAR EXTRACTION

For many children the needling procedure alone proved to be inadequate. The remaining lens material did not absorb completely and often produced an inflammatory reaction. The removal of lens substance with irrigation was sometimes performed at the same time as the needling procedure (one-stage procedure) or a week or more later (two-stage procedure). In children <6 years old, the needling and removal of lens substance could be performed as a one-stage procedure. However, in older children a preliminary needling was preferred, to allow greater mixing of the lens cortex and aqueous. This permitted the lens cortex to fluff up and become flocculent, thus easing the irrigation of lens material from the anterior chamber out, through a wound made at the limbus.

In the first half of the twentieth century this needling plus irrigation procedure was the most common procedure for surgery on congenital cataracts.[8] Gibson is credited for the technique based on a description in 1811. It was subsequently popularized as linear extraction (quoted in Ref. 2). Gibson's original technique involved using a couching needle to rupture the anterior capsule. The eye was left to settle over a period of 2 or 3 weeks. An incision was then made "by a corneal knife of the largest size" and was used to extract the cataract; as the knife was withdrawn, aqueous and some of the lens tissue evacuated spontaneously or was helped by a curette (quoted in Ref. 4). Many modifications of Gibson's technique were used. A capsule forceps was sometimes introduced into the anterior chamber to express dense opaque lens material. A hook or curette was also sometimes used to massage the cornea to express this material without the introduction of an instrument into the anterior chamber. An irrigation needle was often inserted into the anterior chamber and the saline irrigation flushed the remaining fragments of the lens from the chamber through the corneal wound.

In 1965, Ryan et al.[9] reported better results with linear extraction compared to repeated discissions. Chandler[5] reported that the results of linear extraction and iridectomy were poor if the operation was done in infancy. An updrawn pupil and dense secondary membranes formed. Most of the eyes were lost.

ASPIRATION OF CATARACTS

In the early 1960s, the aspiration procedure was popularized by Scheie. With the widespread use of the operating microscope, the Scheie procedure became the accepted technique for extracting cataracts in infants and children. In 1977, Scheie and Ewing[3] described the history of the technique. Rhazes, a Persian physician and philosopher, mentioned aspiration, as did Antillus (a contemporary of Galen), in the fourth century AD. Aspiration was also practiced in Japan in the fifteenth century, in Italy in 1829, and by Laugier in 1847. Although described as early as the fourth century, Scheie's report in 1960[2] reawakened ophthalmologists' interest in the aspiration technique and repopularized it.[9,10]

Scheie[2,3,11,12] reported that the aspiration technique could be performed as a one-stage procedure in eyes with complete cataract or as a two-stage procedure in eyes with partial cataract. The first step was to open the anterior capsule widely and the second step was to aspirate the lens material via the same puncture site using a large-bore, 19-gauge needle and a 2-mL syringe. Many ophthalmologists later reported that the two-stage procedure was unnecessary and also dangerous, since it led to a higher incidence of glaucoma.[13]

Parks[13] reported modifications of the aspiration technique. This technique combined the aspiration principle, however, it differed in that it aspirated the lens cortex while leaving the lens capsule intact except for a 2-mm opening in the anterior capsule near the superior pupillary margin. The coaptation of the collapsed anterior and posterior lens capsule provided a framework for the regrowth of a sheet of new lens fiber, almost always needing secondary postcataract surgery within a few months. The secondary surgery could be avoided by creating a 5-mm central opening in the coapted anterior and posterior lens capsule after the aspiration of the cortex was completed.

The aspiration technique was simple and safe. However, since the cortex removal was often incomplete and the posterior capsule was left intact by most surgeons, secondary opacification of the visual axis occurred frequently and multiple additional procedures were often required.

IRRIGATION–ASPIRATION TECHNIQUE

In the mid-1960s, a double-barreled cannula was introduced, with one barrel for aspiration and one for irrigation. The dual irrigation–aspiration technique enabled the ophthalmologist to maintain the anterior chamber depth during cataract aspiration.

INTRACAPSULAR EXTRACTION

Classic intracapsular surgery found disfavor among most ophthalmologists for children because of the higher risk of vitreous loss caused by the forces required to rupture the tough zonules in young patients.[2,9] A large incision was also needed, which led to wound-related complications.

AUTOMATED VITRECTOR

In the first two thirds of the twentieth century pediatric cataract surgery was completely nonautomated. The advent of vitreous suction cutting devices in the mid-1970s revolutionized pediatric cataract surgery.[14–18] Using this new device, Taylor[19] and Parks[20] began cautiously removing the center of the posterior capsule and a portion of the anterior vitreous during the initial surgery in young children. Removal of all but 2 mm of the peripheral posterior lens capsule with a vitreous suction cutter was recommended, in addition to a generous anterior vitrectomy. In 1981 Taylor[19] reported needing no reoperations in 23 infantile eyes operated with the new method of lensectomy with posterior capsulectomy and anterior vitrectomy. In contrast, of the 28 eyes in which the posterior capsule was left intact, 19 required reoperations a total of 32 times to keep the visual axis clear.

In addition to its use as a cutting device, the vitreous suction cutting instrument was used for automated irriga-

tion/aspiration of lens cortex and nucleus. The often thick and gummy lens material found in children was more easily aspirated using this instrument as opposed to manual irrigation and aspiration. Also, bursts of cutting could be used for any lens material that was initially resistant to aspiration. Later, machines capable of supporting a vitrector handpiece were also fit with separate (noncutting) irrigation/aspiration handpieces designed specifically for removal of the lens cortex.

PHACOEMULSIFICATION

In the 1970s, phacoemulsification was used in pediatric cataract surgery for the first time.[21] At most, only short bursts of ultrasound power were used in pediatric eyes. However, even without ultrasound power, the phacoemulsification handpiece was an effective irrigation/aspiration device. If any hard material was encountered, ultrasound power was available to help remove it. Hiles et al.[22] and Callahan[23] recommended phacoemulsification as a useful extension of the aspiration technique in children since the softness of the lens material can vary greatly from case to case.

INTRAOCULAR LENS (IOL) IMPLANTATION

Details of IOL implantation in children are discussed in Section IV. After the successful implantation of an IOL in an adult by Sir Harold Ridley in 1949,[24–27] Epstein placed an IOL in the eye of a child as early as 1951 (cited in Ref. 28). Peter Choyce[29] reported the implantation of an IOL in a 10-year-old child in 1955. Binkhorst and coworkers[30,31] implanted iridocapsular fixated IOLs in children in 1959. Hiles advocated IOL implantation in children and published many articles related to his experience.[32–36] Sinskey and Patel,[37] BenEzra and Paez,[38] and Dahan and Salmenson[39] were also early advocates of IOLs implantation in children.

However, the use of IOLs in children has evolved slowly and was not truly popularized until a decade ago. Early attempts at IOL implantation in children resulted in frequent complications secondary to poor lens design and the greater inflammatory response that occurs in a child's eye after intraocular surgery. As a result, IOL implantation at the time of cataract surgery in children did not become common practice until the 1990s. Table 8-1 describes the various techniques advocated historically in the evolution of pediatric cataract surgery.[2,3,14–22,28–37,40–72]

To summarize, automation and IOLs have brought pediatric cataract surgery into the modern age and the resulting outcomes are much improved. The evolution of this surgery continues, with many adult cataract surgery

▶ **TABLE 8-1** Evolution of Pediatric Cataract Surgery

Advance	Year	Author(s)
First implant in a child for aphakic correction	1958	Epstein/Choyce
Manual aspiration of congenital/juvenile cataract	1960	Scheie
Iridocapsular implant	1969	Binkhorst
Advancement in vitreous cutting instrument	1972	Machemer
Binkhorst intraocular lenses (IOLs)	1977–1982	Hiles
Posterior chamber IOLs	1982	Hiles
Iris-claw lenses	1983	Singh
Pathophysiology of amblyopia	1977–1985	Weisel/Raviola
Posterior chamber IOLs	1983–1993	Sinskey/Hiles
Posterior capsulotomy/anterior vitrectomy	1983	Parks
Epikeratophakia	1986	Morgan
Epilenticular IOL/pars plana endocapsular lensectomy	1988	Tablante
Retropseudophakic Vitrectomy via limbus	1991	Mackool/Chhatiawala
Pars plana posterior capsulectomy and vitrectomy	1993	Buckley et al.
Primary posterior capsulorhexis/optic capture	1994	Gimbel/DeBroff
IOL biomaterials/Designs/sizing in children	1994	Wilson et al.
Primary posterior capsulotomy & anterior vitrectomy	1994–2000	BenEzra/Cohen Vasavada/Desai/Trivedi
Anterior capsulotomy for pediatric cataract surgery (vitrectorhexis)	1994	Wilson et al.
Heparin in BSS to decrease postoperative inflammation	1995	Brady et al.
Dye-enhanced pediatric cataract surgery	2000–2002	Pandey et al.

BSS, balanced salt solution.

techniques being applied to older children with only minor technical adjustments. In addition, new techniques designed specifically for children have emerged. In very young children, automated posterior capsulotomy and anterior vitrectomy, developed specifically for the pediatric eye, continues to provide the best long-term outcomes, with fewer reoperations and complications compared to older methods described in this chapter.

REFERENCES

1. Costenbader F, Albert D. Conservatism in the management of congenital cataract. *Arch Ophthalmol* 1957;58:426–430.
2. Scheie HG. Aspiration of congenital or soft cataracts: a new technique. *Am J Ophthalmol* 1960;50:1048–1056.
3. Scheie HG, Ewing MQ. Aspiration of soft cataracts. *Int Ophthalmol Clin* 1977;17:51–58.
4. Taylor D. The Doyne lecture. Congenital cataract: the history, the nature and the practice. *Eye* 1998;12:9–36.
5. Chandler PA. Surgery of congenital cataract. *Trans Am Acad Ophthalmol Otolaryngol* 1968;72:341–354.
6. Chandler PA. Surgery of congenital cataract. *Am J Ophthalmol* 1968;65:663–674.
7. Ziegler SL. Complete dicission of the lens by the V-shaped method. *JAMA* 1921;77:1100–1102.
8. McCaslin MF. Discissions and linear extractions. *Int Ophthalmol Clin* 1977;17:47–49.
9. Ryan SJ, Blanton FM, von Noorden GK. Surgery of congenital cataract. *Am J Ophthalmol* 1965;60:583–587.
10. Hogan MJ. Congenital cataract surgery. *Trans Am Ophthalmol Soc* 1966;64:311–318.
11. Scheie HG, Rubenstein RA, Kent RB. Aspiration of congenital or soft cataracts: further experience. *Trans Am Ophthalmol Soc* 1966;64:319–330.
12. Scheie HG, Rubenstein RA, Kent RB. Aspiration of congenital or soft cataracts: further experience. *Am J Ophthalmol* 1967;63:3–8.
13. Parks MM. Intracapsular aspiration. *Int Ophthalmol Clin* 1977;17:59–74.
14. Machemer R. A new concept for vitreous surgery. 7. Two instrument techniques in pars plana vitrectomy. *Arch Ophthalmol* 1974;92:407–412.
15. Parel JM, Machemer R, Aumayr W. A new concept for vitreous surgery. 4. Improvements in instrumentation and illumination. *Am J Ophthalmol* 1974;77:6–12.
16. Machemer R, Norton EW. A new concept for vitreous surgery. 3. Indications and results. *Am J Ophthalmol* 1972;74:1034–1056.

17. Machemer R. A new concept for vitreous surgery. 2. Surgical technique and complications. *Am J Ophthalmol* 1972;74:1022–1033.
18. Machemer R, Parel JM, Buettner H. A new concept for vitreous surgery. I. Instrumentation. *Am J Ophthalmol* 1972;73:1–7.
19. Taylor DSI. Choice of surgical technique in the management of congenital cataract. *Trans Ophthalmol Soc UK* 1981;101:114–117.
20. Parks MM. Posterior lens capsulectomy during primary cataract surgery in children. *Ophthalmology* 1983;90:344–345.
21. Hiles DA, Hurite FG. Results of the first year's experience with phacoemulsification. *Am J Ophthalmol* 1973;75:473–477.
22. Hiles DA, Carter BT, Chotiner B. Phacoemulsification of infantile cataracts. *Trans Pa Acad Ophthalmol Otolaryngol* 1978;31:30–37.
23. Callahan MA. Technique of congenital cataract surgery with the Kelman Cavitron phacoemulsifier. *Ophthalmology* 1979;86:1994–1998.
24. Ridley H. Intra-ocular acrylic lenses. *Trans Ophthalmol Soc UK* 1951;71:617–621.
25. Ridley H. Intra-ocular acrylic lenses: A recent development in the surgery of cataract. *Br J Ophthalmol* 1952;36:113–122.
26. Ridley H. Further observations on intraocular acrylic lenses in cataract surgery. *Trans Am Acad Ophthalmol Otolaryngol* 1953;57:98–106.
27. Apple DJ, Trivedi RH, Ridley NH. Contributions in addition to the intraocular lens. *Arch Ophthalmol* 2002;120:1198–1202.
28. Letocha CE, Pavlin CJ. Follow-up of 3 patients with Ridley intraocular lens implantation. *J Cataract Refract Surg* 1999;25:587–591.
29. Choyce DP. Correction of uniocular aphakia by means of anterior chamber acrylic implants. *Trans Ophthalmol Soc UK* 1958;78:459–470.
30. Binkhorst CD, Gobin MH. Injuries to the eye with lens opacity in young children. *Ophthalmologica* 1964;148:169–183.
31. Binkhorst CD, Greaves B, Kats A, Bermingham AK. Lens injury in children treated with irido-capsular supported intra-ocular lenses. *J Am Intraocul Implant Soc* 1978;4:34–49.
32. Hiles DA. Intraocular lenses in children. *Int Ophthalmol Clin* 1977;17:221–242.
33. Hiles DA. Visual acuities of monocular IOL and non-IOL aphakic children. *Ophthalmology* 1980;87:1296–1300.
34. Hiles DA. Intraocular lens implantation in children with monocular cataracts, 1974–1983. *Ophthalmology* 1984;91:1231–1237.
35. Hiles DA, Hered RW. Modern intraocular lens implants in children with new age limitations. *J Cataract Refract Surg* 1987;13:493–497.
36. Hiles DA. Visual rehabilitation of aphakic children. III. Intraocular lenses. *Surv Ophthalmol* 1990;34:371–379.
37. Sinskey RM, Patel J. Posterior chamber intraocular lens implants in children: report of a series. *J Am Intraocul Implant Soc* 1983;9:157–160.
38. BenEzra D, Paez JH. Congenital cataract and intraocular lenses. *Am J Ophthalmol* 1983;96:311–314.
39. Dahan E, Salmenson BD. Pseudophakia in children: precautions, technique, and feasibility. *J Cataract Refract Surg* 1990;16:75–82.
40. Binkhorst CD, Gobin MH, Leonard PA. Post-traumatic artificial lens implants (pseudophakoi) in children. *Br J Ophthalmol* 1969;53:518–529.
41. Binkhorst CD, Gobin MH, Leonard PA. Post-traumatic pseudophakia in children. *Ophthalmologica* 1968;158(Suppl):284–291.
42. Binkhorst CD. Five hundred planned extracapsular extractions with irido-capsular and iris clip lens implantation in senile cataract. *Ophthalmic Surg* 1977;8:37–44.
43. Binkhorst CD, Greaves B, Katz A, Bermingham AK. Lens injury in children treated with irido-capsular supported intra-ocular lenses. *J Am Intraocul Implant Soc* 1978;4:34–49.
44. Binkhorst CD, Greaves B, Kats A, Bermingham AK. Lens injury in children treated with iridocapsular supported intra-ocular lenses. *Doc Ophthalmol* 1979;46:241–277.
45. Binkhorst CD. Iris-clip and irido-capsular implants (pseudophakoi); personal techniques of pseudophakia. *Br J Ophthalmol* 1967;51:767–771.
46. Hiles DA, Wallar PH, Biglan AW. The surgery and results following traumatic cataracts in children. *J Pediatr Ophthalmol* 1976;13:319–325.
47. Hiles DA, Watson BA. Complications of implant surgery in children. *J Am Intra-Ocular Implant Soc* 1979;5:24–32.
48. Hiles DA. Implant surgery in children. *Int Ophthalmol Clin* 1979;19:95–123.
49. Hiles DA. Intraocular lens implantation in children. *Ann Ophthalmol* 1977;9:789–797.
50. Hiles DA. Peripheral iris erosions associated with pediatric intraocular lens implants. *J Am Intra-Ocular Implant Soc* 1979;5:210–212.
51. Hiles DA. The need for intraocular lens implantation in children. *Ophthal Surg* 1977;8:162–169.
52. Hiles DA. Visual acuities of monocular IOL and non-IOL aphakic children. *Ophthalmology* 1980;87:1296–1300.
53. Singh D. Intraocular lenses in children. *Indian J Ophthalmol* 1984;32:499–500.
54. Singh D. Intraocular lenses in children. *Indian J Ophthalmol* 1987;35:249–250.
55. Weisel TN, Raviola E. Myopia and eye enlargement after neonatal lid fusion in monkeys. *Nature* 1977;266:66–68.
56. Sinskey RM, Amin PA, Stoppel J. Intraocular lens implantation in microphthalmic patients. *J Cataract Refract Surg* 1992;18:480–484.
57. Sinskey RM, Karel F, Dal Ri E. Management of cataracts in children. *J Cataract Refract Surg* 1989;15:196–200.
58. Sinskey RM, Stoppel JO, Amin PA. Long-term results of intraocular lens implantation in pediatric patients. *J Cataract Refract Surg* 1993;19:405–408.
59. Morgan KS. Visual rehabilitation of aphakic children. IV. Epikeratophakia. *Surv Ophthalmol* 1990;34:379–384.
60. Tablante RT, Cruz EDG, Lapus JV, Santos AM. A new technique of congenital cataract surgery with primary posterior chamber intraocular lens implantation. *J Cataract Refract Surg* 1988;14:149–157.
61. Mackool RJ, Chhatiawala H. Pediatric cataract surgery and intraocular lens implantation: a new technique for preventing or excising postoperative secondary membranes. *J Cataract Refract Surg* 1991;17:62–66.
62. Buckley EG, Klombers LA, Seaber JH, et al. Management of the posterior capsule during pediatric intraocular lens implantation. *Am J Ophthalmol* 1993;115:722–728.
63. Gimbel HV, DeBroff DM. Posterior capsulorhexis with optic capture: maintaining a clear visual axis after pediatric cataract surgery. *J Cataract Refract Surg* 1994;20:658–664.
64. Wilson ME, Apple DJ, Bluestein EC, Wang XH. Intraocular lenses for pediatric implantation: biomaterials, designs and sizing. *J Cataract Refract Surg* 1994;20:584–591.
65. BenEzra D, Cohen E. Posterior capsulectomy in pediatric cataract surgery: the necessity of a choice. *Ophthalmology* 1997;104:2168–2174.
66. Vasavada A, Desai J. Primary posterior capsulorhexis with and without anterior vitrectomy in congenital cataracts. *J Cataract Refract Surg* 1997;23(Suppl):647–651.
67. Vasavada AR, Trivedi RH. Role of optic capture in congenital cataract and intraocular lens surgery in children. *J Cataract Refract Surg* 2000;26:824–831.
68. Vasavada AR, Trivedi RH, Singh R. Necessity of vitrectomy when optic capture is performed in children older than 5 years. *J Cataract Refract Surg* 2001;27:1185–1193.
69. Wilson ME, Bluestein EC, Wang XH, et al. Comparison of mechanized anterior capsulectomy and manual continuous capsulorhexis in pediatric eyes. *J Cataract Refract Surg* 1994;20:602–606.
70. Brady KM, Atkinson CS, Kilty LA, et al. Cataract surgery and intraocular lens implantation in children. *Am J Ophthalmol* 1995;120:1–9.
71. Pandey SK, Werner L, Escobar-Gomez M, Werner LP, Apple DJ. Dye-enhanced cataract surgery. Part 3: Posterior capsule staining to learn posterior continuous curvilinear capsulorhexis. *J Cataract Refract Surg* 2000;26:1066–1071.
72. Pandey SK, Werner L, Apple DJ, Wilson ME. Dye-enhanced adult and pediatric cataract surgery. In: Buratto L, Werner L, Zanini M, Apple DJ, eds. *Phacoemulsification: Principles and Techniques.* Thorofare, NJ: Slack, 2002:chap 41.

Planning Pediatric Cataract Surgery: Diverse Issues

Rupal H. Trivedi and M. Edward Wilson, Jr.

The management of cataracts in children is not only complex and tedious, but also controversial. Before planning cataract surgery in children several questions need to be addressed. In this chapter we highlight some of these issues that are not covered as individual chapters in the book:

1. Who should perform pediatric cataract surgery: pediatric ophthalmologists or adult cataract surgeons?
2. How does pediatric cataract surgery differ from adult cataract surgery?
3. Does conservative management have a place in pediatric cataract surgery?
4. Unilateral cataract: Should it be pursued surgically or treated conservatively?
5. Is simultaneous bilateral surgery for pediatric cataracts a reasonable option?

WHO SHOULD PERFORM PEDIATRIC CATARACT SURGERY: PEDIATRIC OPHTHALMOLOGISTS OR ADULT CATARACT SURGEONS?

The incidence of pediatric cataracts is not high enough to allow many surgeons to devote their entire careers to *pediatric cataract surgery*. The result of our worldwide survey revealed that more than 71.5% of American Society of Cataract and Refractive Surgeon respondees performed <10 pediatric cataract surgeries (PCS) per year, while the majority of American Association of Pediatric Ophthalmologist and Strabismus (AAPOS) respondees (85.0%) indicated <20 PCSs performed per year.[1] In most cases, either pediatric ophthalmologists or cataract surgeons (primarily performing adult cataract surgery) cultivate the interest in pediatric cataract surgery. In 2000, Wood and Ogawa[2] wrote, "Given the overall paucity of clinical experience in pediatric patients and its hazardous nature, who should be performing pediatric cataract surgery in the first place? Is this the realm of the pediatric ophthalmologist, the adult cataract surgeon, or perhaps both?"

The question is still debatable: Who should perform pediatric cataract surgery? Is it best performed by pediatric ophthalmologists, who deal with children exclusively, or cataract surgeons, who frequently perform adult cataract surgery?[3] We raised this question in our survey (see Chapter 55) and found that 77.4% of physicians not performing pediatric cataract surgery referred patients to a pediatric ophthalmologist.[1] Among physicians performing pediatric cataract surgery, more than half (52.6%) stated that either a pediatric ophthalmologist or an adult cataract surgeon should perform this procedure.[1]

We believe that this issue may depend on "local" situations and there is no "must" here. In our opinion, the surgeon with the most experience and interest in pediatric cataract surgery should be sent the surgical cases from the locale.[4] Comanagement among ophthalmologists works well in this setting. In the United States, pediatric ophthalmologists are more likely to be the most experienced, however, outside the United States, adult cataract surgeons generally lead the field. Pediatric ophthalmologists are much more aware of the anatomy and functional parameters of pediatric eyes. They have much to teach adult cataract surgeons about operating on the infant eye and various functional issues in postoperative management. Conversely, cataract surgeons (primarily performing adult cataract surgery) are much more experienced in surgical technique such as capsulorhexis and innovations in intraocular lens (IOL)–related technology, and they also have much to teach pediatric ophthalmologists about adult surgical advances that should be applied to children.[4]

In our opinion, the surgeon must have enough experience to feel comfortable with the specific difficulties of the pediatric eye. Children with cataracts often have other associated health problems that increase anesthesia risks. They require close monitoring pre- and postoperatively by staff with expertise in pediatric anesthesia and recovery. It is mandatory to have appropriate backup in case of intraoperative or postoperative anesthetic complications. These cases are best handled at a pediatric care center. Whoever performs pediatric cataract surgery must understand the importance of *teamwork*. A pediatric ophthalmologist should generally be following these eyes during the postoperative course for strabismus, amblyopia, and other functionally related issues.

However, for each region a solution has to be individually tailored based on the resources available and the willingness of pediatric and adult cataract surgeons to continue to learn from each other and to work together to provide good care.

HOW DOES PEDIATRIC CATARACT SURGERY DIFFER FROM ADULT CATARACT SURGERY?

Children are not miniature adults; they have unique anatomy, physiology, psychology, and social status. Not only are children's eyes smaller than adults', but also their tissues are much softer. A cataract in an adult reduces visual acuity, while in a child it may also interfere with normal visual (brain) development. In a young child, a cataract blurs the image received by the retina and disrupts the development of the visual pathways in the central nervous system. The *timing of surgery, the surgical technique, the choice of aphakic correction, and the amblyopia management* are of utmost importance in achieving good and long-lasting results in children.

The management of pediatric cataracts is far more complex than the management of cataracts in adults. Differences and difficulties encountered during the preoperative, intraoperative, and postoperative periods are listed below.

Preoperative Period

1. Difficult and often delayed diagnosis
2. Timing of surgery: In sharp contrast to the treatment of adult cataracts, the timing of cataract surgery in children is of paramount importance. It affects the visual result to a much greater extent than the surgical technique or method of postoperative optical correction used by the surgeon.
3. High incidence of associated ocular and systemic anomalies and prematurity
4. Setup for pediatric general anesthesia a prerequisite
5. Apprehension about general anesthesia

6. Examination under anesthesia: necessary sometimes even to diagnose cataract and for preoperative assessment
7. Need for automated keratometer and A-scan in operating room
8. Difficulty in calculating IOL power
9. Psychologic issues and preoperative counseling of parents

Intraoperative Period

1. Risks of general anesthesia
2. Smaller size of the eye
3. Poor dilation of pupil more often associated in pediatric eyes
4. Low scleral rigidity
5. Relative size of the pars plana: The pars plana region in the infant eye is incompletely developed, so the anterior retina lies just behind the pars plicata (see Chapter 16).
6. Incision and suturing: As opposed to adult eyes, a superior tunnel is preferable in pediatric eyes (as it provides better protection and, in general, children do not have deep-seated eyes, which would require temporal incision). It is preferable to suture even a "self-seal" tunnel incision in children as opposed to adults (see Chapter 11).
7. Need for high-viscosity viscoelastic for capsular management
8. Difficulty in performing an anterior capsulorhexis associated with a highly elastic anterior capsule and increased intralenticular and intravitreal pressure
9. Dense formed vitreous and scleral collapse contributing to vitreous upthrust giving rise to raised intravitreal and lenticular pressure, making anterior and posterior capsular management difficult
10. Removal of lens substance rarely requires phacoemulsification, but the cortex is stickier and gummier than in adults
11. Need for primary posterior capsule management
12. Need for vitrectomy instrumentation
13. Difficult IOL implantation

Postoperative Period

1. Higher risk for opacification of the visual axis
2. Propensity for increased postoperative inflammation
3. Compliance with the use of topical postoperative medications difficult
4. Requirement for frequent correction of residual refractive error, as it is constantly changing due to growth of the eye
5. Difficulty in documenting anatomic, refractive, and visual acuity changes due to poor compliance

6. Examination possibly requiring repeated brief anesthesia
7. Tendency to develop amblyopia and need for patching
8. Long-term follow-up important but not always easily achieved

DOES CONSERVATIVE MANAGEMENT HAVE A PLACE IN PEDIATRIC CATARACT SURGERY?

Poor anatomical and functional outcomes of cataract surgery in children have prompted many surgeons to try conservative treatment such as the use of mydriatic drops.[5-8] Chandler[5,6] noted in the 24th Edward Jackson Memorial Lecture that "the fact that so many eyes are lost after surgery for congenital cataract is the reason why operation is not advised unless the vision is quite low." DeVoe[8] stated that "it is better to have 20/50 vision with accommodation than 20/20 vision without accommodation."

A conservative approach is most commonly indicated for a unilateral partial cataract. However, many conservative surgeons have also stated that bilateral partial cataracts should not be extracted if the visual acuity is better than 20/50 to 20/70.[5,6] But it is not possible to measure visual acuity in infants with these partial cataracts. Difficulties in documenting visual acuity in infants with incomplete, but visually significant, cataracts may unnecessarily defer surgery in these patients, leading to irreversible damage because of amblyopia. In earlier years it was believed that no surgery should be considered if the fundus can

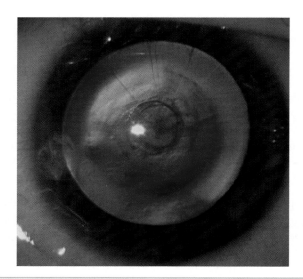

FIGURE 9-2. Central unilateral lens opacity in a 7-week-old child. Should surgery be performed without delay or is a conservative approach indicated? These decisions can be very difficult. This opacity worsened slowly over time and was eventually operated. Patching and observation worked well initially, however.

be viewed around that cataract, and therefore, conservative treatment should be used in eyes with central opacity[7] (Figs. 9-1 and 9-2). When treating eyes with a conservative approach, it is important to prescribe appropriate amblyopia therapy.

Use of mydriatic drops necessitates the patient's wearing glasses for reading if any cycloplegic effect is induced. This has not found widespread acceptance. Associated glare and loss of accommodation are the most common obstacles. Visual outcome has also been unimpressive. Despite these limitations, the use of mydriatics drops can be kept in reserve in eyes with slowly progressive cataracts (for example, steroid-induced cataracts) or central cataracts and, especially, in patients for whom cataract surgery needs to be deferred for any reason—be it medical (high risk for anesthesia), social, or economic.

DENSE UNILATERAL CATARACT: SHOULD IT BE PURSUED SURGICALLY OR TREATED CONSERVATIVELY?

Dense unilateral congenital cataract was once regarded to have a dismal visual prognosis. Children with unilateral congenital cataracts remain challenging, and their visual outcomes are still often disappointing. In 1957, Costenbader and Albert[7] stated that they had not seen a single child with a monocular congenital cataract who had benefited from surgical removal of the lens opacity. They noted that it was best not to operate on eyes with a congenital

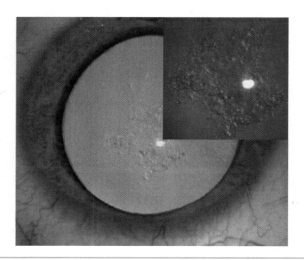

FIGURE 9-1. Posterior subcapsular cataract in an 11-year-old girl who received a bone marrow transplantation for multiple histiocytic cysts. Vision is reduced only to 20/40 but glare is a problem in some lighting conditions. Deciding between surgery and observation can be difficult in cases like this.

monocular cataract because of morbidity and a poor visual result. They[7] further noted that

> ...*since visual acuity is not improved, strabismus is not favorable influenced, and photophobia is not alleviated, we would unequivocally advise against surgery in unilateral congenital cataract unless the cataract is becoming hypermature. The appearance of the eye is usually not improved; function has not been helped, and the eye has been jeopardized if surgery is performed.* ... (p. 428)

In 1979, Francois[9] noted that everyone knows the uselessness of operating on unilateral congenital cataracts, as the functional result is always very bad. Taylor,[10] in his Doyne Memorial Lecture published in 1998, points out that unilateral congenital cataract is not a socially significant disease since it must be a coincidence of considerable rarity when a person who has such a cataract treated successfully (creating a spare eye) blinds the phakic eye. He points out that if days off work, long-distance travel, repeated clinic visits, fees, and all other disturbances are taken into account, the costs and the disturbance to the daily lives of patients and their parents are very substantial.[10] He points out that even at major referral centers, a good functional result (e.g., driving vision) is unlikely to be achieved in more than 50% of patients presenting with unilateral congenital cataract. Taylor[10] acknowledges, however, that an increasing number of cases with some degree of binocular vision is being reported; this has functional benefits of its own and, also, reduces the normally very high incidence of strabismus.

In the past 20 years, recent advances in surgical techniques and aphakic correction have left amblyopia as the major determinant of the ultimate visual outcome of pediatric cataract surgery. With the evolution of cataract surgery and the ability to provide early, effective, and constant optical rehabilitation, several authors[11-13] have reported achieving good vision in the affected eye of children with monocular cataract. To the best of our knowledge, Frey and coworkers,[11] in 1973, were the first to report that "...*some children with monocular cataract can achieve useful central vision*" and were the first to advocate that "*the dictum of extreme conservatism in the management of monocular cataracts in children needs to be re-evaluated*" (p. 388). Subsequently, Bellar et al.[12] in 1981, demonstrated that excellent visual results could be obtained in selected children with monocular congenital cataracts with early treatment and compliant contact lens wear and patching. They emphasized the importance of early treatment during the sensitive period of vision development. They further noted,[12] "... We believe that surgery during the neonatal period is not only justified but probably essential in any successful treatment of monocular congenital cataract..."[4] (p. 564). A review of the literature since 1980 reveals that 37% of infants with early surgery achieved a

visual acuity outcome of 20/80 or better after surgery for dense unilateral congenital cataract.[14] Birch and Stager[15] have reported that there exists a *6-week window of time, beginning at birth*, during which treatment of a dense congenital unilateral cataract is maximally effective. If treatment is initiated during this period and the child is compliant with contact lens wear and occlusion therapy, an excellent visual acuity outcome can be obtained. Early treatment with good compliance is also associated with a lower prevalence of strabismus and a higher prevalence of fusion and stereopsis.

In a recent article, Wright[16] stated, "Not all children treated aggressively will obtain that lofty goal of good visual acuity and binocular vision, but it is guaranteed that without aggressive treatment virtually all children with a visually significant cataract at birth will end up with a blind eye and strabismus ..." (p. 1122). Amaya[17] would say to treat unilateral congenital cataracts aggressively "sometimes!" (p. 1123).

We concur with Wright's view in our practice. We have recently reported the effects of surgical timing and patching compliance on the visual outcomes of children with dense congenital monocular cataracts.[13] The median visual acuity of eyes operated on before 6 weeks of age was 20/40, compared to 20/400 when surgery was performed after 6 weeks of age ($P = .0077$). The median visual acuity of children deemed compliant with patching for amblyopia was 20/40, compared to 20/800 for those deemed noncompliant ($P = .02$). Compliance to amblyopia therapy was one of the frustrating factors in the management of monocular congenital cataracts.

Strabismus was noted preoperatively in 50% (22 of 44) of the children, but in 7 of these the strabismus was not observed after surgery. However, new strabismus was noted in 5 patients after cataract surgery, giving a postoperative overall incidence of 45% (20 of 44). Strabismus is a frequent accompaniment of congenital monocular cataract. We found strabismus in 50% of our patients preoperatively, while it occurred in 45% of patients after cataract surgery. The incidence of strabismus reported by various investigators since 1980 reveals that strabismus was present in 33.3% of their patients preoperatively and in 78.1% postoperatively.[12,13,18-22] The higher incidence of strabismus after treatment than before may reflect the intensity of the occlusion prescribed, the ongoing susceptibility of the infantile eye to amblyopia owing to an uncorrected refractive error, or the easier detection of strabismus in older children. Preoperative strabismus was especially common among older patients at the time of surgery.

Early surgery (before 6 weeks of age) and compliance with patching are important factors for achieving a good visual outcome following monocular congenital cataract surgery. However, if compliance to patching is good during the first year of life, a good visual outcome can result.

Although "temporary patching failure" is likely between 18 and 30 months, we recommend continued patching as much as possible, with the resumption of more aggressive patching as the child ages beyond 30 months. Encourage the parents not to give up, especially if compliance with patching was present during the first year of the child's life.

There exists a 6-week window of time, beginning at birth, during which treatment of dense congenital cataracts is maximally effective.[15] If treatment is initiated during this period and the child is compliant with optical correction and occlusion therapy, frequently an excellent visual acuity outcome can be obtained. In addition, frequently better contrast sensitivity and vernier acuity outcomes can also be obtained.[15]

In a nutshell, during the past 20 years, dense monocular infantile cataract has changed from a "hopeless" disease to a treatable, although frustrating, condition. And again, we concur with the view that "not all children treated aggressively will obtain that lofty goal of good visual acuity and binocular vision, but it is guaranteed that without aggressive treatment virtually all children with a visually significant cataract at birth will end up with a blind eye and strabismus,"[16] and we continue treating these eyes aggressively.

IS SIMULTANEOUS BILATERAL SURGERY FOR PEDIATRIC CATARACTS A REASONABLE OPTION?

Sequential cataract surgery, more popularly known as simultaneous bilateral cataract surgery (SBCS), remains controversial. Almost every discussion on SBCS either starts or ends with a comment on the disagreement surrounding its use.[23–35] There are obvious reasons for the historical reluctance regarding bilateral surgery. Can the benefits of SBCS justify the risk of simultaneous bilateral complications, in particular, endophthalmitis? The important question here is not "Can it be done?" but, more properly, "Should it be done?"

Surgical management of bilateral adult and pediatric cataracts has traditionally been performed during separate sessions separated by different intervals depending on the surgeon's preference, patient's/parent's preference, outcome of the first procedure, and patient's general health. Advantages and disadvantages of SBCS are summarized in Table 9-1. Before proceeding with simultaneous surgery one should consider the questions listed in Table 9-2. Once the decision is made to move forward with this option, techniques should be chosen throughout to minimize the associated risk (see Table 9-3).

Although SBCS remains controversial, some believe that there is a limited place for this approach in a selected group of patients, particularly those for whom general anesthesia poses more than average risks.[27] Several authors have proposed that this is a feasible approach in children undergoing cataract surgery.[27,36,37]

Fear of endophthalmitis occurring in both eyes, leading to blindness, is the most important factor deterring ophthalmologists from performing SBCS.[31,38] In 1978, BenEzra and Chirambo[39] reported a single case of simultaneous bilateral endophthalmitis after intracapsular surgery among 448 patients. It occurred in a patient who had bacteremia and dysentery. After intensive therapy both eyes still perceived hand movement only.[39] Uniocular endophthalmitis after bilateral surgery[32] has also been reported. Arshinoff et al.[24] noted, "We found no published reports of bilateral endophthalmitis after ECCE [extracapsular cataract extraction] or phacoemulsification. However, after we presented our bilateral results at a meeting, 1 audience member presented an anecdotal unpublished case of severe bilateral endophthalmitis after bilateral phacoemulsification."

▶ **TABLE 9-1 Simultaneous Bilateral Cataract Surgery**

Pros	Reduction in mortality and morbidity associated with risk of two sessions of general anesthesia
	Immediate improved visual acuity and early binocular vision
	Only one admission for surgery and fewer hospital visits
	Less surgical stress
Cons	Concern with the risk of bilateral postoperative complications, especially endophthalmitis
	Difficult to defend medicolegally, especially if serious complications arise
	Loss of ability to adjust surgical plans for second eye that are based on results from first eye surgery

▶ **TABLE 9-2 Questions That Need to Be Answered Before Proceeding with Simultaneous Bilateral Cataract Surgery**

- What is the risk of endophthalmitis?
- What do we achieve by doing simultaneous surgery?
- What are the risks of anesthesia, in particular, those of two anesthesias within a period of a few days or weeks, compared with lengthening the duration of one anesthesia?
- What are the chances that the patient will not come for follow-up?
- Do both eyes have a significant cataract?
- Has there been a careful checkup for evidence of conjunctivitis, nasolacrimal duct obstruction, or upper respiratory tract infection?
- Is there a history of intake of immunosuppressive agents?
- Have the parents or caregiver received appropriate information and have they provided informed consent?

▶ **TABLE 9-3** **Precautions for Simultaneous Bilateral Cataract Surgery**

- Consider treating the second eye as a separate case (scrub in between the surgeries, use a separate instrument set and separate intraocular medications) but recognize that doing so have not been proven to reduce the risk of bilateral endophthalmitis.
- Use of intraocular substances such as viscoelastic materials and BSS (balanced salt solution) made by different manufacturers, or from different batches if from the same manufacturer, for each of the two eyes is recommended.[24]
- Defer the second eye if any intraoperative complication occurs with the first eye.

In larger series of patients, Javitt et al.[40] and Menikoff and coauthors[41] found an increased risk of endophthalmitis when an anterior vitrectomy is performed. These data, however, were collected in adults with inadvertent rupture of the posterior capsule, leading to a longer surgery time and often other complications. Whether pediatric posterior capsulotomy and anterior vitrectomy increase the risk of endophthalmitis is not known.

The American Academy of Ophthalmology preferred practice pattern (AAO PPP) 2001 does not support routine SBCS, although in contrast to 1996, the more recent AAO PPP includes some indications for SBCS. This may reflect an attitude shift toward acceptance of the procedure. The 2001 AAO PPP for adult cataract surgery states,

> *Surgery should not be routinely performed in both eyes at the same time because of the potential for bilateral visual impairment and loss of the ability to adjust surgical plans for the second eye that are based on results from first eye surgery. However, there are occasional circumstances under which bilateral surgery may be indicated, but the potential benefits and risks to the patient should be critically considered.*[42]

The February 2001 Royal College of Ophthalmologists cataract surgery guidelines (www.rcophth.ac.uk/pdf/cataract.pdf) also include *relative indications* and *precautions* for bilateral cataract surgery. One of the relative indication is "when a general anesthesia (GA) is necessary to perform the cataract surgery safely and repeated GAs are contraindicated on general health grounds." The precautions listed are as follows:

> *The operation on each eye must be treated as a completely separate procedure. If complications occur with the first eye, careful consideration should be given before proceeding with surgery on the second eye. Instructions should be given on using separate drop bottles for each eye postoperatively and washing hands before instilling eyedrops into the second eye. Every effort should be made to reduce the*

possibility of serial infection by using instruments, fluids and intraocular lenses prepared in different batches.

They further note that the *"ophthalmologist should be prepared to justify a decision to perform bilateral cataract surgery."*

Zwaan[27] have reported their experience with simultaneous bilateral surgery for pediatric cataracts. Although the authors reported no complications in their series, they conclude that

> *data in the current literature on endophthalmitis after cataract surgery and on the risks of repetitive anesthesia are inadequate to weigh the risk of bilateral endophthalmitis against the reduced risk of one anesthetics versus two and the advantages of simultaneous early visual rehabilitation. Until such information becomes available, simultaneous removal of bilateral infantile cataracts should probably be reserved for selected cases where the anesthetic risk is higher than average.*

The systemic diseases associated with congenital/infantile cataracts in which anesthetic difficulties are higher than average are also described by Zwann et al.:[27] rubella syndrome (congenital heart defects), Lowe's syndrome (hypocalcemia, acidosis, renal failure), homocystinuria (thromboembolic episodes), Marfan's syndrome (cardiovascular and respiratory problems), prematurity (respiratory problems), and craniosynostoses (difficult intubation, increased intracranial pressure, associated heart defects, respiratory problems), among others. Mortality and morbidity statistics related to anesthesia are difficult to obtain. However, various literature has reported that the overall complication rate is much higher in infants (43/10,000) than in older children (5/10,000).[43]

SBCS is a reasonable option in the developing world setting and can help to manage the backlog of cataract blindness. In the developing world, the cautious approach of avoiding SBCS may not be practical. To avoid the risks and costs of a second anesthesia and to make maximal use of the vitrector tubing and cutter, SBCS on children should be given strong consideration.[44]

To summarize, this should be a joint decision among the anesthetist, the ophthalmic surgeon, and the parents. The concept of SBCS is still controversial. Although the number of surgeons who report performing this procedure has increased, most appear to oppose the concept except in exceptional circumstances. This technique should be reserved for confident, experienced surgeons who have studied their complication rates, and the accuracy of their biometry, and are certain that complications occur extremely rarely in their hands. Although theoretically we support the conservative approach and vote against SBCS in children, in real life we may apply this approach when anesthesia is contraindicated for medical reasons or the patient lives far away and a visit for surgery on the second eye would be difficult.

REFERENCES

1. Wilson ME Jr, Bartholomew LR, Trivedi RH. Pediatric cataract surgery and intraocular lens implantation: Practice preferences of the 2001 ASCRS and AAPOS memberships. *J Cataract Refract Surg* 2003;29:1811–1820.
2. Wood MG, Ogawa GS. The challenge of pediatric cataract surgery. *J AAPOS* 2000;4:323.
3. Astle WF, Gimbel HV, Levin AV. Who should perform pediatric cataract surgery? *Can J Ophthalmol* 1998;33:132–133.
4. Wilson ME. The challenge of pediatric cataract surgery. *J AAPOS* 2001;5:265–266.
5. Chandler PA. Surgery of congenital cataract. *Trans Am Acad Ophthalmol Otolaryngol* 1968;72:341–354.
6. Chandler PA. Surgery of congenital cataract. *Am J Ophthalmol* 1968;65:663–674.
7. Costenbader F, Albert D. Conservatism in the management of congenital cataract. *Arch Ophthalmol* 1957;58:426–430.
8. DeVoe AG. The management of congenital cataract. *Trans Pac Coast Otoophthalmol Soc Annu Meet* 1965;46:201–209.
9. Francois J. Late results of congenital cataract surgery. *Ophthalmology* 1979;86:1586–1598.
10. Taylor D. The Doyne Lecture. Congenital cataract: the history, the nature and the practice. *Eye* 1998;12:9–36.
11. Frey T, Friendly D, Wyatt D. Re-evaluation of monocular cataracts in children. *Am J Ophthalmol* 1973;76:381–388.
12. Beller R, Hoyt CS, Marg E, Odom JV. Good visual function after neonatal surgery for congenital monocular cataracts. *Am J Ophthalmol* 1981;91:559–565.
13. Wilson ME, Trivedi RH, Hoxie JP, Bartholomew LR. Treatment outcomes of congenital monocular cataracts: the effects of surgical timing and patching compliance. *J Pediatr Ophthalmol Strabismus* 2003;40:323–329.
14. Birch EE, Swanson WH, Stager DR, Woody M, Everett M. Outcome after very early treatment of dense congenital unilateral cataract. *Invest Ophthalmol Vis Sci* 1993;34:3687–3699.
15. Birch EE, Stager DR. The critical period for surgical treatment of dense congenital unilateral cataract. *Invest Ophthalmol Vis Sci* 1996;37:1532–1538.
16. Wright KW. Should we aggressively treat unilateral congenital cataracts? View 1. *Br J Ophthalmol* 2001;85:1120–1122.
17. Amaya L. Should we aggressively treat unilateral congenital cataracts? View 2. *Br J Ophthalmol* 2001;85:1122–1125.
18. Cheng KP, Hiles DA, Biglan AW, Pettapiece MC. Visual results after early surgical treatment of unilateral congenital cataracts. *Ophthalmology* 1991;98:903–910.
19. BenEzra D, Paez JH. Congenital cataract and intraocular lenses. *Am J Ophthalmol* 1983;96:311–314.
20. France TD, Frank JW. The association of strabismus and aphakia in children. *J Pediatr Ophthalmol Strabismus* 1984;21:223–226.
21. Pratt-Johnson JA, Tillson G. Unilateral congenital cataract: binocular status after treatment. *J Pediatr Ophthalmol Strabismus* 1989;26:72–75.
22. Awner S, Buckley EG, DeVaro JM, Seaber JH. Unilateral pseudophakia in children under 4 years. *J Pediatr Ophthalmol Strabismus* 1996;33:230–236.
23. Arshinoff S. Simultaneous bilateral cataract surgery. *J Cataract Refract Surg* 1998;24:1015–1016.
24. Arshinoff SA, Strube YN, Yagev R. Simultaneous bilateral cataract surgery. *J Cataract Refract Surg* 2003;29:1281–1291.
25. Sharma TK, Worstmann T. Simultaneous bilateral cataract extraction. *J Cataract Refract Surg* 2001;27:741–744.
26. Tyagi AK, McDonnell PJ. Visual impairment due to bilateral corneal endothelial failure following simultaneous bilateral cataract surgery. *Br J Ophthalmol* 1998;82:1341–1342.
27. Zwaan J. Simultaneous surgery for bilateral pediatric cataracts. *Ophthal Surg Lasers* 1996;27:15–20.
28. Kontkanen M, Kaipiainen S. Simultaneous bilateral cataract extraction: a positive view. *J Cataract Refract Surg* 2002;28:2060–2061.
29. Khokhar S, Pangtey MS, Soni A. Misgivings about simultaneous bilateral cataract extraction. *J Cataract Refract Surg* 2002;28:
30. Nachiketa N, Munshi V. Ethical issue in simultaneous bilateral cataract extractions [comment]. *J Cataract Refract Surg* 2002;28:3–4.
31. Kushner BT. Discussion (Simultaneous Surgery for Bilateral Congenital Cataracts). *J Pediatr Ophthalmol Strabismus* 1990;27:26–27.
32. Bayramlar H, Keskin UC. Unilateral endophthalmitis after simultaneous bilateral cataract surgery. *J Cataract Refract Surg* 2002;28:1502.
33. McDonnell PJ. Bilateral corneal decompensation after bilateral simultaneous cataract surgery. *J Cataract Refract Surg* 1999;25:1038.
34. Chang DF. Simultaneous bilateral cataract surgery. *Br J Ophthalmol* 2003;87:253–254.
35. Masket S. Consultation section: cataract surgical problems. *J Cataract Refract Surg* 1997;23:1437–1441.
36. Guo S, Nelson LB, Calhoun J, Levin A. Simultaneous surgery for bilateral congenital cataracts. *J Pediatr Ophthalmol Strabismus* 1990;27:23–25.
37. Yagasaki T, Sato M, Awaya S, Nakamura N. Changes in nystagmus after simultaneous surgery for bilateral congenital cataracts. *Jap J Ophthalmol* 1993;37:330–338.
38. Good WV, Hing S, Irvine AR, Hoyt CS, Taylor DS. Postoperative endophthalmitis in children following cataract surgery. *J Pediatr Ophthalmol Strabismus* 1990;27:283–285.
39. BenEzra D, Chirambo MC. Bilateral versus unilateral cataract extraction: advantages and complications. *Br J Ophthalmol* 1978;62:770–773.
40. Javitt JC, Vitale S, Canner JK, et al. National outcomes of cataract extraction. Endophthalmitis following inpatient surgery. *Arch Ophthalmol* 1085;109:1085–1089.
41. Menikoff JA, Speaker MG, Marmor M, Raskin EM. A case-control study of risk factors for postoperative endophthalmitis [comment]. *Ophthalmology* 1761;98:1761–1768.
42. AAO. *Preferred Practice Patterns: Cataract in the Adult Eye.* San Francisco: American Academy of Ophthalmology, 2001.
43. Tiret L, Nivoche Y, Hatton F, Desmonts JM, Vourc'h G. Complications related to anaesthesia in infants and children. A prospective survey of 40240 anaesthetics. *BJA Br J Anaesth* 1988;61:263–269.
44. Wilson ME, Pandey SK, Thakur J. Paediatric cataract blindness in the developing world: surgical techniques and intraocular lenses in the new millennium. *Br J Ophthalmol* 2003;87:14–19.

Anesthetic Management of the Pediatric Patient with Cataracts

Linda S. Dancy and Charles T. Wallace

Satisfactory anesthesia for the pediatric ophthalmic patient presents many special challenges. These include control of the intraocular pressure (IOP), awareness of the oculocardiac reflex, thorough knowledge of drug interactions, smooth anesthetic maintenance and emergence, and control or prevention of postoperative nausea and vomiting (PONV).

PERIOPERATIVE ROUTINE AND SELECTION OF ANESTHETIC AGENTS

Stringent fasting guidelines and separation from parents make the perioperative period an anxious time for small children. New directions for the optimal fasting time for children suggest that they may receive clear liquids 2 to 3 hr before surgery without increasing the risk of aspiration.[1] Adequate preoperative hydration decreases the incidence of intraoperative hypoglycemia and hypovolemia and PONV. These new guidelines have greatly increased patient and parent satisfaction. Parental separation and fears of pain and blindness after surgery can be effectively addressed with preoperative interview and appropriate anxiolysis. Many institutions routinely use premedication for young children (between 18 months and 5 years of age) before ophthalmic procedures. Midazolam, 0.5 mg/kg, as an oral premedicant combined with an acetaminophen elixir or ibuprofen elixir alleviates separation anxiety and eases the induction of general anesthesia.

Both inhalational and intravenous general anesthetic techniques have been used successfully for pediatric cataract surgery. However, with the exception of pediatric patients with a history or a family history of malignant hyperthermia, most general anesthesia in young children undergoing cataract surgery is done with an inhalational agent. Sevoflurane has widely replaced halothane as the induction agent of choice in children. It possesses a less offensive odor than other volatile agents, is less stimulating to the airway, and lacks the arrhythmogenic properties of halothane. General anesthesia may be maintained with sevoflurane, isoflurane, or desflurane in air and oxygen. Desflurane possesses an extremely low blood-gas coefficient that allows for a rapid induction of and emergence from general anesthesia. Desflurane has been associated with increased airway irritability when used for induction. However, it is widely used for maintenance of general anesthesia. Nitrous oxide, traditionally used with volatile anesthetics, may increase postoperative nausea and vomiting. The cause-and-effect relationship between nausea/vomiting and nitrous oxide remains controversial. However, in patients with a known high risk for perioperative emesis, such as ophthalmic procedures, a mixture of air/oxygen or oxygen can be used in place of nitrous oxide.

Propofol is the intravenous induction agent of choice for cataract surgery in older pediatric patients and those with preoperative intravenous access. Propofol is an isopropyl phenol that has a rapid onset and offset of action. It is used for the induction and maintenance of anesthesia or sedation. Intravenous injection of a therapeutic dose of propofol produces hypnosis rapidly with minimal excitation. Propofol is also believed to have antiemetic properties. It effectively produces hypnosis of short duration with minimal "hangover."

Ketamine hydrochloride, a dissociative anesthetic that can be used for the induction and maintenance of anesthesia, is occasionally utilized for pediatric patients undergoing short procedures, such as an examination under anesthesia. An intramuscular injection of 5 to 7 mg/kg will provide approximately 30 min of anesthesia. Additional doses at one half of the initial dose should be given intravenously. There is a prolongation of emergence with repeated doses. Some of the principal adverse reactions include tachycardia, hypertension, respiratory depression, apnea, laryngospasm, tonic–clonic movements, hypersalivation, nausea and vomiting, diplopia, nystagmus, and an elevation in IOP. For pediatric patients having only an examination under anesthesia, ketamine hydrochloride is a suitable agent, but one must remember that it causes an increase in IOP, which should be kept in mind when following patients with glaucoma.

During anesthesia, even in patients whose IOP is usually normal, an increase in pressure can produce permanent visual loss. If penetration of the globe occurs when the IOP is excessively high, blood vessel rupture with subsequent hemorrhage may transpire. The IOP becomes atmospheric when the eye cavity has been entered, and any sudden increase in pressure may lead to prolapse of the iris and lens and loss of vitreous. Therefore, proper control of IOP is critical during such delicate intraocular procedures as in pediatric cataract surgery.

In some developing world settings, where inhalation agents are not available, ketamine is used for pediatric cataract surgery. After ketamine induction, a peribulbar injection of lidocaine is usually given and combined with ocular massage before entering the eye.[2]

Bell's phenomenon can be seen at any time during anesthesia when the patient's depth of anesthesia has changed. It manifests as upward (or sometime downward) movement of the eye. It is usually a sign of being *light*, although the patient is not *awake*. This phenomenon can make exams under anesthesia, corneal measurements, and A and B scans difficult or impossible to perform. The anesthesia provider should be aware of this reaction and be prepared to "deepen" the anesthesia to facilitate these procedures.

OCULOCARDIAC REFLEX

The oculocardiac reflex is triggered by pressure on the globe and by traction on the extraocular muscles, the conjunctiva, or the orbital structures. The afferent limb is trigeminal and the efferent limb is vagal. Although the oculocardiac reflex is commonly associated with bradycardia, virtually any dysrhythmia, including ventricular tachycardia and asystole, may be seen.[3,4] Children have increased vagal tone and, therefore, are more apt to manifest this problem. If a dysrhythmia appears, the initial treatment is to ask the surgeon to cease the manipulation. At this point, the anesthesia provider should determine that the depth of anesthesia and ventilatory status are adequate. Commonly, the heart rate and rhythm return to baseline within 20 sec. Usually, the reflex fatigues with repeated manipulations, and if it does occur again, it is not as dramatic. If the reflex becomes a problem, atropine should be given intravenously.

PREVENTION AND TREATMENT OF POSTOPERATIVE PAIN

Excessive postoperative pain causes postoperative nausea, emotional distress, and delays in recovery room discharge. Narcotics are traditionally used for the prevention and treatment of pain. The additional nausea and vomiting associated with narcotic use are a problem. Narcotics can also excessively sedate patients, cause respiratory depression, and also delay discharge. There have been multiple studies demonstrating the successful treatment of perioperative pain in pediatric patients with nonopioid medications including acetaminophen, ibuprofen, and ketorolac.[5,6] Commonly prescribed doses of these drugs are 10 to 20 mg/kg acetaminophen orally, 10 mg/kg ibuprofen orally, and 0.5 mg/kg ketorolac intravenously. Oral preparations of acetaminophen or ibuprofen may be administered with midazolam (0.5 mg/kg) approximately 30 min before the surgical procedure as a preoperative medication. Ketorolac is a nonsteroidal anti-inflammatory drug that interferes with prostaglandin production by blocking the cyclooxygenase pathway. Ketorolac is effective within approximately 45 min when administered intravenously and has an analgesic half-life of approximately 6 hr.

ISSUES RELATED TO POSTOPERATIVE OPERATING ROOM TURNOVER

Multiple factors contribute to the efficiency of operating room turnover. Many people and departments are involved in the process. Ideally, the history, physical examination, and informed consent should be done before the patient's arrival at the hospital. If there is a preoperative clinic, the patient should also have the anesthesia workup done there, and any additional examination/investigations can be addressed there before the day of surgery. Paperwork not done ahead of time slows down an otherwise efficient process.

In the past, surgeons were asked to give the anesthesia provider a 10- to 15-min notice that surgery was ending, to begin the process of decreasing the depth of anesthesia. However, the newer anesthetic agents can be eliminated much more rapidly. A 10-min *notification* before the end of surgery is still desirable so that the anesthesia provider can perform other duties. This notification is now used to get the patient back to spontaneous respiration, discontinue the air warming unit, tally the amount of intravenous fluids, and administer any antiemetics not already given. This would also be the appropriate time frame in which to premedicate the next patient. If there are no anesthesia technicians working in the department, the anesthesia provider should prepare for the next patient by opening syringes, an endotracheal tube or laryngeal mask airway, and intravenous fluids. The other part of the turnover issue is housekeeping. By having enough housekeeping staff to expedite room cleaning, the operating room staff can quickly prepare the room for the next surgery.

The need for a rapid operating room turnaround time should never jeopardize patient safety. Patient safety is paramount. Sometimes a patient will require additional attention from the anesthesia provider in the recovery room/postoperative acute care unit following surgery. All patients should be stable, comfortable, and left with a competent RN to monitor their continuing emergence from the effects of general anesthesia.

PREVENTION AND TREATMENT OF POSTOPERATIVE NAUSEA AND VOMITING

The incidence of PONV over all patient populations is 10 to 20% and is influenced by many factors, including anesthetic technique, patient age, gender, surgical procedure, and underlying diseases.[7] Multiple factors increase the incidence of PONV in the ophthalmic patient, including an alteration in visual perception, anesthetic technique, and the oculocardiac reflex.[3] Commonly used drugs for the prevention and treatment of PONV include droperidol, metoclopramide, and ondansetron. Droperidol is a butyrophenone that possesses antiemetic activity as a result of its central antagonism of dopamine receptors in the chemoreceptor trigger zone.[8] Effective intravenous doses of droperidol range from 50 to 75 μg/kg. Potential side effects from the use of droperidol include sedation and delayed emergence from anesthesia, extrapyramidal side effects, restlessness, and anxiety.[9] Metoclopramide, a benzamide, acts as a central dopaminergic antagonist and acts peripherally to increase lower esophageal sphincter tone and gastric motility.[10] Conventional antiemetic doses range from 0.1 to 0.2 mg/kg. Potential side effects include sedation and extrapyramidal side effects. Ondansetron is a centrally acting serotonin antagonist at the 5-hydroxytryptamine$_3$ (5-HT$_3$) receptor. Effective intravenous doses are 0.15 mg/kg but not >4.0 mg/kg.[11,12] Its use is associated with minimal side effects and it lacks the sedative and extrapyramidal side effects of droperidol and metoclopramide.[13] Granisetron HCl is a 5-HT$_3$ antagonist recently approved by the U.S. Food and Drug Administration for use in surgery to prevent PONV. The dose ranges from 0.1 to

1 mg given intravenously over 30 sec at the end of the surgical procedure. It has little effect on blood pressure, heart rate, or heart rhythm, but its safety and efficacy in children <2 years of age have not been established.[14] Dolasetron mesylate is also a 5-HT$_3$ antagonist, with a dose range of 0.35 to 12.5 mg/kg given intravenously 15 min before the end of surgery. Its safety and efficacy in children <2 years of age have not been established.[15] As with all antiemetics, routine prophylaxis is not recommended for patients for whom there is little expectation that PONV will occur.[10,11,14,15]

To summarize, recent protocols and techniques and the use of newer agents will result in a dramatic improvement in patient and parent satisfaction. Effective use of antiemetics, careful anesthetic selection, and relaxed fasting guidelines will result in a very low incidence of both PONV and unanticipated hospital admissions.

REFERENCES

1. Cote CJ. NPO guidelines: children and adults. In: McGoldrick KE, ed. *Ambulatory Anesthesiology.* Baltimore: Williams & Wilkins, 1995: 20–32.
2. Pun MS, Thakur J, Poudyal G, et al. Ketamine anaesthesia for paediatric ophthalmology surgery. *Br J Ophthalmol* 2003;87(5):535–537.
3. Van den Berg AA, Lambourne A, Clyburn PR. The oculoemetic reflex: a rationalization of postophthalmic anaesthesia vomiting. *Anaesthesia* 1989;44:110–117.
4. Bosomworth PP, Ziegler CH. Oculocardiac reflex in eye muscle surgery. *Anesthesiology* 1958;19:7.
5. Gold BS, Kitz DS, Lecky JH, Neuhaus JM. Unanticipated admission to the hospital following ambulatory surgery. *JAMA* 1989;262:3008–3010.
6. McGoldrick KE, Mardirossian J. Ophthalmic surgery. In: McGoldrick KE, ed. *Ambulatory Anesthesiology—A Problem Oriented Approach.* Baltimore: Williams & Wilkins, 1995:507–535.
7. Rowley MP, Brown TCK. Postoperative vomiting in children. *Anaesth Intensive Care* 1982;10:309–313.
8. Droperidol [package insert]. Abbott Park, IL: Abbott Laboratories, 2000.
9. FDA strengthens warnings for droperidol. Available at http://www.fda.gov/bbs/topics/ANSWERS/2001/ANS01123.html.
10. Metoclopramide HCL [package insert]. Madison, NJ: Whitehall–Robins Healthcare, 2003.
11. Ondansetron HCL [package insert]. Research Triangle Park, NC: GlaxoSmithKline Pharmaceuticals, 2003.
12. Watcha MF, Bras PJ, Cieslak GD, Pennant JH. The dose-response relationship of ondansetron in preventing postoperative emesis in pediatric patients undergoing ambulatory surgery. *Anesthesiology* 1995;82:47.
13. Polati E, Verlato G, Finco G, et al. Ondansetron versus metoclopramide in the treatment of postoperative nausea and vomiting. *Anesth Analg* 1997;85:395–399.
14. Granisetron HCl [package insert]. Nutley, NJ: Roche Laboratories, 2003.
15. Dolasetron [package insert]. Bridgewater, NJ: Aventis Pharmaceuticals, 2003.

Principles of Incision Construction in Pediatric Cataract Surgery

Rupal H. Trivedi and M. Edward Wilson, Jr.

In general, "incision construction" in pediatric cataract surgery follows the techniques and innovations developed for adult cataract surgery.[1] Tunnel incisions have replaced limbal incisions made with corneoscleral scissors in children, just as in adults. Foldable intraocular lenses (IOLs) have allowed tunnel incisions to become smaller. Placing an IOL through an incision <3 mm long using an injector device has become the norm. Pediatric surgeons have been less inclined, however, to follow the adult trend toward temporal, rather than superior, tunnel location. They also prefer to suture the tunnel incision, in contrast to the adult trend. This and other trends are discussed here.

The most immediate goal when planning the incision strategy is to aid intraoperative maneuvering. However, the ultimate goal is mainly to decrease astigmatism. This is especially important in children. Astigmatism may complicate the management of amblyopia. A recent report concluded that the outcome of amblyopia treatment is less favorable in patients with against-the-rule astigmatism.[2]

Advantages of small tunnel incisions include *less iris prolapse, better anterior chamber stability (less anterior chamber fluctuation), less postoperative astigmatism, less chance of damage from postoperative trauma, and less inflammation overall.*

Tunnel incisions constructed with an equal length and width (square incision) are self-sealing in adults.[3] These "square" tunnels are astigmatically neutral and allow better stability of the anterior chamber and no iris prolapse. However, low scleral and corneal rigidity in children promote leaking. Suture closure is usually needed, especially since children rub the eye after surgery more often than adults.

Before moving forward, it is important to remember the applied anatomy of the child's eye and how it is different from the adult eye in relation to the construction of the incision. The cornea in premature and full-term babies is thick and reaches adult levels within the first 2–4 years of life.[4] The sclera has a low rigidity and is not as thick. The anterior chamber is shallower in infant eyes compared to adult eyes. It is now generally agreed that there is a higher prevalence of against-the-rule astigmatism during infancy, which decreases with increasing age, while the prevalence of with-the-rule astigmatism increases.[2,5,6]

TUNNEL INCISION ARCHITECTURE

Location

Superior/Temporal/Meridian of Steepest Curvature

Most adult cataract surgeons have moved toward the temporal side as the "preferred location" for a cataract surgical incision. The temporal wound presents similar advantages in children as it does in adults. However, the superior approach allows the wound to be protected by the brow and Bell's phenomenon in the trauma-prone childhood years. Both scleral tunnels and corneal tunnels can be easily made from a superior approach since children rarely have deep-set orbits or overhanging brows. Our recent survey indicated that 63.6% of ASCRS and 84.3% of AAPOS members prefer the superior location for incisions in pediatric cataract surgery.[7]

Theoretically, an incision at the steepest meridian would help decrease surgically induced astigmatism.[8,9] However, in eyes with pediatric cataracts, it may be difficult to accurately document the steep corneal axis. Refraction by retinoscopy is difficult when a cataract is present. The reliability of handheld autokeratometers, while reasonably good for sphere measurement, may be dubious for the purpose of axis measurement.[10] Corneal topography requires cooperation and fixation. Also, pediatric eyes undergo changes in astigmatism with growth. Since it is likely that children will wear glasses after cataract surgery

▶ TABLE 11-1 Corneal Tunnel Incision

Pros

Avoids conjuctival peritomy and subsequent cauterization

Avoids occasional hyphema and conjuctival ballooning encountered with scleral tunnel

Ease of intraoperative maneuvering

Cosmetically better

Future filtration surgery—better outcome with untouched conjunctivae[11]

Indicated in eyes undergoing coagulant therapy and patients with insufficient platelet count

Decreased early postoperative breakdown in blood–aqueous barrier[18]

May reduce the risk of inadvertent conjuctival implantation of viable tumor cells and may allow for direct inspection of the incision site for tumor recurrence[19]

Cons

Higher rate of surgically induced astigmatism

Poor stability, especially if larger incision required

Increased risk of endophthalmitis[12,20]

Higher rate of endothelial cell loss[21]

Because an avascular structure, healing possibly delayed compared to that with a vascular scleral tunnel

Presence of radial keratotomy incision challenges the clear corneal incision if cataract surgery needed in an eye that underwent radial keratotomy

---

to correct for residual refractive error or at least for reading, less emphasis has been given in children to surgical maneuvers designed to treat preexisting astigmatism.

Scleral/Corneal

The pendulum has swung historically from a corneal to a scleral and back to a corneal location for the tunnel incision. Pros and cons of a corneal tunnel are listed in Table 11-1.

Eyes operated on for cataracts in children may be at increased risk for glaucoma (see Chapter 44). A scleral incision involving the conjunctiva increases the number of conjuctival fibroblasts and inflammatory cells. This may account for the increased risk of trabeculectomy failure.[11] Most adult cataract surgeons prefer a corneal tunnel as opposed to a scleral tunnel. However, our recent survey indicated that only 37.8% of ASCRS respondees and 26.9% of AAPOS respondees preferred a corneal tunnel when performing pediatric cataract surgery.[7] In addition, a recent article on adults found clear corneal incisions to be a statistically significant risk factor for acute post–cataract surgery endophthalmitis when compared to scleral tunnel incisions.[12] It is unclear whether the added risk of corneal tunnels in adults would be found if the study were conducted using children. Most of the adult corneal tunnels were left unsutured and pediatric corneal tunnels are usually sutured. The additional risk of endophthalmitis may

diminish or disappear when suture closure is added to the corneal incision location.

When inserting a foldable IOL, we generally prefer a corneal tunnel in older children and a scleral tunnel in infants. We have observed that infant corneal tissue opacifies easily at the sight of the tunnel and can appear unsightly after healing. Scleral tunnels are thus now preferred for use in infants. Other situations in which we use a scleral tunnel include the following. (1) When it is not possible to implant a foldable lens and a rigid one has to be used, the increased width of the incision—generally between 5 and 7 mm—favors a scleral location. (2) When we are not certain which IOL we are going to implant—foldable or polymethylmethacrylate (PMMA)—we prefer a scleral tunnel, as it is easy to enlarge if the need arises. This is mostly observed in eyes with traumatic cataract or when ciliary sulcus fixation is anticipated. (3) When a pars plana entry site will be used for the posterior capsulotomy and anterior vitrectomy, we often use a scleral tunnel even with a foldable IOL since the conjunctivae will need to be opened anyway to prepare the pars plana entry site.

Shape of the Incision: Straight/Frown/Circumlimbal

Straight or circumlimbal incisions are widely used in children. All of the listed shapes are acceptable and all have their proponents.

ARCHITECTURE OF A PARACENTESIS

Preparation of paracentesis incisions is very important in pediatric cataract surgery. If IOL implantation is not planned, the pediatric cataract can be aspirated through two paracentesis incisions. Paracentesis incisions are useful for

1. performing bimanual maneuvering (irrigation/cutting/aspiration);
2. injecting intraocular solutions and ophthalmic viscosurgical devices—without losing the chamber;
3. stabilizing the globe;
4. controlling the movements of instruments;
5. facilitating implantation of the lens; and
6. facilitating the use of iris retractors if needed.

TECHNIQUE

Diamond/Steel Knife

For years, steel blades have been considered the standard instrument in the construction of incisions. Diamond knives have several advantages over steel knives. However, several disadvantages of diamond knives have

▶ **TABLE 11-2 Pros and Cons of Diamond Knife Compared to Metal Knife**

Pros
Great cutting precision
Less pressure required while cutting
Less friction on tissue being cut
Cutting edge remains sharp after repeated use

Cons
Expensive
Extreme attention required for cleaning and repositioning by
  operating assistants
Lower tendency to forgive a surgeon's mistake

led many physicians to use disposable steel knives instead (Table 11-2).

The need for instruments with perfect cutting edges becomes more obvious when enlarging an incision (for IOL placement) in soft vitrectomized eyes.

Surgical Technique

Conjuctival Opening

For a scleral tunnel, a fornix base conjunctival flap measuring 6 to 7 mm is made with Westcott scissors and 0.3-mm forceps. Vertical relaxing incisions should be placed in the conjunctivae and Tenon's fascia, at both ends. The subtenon space is bluntly dissected with a scissors.

Cauterization

For scleral tunnel incision, after conjuctival peritomy is performed, cauterization must be done. Mild bipolar cautery (using an eraser tip) is performed near the limbus. Posteriorly, however, heavier cautery is used. The large vessels emanating from the rectus muscles and perforating the sclera between the muscle and the beginning of the tunnels are cauterized directly and adequately.[1]

Groove

The desired width (depends mainly on the type of IOL—rigid or flexible—and size of the optic) of the incision is marked (stamped at the tip with a marking pen) using a caliper: for a scleral tunnel, 1.5 mm from the insertion of the conjunctivae; and for a corneal tunnel—clear corneal, limbal, or sclerocorneal, depending on the preference of the surgeon—the globe is fixed with a forceps and the sclera/cornea is cut perpendicularly to make a groove.

Dissection

Starting above the base of the groove and remaining at half of the scleral/corneal thickness with a bevel-up blade (crescent knife), the tunnel should be dissected. Right-to-left

lateral movement should be performed while progressing forward. Superficial incisions tend to be fragile and may tear during the surgery. If the dissection is too deep, the anterior chamber may be entered prematurely. As the limbus is crossed, the plane of the dissection is slightly anterior so that the appropriate corneal plane is maintained. If the scleral dissection plane is maintained across the limbus, the anterior chamber will be entered or the internal corneal lip will be thin.

Anterior Chamber Entry

Anterior chamber entry is made at an angle of 45 degrees with a "dimple-down" maneuver. After entering the anterior chamber the direction of the knife should be changed and moved to the iris plane to avoid injuring the iris or the capsule.

Paracentesis

Paracentesis is performed in front of the limbal vascular arcade, about 70° to the left of the primary incision (for the right-handed surgeon, and vice versa). Two paracentesis incisions are sometimes made at the 2 o'clock and the 10 o'clock positions to help assist bimanual maneuvering. As the corneal tissue is entered, it may prove useful to exert light counter-pressure on the opposite side with forceps. The paracentesis should measure approximately 1 mm and run parallel to the iris plane, to facilitate sealing at the end of surgery. For instance, a micro vitreoretinal blade with a 20-gauge (0.9-mm) opening that provides a precise incision for insertion of a 0.9 mm (20-gauge) cannula is ideal for a 20-gauge vitrector/aspirator to enter the anterior chamber. A 20-gauge, blunt-tipped irrigating cannula can also be used through a separate micro vitreoretinal blade stab incision. If the instrument positions need to be reversed, the snug fit is maintained. We generally use a 20-gauge (0.9-mm) micro vitreoretinal blade, which gives a tight incision for the 20-gauge cannula that we are using for irrigation/aspiration/cutter. A second sideport incision, as described above, is used, particularly when aspiration of the cortical material is performed with two separate handpieces. Although these incisions are referred to as "stab" incisions, they take on a tunnel shape. If a tunnel is not formed, leakage is immediate when the instruments are removed, even in older children. However, if the tunnel is too long, the instruments cannot be maneuvered in the anterior chamber well because of "oar locking."

Enlargement of the Incision (Internal Entry) for IOL Implantation

The internal entry needs to be enlarged for smooth maneuvering in IOL implantation. The size of the internal entry selected depends on the type of IOL.

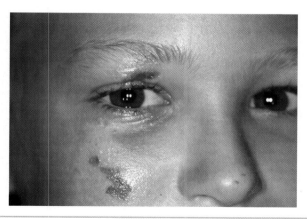

FIGURE 11-1. Ocular trauma in an eye 1 week postoperatively.

Suturing

Unlike in adults, tunnel incisions do not often self-seal in children. We feel it is important to suture the incision during the trauma-prone years of childhood (Fig. 11-1). Our recent survey indicated that only 19.8% of ASCRS respondees left both (tunnel and paracentesis) incisions unsutured. The figure for AAPOS respondees was 2.8%.[7] A higher dose of steroid drops is used for cataract surgery in children compared to adults. This may be another reason to suture the wounds since the steroids can theoretically postpone the healing. The elasticity of the pediatric eye wall tends to promote leakage from scleral tunnel incisions that would not leak in adults. It can be difficult to perform detailed examinations in the immediate postoperative period, making identification of a small leak, a slightly shallow anterior chamber, or a subnormal intraocular pressure difficult. For these reasons, the security of a well-sutured incision is preferred in children. According to the study by Basti et al.,[13] self-sealing wounds failed to remain watertight in children <11 years of age, especially when an anterior vitrectomy was combined with cataract extraction. Vitrectomy collapses the sclera, making the already relatively elastic sclera of children even less rigid. The authors attributed this to low scleral rigidity resulting in fish-mouthing of the wound, leading to poor approximation of the internal corneal valve to the overlying stroma. Brown et al.[14] have also recommended tight suturing in pediatric eyes.

Table 11-3 summarizes basic surgical principles for suturing the incision. We use 10/0 vicryl (polyglactic acid suture) absorbable suture (synthetic braided), which takes 60 to 90 days to completely absorb. Bourne et al.[15] reported that the in vivo half-life tensile strength of polyglactin is 2 weeks. Recently Ethicon received FDA clearance to market Vicryl Plus antibacterial suture, designed to reduce bacterial colonization on the suture.[16] Rothenburger et al.[17] have reported that coated polyglactin 910 suture with triclocan provides an antimicrobial effect sufficient to pre-

▶ TABLE 11-3 Basic General Surgical Principles to Keep in Mind While Performing Suturing

- Lower microscope magnification
- Equidistant needle entries from wound edge
- Uniform closure tension
- Placed at same depth
- Length of suture: must not be too far forward or too far back
- Suture must be applied with the globe as close to the physiologic volume as possible
- Knots should be embedded or at least tucked snuggly on the scleral side

vent in vitro colonization by *Staphylococcus aureus* and *S. epidermidis*. The agent is known to be effective against *S. aureus*, *S. epidermidis*, and methicillin-resistant strains of *Staphylococcus*.

We generally do not close conjunctiva with the sutures. However, after apposition of conjunctiva we do use subconjuctival injection of antibiotics and steroid injection and try to cover the incision site with the subconjunctival injection.

CONCLUSION

To summarize, adult cataract surgeons have developed wound construction techniques that require no or minimal suturing and induce little astigmatism in the immediate postoperative period. Although appealing, these techniques are not without added risk when applied to pediatric eyes, which are more elastic than adult eyes. A return to the operating room may be required to detect and treat a leaking wound. Surgeons desiring uncomplicated postoperative wound management may prefer to suture the wounds.

REFERENCES

1. Fine HI, Hoffman RS, Packer M. Incision construction. In: Steinert RF, ed. *Cataract Surgery: Technique, Complications, Management.* Philadelphia: Saunders, 2004.
2. Somer D, Budak K, Demirci S, Duman S. Against-the-rule (ATR) astigmatism as a predicting factor for the outcome of amblyopia treatment. *Am J Ophthalmol* 2002;133:741–745.
3. Ernest PH, Lavery KT, Kiessling LA. Relative strength of scleral corneal and clear corneal incisions constructed in cadaver eyes. *J Cataract Refract Surg* 1994;20:626–629.
4. Ehlers N, Sorensen T, Bramsen T, Poulsen EH. Central corneal thickness in newborns and children. *Acta Ophthalmol (Copenh)* 1976;54:285–290.
5. Dobson V, Miller JM, Harvey EM, Mohan KM. Amblyopia in astigmatic preschool children. *Vision Res* 2003;43:1081–1090.
6. Montes-Mico R. Astigmatism in infancy and childhood. *J Pediatr Ophthalmol Strabismus* 2000;37:349–353.
7. Wilson Jr ME, Bartholomew LR, Trivedi RH. Pediatric cataract surgery and intraocular lens implantation: practice preferences of

the 2001 ASCRS and AAPOS memberships. *J Cataract Refract Surg* 2003;29:1811–1820.

8. Oshika T, Sugita G, Tanabe T, Tomidokoro A, Amano S. Regular and irregular astigmatism after superior versus temporal scleral incision cataract surgery. *Ophthalmology* 2000;107:2049–2053.

9. Matsumoto Y, Hara T, Chiba K, Chikuda M. Optimal incision sites to obtain an astigmatism-free cornea after cataract surgery with a 3.2 mm sutureless incision. *J Cataract Refract Surg* 2001;27:1615–1619.

10. Noonan CP, Rao GP, Kaye SB, Green JR, Chandna A. Validation of a handheld automated keratometer in adults. *J Cataract Refract Surg* 1998;24:411–414.

11. Broadway DC, Grierson I, Hitchings RA. Local effects of previous conjunctival incisional surgery and the subsequent outcome of filtration surgery. *Am J Ophthalmol* 1998;125:805–818.

12. Cooper BA, Holekamp NM, Bohigian G, Thompson PA. Case-control study of endophthalmitis after cataract surgery comparing scleral tunnel and clear corneal wounds. *Am J Ophthalmol* 2003;136:300–305.

13. Basti S, Krishnamachary M, Gupta S. Results of sutureless wound construction in children undergoing cataract extraction. *J Pediatr Ophthalmol Strabismus* 1996;33:52–54.

14. Brown SM, Hodges MR, Corona J. Relaxation of postoperative astigmatism after lens implantation through a 6.25 mm scleral wound in children. *J Cataract Refract Surg* 2001;27:2012–2016.

15. Bourne RB, Bitar H, Andreae PR, Martin LM, Finlay JB, Marquis F. In-vivo comparison of four absorbable sutures: Vicryl, Dexon Plus, Maxon and PDS. *Can J Surg* 1988;31:43–45.

16. Ethicon receives FDA clearance to Market Vicryl Plus, first-ever antibacterial suture. Retrieved at www.infectioncontroltoday.com, 2002.

17. Rothenburger S, Spangler D, Bhende S, Burkley D. In vitro antimicrobial evaluation of Coated VICRYL* Plus Antibacterial Suture (coated polyglactin 910 with triclosan) using zone of inhibition assays. *Surg Infect (Larchmt)* 2002;3 (Suppl 1):S79–S87.

18. Dick HB, Schwenn O, Krummenauer F, Krist R, Pfeiffer N. Inflammation after sclerocorneal versus clear corneal tunnel phacoemulsification. *Ophthalmology* 2000;107:241–247.

19. Honavar SG, Shields CL, Shields JA, Demirci H, Naduvilath TJ. Intraocular surgery after treatment of retinoblastoma. *Arch Ophthalmol* 2001;119:1613–1621.

20. Nagaki Y, Hayasaka S, Kadoi C, Matsumoto M, Yanagisawa S, Watanabe K, et al. Bacterial endophthalmitis after small-incision cataract surgery. effect of incision placement and intraocular lens type. *J Cataract Refract Surg* 2003;29:20–26.

21. Beltrame G, Salvetat ML, Driussi G, Chizzolini M. Effect of incision size and site on corneal endothelial changes in cataract surgery. *J Cataract Refract Surg* 2002;28:118–125.

Ophthalmic Viscosurgical Devices

Rupal H. Trivedi and M. Edward Wilson, Jr.

The aim of surgery using *viscoelastic agents,* or *visco-surgery,* is to provide greater protection to intraocular tissue from mechanical damage, while increasing the space available for surgical manipulation. The use of viscoelastic substances has become an integral part of ophthalmic surgery, particularly anterior segment surgery. Although the term *viscoelastics* has made its way into the ophthalmic lexicon, surgeons have recognized that *viscoelastic* is an imprecise term that refers to the substances, since viscous products are not always elastic. Recently, the term *ophthalmic viscosurgical devices* (OVDs) was introduced.[1] OVD more clearly implies the intended surgical role of these substances, viscosurgery. A variety of OVDs is now available, each possessing specific chemical and physical properties and leading to different intraoperative behaviors. Only with a better understanding of this advancing area of technology can pediatric cataract surgeons optimize the use of these agents to improve outcomes.

Using high-viscosity cohesive agents seems to us a *necessity rather than a choice* during pediatric cataract surgery. However, to our surprise, fewer than 20% of physicians surveyed worldwide reported using this type of OVD during pediatric cataract surgery.[2]

Since an understanding of the basic properties of OVDs is essential for understanding their use, our initial emphasis here is on the physical and chemical properties of various OVDs and the available materials used in the manufacture of these agents. Next, we address the anatomical challenges posed by childhood cataracts and how OVDs help to overcome some of them. Finally, we specifically address the indispensable role that OVDs play in special situations during pediatric cataract surgery.

A GLOSSARY OF OVD TERMS AND PROPERTIES

Rheology is the study of the relationship between the deformation of physical bodies and the forces generated within them. The major physical properties of OVDs that affect their rheological function are viscosity, elasticity, pseudoplasticity, surface tension, and cohesiveness.[3–5]

Viscosity can be defined as the internal friction caused by molecular attraction that leads to a solution's resistance to flow. Viscosity denotes the protective and lubricating property of the material. Increasing either the concentration or the molecular weight of a solution can increase the viscosity and make the material more resistant to flow. Viscosity depends on the degree of molecular movement within a solution (also known as the *shear rate*) and it varies inversely with temperature. This is the reason why it is essential to state the temperature at which viscosity is being measured. Fluids that have the same viscosity at low shear rates and at high shear rates (i.e., when the viscosity is independent of shear rates) are referred to as *Newtonian fluids*. Chondroitin sulfate is such an example. Fluids exhibiting a decrease in viscosity at high shear rates are referred to as *non-Newtonian fluids*. Sodium hyaluronate (Na–Ha) is one such example.

Very low shear rates are present when the ocular structures are stationary and an OVD is simply expanding space during the surgical procedure. Zero-shear viscosity correlates with the molecular weight of a rheologically active OVD and can be used to rank and classify these agents. *High viscosity at low shear rates* maintains space and protects intraocular tissues.

Medium shear rates correspond to the velocities at which the surgeon moves objects through the eye, such as during an intraocular lens (IOL) implantation. *Moderate viscosity at medium shear rates* allows movement of surgical instruments, thus assisting IOL implantation.

Very high shear rates are operative when an OVD is being injected through a cannula. *Low viscosity at high shear rates* allows for easy introduction into the eye through a small cannula. Although the zero-shear viscosity of viscoelastic substances is a composite function of the concentration, molecular weight, and size of the flexible random coils, at high shear rates the viscosity is lowered. At high shear rates, the viscosity is related mostly to concentration and rarely depends on the molecular weight.

Elasticity is the tendency of a material to return to its original size and shape after having been deformed (i.e., stretched or compressed). Long-chain molecules such as Na–Ha tend to be more elastic than short-chain molecules.

Plasticity can be defined as the initial resistance to flow. The resistance decreases once a fluid begins to move. The more plastic a substance, the less force is required to initiate this movement.

Pseudoplasticity refers to a solution's ability to transform when under pressure from a gel-like state to a more liquid state.

Cohesiveness is the degree to which a material adheres to itself. It is a function of molecular weight and elasticity. Long-stranded OVDs with a high molecular weight become entangled and tend to remain as a single mass. *Superviscous cohesive* OVDs have zero-shear viscosities exceeding 1,000,000 mPs (milli–pascal seconds), while *viscous cohesive* agents have zero-shear viscosities between 100,000 and 1,000,000 mPs.

Dispersiveness is the tendency of a material to disperse when it is injected into the anterior chamber (AC). *Dispersive* agents commonly have low molecular weights and shorter molecular chains. In agents that have lower zero-shear viscosities, molecular chain entanglements become far less important and cohesion tends to be significantly weaker, resulting in a tendency to disperse when injected into the AC. *Medium-viscosity dispersive* OVDs possess zero-shear viscosities between 10,000 and 100,000 mPs. *Very-low-viscosity dispersive* agents include all of the unmodified hydroxypropylmethylcellulose (HPMC) agents.

Coatability refers to the ability of an OVD to adhere to the surface of tissues, instruments, and implants. A lower surface tension and a lower contact angle indicate a better ability to coat. In addition, the molecular charge of the viscoelastic substance may influence its coating ability.

AVAILABLE MATERIALS

Table 12-1 lists OVDs classified as high-viscosity cohesive and low-viscosity dispersive agents.

Balanced salt solutions and **air,** while not technically viscosurgical materials, were the first substances used as protective agents. Both are readily lost once the cornea is retracted or during difficult surgical manipulations in the AC.

HPMC is synthesized from methylcellulose as a raw wood pulp product of medical grade. Methylcellulose, in a 1% solution, was used to coat IOLs prior to implantation and later 2% methylcellulose was used to maintain the AC.[6] HPMC (2%) consists of a long chain of glucose molecules with replacement of the hydroxy groups by methoxypropyl and hydroxypropyl side chains. This

▶ **TABLE 12-1 Ophthalmic Viscosurgical Devices (OVDs)**

Viscosurgical Agent	Manufacturer	Viscosity (%)
Higher-Viscosity Cohesive OVDs		
Fracturable		
I-Visc Phaco	I-Med Pharma	2.5 Na–Ha
Microvisc Phaco	Bohus Biotech	2.5 Na–Ha
Healon-5	Advanced Medical Optics (AMO)	2.3 Na–Ha
Superviscous		
Oculocrom	Croma Pharama	2.0 Na–Ha
I-Visc Plus	I-Med Pharma	1.4 Na–Ha
MicroVisc-Plus	Bohus Biotech	1.4 Na–Ha
Healon-GV	AMO	1.4 Na–Ha
Viscous OVDs		
I-Visc	I-Med Pharma	1.0 Na–Ha
MicroVisc	Bohus Biotech	1.0 Na–Ha
Healon	AMO	1.0 Na–Ha
Provics	Alcon Laboratories	1.0 Na–Ha
BioLon	Bio-technology General Corp.	1.0 Na–Ha
Amvisc Plus	IOLAB (B & L Surgical)	1.6 Na–Ha
Amvisc	IOLAB (B & L Surgical)	1.2 Na–Ha
Viscornéal Plus	Corneal	1.4 Na–Ha
Viscornéal	Corneal	1.0 Na–Ha
Ophthalin	Ciba	1.0 Na–Ha
Ophthalin-Plus	Ciba	1.5 Na–Ha
Lower-Viscosity Dispersive OVDs		
Medium viscosity		
Viscoat	Alcon Laboratories	3.0 Na–Ha 4.0 CDS
Vitrax	Allergan Inc.	3.0 Na–Ha
Cellugel	Vision Biology (Alcon)	2.0 chemically modified HPMC
Low viscosity		
OcuCoat	Storz (B & L Surgical)	2.0 HPMC
Ocuvis	CIMA Technology	2.0 HPMC
Visilon	Shah & Shah	2.0 HPMC
Viscomet	Milmet Ophth Laboratories	2.0 HPMC
I-Cel	I-Med Pharma	2.0 HPMC
Visicrom	Croma Pharma	2.0 HPMC
Celoftal	Alcon Laboratories	2.0 HPMC
Combined package OVDs		
Duovisc (Viscoat and Provisc)	Alcon Laboratories	3.0 Na–Ha, 4.0 CDS and 1.0 Na–Ha
Duo Plus (I-Visc-Plus and I-Cel)	I-Med Pharma	1.4 Na–Ha and 2.0 HPMC

Na–Ha, sodium hyaluronate; CDS, chondroitin sulfate; HPMC, hydroxypropylmethylcellulose.

polymeric backbone is cellulose, a carbohydrate that is not a natural component of animals or humans, and so its fate in the eye remains unknown. The physical properties of HPMC require that a large-bore cannula with increased infusion pressure be used for injection. It is relatively difficult to completely remove HPMC from the eye. The primary advantages of HPMC are its ability to coat, availability, ease of preparation, room-temperature storage, ability to withstand autoclaving, and low cost compared with other OVDs.[3] Its safety and efficacy in intraocular surgery have been reported.[6,7] Cellugel, OcuCoat, Viscomet, Visilon, and I-Cell are some of the commercially available HPMC OVDs.

Sodium hyaluronate (Na–Ha), a viscous substance, was used in animal implant experiments as early as 1977[8] and in human implant experiments beginning in 1979.[9] It is a naturally occurring lubricant and shock absorber present in nearly all vertebrate connective tissue matrices. In the eye, Na–Ha is found at high concentrations in the vitreous and connective tissue of the trabecular angle and at low concentrations in the aqueous humor and covering the corneal endothelium.[10] Importantly, the use of this product in surgical situations does not represent the introduction of a "foreign" material. All Na–Ha products require refrigeration, with subsequent acclimation to room temperature prior to use. The prime advantages of Na–Ha products are its creation and maintenance of space in the AC, its ease of insertion and removal, and the fact that it is a natural product of the eye. The disadvantages are its poor coating ability, its removal as a mass during high-turbulence situations, and the necessity to refrigerate it. Manufacturers emphasize the importance of the product's purity, with various proprietary methods used to ensure this quality. It has been extracted from a variety of sources, including the dermis of rooster combs, umbilical cords, and cultures of streptococci.[3] Although highly purified Na–Ha from each of these sources has the same structure, the molecular weight can vary. Healon, Healon-GV, Healon-5, Amvisc, Amvisc-plus, and Biolon are some of the available Na–Ha products (Table 12-1).

Chondroitin sulfate at low concentrations is useful for coating tissue but poor for maintaining space because of its low viscosity. Increasing its concentration to 50% improves the viscosity but causes endothelial dehydration and cell damage. Viscoat is a 1:3 mixture of 4% chondroitin sulfate and 3% Na–Ha. The Na–Ha in Viscoat is produced by bacterial fermentation through genetic engineering techniques, and the chondroitin sulfate is obtained from shark fin cartilage. The combination of two biological polymers creates a unique chemical structure with a relatively high viscosity and perhaps increases its coating ability and cell protection, because of the additional presence of a negative charge. Viscoat requires refrigeration, with subsequent acclimation to room temperature prior to use. Ocugel is a combination of chondroitin sulfate and HPMC.

Polyacrylamide[11,12] and **collagen**[13] are also described in the literature as other available OVDs.

HIGH-VISCOSITY COHESIVE VISCOELASTIC AGENTS

Cohesive viscoelastic agents with high zero-shear viscosities are better for creating space compared to dispersive OVDs. This is especially important when expanding a shallow AC in an infantile eye. They are also useful when it is desirable to pressurize the AC to a level equal to the posterior pressure. This pressure equalization during cataract surgery is especially helpful for capsulorhexis, because it flattens the lens capsule. Cohesive OVDs can also be used to enlarge a small pupil, to dissect adhesions, and to aid IOL implantation. The high cohesiveness of viscous and superviscous material results in easy removal at the end of the surgical procedure. However, because of this same cohesive behavior, these agents also rapidly leave the AC during surgery.

Some surgeons find that the extremely high zero-shear viscosity of superviscous cohesive materials make them initially somewhat difficult to work with. When using these agents, surgeons must be more precise in their movements, as things moved into the wrong place tend to stay there (e.g., folds of the capsular flap when creating a capsulorhexis). However, with practice, the benefits of these materials quickly become apparent to the surgeon, and many have come to prefer them as their primary viscoelastic agents in pediatric cataract surgery, unless a dispersive material is surgically indicated.

LOWER-VISCOSITY DISPERSIVE VISCOELASTIC AGENTS

The most useful properties of dispersive OVDs are their resistance to aspiration and their ability to partition spaces. Their dispersive nature, a negative electrical charge and the presence of hyaluronic acid that can bind to specific binding sites on the corneal endothelium, improves the retention of these agents within the AC throughout the surgery. Thus, these agents are capable of partitioning the AC into an OVD-occupied space and a surgical zone in which irrigation/aspiration can be continued, without the two areas mixing. This is referred to as surgical *compartmentalization*. Therefore, their use is even more beneficial in eyes in which a compromised endothelium is suspected. Dispersive OVDs can also selectively move or isolate a single intraocular structure within the AC (e.g., holding back vitreous at an area of zonule disinsertion or at a small hole in the posterior capsule).

As we know, prevention of posterior capsule opacification remains an important goal in cataract surgery, especially pediatric cataract surgery. Posterior capsule opacification is caused mainly by the proliferation of lens epithelial cells. Recently, Budo et al.[14] investigated the morphological effects of Viscoat on lens epithelial cells. They conclude that

> light microscopy and transmission electron microscopy of human lens capsule suggest that Viscoat induces significant morphological changes in LECs [lens epithelial cells] during cataract surgery. The changes may underlie the improved visualization of these cells that has been reported during cataract surgery. Studies in a rabbit model suggest that the hyperosmolarity of Viscoat may play a partial role in the LEC changes.

The major drawback of lower-viscosity dispersive OVDs is their relatively low viscosity and elasticity, which do not allow them to maintain or stabilize spaces as well as higher-viscosity cohesive OVDs (e.g., in the performance of capsulorhexis or IOL implantation). They tend to be aspirated in small fragments during irrigation/aspiration, which leads to an irregular viscoelastic–aqueous interface that partially obscures the surgeon's view of the posterior capsule during surgery. The microbubbles that can form during surgery also tend to become trapped at this irregular interface, further obscuring visibility and making surgical maneuvers in the posterior chamber even more difficult. Because of low cohesion, lower-viscosity dispersive OVDs are more difficult to remove at the end of surgery.

As mentioned earlier, cohesive agents are best at creating and preserving space, while lower-viscosity dispersive agents are retained better in the AC and are capable of partitioning spaces. High zero-shear viscosity agents tend to leave the AC rapidly during the turbulent surgical outflow. Although zero-shear low-viscosity OVDs remain in the AC during surgery, they are not of use in pressure-equalized surgery, and they are more difficult to remove. The so-called *soft-shell technique* has been described in the literature; it maximizes the advantages and minimize the disadvantages of both cohesive and dispersive OVDs by using them together.[5] Healon-5 is a product attempting to combine the best of the cohesive and dispersive agents into a single agent.[15,16]

SOFT-SHELL TECHNIQUE

A lower-viscosity dispersive agent is first injected into the AC. Then a high-viscosity cohesive agent is injected into the posterior center of the dispersive agent. This combination of agents gives corneal endothelial cell protection throughout most of the lens removal, since the dispersive agent retains its attachment to the cornea even at higher turbulence.[5]

After the lens substance has been removed, these same two OVDs are injected, but in a reversed manner. That is, the high-viscosity cohesive agent is injected first, and then the lower-viscosity dispersive agent is injected into the center of the cohesive agent. This allows free movement of the incoming IOL through the dispersive agent, with better stabilization of the surrounding iris and capsular bag by the higher-viscosity cohesive agent. Removal of OVDs at the end of surgery can be easily accomplished, since the lower-viscosity dispersive OVD (more difficult to remove) can be aspirated from the central anterior segment first, followed by the easier-to-remove high-viscosity cohesive agent.

VISCOADAPTIVE AGENTS

Healon-5 is the first OVD to be referred to as *viscoadaptive*, denoting its adaptability to the surgical environment. This adaptability was accomplished by modifying the Na–Ha molecule to a log unit higher viscosity than most viscous products available to date. Theoretically, such a cohesive substance will become dispersive by fracturing under turbulent energetic conditions while, at the same time, remaining as a shield to protect the corneal endothelium. This ability to alter its viscosity during various manipulations is an important property of viscoadaptive agents. Healon-5 has a molecular weight of 4 million daltons, which is similar to that of Healon. However, the concentration of Na–Ha in Healon-5 is 23 mg/mL, compared to 14 mg/mL in Healon-GV and 12 mg/mL in Healon. Healon-5 has a higher viscosity at the zero-shear rate than any currently available OVD. In the midshear range (e.g., when being manipulated with instruments), it behaves very similarly to Healon-GV. At high shear rates (e.g., during injection), it flows very easily through a 25- to 27-gauge cannula, thus allowing surgeons to use their fingertips to sense the inflation pressure in the eye, rather than the resistance in the cannula.

The rheological features of Healon-5 are both cohesive and dispersive. At low shear rates it has the properties of a cohesive viscoelastic, while at high shear rates, because it can be fractured, it acts like a dispersive agent. Thus, the agent can adapt to different surgical needs and turbulence. The adaptive character of Healon-5 may be the result of its molecular structure. At low turbulence, long molecular chains become entangled and maintain space (as cohesive OVDs do). Thus, Healon-5 stays in the AC during capsulorhexis (a nonturbulent situation). During lens substance removal, and the accompanying increase in turbulence at that time, the agent fractures into smaller pieces and starts behaving as a dispersive OVD. During lens substance removal, Healon-5 partially remains in the AC, whereas a cohesive OVD such as Healon-GV has a tendency to leave the eye immediately. The cohesive qualities of Healon-5 allow expansion of the operating space and protection of the intraocular tissue, yet its dispersive qualities allow surgeons to easily remove the product upon completion of the procedure. During IOL implantation Healon-5 minimizes the problems that can be caused by positive vitreous pressure. It is easy to inject, like a cohesive agent, and it remains in the AC during surgery, like a dispersive agent. It flattens the anterior lens capsule (ALC) for controlled tearing, and it reduces the risk of peripheral extension. However, like any other new aid, it has its own learning curve.

APPLIED ANATOMY—USING OVDs IN PEDIATRIC SURGERY

With this understanding of the physiochemical characteristics of OVDs in mind, a discussion of how children's eyes differ anatomically from adult eyes, and the role of specific OVDs at different stages of pediatric cataract surgery, follows.

As we know, pediatric cataract surgery is performed by pediatric ophthalmologists as well as by adult cataract surgeons.[17] Pediatric ophthalmologists are often more familiar with the anatomical challenges encountered in small eyes, while adult cataract surgeons may be more familiar with the challenges posed by IOL implantation. However, it is important for both physicians to understand the following differences between the pediatric eye and the adult eye as they relate to surgery within the anterior segment.

Small Pupil

In the newborn or infant, the pupils are miotic and remain that way through the first year of life. The pupil also dilates poorly in infantile eyes. At birth, the dilator muscle is poorly developed, which explains the difficulty in obtaining good mydriasis with sympathomimetic agents.[18] Superviscous and viscous cohesive OVDs can help to dilate the pupil as an adjunct to mydriatic agents.

Corneal Endothelium

An obligatory level of endothelial cell loss occurs during growth and with aging.[19] In addition, operated eyes continue to lose endothelial cells at a higher rate (2.5% per year) for several years after cataract surgery.[20] Since the eyes of a child will need to function for many more years after surgery compared to those of an adult, it is very important to protect the corneal endothelium in these small eyes. OVDs play an important role in this regard.

Shallow Anterior Chamber

The depth of the AC is at its minimum in the newborn eye. The anterior chamber depth shows a rapid increase early in life, reaching its final adult depth at between 8 and

12 years. However, the depth will decrease in the presence of advanced intumescent infantile or childhood cataracts. OVDs can deepen the AC in these small eyes, allowing safer surgical maneuvering within the anterior segment.

Anterior Lens Capsule

Clinically, it has become evident that the pediatric ALC is more elastic than that in adults, because more force is required to initiate tearing during surgery. Laboratory investigations have verified a markedly higher fracture toughness and extensibility in the pediatric ALC compared to that of elderly adults.[21] The ALC is thin in pediatric eyes, which also adds to the difficulty encountered during capsulorhexis. Capsulorhexis is made easier by using OVDs to fill the ALC and flatten the ALC surface. Vitreous upthrust from low scleral rigidity promotes a taut ALC surface. This taut surface encourages radial tearing and the so-called *run-away rhexis*.[22] OVDs can flatten the ALC surface and create a less taut surface for a more controlled capsulorhexis. We recommend high-viscosity viscoelastic at this stage for pediatric cataract surgery (Fig. 12-1). In general, we do not need any OVD prior to the vitrectorhexis technique. However, if the anterior chamber collapses (due to aqueous outflow, subsequent to entry in the anterior chamber), we use a high-viscosity OVD to maintain the anterior chamber depth.

Low Scleral Rigidity

Low scleral rigidity increases fluctuations of the AC during high surgical turbulence. Maintaining a tight fit when instruments enter the eye, as well as using OVDs,

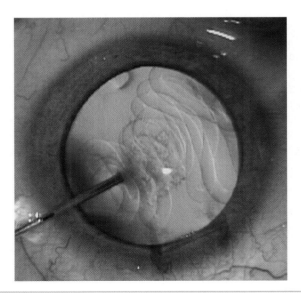

FIGURE 12-1. Injection of a high-viscosity viscoelastic before anterior capsulorhexis.

promotes AC stability and avoids collapse during surgical manipulation.

Posterior Capsule

Management of the posterior capsule is very important in children.[23] Integrity of the posterior capsule opening is essential in long-term stability of the IOL. OVDs can stabilize the posterior chamber and push back the vitreous face during posterior capsulorhexis.

Increased Intravitreal Pressure

Lifelong changes are also a characteristic of the vitreous. Although the vitreous probably has a very small liquid component at birth, the liquid fraction is measurable by the age of 3 years and increases steadily in volume thereafter, eventually making up just over half of the vitreous volume. As the liquid fraction increases, the collagens in the gel apparently aggregate. This solid vitreous, combined with the low scleral rigidity, increases the vitreous pressure and adds to the difficulties encountered during anterior capsulorhexis, posterior capsulorhexis, and also IOL implantation. OVDs allow surgeons to neutralize the posterior vitreous pressure during pediatric cataract surgery.

SPECIAL CONSIDERATIONS

Poor Corneal Visibility

Poor corneal visibility during surgery is more common in pediatric cataract surgery than its adult counterpart. Often in young children a complete examination under anesthesia, as well as keratometry and "A-scan" ultrasound, is performed before the surgery begins. Corneal drying and epithelial damage can occur during these examinations. Exposure keratopathy during the induction of general anesthesia may aggravate this situation. Visualization through the cornea may deteriorate further as the surgery progresses. Sometimes it is helpful to cover the cornea with dispersive lubricating OVDs. The lubricating effect of the OVD helps to improve clarity by maintaining corneal moisture throughout the surgery.

Hydrodissection

Hydrodissection is often performed in older children just prior to lens aspiration. Care should be taken not to inject too much of the highly viscous OVD before hydrodissection. The OVD will not evacuate from the AC during hydrodissection. The injected fluid, combined with an already overfilled AC, can markedly raise the intraocular pressure and increase the risk of posterior capsule rupture during hydrodissection.

Posterior Capsule Rupture with Vitreous Herniation

To avoid widening the posterior capsular opening, OVDs can be injected into the AC and the capsular bag as soon as a posterior capsule rupture is detected. Using low-flow aspiration, the remaining cortex can be carefully removed. A vitrectomy can be done under dry conditions beneath the OVD, thus avoiding an uncontrolled extension of the posterior capsular tear.

Preexisting Posterior Capsule Defect

A preexisting posterior capsule defect may be present in children presenting with a white, complete cataract (see Chapter 34). This is seen most often with posterior lentiglobus or trauma. Care must be taken to avoid an uncontrolled extension of any posterior capsule defect at the end of the lens aspiration. The AC may collapse during the withdrawal of the aspiration probe, allowing the vitreous face to bulge forward, extending the posterior capsular defect. To prevent this, a high-viscosity OVD is injected through the paracentesis incision. The irrigation probe is pulled out only when the majority of the chamber is filled with viscoelastic. This aids in keeping the vitreous in the posterior segment and may prevent the defect from extending further. The surgeon may need to reenter the eye for further cortex removal or for vitrectomy. However, every time the ports are exchanged it is necessary to repeat the procedure described above to maintain the anterior chamber. With the help of OVDs, posterior capsule support can usually be maintained, thus facilitating an in-the-bag placement of the IOL.

Posterior Capsule Plaque

It is not uncommon to observe a plaque on the posterior capsule. If the opacity cannot be removed completely during lens aspiration, a posterior capsulorhexis will be needed. In older children, OVDs can assist in the performance of a manual posterior capsulorhexis to remove the plaque without disturbing the vitreous face. A cystitome is used to puncture the posterior capsule, peripheral to the plaque. A viscous OVD is injected slowly through the puncture to push the intact vitreous face posteriorly. Capsulorhexis forceps can then be used to complete a posterior capsulorhexis that incorporates the plaque and removes it completely. Although the OVD is removed from the anterior segment and from the capsular bag after IOL

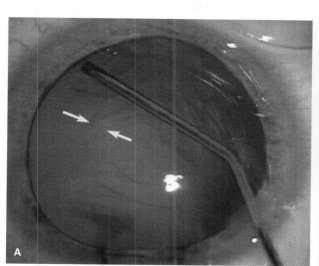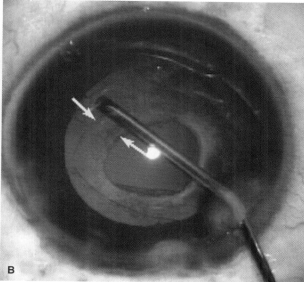

FIGURE 12-2. Injection of OVDs into the capsular fornices (between the anterior and the posterior capsules). **A.** Primary IOL implantation. **B.** Secondary IOL implantation.

insertion, OVD in the vitreous cavity can be left in place. If desired, the use of OVDs can thus help avoid a vitrectomy in older children, even when a posterior capsulorhexis is performed.

IOL Implantation

When using OVDs before IOL implantation, it is important to remember the site of fixation. *State-of-the-art* "in-the-bag" fixation requires injection of OVDs into the capsule fornices (between the anterior capsule and the posterior capsule) (Figs. 12-2A and B).

Congenital Subluxated Crystalline Lens

A lower-viscosity dispersive OVD can be placed over the area of the weakened zonules to tamponade the vitreous. A high-viscosity cohesive OVD can then be placed over the crystalline lens to help when performing the capsulorhexis. Low-flow aspiration of the lens contents can be accomplished with retention of the dispersive OVD placed over the exposed vitreous.

Uveitis

In eyes with uveitis, the surgeon often needs to deal with a miotic pupil associated with synechiae. OVDs can facilitate synechiolysis and add to dilation of the pupil (Fig. 12-3).

Secondary IOL Implantation

OVDs can assist with a more atraumatic lysis of posterior synechiae. Viscodissection, combined with gentle instrument dissection, can clear the ciliary sulcus in preparation for placement of an IOL, thus avoiding lens implant decentration that can result from incomplete synechiolysis. When attempting secondary IOL implantation in-the-bag,

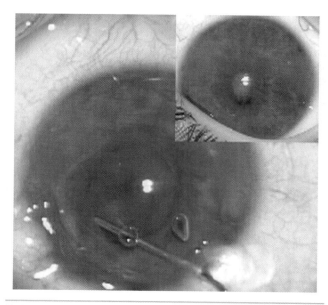

FIGURE 12-3. An eye with uveitis in a 7-year-old child with juvenile rheumatoid arthritis. *Inset:* Preoperative appearance.

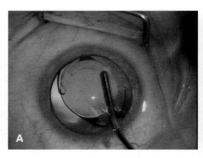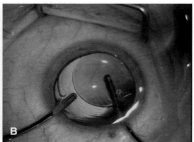

FIGURE 12-4. Removal of OVDs (**A** and **B**). Note that sometimes it is also necessary to go behind the IOL optic for thorough removal of OVDs (**B**).

again it is important to inject OVDs into the capsular fornices (between the anterior capsule and the posterior capsule) (Fig. 12-3B).

REMOVAL OF OVDs

As in adults, retained viscous OVDs can cause a marked postoperative intraocular pressure elevation after surgery for childhood cataracts. Englert and Wilson[24] have suggested the need for more meticulous removal of OVDs. Recent studies have verified that cohesive OVDs, while responsible for most intraocular pressure spikes, are easier to remove than dispersive OVDs. As discussed previously, most high-viscosity cohesive OVDs are made from Na–Ha. Na–Ha is not metabolized in the eye. It passes through the trabecular meshwork as a voluminous molecule, such that AC clearance depends mostly on the viscosity and the amount of OVD injected. In contrast, HPMC, found mostly in dispersive OVDs, may be partially metabolized prior to its exit from the eye.

Na–Ha stays in the vitreous much longer than in the aqueous, and its residence in the vitreous depends on the concentration, the viscosity, the volume, the presence of a lens capsule, and inflammation of the vitreous and on the thickness, density, and structural integrity of the cortical gel. The vitreous may not tolerate HPMC as well as it tolerates Na–Ha, however. With the former, white precipitates, vitreous bands, and inflammation have been reported in rabbit eyes.[25]

OVDs can be removed with irrigation/aspiration using a small bimanual handpiece or the vitrector handpiece. Although posterior capsular striae have been reported as a sign of complete removal of the OVD in adult eyes, striae may not appear in the young eye, even with an intact posterior capsule.[26,27] It is relatively easy to remove OVDs in an eye with an intact capsule (Figs. 12-4A and B). When planning to do posterior capsulectomy and anterior vitrectomy, from the *OVD removal* point of view, the pars plana approach (after OVD removal) is better. With the limbal approach it is sometimes difficult to achieve complete removal of OVDs (see Chapter 16).

RECOMMENDATIONS

We recommend using viscoadaptive agents or superviscous OVDs during pediatric cataract surgery to facilitate the difficult intraocular manipulations that must be performed. These cohesive OVDs help maintain space, promote AC stability, and offset somewhat the low scleral rigidity and increased vitreous upthrust found in pediatric eyes. Although superviscous and viscous cohesive OVDs are costly, which may prevent their use in developing countries, we recommend their use whenever possible.

In special situations (e.g., compromised corneal endothelium), it may be advantageous to use a lower-viscosity dispersive agent in combination with cohesive OVDs as discussed in more detail under "soft-shell technique." Also, during subluxated lens removal, it is advisable to use dispersive OVDs to place over the area of the weakened zonules to tamponade the vitreous. Recent advances in OVDs hold the promise of making surgical maneuvers easier within the small, often unstable AC of young children. More reports are emerging as surgeons gain experience with these new OVDs.[28]

ACKNOWLEDGMENTS

We acknowledge the help of Luanna Bartholomew, PhD, Liliana Werner, MD, PhD, and Suresh K. Pandey, MD.

REFERENCES

1. Arshinoff S. New terminology: ophthalmic viscosurgical devices. *J Cataract Refract Surg* 2000;26:627–628.
2. Wilson ME Jr, Bartholomew LR, Trivedi RH. Pediatric cataract surgery and intraocular lens implantation: practice preferences of the 2001 ASCRS and AAPOS memberships. *J Cataract Refract Surg* 2003;29:1811–1820.
3. Liesegang TJ. Viscoelastic substances in ophthalmology. *Surv Ophthalmol* 1990;34:268–293.
4. Arshinoff S. Dispersive and cohesive viscoelastic materials in phacoemulsification revisited 1998. *Ophthal Pract* 1998;16:24–32.
5. Arshinoff SA. Dispersive-cohesive viscoelastic soft shell technique. *J Cataract Refract Surg* 1999;25:167–173.
6. Fechner PU, Rimpler M. Comparison of hydroxypropyl methylcellulose 2% (Adatocel) and hyaluronic acid 1% (Healon). *J Cataract Refract Surg* 1989;15:685–688.

7. Mac Rae SM, Edelhauser HF, Hyndiuk RA, Burd EM, Schultz RO. The effects of sodium hyaluronate, chondroitin sulfate, and methylcellulose on the corneal endothelium and intraocular pressure. *Am J Ophthalmol* 1983;95:332–341.

8. Miller D, O'Connor P, Williams J. Use of Na-hyaluronate during intraocular lens implantation in rabbits. *Ophthal Surg* 1977;8:58–61.

9. Miller D, Stegmann R. Use of sodium hyaluronate in human IOL implantation. *Ann Ophthalmol* 1981;13:811–815.

10. Laurent UB, Granath KA. The molecular weight of hyaluronate in the aqueous humour and vitreous body of rabbit and cattle eyes. *Exp Eye Res* 1983;36:481–492.

11. Laflamme MY, Swieca R. A prospective comparison of 4% polyacrylamide (Orcolon) and 1% sodium hyaluronate (Healon) in cataract and intraocular lens implant surgery. *Can J Ophthalmol* 1990;25:229–233.

12. Mortimer C, Sutton H, Henderson C. Efficacy of polyacrylamide vs. sodium hyaluronate in cataract surgery. *Can J Ophthalmol* 1991;26:144–147.

13. Bleckmann H, Vogt R, Garus HJ. Collagel—A new viscoelastic substance for ophthalmic surgery. *J Cataract Refract Surg* 1992;18:20–26.

14. Budo C GG, Bellotto D, Petroll WM. Effect of ophthalmic viscosurgical devices on lens epithelial cells: a morphological study. *J Cataract Refract Surg* 2003;29:2411–2418.

15. Holzer MP, Tetz MR, Auffarth GU, Welt R, Volcker HE. Effect of Healon5 and 4 other viscoelastic substances on intraocular pressure and endothelium after cataract surgery. *J Cataract Refract Surg* 2001;27:213–218.

16. Tetz MR, Holzer MP, Lundberg K, Auffarth GU, Burk RO, Kruse FE. Clinical results of phacoemulsification with the use of Healon5 or Viscoat. *J Cataract Refract Surg* 2001;27:416–420.

17. Astle WF, Gimbel HV, Levin AV. Who should perform pediatric cataract surgery? *Can J Ophthalmol* 1998;33:132–133; discussion, 133–134.

18. Zinn KM. *The Pupil.* Springfield, IL: Charles C Thomas, 1972.

19. Yee RW, Matsuda M, Schultz RO, Edelhauser HF. Changes in the normal corneal endothelial cellular pattern as a function of age. *Curr Eye Res* 1985;4:671–678.

20. Bourne WM, Nelson LR, Hodge DO. Continued endothelial cell loss ten years after lens implantation. *Ophthalmology* 1994;101:1014–1022; discussion, 1022–1023.

21. Auffarth GU, Wesendahl TA, Newland TJ, Apple DJ. Capsulorhexis in the rabbit eye as a model for pediatric capsulectomy. *J Cataract Refract Surg* 1994;20:188–191.

22. Wilson ME. Anterior capsule management for pediatric intraocular lens implantation. *J Pediatr Ophthalmol Strabismus* 1999;36:314–319.

23. Parks MM. Posterior lens capsulectomy during primary cataract surgery in children. *Ophthalmology* 1983;90:344–345.

24. Englert JA, Wilson ME. Postoperative intraocular pressure elevation after the use of Healon GV in pediatric cataract surgery. *J AAPOS* 2000;4:60–61.

25. Koster R, Stilma JS. Comparison of vitreous replacement with Healon and with HPMC in rabbits' eyes. *Doc Ophthalmol* 1986;61:247–253.

26. Vasavada AR, Trivedi RH. Posterior capsule striae. *J Cataract Refract Surg* 1999;25:1527–1531.

27. Durak I, Oner FH. Clue to complete removal of OVD during phacoemulsification. *J Cataract Refract Surg* 2000;26:633–634.

28. Jeng BH, Hoyt CS, McLeod SD. Completion rate of continuous curvilinear capsulorhexis in pediatric cataract surgery using different viscoelastic materials. *J Cataract Refract Surg* 2004;30:85–88.

Anterior Capsule Management

M. Edward Wilson, Jr. and Suresh K. Pandey

An intact anterior capsulotomy supports all the subsequent steps of lens aspiration and introcular lens (IOL) implantation. Its shape, size, and edge integrity are also important for long-term centration of a capsular-bag fixated IOL. Anterior capsulotomy, specifically a continuous curvilinear capsulorhexis (CCC), is notoriously difficult in infants and young children because of the extreme elasticity of the anterior capsule, positive vitreous pressure, and at times, poor dilatation of the pupil.[1] The availability of better operating microscopes and microsurgical instruments combined with higher-viscosity ophthalmic viscosurgical devices (OVDs) is helpful, but the creation of an intact capsulorhexis in infants remains a challenge.[2–5] Experienced surgeons and researchers have tested various alternative techniques for pediatric anterior capsulotomy, clinically and using animal models. Several of these methods have been proposed for successful management of the anterior lens capsule during pediatric cataract surgery and IOL implantation.[6] In addition, specific modifications of the adult CCC technique have been proposed specifically for the elastic capsule of children.

PEDIATRIC ANTERIOR CAPSULOTOMY TECHNIQUES

Evolution

Table 13-1 reports the evolution of the anterior capsulotomy technique. The first anterior capsulotomy technique associated with an IOL implantation, performed by Sir Harold Ridley in the 1950s, was an uncontrolled tear using forceps without the aid of microscope magnification.[7] It served only as a means to gain access to the lens contents. Complete removal of the anterior capsule was desired. If remnants or tags were seen after nucleus expression, they were torn with smooth-bladed capsule forceps. This maneuver at times resulted in the entire posterior capsule's also being delivered from the eye, effecting an un-

planned intracapsular surgery. Within 10 years after its introduction, Ridley's extracapsular IOL implantation technique for adult cataract extraction and IOL implantation was replaced by intracapsular cataract extraction, with which capsulotomies were unnecessary and the IOL was placed in the anterior chamber.[8] During this time (in 1958) D. Peter Choyce implanted an anterior chamber IOL in a child following removal of a traumatic cataract.[9] Years later, the return to extracapsular cataract extraction and posterior chamber IOLs in adults again required the anterior capsule to be opened. To reduce the stress on the zonule and produce a more round capsulotomy with fewer tags, the multipuncture or "can-opener" capsulotomy came into common use. This technique has been ascribed to Pearce and, alternatively, to Little (cited in references 10 and 11). A capsulotomy was made by punching a bent-needle cystotome repeatedly through the anterior capsule in a postage stamp or can-opener fashion and connecting the punches to form a circular opening. A. Galand and G. Baikoff proposed a horizontal (envelope) anterior capsulotomy for adult cataract surgery.[12] The anterior capsule flap was first opened in a horizontal direction and the residual part was later removed after the IOL insertion.

Ironically, the first continuous circular anterior capsulotomy was formed for both the anterior and the posterior capsules in pediatric cataract surgery, beginning about 1976.[13] Although IOL placement would not become commonplace in children until much later, the pediatric cataract extraction technique had evolved into a mechanized small incision procedure at a time when cataract surgery in adults involved removal of the entire lens using a cryoprobe through a large limbal opening. Most of the pediatric cataract surgeon trainees beginning in the late 1970s were taught to perform a large, round, mechanized anterior capsulectomy followed by aspiration of the lens contents, a posterior capsulectomy identical in size to the anterior opening, and an anterior vitrectomy without removing the instruments from the eye. No viscoelastic substances were needed.

▶ TABLE 13-1 Evolution of Anterior Capsulotomy Techniques

Technique	Year	Author/Surgeon
Anterior capsulotomy & IOL	1949	Sir Harold Ridley
Can-opener capsulotomy	Unknown	Little and Pearce
Envelope (horizontal)	1979	Galand/Baikoff
CCC for adults	1992	Gimbel & Neuhann
Vitrectorhexis	1994	Wilson et al.
Push–pull CCC in rabbit model	1994	Auffarth et al.
Radiofrequency diathermy	1994	Kloti
Fugo plasma blade	1999	R. Fugo
Dye-enhanced CCC/ cataract surgery	2000	Pandey/Werner/Apple/ Wilson (lab. studies)

Many of the children left aphakic during those years have now presented for secondary IOL implantation as older children or young adults. Time and again, a round, intact, smooth anterior capsular edge has been noted, providing circumferential support for the secondary implant. Unfortunately, in an attempt to decrease inflammation and the incidence of synechiae between the capsule remnants and the iris, some pediatric surgeons advocated mechanized removal of as much of the equatorial capsular remnants as possible. This procedure eliminated posterior synechiae but left no support for a secondary implant. During the late 1980s and the early 1990s, nonimplanting pediatric surgeons nearly uniformly recognized the need for a capsular rim to support an IOL later. Mechanized, anterior capsular openings evolved to a size small enough to leave an adequate capsular ring to support a secondary IOL, yet large enough to prevent frequent closure of the opening by secondary membrane formation. At the time of secondary IOL implantation, the anterior capsular opening is characteristically round, smooth-edged, and fused to the posterior capsule.

SURGICAL TECHNIQUES

Manual CCC

Gimbel and Neuhann[14] advocated the continuous tear anterior capsulotomy or CCC technique for small-incision adult cataract surgery in the mid-1990s. During the same time, capsular bag fixation of a posterior chamber IOL placed at the time of cataract surgery became commonplace for children beyond age 2.[15] Because manual CCC had become the standard anterior capsulotomy technique in adults, it was naturally also applied to the pediatric age group, but with mixed success.

Clinically, it became evident that the pediatric lens capsule is more elastic than in adults and requires increased force before tearing begins. Laboratory investigations have now verified a markedly higher fracture toughness and extensibility in the pediatric anterior capsule compared to that of elderly adults.[16] In addition, reduced scleral rigidity results in posterior vitreous upthrust when the eye is entered. This vitreous "pressure" pushes the lens anteriorly and keeps the anterior lens capsule taut. Surgeons encountered more difficulty completing an intact circular capsulotomy. The so-called "runaway rhexis" became all too common. In addition, a capsulotomy that started out small would end up much larger than intended. This result was also due to the marked elasticity of the child's anterior capsule. Performing an intact CCC is challenging in young children even for an experienced surgeon as reported by Vasavada and Chauhan,[17] in a series of 21 eyes of 13 infants, in which the authors failed to create an intact CCC using manual techniques in as many as 80% of the cases.

Modified CCC Technique in a Rabbit Model

Auffarth and colleagues[16] developed a modified CCC technique for use in experiments on eyes of young albino rabbits. These animals have very elastic lens capsules reminiscent of the pediatric human lens capsule. The technique begins with a puncture of the lens capsule at the superior border of the intended capsulotomy using a 27-gauge needle. Capsulorhexis forceps are then used to grasp the anterior capsule centrally. The capsular flap is torn toward the 6 o'clock position until a half-circle is completed. The force is then reversed toward 12 o'clock, pulling with equal force to both tearing edges. This technique was used in an experimental study with 16 rabbits (32 eyes). The authors reported radial tears in only 2 of 32 eyes. Although this technique has become the standard for rabbit capsulotomies in studies performed at the Storm Eye Institute and elsewhere, it has not been adequately studied in human clinical cases.

Small Peripheral Anterior CCC in a Rabbit Model

Researchers at Bascom Palmer Eye Institute recently described a manual surgical technique for performing a small (<1.5-mm-diameter) anterior CCC.[18] This technique's applications extend from Phaco-Ersatz, a cataract surgical technique designed to restore accommodation. The researchers conducted an experimental rabbit study to determine the feasibility of the technique. A 30-gauge needle and Utrata capsulorhexis forceps were used to construct the CCC. The authors were able to make up to nine small peripheral anterior CCCs in the same lens capsule without the capsule tearing. The mean diameter of the CCCs was 1.1 ± 0.3 mm (SD). This technique, according to the researchers, shows promise for the successful performance

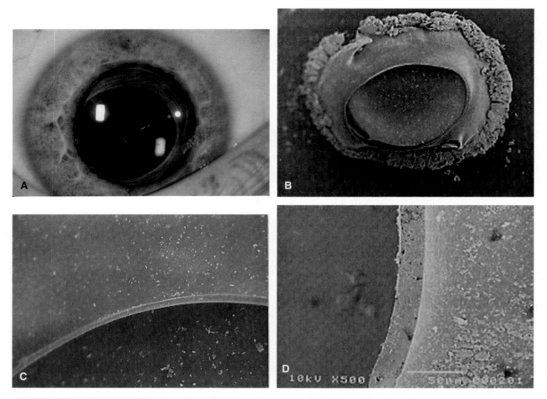

FIGURE 13-1. Manual continuous curvilinear capsulorhexis (CCC) is the gold standard when it can be successfully completed. **A.** A manual CCC is shown 4 years postoperative. The child was 10 years old at the times of surgery. A manual tear capsulorhexis was easily accomplished. The posterior capsule was left intact but has now received a YAG laser application. **B–D.** Scanning electron micrographs of the capsule edge after a manual CCC and implantation of a posterior chamber IOL in the capsular bag. Note the smooth edge of the anterior capsule edge following the manual CCC (original magnifications [B] ×5, [C] ×100, [D] ×500).

of small CCCs in Phaco-Ersatz procedures and pediatric cataract surgery.[18]

How to Create an Intact Manual CCC in Pediatric Eyes

Figures 13-1A–D present clinical and scanning electron microscopic appearance of the manual CCC technique, based on clinical and laboratory studies done at the Storm Eye Institute. To maximize successful completion of a CCC in a child's eye, the following caveats are offered. Use a high molecular weight OVD (Healon-GV or Healon-5; AMO Inc., Santa Ana, CA.) to push the anterior capsule back and deepen the anterior chamber. This will create laxity in the anterior capsule and combat the effects of vitreous upthrust caused by scleral collapse. Aim to make a slightly smaller CCC in children than in adults. With the stretch in the anterior capsule, the opening is nearly always larger at completion than it appears during the active tearing. When creating the CCC, frequently release the capsular flap and inspect the size, shape, and direction of

the tear. Regrasp near the site of the continuous tear and readjust the direction of pull if needed to keep the capsulotomy on the planned course. Often, more pull is needed toward the center of the pupil (centripetally) to avoid an extension of the CCC out to the lens equator. Additional OVD should be added as needed to keep the capsule lax during the tearing. Lenticular contents may escape into the anterior chamber during the CCC as a result of increased intralenticular pressure from vitreous upthrust. If this happens, aspiration of a portion of the lens contents (cortical "milk") may be needed before completing the CCC.

Can-Opener Anterior Capsulotomy

To avoid the difficulties of CCC in children, some surgeons have returned to the can-opener style capsulotomy when operating on children (Fig. 13-2A). Wood and Schelonka[19] compared the strength and safety of a CCC with those of a can-opener capsulotomy in a porcine model that closely resembles the high elasticity of the human pediatric lens

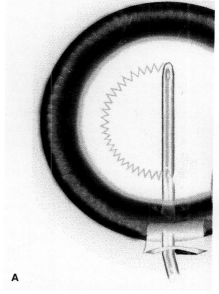

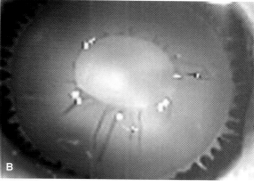

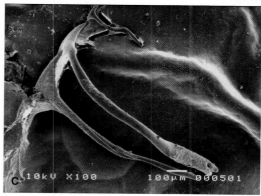

FIGURE 13-2. A can-opener anterior capsulotomy has also been proposed by some investigators as an alternative to the manual CCC technique. **A.** A can-opener capsulotomy is illustrated. A bent-needle cystotome is used to make jagged punctures in the capsule. As these punctures are connected, they form a circular opening. Capsular tags are created that can promote radial tears. The sharp apex of each capsular tag that points outward away from the center of the circle has been shown to be an area of high-stress accumulation, making radial tear formation likely. **B.** Can-opener anterior capsulotomy in the human eye obtained postmortem. Note the presence of capsular tags (arrow), which can lead to radial tear formation, jeopardizing successful in-the-bag fixation. The capsular bag was stained using 0.1% trypan blue dye to enhance visualization of the anterior capsular flap. Experimental surgery performed by the authors at The Center for Research on Ocular Therapeutics and Biodevices, Storm Eye Institute, MUSC, Charleston, South Carolina. **C.** Scanning electron microscopy of the anterior capsulotomy margin showing the presence of a capsular tag (original magnification ×100).

capsule. A CCC and a can-opener capsulotomy were performed inside the anterior chamber of fresh pig eyes. Any uncontrolled tears were noted. According to these authors, the porcine capsule is more reliably opened, with fewer uncontrolled tears, by a can-opener capsulotomy than by a CCC. Based on their study, the authors predict that pediatric capsules can be opened safely (i.e., few radial tears) with a can-opener capsulotomy.

In a preliminary study performed on postmortem pediatric human eyes at the Storm Eye Institute, we successfully performed a lens aspiration and IOL implantation without radial tear formation after opening the anterior capsule in a can-opener fashion (unpublished data) (Fig. 13-2B). Scanning electron microscopy revealed anterior capsule tags after these can-opener anterior capsulotomies (Fig. 13-2C). It is difficult to draw a firm conclusion about the can-opener anterior capsulotomy in pediatric eyes, especially with regard to performance and radial tear formation. However, radial tears have been documented in nearly 100% of adult eyes when the can-opener capsulotomy is used.[20] The radial tear rate may be lower with the highly elastic capsules of children but this has not been adequately studied. Based on the work of Krag et al.,[21] can-opener cuts at the edge of a capsulotomy would be expected to tear easily. These authors used the finite element method to document areas of high stress accumulation at each puncture made by the cystotome when performing a can-opener style capsulotomy. In contrast, a CCC demonstrated a low and uniform stress distribution, with a reduced risk of radial tears. It is well known that radial tears extending outward from the anterior capsulotomy margin can promote IOL decentration by allowing one of the haptics to exit the capsular bag and become fixated in the ciliary sulcus.[22] Decentration has been documented pathologically in up to 50% of adult eyes implanted after a can-opener style anterior capsulotomy.[23] Since children have much greater tissue reactivity and more intense equatorial capsular fibrosis, asymmetric loop fixation would be expected to cause decentration at a higher rate in children than in adults.

Vitrector-Cut Anterior Capsulectomy (Vitrectorhexis)

An ideal anterior capsulotomy for children would be easy to perform and yet have a low rate of radial tear formation even as it is stretched and deformed during cataract aspiration and IOL placement. The manual CCC remains the gold standard for resistance to tearing and should be accomplished when possible. However, its difficult completion in children has prompted the development and investigation of alternative techniques.

Laboratory and Clinical Studies in Human Pediatric Eyes

Wilson and coworkers have tested a mechanized circular anterior capsulectomy in both laboratory and clinical settings.[24,25] It has proven to be a very good alternative to CCC for young children in whom the CCC may be difficult to control. This technique, known as *vitrectorhexis*, is best performed using a vitrector tip attached to a Venturi pump irrigation and aspiration system. The capsulectomy need not be started with a bent-needle cystotome. Rather, the vitrector tip is placed through a tight-fit stab incision at the limbus or through a scleral tunnel. Irrigation is provided by a sleeve surrounding the vitrector or through a separate stab incision. A cut rate of 150 cycles/min is recommended. With the cutting port oriented posteriorly, the center of the anterior capsule is aspirated into the cutting port to create an initial opening. Any nuclear or cortical material that spontaneously exits the capsular bag anteriorly is easily aspirated without interrupting the capsulectomy technique. The capsular opening is enlarged using the cutter in a gentle circular fashion. The cutter is kept just anterior to the capsular edge, aspirating the capsule up into the cutting port rather than engaging the capsular edge directly. Visualization of the capsular edge during enlargement of the capsulectomy is excellent because the aspirating capability of the vitrector continuously removes lens cortex as it enters.

Vitrectorhexis, or a mechanized, vitrector-cut anterior capsulotomy (Figs. 13-3A to E), compared favorably to manual CCC in a direct comparison using fresh pediatric autopsy eyes.[24] It was easier to perform and resisted tearing during IOL placement. A prospective clinical series was subsequently published containing data on 20 eyes of 17 patients.[25] Two patients, both age 11, were noted to have radial tears in the anterior capsule after IOL insertion. None of the children younger than age 11 developed radial tears. The senior author (M.E.W.) has performed more than 250 successful anterior capsulectomies in children using this technique and it has become the capsulotomy technique of choice for children ≤4 years old. After an initial learning curve, radial tears are very rare with this technique. Manual CCC, while still difficult, begins to resemble the adult technique when operating on older children.

How to Create a Successful Vitrectorhexis in Pediatric Eyes

For creating a vitrectorhexis, the following surgical caveats are offered. Use a vitrector supported by a Venturi pump. Peristaltic pump systems will not cut the anterior capsule as easily. Use an infusion sleeve or a separate infusion port, but with either approach, maintain a snug fit of the instruments in the incisions through which they are placed. The anterior chamber of these soft eyes will collapse readily if leakage occurs around the instruments, making the vitrectorhexis more difficult to complete.

A micro vitreoretinal blade can be used to enter the eye. The vitrector and the blunt-tip irrigating cannula (Nichamin cannula; Storz) (or Alcon/Grieshaber irrigation hand-piece) fit snugly into the micro vitreoretinal blade openings. Do not begin the capsulotomy with a bent-needle cystotome. Merely place the vitrector, with its cutting port positioned posteriorly, in contact with the center of the intact anterior capsule. Turn the cutter on and increase the suction using the foot pedal until the capsule is engaged and opened. A cutting rate of 150 to 300 cuts/min and an aspiration maximum of 150 to 250 are recommended (these settings are for the Alcon Accurus and the Storz Premier—adjustments may be needed for other machines). With the cutting port facing down against the capsule, the authors then enlarge the round capsular opening to the desired shape and size. Any lens cortex that escapes into the anterior chamber during the vitrectorhexis is aspirated easily without interrupting the capsulotomy technique. Care should be taken to avoid leaving any right-angle edges, which could predispose to radial tear formation. The completed vitrectorhexis should be slightly smaller than the size of the IOL optic being implanted. The vitrector creates a slightly scalloped edge but inspection under both the dissecting microscope and the scanning electron microscope has revealed that the scallops roll outward to leave a smooth edge (Figs. 13-3D–E).[26] Any capsular tags or points created at the apex of a scalloped cut from the vitrector are located in an area of low biomechanical stress much like in an irregular outside-in completion of a CCC. These tags do not predispose to radial tear formation as demonstrated by finite element method computer modeling.

Bipolar Radiofrequency Capsulotomy

Radiofrequency diathermy capsulotomy, developed by Kloti et al.,[27–29] has been used as an alternative to CCC for intumescent adult cataracts[30,31] and for cataract surgery in children.[32] The Kloti device cuts the anterior capsule with a platinum alloy–tipped probe (Fig. 13-4) using a high-frequency current of 500 kHz. The probe tip is heated to about 160°C and produces a thermal capsulotomy as it is moved, under viscoelastic, in a circular path across the anterior capsule. Small gas bubbles are formed while the tip is active, but these do not usually interfere with visibility during the capsulotomy. Gentle pressure must be

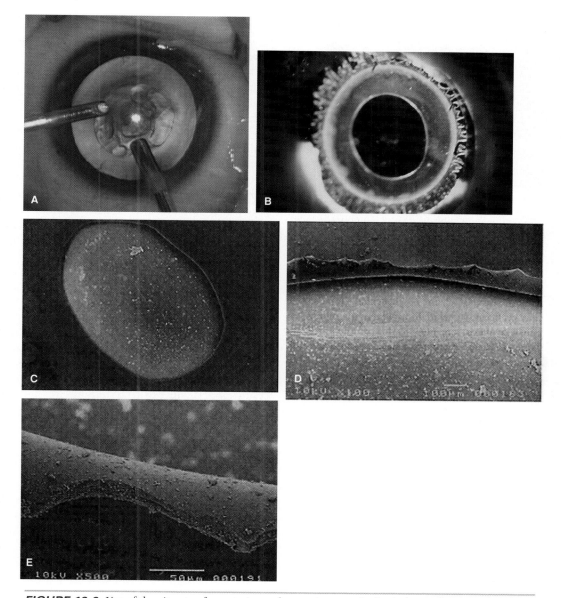

FIGURE 13-3. Use of the vitrector for anterior and posterior capsulorhexis (termed *vitrectorhexis*) has been extensively studied in both clinical and laboratory settings. **A.** Intraoperative photograph illustrating vitrector-cut anterior capsulectomy ("vitrectorhexis") being performed in a case of pediatric cataract. **B.** A vitrector-cut anterior capsulectomy is shown in this pediatric autopsy eye from the Miyake–Apple posterior view. **C–E.** Scanning electron micrographs of the vitrectorhexis capsule edge. Note the scalloped edges, but smooth internal surface (original magnifications [D] ×5, [E] ×100, [F] ×500).

maintained on the capsule with the tip as it moves either clockwise or counterclockwise. If contact is too light or movement too fast, skipped areas will result. If contact is too firm or movement too slow, the tip will burn through the capsule and enter the lens cortex. Subsequent tip movement drags the capsulotomy edge rather than cutting it, which may cause radial tearing. However, the preferred rate of movement and firmness of capsule contact are quickly learned after a few cases. Even when performed perfectly, a diathermy-cut capsulotomy can be seen to have coagulated capsular debris along the circular edge. In addition, this edge has been shown experimentally to be less

elastic than a comparable CCC edge.[33–35] Since the stretching force needed to break the edge of a diathermy-cut capsulotomy is much reduced compared to a CCC edge, surgical manipulations needed to remove a cataract and place an IOL may result in more radial tears when the diathermy is used. However, the experimental measurements were all made on adult autopsy globes. It is well known that the pediatric capsule responds differently. In fact, Comer et al.[32] reported no radial tears when using the diathermy-cut capsulotomy in 14 eyes of 7 children whose mean age was 23 months. Clinically, the diathermy device is useful in children for both the anterior and the posterior capsules.

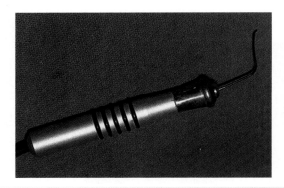

FIGURE 13-4. Kloti radiofrequency diathermy needle handpiece. The platinum alloy–tipped probe directs a high-frequency current of 500 kHz. Under viscoelastic, the probe tip is placed in contact with the intact anterior capsule and moved in a circular path to create a round opening.

Fugo Plasma Blade Anterior Capsulotomy

The Fugo plasma blade has also recently been introduced as a cutting unit that can be used to perform an anterior capsulectomy. The Fugo Blade capsulotomy unit is a portable electronic system that operates on rechargeable batteries and provides an alternative to manual capsulorhexis (see Chapter 18 for details on the Fugo blade). The Fugo Blade provides an anterior capsulotomy that requires no red reflex and usually requires <10 sec to perform. The instrument developer reports that the Fugo Blade is easy to use and does not have a steep learning curve.[36]

The Fugo Blade may be particularly suited for the highly elastic capsule of children. Because it cuts the capsule with a "plasma blade," it may not suffer from the tendency for skip areas seen with the Kloti radiofrequency device. However, the edge of the Fugo Blade capsulotomies we have performed clinically, thus far, have not been more resistant to tearing than the Kloti diathermy.

ANTERIOR CAPSULE MANAGEMENT IN SPECIFIC CASES

Anterior Capsulorhexis in White Pediatric Cataracts

As emphasized earlier, a manual CCC creates an opening in the anterior capsule of the crystalline lens that is resistant to tear during cataract removal and ensures in-the-bag implantation of an IOL. The retroillumination produced by the operating microscope is important in visualizing the anterior capsule while performing CCC. It is difficult to distinguish the anterior capsule from the underlying cortex in total, advanced/white cataracts and in patients with pigmented fundi or vitreous disease, owing to the absence of the red reflex.[37,38] Poor visualization of the capsule results in an inadequate CCC, with a high risk of radial tears

toward or beyond the lens equator and associated complications, such as zonular and posterior capsular rupture, vitreous loss, and IOL displacement.

Methods used to enhance the visualization of the anterior capsule during CCC in white cataracts have been discussed in detail elsewhere.[37,38] These include side illumination with an endoilluminator, injection of an air bubble in the anterior chamber, hemocoloration of the capsule with the patient's autologous blood, and the two-step CCC method, which involves creating a small CCC followed by a second CCC to enlarge the initial capsular opening. Other techniques to facilitate performing CCC in the aforementioned cases include dimming the room lights, increasing the optical magnification of the operating microscope, using a high-frequency diathermy probe, using high-density viscoelastic agents, performing a vitrectorhexis, and aspirating cortical material in liquefied cataracts. Recently, various capsular dyes such as fluorescein sodium (staining from above, under an air bubble, or intracameral subcapsular injection), indocyanine green, and trypan blue have been successfully used for staining the anterior capsule for performing a CCC. Clinical and laboratory studies done in adult cataracts (with poor or no red reflex) using capsular dyes for anterior capsule staining have shown encouraging results.[37,38] However, further studies are needed to evaluate their performance and safety in pediatric eyes presenting with white cataracts.

Anterior Capsulorhexis in Pediatric Traumatic Cataracts

Visualization of the anterior lens capsule in pediatric traumatic cataract cases may be difficult due to a ruptured lens capsule with flocculent lens matter in the anterior chamber.[39] Creation of an intact capsulorhexis may be difficult in such a situation. A vitrectorhexis is a good alternative to manual capsulorhexis. Staining of the anterior lens capsule may be helpful to enhance visibility in these eyes with a "torn anterior capsule" or "white cataract."[40] Based on the laboratory and clinical experience, anterior capsule staining can be successfully done using nontoxic capsular dyes such as 0.5% indocyanine green or 0.1% trypan blue.

SUMMARY, RECOMMENDATIONS, AND GUIDELINES FOR SURGEONS

The anterior capsule is highly elastic in the pediatric patient and poses challenges in the creation of the capsulotomy.[41] Table 13-2 lists advantages of, disadvantages of, and recommendations for various anterior capsulotomy techniques. While a manual CCC is ideal for adults, it is more difficult to perform in infantile eyes with cataracts. However, it is still the gold standard since it resists tearing

▶ **TABLE 13-2** Advantages, Disadvantages, and Recommendations of Various Anterior Capsulotomy Techniques

Capsulorhexis: *Preferred at >4 yr*	*Vitrectorhexis:* *Preferred at ≤4 yr*	*Bipolar Radiofrequency:* *Alternative at All Ages*
Difficult to perform	Relatively easy to perform	Relatively easy to perform
Best resistant to tear	Next-best resistant to tear	Least resistant to radial tear
"Runaway rhexis" common	"Runaway rhexis" less common	"Runaway rhexis" less common

once completed successfully. Because of the increased elasticity of the pediatric anterior capsule, more force is required when pulling on the capsular flap before tearing begins. Control of the capsulectomy and prevention of extensions out toward the lens equator are inversely related to the force needed to generate the tear. As a result, inadvertent extensions out to the lens equator (known as the "runaway" rhexis) are common in children. When performing a manual CCC in a child, the following technical recommendations are offered.

- Use highly viscous OVDs to fill the anterior chamber and flatten the anterior capsule. A slack anterior capsule will be easier to tear in a controlled fashion.
- Regrasp the capsulorhexis edge frequently and begin with a smaller capsulotomy than desired. Because of the elasticity, the opening will be larger than it appears once the forceps release the capsule flap.
- Force when tearing must often be directed toward the center of the pupil to control the turning of the CCC edge along a circular path.
- If the capsule begins to extend peripherally, stop before the edge is out of sight under the iris. Converting to a vitrector-cut capsulotomy or a radiofrequency diathermy capsulotomy is recommended when this occurs.

The anterior vitrectorhexis technique is recommended for young children whenever a posterior capsulectomy and anterior vitrectomy are planned. Since the vitrectomy will require a mechanical cutting instrument, it will be very convenient to simply use the device on the anterior and posterior capsule also. When performing anterior vitrectorhexis in a child, the following technical recommendations are offered.

- Use a micro vitreoretinal blade to enter the eye.
- Place the vitrector, with its cutting port positioned posteriorly, in contact with the center of the intact anterior capsule.
- Turn the cutter on and increase the suction using the foot pedals until the capsule is engaged and opened.
- Use a cutting rate of 150 to 300 cuts/min and an aspiration maximum of 150 to 250.
- With the cutting port facing down against the capsule, enlarge the round capsular opening to the desired shape and size.

- Aspirate any lens cortex that escapes into the anterior chamber during the vitrectorhexis.
- Avoid leaving any right-angle edges, which could predispose to radial tear formation.

REFERENCES

1. Wilson ME. The challenge of pediatric cataract surgery. *J AAPOS* 2001;5:265–266.
2. Wilson ME, Pandey SK, Werner L, et al. Pediatric cataract surgery: current techniques, complications and management. In: Agarwal S, Agarwal A, Sachdev MS, Mehta KR, Fine IH, Agarwal A, eds. *Phacoemulsification, Laser Cataract Surgery and Foldable IOLs.* New Delhi, India: Jaypee Brothers Medical, 2000:369–388.
3. Pandey SK, Wilson ME, Trivedi RH, et al. Pediatric cataract surgery and intraocular lens implantation: current techniques, complications and management. *Int Ophthalmol Clin* 2001;41:175–196.
4. Ram J, Pandey SK. Infantile cataract surgery: Current techniques, complications and their management. In: Dutta LC, ed. *Modern Ophthalmology.* New Delhi, India: Jaypee Brothers, 2000:378–384.
5. Wilson ME. Pediatric cataract surgery. In: Spaeth GL, ed. *Ophthalmic Surgery, Principles and Practices.* Philadelphia: Saunders, 2003:103–107.
6. Wilson ME. Anterior capsule management for pediatric intraocular lens implantation. *J Pediatr Ophthalmol Strabismus* 1999;36:1–6.
7. Ridley H. Intraocular acrylic lenses: a recent development in the surgery of cataracts. *Br J Ophthalmol* 1952;36:113–122.
8. Ridley H. Intraocular acrylic lenses: 10 years development. *Br J Ophthalmol* 1960;44:705–712.
9. Choyce DP. Correction of uniocular aphakia by means of anterior chamber acrylic implants. *Trans Ophthalmol Soc UK* 1958;78:459–470.
10. Rosen E. Capsular surgery. *Eur J Implant Ref Surg* 1990;2:1–4.
11. Gimbel HV. Advanced capsulotomy. In: Gills JP, Fenzl R, Martin RG, eds. *Cataract Surgery: State of the Art.* Thorofare, NJ: Slack, 1998:69–74.
12. Galand A. A simple method of implantation within the capsular bag. *J Am Intraocular Implant Soc* 1983;9:330–332.
13. Parks MM. Posterior lens capsulectomy during primary cataract surgery in children. *Ophthalmology* 1983;90:344–345.
14. Gimbel HV, Neuhann T. Development, advantage, and methods of the continuous circular capsulorhexis technique. *J Cataract Refract Surg* 1990;16:31–37.
15. Wilson ME. Intraocular lens implantation: has it become the standard of care for children? *Ophthalmology* 1996;103:1719–1720.
16. Auffarth GU, Wesendahl TA, Newland TJ, Apple DJ. Capsulorhexis in the rabbit eye as a model for pediatric capsulectomy. *J Cataract Refract Surg* 1994;20:188–191.
17. Vasavada A, Chauhan H. Intraocular lens implantation in infants with congenital cataracts. *J Cataract Refract Surg* 1994;20:592–597.
18. Tahi H, Fantes F, Hamaoui M, Parel JM. Small peripheral anterior continuous curvilinear capsulorhexis. *J Cataract Refract Surg* 1999;25:744–747.
19. Wood MG, Schelonka LP. A porcine model predicts a can opener capsulotomy can be done safely in pediatric patients. *J AAPOS* 1999;3:356–362.

20. Wasserman D, Apple DJ, Castaneda VE, et al. Anterior capsular tears and loop fixation of posterior chamber intraocular lenses. *Ophthalmology* 1991;98:425–431.
21. Krag S, Thim K, Corydon L, Cyster B. Biomechanical aspects of the anterior capsulotomy. *J Cataract Refract Surg* 1994;20:410–416.
22. Apple DJ, Assia EI, Wasserman D, et al. Evidence and support of the continuous tear anterior capsulectomy (capsulorhexis technique). In: Cangelosi GC, ed. *Advances in Cataract Surgery.* New Orleans Academy of Ophthalmology. Thorofare, NJ: SLACK, 1991: 21–47.
23. Assia EI, Leglar UFC, Merrill C, et al. Clinical pathologic study of the effect of radial tears and loop fixation on intraocular lens decentration. *Ophthalmology* 1993;100:153–158.
24. Wilson ME, Bluestein EC, Wang XH, Apple DJ. Comparison of mechanized anterior capsulectomy and manual continuous capsulorhexis in pediatric eyes. *J Cataract Refract Surg* 1994;20:602–606.
25. Wilson ME, Saunders RA, Roberts EL, Apple DJ. Mechanized anterior capsulectomy as an alternative to manual capsulorhexis in children undergoing intraocular lens implantation. *J Pediatr Ophthalmol Strabismus* 1996;33:237–240.
26. Andreo LK, Wilson ME, Apple DJ. Elastic properties and scanning electron microscopic appearance of manual continuous curvilinear capsulorhexis and vitrectorhexis in an animal model of pediatric cataract. *J Cataract Refract Surg* 1999;25:534–539.
27. Kloti R. Bipolar wet field diathermy in microsurgery. *Klin Monatsbl Augenheilkd* 1984;184:442–444.
28. Kloti R. Anterior high-frequency (HF) capsulotomy. Part I: Experimental study. *Klin Monatsbl Augenheilkd* 1992;200:507–510.
29. Coester C, Kloti R, Speiser P. Anterior high-frequency (HF) capsulotomy. Part II. Clinical surgical experience. *Klin Monatsbl Augenheilkd* 1992;200:511–514.
30. Hausman N, Richard CT. Investigations on diathermy for anterior capsulotomy. *Invest Ophthalmol Vis Sci* 1991;32:2155–2159.
31. Delcoigne CD, Hennekes R. Circular continuous anterior capsulotomy with high-frequency diathermy. *Bull Soc Belge Ophthalmol* 1993;249:67–72.
32. Comer RM, Abdulla N, O'Keefe M. Radiofrequency diathermy capsulorhexis of the anterior and posterior capsules in pediatric cataract surgery: preliminary studies. *J Cataract Refract Surg* 1997;23: 641–644.
33. Morgan JE, Ellingham RB, Young RD, Tumal GJ. Mechanical properties of a human lens capsule following capsulorhexis or radiofrequency diathermy capsulotomy. *Arch Ophthalmol* 1996;114:1110–1115.
34. Luck J, Brahma AK, Noble BA. A comparative study of the elastic properties of continuous tear curvilinear capsulorhexis versus capsulorhexis produced by radiofrequency endodiathermy. *Br J Ophthalmol* 1994;78:392–396.
35. Krag S, Kirsten T, Leif C. Diathermic capsulotomy versus capsulorhexis: a biochemical study. *J Cataract Refract Surg* 1997;23: 86–90.
36. Fugo RJ, Coccio D, McGrann D, Becht L, DelCampo D. The Fugo Blade. . . the next step after capsulorhexis. Presented at the American Society of Cataract and Refractive Surgery Symposium on Cataract, IOL and Refractive Surgery, Congress on Ophthalmic Practice Management, Boston, 2001.
37. Pandey SK, Werner L, Apple DJ, Wilson ME. Ophthalmic dye-enhanced adult and pediatric cataract surgery. In: Agarwal S, Agarwal A, Agarwal A (Eds). *Phaco, Phakonit, and Laser Phaco: A guest for the best.* Panama: Highlights of Ophthalmology International, 2002, pp 179–204.
38. Pandey SK, Werner L, Escobar-Gomez M, et al. Dye-enhanced cataract surgery. I. Anterior capsule staining for capsulorhexis in advanced/white cataracts. *J Cataract Refract Surg* 2000;26:1052–1059.
39. Pandey SK, Ram J, Werner L, et al. Visual results and postoperative complications of capsular bag versus sulcus fixation of posterior chamber intraocular lenses for traumatic cataract in children. *J Cataract Refract Surg* 1999;25:1576–1584.
40. Newsom TH, Oetting TN. Indocyanine green staining in traumatic cataract. *J Cataract Refract Surg* 2000;26:1691–1693.
41. Wilson ME. Anterior lens capsule management in pediatric cataract surgery. *Trans Am Ophthalmol Soc* 2004;102:391–422.

Chapter 14

Multiquadrant Hydrodissection

Abhay R. Vasavada, Rupal H. Trivedi, and Bharti Nihalani

Cortical-cleaving hydrodissection is recognized as an important surgical step for adult cataract surgery. Several authorities have advocated various forms of interlenticular injection of fluid in adult cataract surgery.[1–6] Faust coined the term *hydrodissection* in 1984.[1] He described it as an injection of fluid designed to separate the lens nucleus from the cortex. In 1992, Fine published his classic description of the "cortical-cleaving hydrodissection" technique.[2] This highly effective procedure enhances the separation of the capsule from the cortex and is widely accepted as a routine surgical step for adult cataract surgery.

Pediatric cataract surgeons have been less inclined, however, to follow the adult trend for hydrodissection. Hydrodissection is often barely mentioned or is glossed over in the management of pediatric cataract surgery. As the main function of hydrodissection is to release the nucleus to facilitate phacoemulsification, which is not usually an issue for pediatric cataract surgeons, it may not prove useful to pediatric cataract surgeons.

Numerous advantages of cortical-cleaving hydrodissection (e.g., ease, safety, and efficacy of nuclear emulsification of adult cataracts) are well established in the literature. Apple et al.[5] reported that the major advantage of hydrodissection lies in the shearing effect of the fluid wave. Direct injection of fluid under the anterior capsule is particularly useful in helping to remove equatorial lens epithelial cells, thereby reducing the incidence of posterior capsule opacification (PCO). When surgeons leave cortical material, which clinically resembles strand or fiber, they actually leave large numbers of mitotically active cells from the equatorial lens bow. These cells have the potential to grow across the visual axis, especially the pearl form. The best means of reducing the incidence of this complication is to remove as many of these cells as possible at the outset.

Since PCO is one of the most frequent and severe complications in pediatric cataract surgery, reports that hydrodissection may decrease the incidence of capsular opacification prompted us to apply this inexpensive, practical, immediately implementable procedure to pediatric cataract surgery.[7]

TECHNIQUE

The technique for performing cortical-cleaving hydrodissection has been well described in the literature. Table 14-1 describes the technique of multiple quadrant hydrodissection. Signs of successful hydrodissection are listed in Table 14-2. We believe that multiple-quadrant hydrodissection is the key to the removal and washout of equatorial lens epithelial cells, and we strongly recommend it in pediatric eyes.

Capsulorhexis size is critical in hydrodissection. A small capsulorhexis provides a broader area of anterior capsule into which the cannula can be inserted (up to an optimal length). However, this may make removal of the lens substance more difficult. Conversely, a large capsulorhexis may hamper endocapsular surgery.

COMPLICATIONS

1. *Anterior capsule tear*. We believe that hydrodissection should not be performed with other forms of capsulotomy (vitrectorhexis, Fugo capsulotomy, radiofrequency diathermy, multipuncture capsulotomy). The edge of the other capsulotomy openings may not be strong enough and may tear during the hydrodissection procedure.

2. *Viscoelastic escape*. Cohesive ophthalmic viscosurgical devices (OVDs) may escape as a bolus if forceful hydrodissection is performed. It is crucial to do a *gentle* hydrodissection when using such OVDs. With any OVD, the surgeon should gently depress the posterior lip of the incision between every one or two injections to permit excess fluid to escape and to allow equilibration of the pressure between the anterior and the posterior chambers.

▶ **TABLE 14-1** **Multiquadrant Hydrodissection Technique for Pediatric Cataract Surgery**

■ Instrument: a 27-gauge cannula attached to a 5-mL syringe filled with balanced salt solution. A J-shaped Binkhorst cannula can be useful for injection at the subincision site.[8] We currently use right-angle cannulas (separate cannulas for right and left side) for multiquadrant hydrodissection (see Fig. 14-1).
■ Technique
  1. After performing capsulorhexis, two paracentesis incisions are made.
  2. The tip of the cannula is inserted under the anterior capsule for a distance of approximately 1 or 2 mm.
  3. Fluid is gently injected after careful tenting of the anterior capsule. Decompress the nucleus after each wave.

Multiple quadrant hydrodissection, of at least three quadrants, is performed, repeating the technique described above.

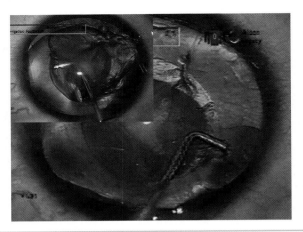

FIGURE 14-1. Multiquadrant hydrodissection with a right-sided right-angle cannula. *Inset:* left-sided right-angled cannula.

3. *Iris prolapse.* It is important to remember that excessive hydrodissection from a paracentesis opening can cause increased fluid pressure behind the iris. This increased pressure can lead to iris prolapse through the incisions.

4. *Nucleus prolapse in the anterior chamber.* An unwanted consequence of continuous and forceful hydrodissection is nucleus prolapse into the anterior chamber. Strong corticocapsular adhesions in children require excessive force to cleave apart from the capsule. This results in prolapse of the nucleus more frequently in eyes with pediatric cataract. Immediate decompression of the nucleus after the injection of fluid prevents this complication.

5. *Posterior capsule rupture.* In the absence of a preexisting defect this is a very rare complication. *Hydrodissection is an absolute contraindication in eyes with a suspected preexisting posterior capsular defect.* Hydrodissection in a total cataract with poor visibility should be done with special caution because the opaque lens substance may camouflage a preexisting posterior capsular defect.

Like any other new technique, hydrodissection has its own learning curve. During the learning phase it may not be possible to consistently achieve thorough hydrodissections.

OUTCOME OF HYDRODISSECTION IN EYES WITH PEDIATRIC CATARACTS

We have designed a prospective, randomized, multicenter clinical trial to evaluate the impact of hydrodissection on intraoperative performance as well as postoperative outcome for pediatric cataract surgery. We have reported that multiquadrant cortical-cleaving hydrodissection decreases the lens substance removal time, lessens the fluid volume used for lens substance removal, and facilitates lens substance removal in pediatric cataract surgery.[7] At the end of lens substance removal, residual cortical fibers on the posterior capsule were noted in 12.5% of the hydrodissection group and 22.5% of the no-hydrodissection group. Although this difference was not statistically significant, we believe that it may eventually affect the postoperative outcome with regard to PCO. We are following these eyes at our center (Iladevi Cataract and IOL Research Center, Ahmedabad, India) and hope to report long-term follow-up of these eyes.

To summarize, hydrodissection is a very simple and inexpensive procedure that allows fast, easy, and safe removal of lens substance during pediatric cataract surgery. It has a definitive influence on intraoperative performance and a possible influence on postoperative outcome in terms of reducing PCO.

▶ **TABLE 14-2 Signs of Successful Hydrodissection**

■ Forward bulge of the nucleus
■ Visible presence of a fluid wave: This is considered a definitive sign of successful hydrodissection, but it may not always be visible in pediatric eyes. Strong corticocapsular adhesions in pediatric eyes may prevent the appearance of a visible fluid wave.
■ Prominence of the capsulorhexis edge
■ Release of trapped fluid from the rhexis margin following decompression of the nucleus

REFERENCES

1. Faust KJ. Hydrodissection of soft nuclei. *J Am Intra-Ocular Implant Soc* 1984;10:75–77.
2. Fine IH. Cortical cleaving hydrodissection. *J Cataract Refract Surg* 1992;18:508–512.

3. Fine IH. Cortical cleaving hydrodissection. *J Cataract Refract Surg* 2000;26:943–944.

4. Gimbel HV. Hydrodissection and hydrodelineation. *Int Ophthalmol Clin* 1994;34:73–90.

5. Apple DJ, Peng Q, Visessook N, Werner L, Pandey SK, Escobar-Gomez M, et al. Surgical prevention of posterior capsule opacification. Part 1: Progress in eliminating this complication of cataract surgery. *J Cataract Refract Surg* 2000;26:180–187.

6. Vasavada AR, Singh R, Apple DJ, Trivedi RH, Pandey SK, Werner L. Effect of hydrodissection on intraoperative performance: randomized study. *J Cataract Refract Surg* 2002;28:1623–1628.

7. Vasavada AR, Trivedi RH, Apple DJ, Ram J, Werner L. Randomized, clinical trial of multiquadrant hydrodissection in pediatric cataract surgery. *Am J Ophthalmol* 2003;135:84–88.

8. Dewey SH. Cortical removal simplified by J-cannula irrigation. *J Cataract Refract Surg* 2002;28:11–14.

Lens Substance Aspiration

Rupal H. Trivedi and M. Edward Wilson, Jr.

Lens substance aspiration has probably received the least interest in the discussion of management of pediatric cataracts. Pediatric cataracts are generally soft and can be aspirated easily. However, our target should be not only to *aspirate the lens substance,* but to *aspirate it thoroughly.* When surgeons leave behind cortical material, which clinically resembles a harmless strand or fiber, they actually leave a large number of mitotically active cells.[1,2] These cells have the potential to grow across the visual axis and cause the proliferative form of visual axis opacification. The best means of reducing the incidence of this complication is to remove as many of these cells as possible at the time of cataract removal.[1,2] Since visual axis opacification is one of the most frequent and severe complications in pediatric cataract surgery, meticulous removal of lens substance is a crucial step in the management of pediatric cataracts.

In most eyes with pediatric cataracts, the lens is not hard enough to require any phacoemulsification power. However, the cortex in these infantile eyes is gummy and is occasionally difficult to aspirate. When using a phacoemulsification machine, in the absence of ultrasonic power, some authors recommend using the term *phacoaspiration* instead of the widely known term *phacoemulsification* for adult cataract emulsification.[3]

In the mid-1960s, the principle of maintaining the anterior chamber (AC) while aspirating the lens cortex was introduced. This was done either using a two-bored needle or through a separate infusion site. This principle is still valid with all the methods described below.

SINGLE-PORT VERSUS BIMANUAL APPROACH

The lens substance can be aspirated through a single port or using a bimanual approach. Single-port irrigation/aspiration (I/A) is an awkward maneuver for subincisional cortex removal.[4] The technique of bimanual I/A was developed to make cortical removal easier. The technique uses two separate cannulas inserted through two sideport incisions. AC stability during bimanual I/A requires the irrigation system to have a flow resistance lower than that of the aspiration system, which can be accomplished by using cannulas with larger lumen diameters and shorter lengths.[5] A J-shaped cannula also helps us to approach the subincisional cortex more easily.[6] However, pediatric eyes are especially appropriate candidates for bimanual I/A because

- Separate irrigation and aspiration help to maintain the anterior chamber and decrease the fluctuation of the AC. This is especially advantageous in pediatric eyes with low scleral rigidity.
- The bimanual approach helps to achieve thorough removal of lens substance (especially subincisional), which, again, is very crucial when performing pediatric cataract surgery.

MANUAL VERSUS AUTOMATED APPROACH

Pediatric cataracts can be aspirated using the manual or the automated approach. In automated removal, either a phacoemulsification machine or a vitrector machine can be used.

Machemer and coworkers developed the vitreous infusion suction cutter in 1970, primarily for removal of the vitreous and vitreous membranes.[7,8] Pediatric cataracts can be aspirated using the cutter-off position of the vitrectomy machine. The advantage of using the vitrector is that it is possible to perform vitrectorhexis, I/A, posterior capsulotomy, and vitrectomy—all with one instrument (the setting needs to be changed) (see Fig. 15-1). This avoids extra manipulation and repeated entry to and exit from the eye. We use Accurus (Alcon Surgical) for this purpose. Although

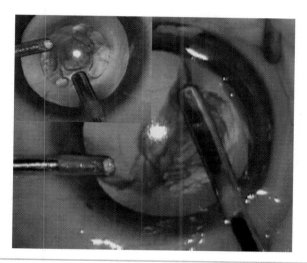

FIGURE 15-1. After vitrectorhexis (inset), without exiting an eye, irrigation/aspiration is being performed with a Nichamin (20 G) cannula and the vitrectomy handpiece set to the cutter-off position.

any machine can be used for I/A, capsulotomy and vitrectomy can be achieved more efficiently with Venturi pump machines. It is important to know your machine well. We recommend referring to the instruction manual provided by the manufacturer to learn the mechanics of the specific machine.

In cases in which intraocular lens implantation is not intended to be the primary procedure, pediatric cataracts can be removed through one or two very small incisions— wide enough to permit entry of the I/A probe only. Incision width is very important—it should be loose enough to insert the instrument but tight enough to avoid any

leakage of fluid. This helps to prevent anterior chamber fluctuation.

Maintenance of the AC is critical when removing lens substances. Aspiration of fluid from the AC must be balanced by adequate infusion. We use a 20-gauge Nichamin cannula irrigation-hand-piece (Alcon/Grieshaber 170-01) for irrigation. The infusion requirements are usually supplied by gravity or positive-pressure irrigation systems. The addition of 0.5 mL of adrenaline to the infusion bottle (1:1,000 for cardiac use) helps to maintain mydriasis. Dada et al.[9,10] have recommended the use of intracameral low molecular weight heparin to inhibit fibrin formation and fibroblast activity after intraocular surgery. Low molecular weight heparin is available as Fragmin (Pharmacia and Upjohn). One vial contains 2,500 IU, and two vials are added in a 500-mL bottle of BSS (balanced salt solution) to yield a concentration of 10 IU/mL for intracameral use.

Before introducing the probe into the AC, it is a good rule of thumb to examine the patency of the cannula and to check that the level of irrigation is adequate. While entering the AC, the irrigation must be on. We prefer to set irrigation to the *irrigation continuous* mode. When the tip is in contact with the cortical material, the pedal is moved to position 2. With peristaltic pump machines, the surgeon must occlude the aspirating orifices to allow an increase in the vacuum level to the maximum preset level. The maximum preset vacuum value is reached with these machines only when the orifice has been occluded. Venturi pump machines allow the aspiration vacuum to be increased using the foot pedal without the need for tip occlusion. The advantage of this approach is that the tip can bring the cortex toward and into the tip even without occlusion.

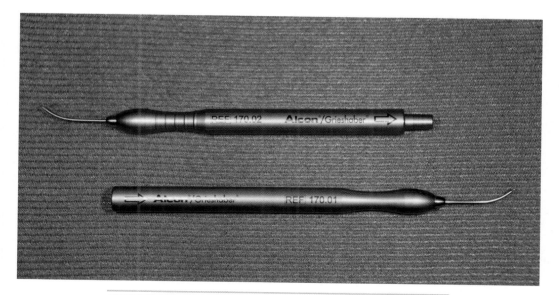

FIGURE 15-2. Irrigation/Aspiration hand piece (Alcon/Grieshaber).

Once the cortical material is engaged, the tip is moved slowly toward the center of the pupil to detach the lens substance progressively from the periphery to the center. At times, in pediatric eyes, the cortex does not strip from the lens periphery easily. In this situation, the aspirating tip is held in the lens periphery while the aspiration vacuum is increased until the cortex is removed. The aspirating orifice of the instrument must always be under the visual control of the operator. This prevents snagging unwanted tissue (anterior capsule, iris, posterior capsule). First, aspirate free-floating material (if any), then remove stratified material, and, finally, remove material adhering to the posterior capsule (if any). In general it is easiest to aspirate more accessible sectors first, that is, the temporal, nasal, and inferior sectors, and then proceed to those that are more difficult to reach, that is, subincisional. The latter area (subincisional cortex) may aspirate more easily if the surgeon switches hands and places the aspiration handpiece through the nondominant sideport incision. If the external diameters of the aspiration and the irrigation handpieces are equal, this reversal of hand positions can be accomplished without creating leakage of fluid around the instruments.

To summarize, we cannot overstress the importance of bimanual I/A technology for lens substance aspiration in pediatric eyes. Either a vitrector probe (cutter-off position) or an aspiration probe we recommend aspiration hand-piece (Alcon/Grieshaber 170-02; Fig. 15-2) can be used for aspiration maneuvering. With either approach, it is crucial to achieve thorough removal of lens substance.

REFERENCES

1. Peng Q, Apple DJ, Visessook N, et al. Surgical prevention of posterior capsule opacification. Part 2: Enhancement of cortical cleanup by focusing on hydrodissection. *J Cataract Refract Surg* 2000;26:188–197.
2. Apple DJ, Peng Q, Visessook N, et al. Surgical prevention of posterior capsule opacification. Part 1: Progress in eliminating this complication of cataract surgery. *J Cataract Refract Surg* 2000;26:180–187.
3. Amaya L, Taylor D, Russell I, Nischall K. Phacoaspiration in children. *J Cataract Refract Surg* 2001;27:1534–1535.
4. Brauweiler P. Bimanual irrigation/aspiration. *J Cataract Refract Surg* 1996;22:1013–1016.
5. Jeng BH, Huang D. Anterior chamber stability during bimanual irrigation and aspiration. Theoretical and experimental analysis. *J Cataract Refract Surg* 2001;27:1670–1678.
6. Dewey SH. Cortical removal simplified by J-cannula irrigation. *J Cataract Refract Surg* 2002;28:11–14.
7. Machemer R, Parel JM, Norton EW. Vitrectomy: a pars plana approach. Technical improvements and further results. *Trans Am Acad Ophthalmol Otolaryngol* 1972;76:462–466.
8. Machemer R, Buettner H, Norton EW, Parel JM. Vitrectomy: a pars plana approach. *Trans Am Acad Ophthalmol Otolaryngol* 1971;75:813–820.
9. Dada T. Intracameral heparin in pediatric cataract surgery. *J Cataract Refract Surg* 2003;29:1056.
10. Dada T, Dada VK, Sharma N, Vajpayee RB. Primary posterior capsulorhexis with optic capture and intracameral heparin in paediatric cataract surgery. *Clin Exp Ophthalmol* 2000;28:361–363.

Posterior Capsulotomy and Anterior Vitrectomy for the Management of Pediatric Cataracts

Rupal H. Trivedi and M. Edward Wilson, Jr.

It is well known that the management of the posterior capsule greatly influences the outcome of pediatric cataract surgery (Figs. 16-1A–C). Visual axis opacification (VAO) is rapid and virtually inevitable in the very young child after pediatric cataract surgery when adult-style surgery, leaving the posterior capsule intact, is performed. The younger the child, the more acute is the problem, because VAO is faster and the amblyogenic effect is greater.

The anterior vitreous face (AVF) is closely linked to the posterior capsule. It is more "reactive" in infants and young children (Figs. 16-2A and B). It acts as a scaffold, not only for lens epithelial cell proliferation, but also for metaplastic pigment epithelial cells, exudates, and cells that result from a break in the blood–aqueous barrier. The inflammatory response in small children is severe and fibrous membranes may form on an intact AVF, resulting in VAO. The need for removal of the anterior vitreous along with the center of the posterior capsule has been well recognized in the literature.[1–6] With the advent of automated vitrectomy techniques in the late 1970s, many pediatric cataract surgeons began to routinely perform primary posterior capsulotomy and vitrectomy with a vitrector.[1,7–10] As of today, primary posterior capsulotomy and anterior vitrectomy are considered "routine surgical steps," especially in younger children.

In earlier years, when handling the posterior capsule, clarity of the visual axis, reduced inflammation, and prevention of synechiae were the goals. Preparation for a secondary intraocular lens (IOL) implantation, at a later date, was not considered. Surgeons recommended removing all but the peripheral 2 mm of the posterior capsule. However, widespread acceptance of IOL implantation in children has forced us to modify this. Treatment of the posterior capsule determines where and how safely the IOL

can be fixed. This requires leaving behind more peripheral posterior capsule support.

Thus, management of the posterior capsule should eliminate or delay the formation of VAO and yet leave sufficient capsular support to achieve desired "in-the-bag" (or ciliary sulcus) fixation of an IOL. Even when IOL implantation is not performed as the primary procedure, it is important to treat and prepare the eye in such a way that secondary implantation can be achieved safely.

Modern high-quality vitrectomy machines, and the improved visualization provided by the optics of the highest-quality operating microscopes, have allowed surgeons to perform posterior capsulotomy and anterior vitrectomy more safely. In addition, a better understanding of the importance of a tight-fitting wound around instruments that enter the eye of a child has helped reduce the anterior chamber instability that can occur during these surgical maneuvers in young eyes. Despite this, various questions for the surgeon remain. When should the posterior capsule be opened and when can it be left intact? When does an anterior vitrectomy need to be added to the posterior capsulotomy and when can manipulation of the vitreous be avoided? Is it best to perform posterior capsulotomy and anterior vitrectomy before or after an IOL is implanted? Is the anterior (limbal) or the posterior (pars plana) approach preferred for posterior capsulectomy and vitrectomy? In this chapter we address some of these controversial issues.

WHEN SHOULD THE POSTERIOR CAPSULE BE LEFT INTACT?

This is perhaps one of the most common and controversial questions. The answer depends on several factors including the age at cataract surgery, the condition of the

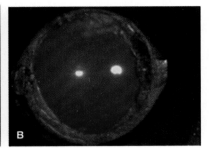

FIGURE 16-1. Note the clear visual axis and well-centered IOL in these two examples of children (**A** + **B**) photographed several years after cataract surgery with primary posterior capsulotomy and vitrectomy.

posterior capsule, and the child's presumed cooperation for YAG laser capsulotomy in the future.

Proponents of primary posterior capsulotomy and anterior vitrectomy argue that performance of these steps is a *necessity* in all children within the amblyopic ages to prevent VAO and worsening amblyopia. However, opponents argue that it is not a safe *choice*. The posterior capsule is a physiologic barrier between the anterior and the posterior segment of the eye and should not be removed. It prevents the vitreous from entering the anterior chamber, and it theoretically preserves the ocular anatomic relationship and the blood–aqueous barrier after cataract surgery. Despite this controversy in the past, as of 2004, we can say confidently that posterior capsulotomy and anterior vitrectomy are necessary steps for the management of cataracts in young children. However, the literature does not provide sufficient evidence to definitively answer the question of when (at what age and in what circumstances) the posterior capsule should be left intact. Visually significant posterior capsule opacification develops most commonly about 18 months to 2 years after surgery when the posterior capsule is left intact. Therefore, it is reasonable to leave the posterior capsule unopened if it is anticipated that the child will be cooperative for a YAG laser capsulotomy 18 months to 2 years after surgery. However, it is now well known that some (one third or more) YAG laser capsulotomies will close spontaneously when performed in young children (<6 years of age or so). The practice of leaving the posterior capsule intact in all children at the time of surgery and bringing them back to the operating room 6 weeks later for a YAG laser capsulotomy has been described, but did not find wide spread acceptance because of the recurrence of VAO. Vertically mounted YAG lasers designed for use in the operating room are now difficult to find because of their infrequent use.

Generally speaking, we recommend leaving the posterior capsule intact when children present for cataract surgery at age 8 years or older (see Fig. 16-3). We will perform a primary posterior capsulotomy at any age if YAG laser availability is in question, a posterior capsule anomaly (plaque, defect, etc.) is present, or the child is developmentally delayed or uncooperative for YAG laser capsulotomy.

DO I NEED TO PERFORM AN ANTERIOR VITRECTOMY WHENEVER I PERFORM A POSTERIOR CAPSULOTOMY?

In general, in patients up to 5 years of age, this is an *essential* step, since vitreous face opacification is likely to occur if an anterior vitrectomy is not performed. However, in children between 5 and 8 years of age, it is an *optional* step since the chances are better that a posterior capsulotomy (posterior capsulorhexis) alone will result in a long-term clear visual axis. Nonetheless, a pars plana anterior vitrectomy may be needed secondary to vitreous face opacification anytime a posterior capsulorhexis is done without an anterior vitrectomy.

FIGURE 16-2. Five and a half-year-old child operated for bilateral cataract and IOL implantation. Right eye received posterior capsulotomy (but no vitrectomy) and left eye received posterior capsulotomy and vitrectomy. At 18 months postoperative period, the right eye was noted to have translucent opacification of the visual axis (**A**) and the left eye was clear (**B**).

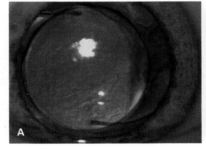
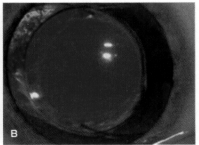

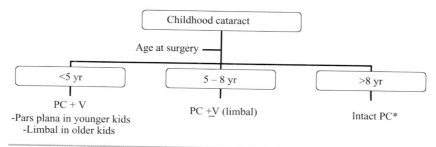

FIGURE 16-3. Schematic diagram showing our recommendation for posterior capsule management. PC, posterior capsulotomy (manual or automated); V, vitrectomy. *Leave intact posterior capsule behind. Eight years is an arbitrary age. It may need to be modified according to the availability of a YAG laser, the child's expected cooperation for YAG approximately 2 years after cataract surgery, or the cataract's being associated with a dense posterior capsule plaque or preexisting posterior capsule defect.

HOW SHOULD I TREAT THE POSTERIOR CAPSULE? SO MANY OPTIONS: WHICH TO CHOOSE?

Various options are available for posterior capsulotomy and vitrectomy in children. Selection among the various technical alternatives is probably best left to the individual surgeon's preference based on the individual case, available facilities, individual circumstances, and personal experience.

1. Primary capsulotomy versus secondary capsulotomy
2. Surgical capsulotomy versus YAG laser capsulotomy
3. Type of surgical opening: Capsulorhexis or capsulotomy?
4. Limbal versus pars plana approach
5. Before versus after IOL implantation
6. Architecture of the posterior capsule opening: size, centricity, and shape
7. Does no-suture vitrectomy technology have a role?
8. Are special aids or techniques for visualization needed?
9. How is the end point of the vitrectomy defined? How much vitreous should be removed?

Primary Capsulotomy Versus Secondary Capsulotomy

Posterior capsulotomy may be performed at the time of cataract removal or secondarily. Most pediatric cataract surgeons now prefer to manage the posterior capsule at the time of cataract surgery. Parks[1,7] was an early proponent of primary posterior capsulotomy and vitrectomy. He stated, "It should be abundantly clear that the best visual acuity in patients with intractable amblyopia is usually far worse than the best acuity in recovered clinically significant cystoid macular oedema (CME)." He further asked, "How can invasion of the vitreous during a secondary procedure to open the translucent membraneous posterior lens capsule be less likely to cause CME than opening the posterior capsule during the primary lens surgery?" CME turned out to occur much less frequently in children after posterior capsulotomy and anterior vitrectomy than originally feared. Remarkably, retinal detachment rates have also been very low after this procedure, owing in part to the formed vitreous of the child's eye. With the advent of higher-quality vitrectomy machines and sharp, high-speed cutting handpieces, the procedure is even safer than when Parks and others popularized it.

We recommend continuing to treat the posterior capsule as a primary procedure in young children until a method is developed to predictably kill residual lens epithelial cells and reduce the likelihood of postoperative VAO.

Surgical Capsulotomy Versus YAG Laser Capsulotomy

Nd–YAG laser capsulotomy can be used as a primary or secondary posterior capsulotomy (Fig. 16-4). Although YAG lasers were most commonly used to perform secondary capsulotomy, it became possible to perform primary

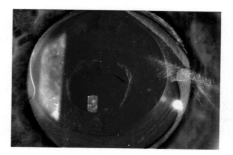

FIGURE 16-4. Nd-YAG laser has been successfully accomplished in this child's eye returning the visual acuity to 20/20.

▶ TABLE 16-1 Surgical Versus Nd–YAG Laser Posterior Capsulotomy

Surgical Capsulotomy	Nd–YAG Laser Capsulotomy
Need anesthesia	Anesthesia can be avoided.
Reopacification rate is lower because it is possible to treat the anterior vitreous face also.	Reopacification rate is high because it is not possible to treat a scaffold of the anterior vitreous face.
Routinely used by most surgeons for primary capsulotomy	Reopacification rate, cost, and availability of YAG laser mounted on operative microscope preclude its routine use in the very young.

capsulotomy with the advent of YAG lasers mounted vertically and used with patients in the supine position. These instruments are rarely used today and are manufactured in small numbers if at all. Table 16-1 lists the pros and cons of both techniques.

In 1985 Maltzman et al.[11] described the outcome of YAG laser capsulotomy for secondary membranes in the pediatric population by using a standard office-based laser delivery system. However, this approach cannot be used for young or uncooperative children. A headrest was designed by Kaufman (cited in Ref. 11) for patients placed in the lateral decubitus position. This headrest allowed for treatment of anesthetized children, but it has not come into wide use. The Microruptor III laser system allows for controlled laser procedures in supine anesthetized patients and offers the advantage of being familiar to most surgeons.

Atkinson and Hiles,[12] in 1994, reported leaving the posterior capsule intact and performing Nd:YAG capsulotomy under a second general anesthesia in the early postoperative period. They reported a 28% recurrence rate with this technique. This method does not address the problem of the remaining intact anterior vitreous face, which is known to provide a scaffolding on which residual lens fibers grow to create secondary opaque membranes. Hutcheson et al.[13] examined the clarity of the visual axis after Nd:YAG laser capsulotomy following cataract extraction and primary IOL implantation in a pediatric population. A group of children who had been treated by primary surgical posterior capsulotomy and anterior vitrectomy (Group 1) was used as the "gold standard," with whom the children treated with Nd:YAG laser capsulotomy (Group 2) were compared. One eye (3%) in Group 1 experienced postoperative VAO. Thirteen (57%) of 23 eyes in Group 2 experienced reopacification, requiring retreatment. Four eyes (17%) treated with Nd:YAG laser required a third treatment.

Stager et al.[14] reported rates of posterior capsule opacification following foldable acrylic IOL implantation. The authors noted that 60% of the eyes developed recurrent opacification following Nd-YAG laser treatment in the younger age group (<4 years), which suggested that surgical capsulotomy combined with an anterior vitrectomy, rather than YAG laser capsulotomy, may be needed in these young children to keep the visual axis clear.

A transient rise in intraocular pressure has been described after use of a YAG laser in pediatric patients.[11] The cost and nonavailability of the instrument in children's hospitals or pediatric ophthalmology offices may be additional barriers to the use of the YAG laser. Many surgeons prefer to perform a surgical procedure initially that will, hopefully, preclude the need for laser capsulotomy.[15]

Type of Surgical Opening: Capsulorhexis or Capsulotomy?

Before moving forward, it is important to recapitulate the applied anatomy and physiology of the posterior lens capsule. Mechanical properties of the human posterior capsule differ in several aspects from those of the anterior capsule.[16]

The posterior lens capsule is substantially *thinner* than the anterior lens capsule. Krag and Andreassen[16] reported that the thickness of the posterior lens capsule ranged from 4 to 9 μm and showed no significant change with age. The posterior capsule was three to five times thinner than the anterior capsule.[16] The *mechanical strength* of the posterior lens capsule (ultimate strain, ultimate load, ultimate elastic stiffness, ultimate stress, and ultimate elastic modulus) was found to decrease markedly with age.[16] The age-related loss of mechanical strength seemed to begin earlier in the posterior lens capsule than in the anterior lens capsule.[16] Extensibility (ultimate strain) of the posterior lens capsule decreased by a factor of two during the lifespan, and the forces required to break the posterior lens capsule were found to decrease by a factor of five.[16]

The posterior capsule opening can be performed with the manual technique (capsulorhexis) or with a vitrector. Primary posterior capsulorhexis makes it possible to achieve an opening with a strong margin that resists peripheral extension of tears and holds the vitreous in place. It allows safe anterior vitrectomy and prevents uncontrolled widening of the opening. The IOL can be supported over the capsule, and if desired, optic capture can be obtained through the opening. When vitrectomy has been planned in addition to posterior capsulotomy, many surgeons prefer to use the vitrector to cut an opening instead of performing a manual posterior continuous curvilinear capsulorhexis (PCCC). The use of radiofrequency diathermy for this purpose has also been reported in the literature.[17] The radiofrequency bipolar unit is not easily manipulated beneath an IOL and is therefore usually performed on the posterior capsule from an anterior approach prior to IOL insertion.

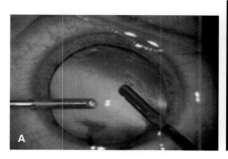
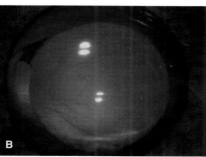

FIGURE 16-5. Limbal-approach posterior capsulectomy and vitrectomy. Note smaller opening of posterior capsule (than anterior capsule) and well-centered IOL.

Limbal Versus Pars Plana Approach

Preference for limbal over pars plana approach depends on several factors—age at surgery, condition of posterior capsule (plaque, defect, vascularization), whether or not IOL implantation is intended (see Figs. 16-5 to 16-10). Surgical approaches through the limbus[18] and pars plicata[8–10,19] have been described in the literature. Pros and cons of these techniques are listed in Table 16-2. Ahmadieh et al.[20] reported that inadequate size of the posterior capsule opening (<3 mm) was three times more common with the limbal route than the pars plana route. They further noted that fibrin formation was more common with the pars plana route than the limbal route (26 versus 21%; $P > .05$).

Our current strategy is to perform posterior capsulotomy and anterior vitrectomy via the limbal approach in children past their fourth birthday, although we think that other surgeons may make a different decision. In younger children, from birth through 3 years, it sometimes becomes particularly difficult to implant an IOL in a soft vitrectomized eye (unless the ciliary sulcus is the intended location of the IOL), and the pars plana approach (after IOL implantation) is preferable. In cases in which IOL implantation has not been targeted, the limbal approach should be used in any age group (Fig. 16-6).

Before Versus After IOL Implantation

There is no agreement on whether the IOL should be implanted before or after the primary posterior capsulectomy and anterior vitrectomy. Some advocate removing the

posterior capsule and anterior vitreous before IOL implantation. Others prefer to have the IOL in place before removing the posterior capsule to allow for an adequate posterior capsulectomy and better anterior vitrectomy.[2,21] The advantage is that the IOL can be safely fixed in the desired plane (Table 16-3).

The common practice is to do the posterior capsulotomy before IOL implantation if the limbal approach has been used (see Fig. 16-5). However, if the pars plana approach is used, in general, the posterior capsulotomy and vitrectomy should be performed after IOL implantation (Figs. 16-7 to 16-9). However, some surgeons prefer to do a limbal-approach retropseudophakic vitrectomy, a technique reported by Mackool and Chhatiawala[22] in 1991. Therefore, after implantation of an IOL, posterior capsulectomy and vitrectomy can be performed via the limbal approach. This approach can be used in primary as well as secondary opacification.

Our current approach is to perform IOL implantation after limbal vitrectomy in older children, beyond their fourth birthday, and IOL implantation before pars plana vitrectomy otherwise. In infantile eyes, the rigidity of the sclera is very low. Squire[23] noted that the thickness of the infantile sclera was 0.4 times, and the coefficient of stretching 0.6 times, that of the adult. IOL implantation is technically difficult in these eyes with low scleral rigidity. Additional vitrectomy adds to the difficulty by making for a softer eye.

However, in the presence of a large posterior capsule plaque, we prefer to implant an IOL before posterior capsulotomy in children of any age (Fig. 16-9). If a large posterior capsule opening is needed to encompass the

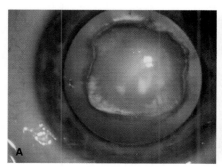
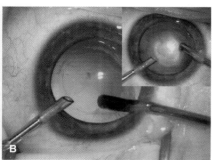

FIGURE 16-6. Three-month-old child operated for cataract surgery **A.** Preoperative appearance. **B.** Surgical photos. Note dense plaque on posterior capsule (B-insert). As IOL implantation was not the intended management for this eye, the limbal approach was used. A large posterior capsulotomy was required to encompass the plaque. If IOL implantation had been intended, we would have used the pars plicata approach in this eye (after IOL implantation).

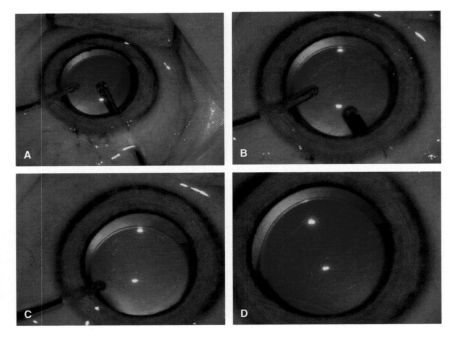

FIGURE 16-7. Pars plana posterior capsulectomy and vitrectomy (after IOL implantation). **A.** The vitrector has been placed 2.5 mm posterior to the limbus. **B.** A round posterior capsulotomy is made with cutting port facing anterior. **C.** Irrigation is from an anterior approach. **D.** The completed surgery reveals a well centered posterior capsulotomy and a capsular-fixated IOL.

plaque, this may hamper secure in-the-bag placement (if IOL implantation is performed after posterior capsulectomy and vitrectomy).

Architecture of the Posterior Capsule Opening: Size, Centricity, and Shape

Ideally one should aim to achieve an optimum-size (ca. 1 to 1.5 mm smaller than the IOL optic) centric, circular opening in the posterior capsule.

During the early 1990s, many pediatric ophthalmologists recommended removing all but 1 or 2 mm of the peripheral posterior lens capsule during pediatric cataract surgery. Caputo et al.[24] described a method of using a small central posterior capsulectomy for pediatric cataracts that is designed to eliminate VAO and to keep open the

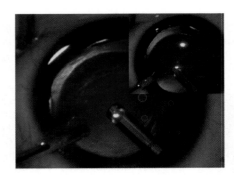

FIGURE 16-8. Pars plana posterior capsulectomy and anterior vitrectomy after IOL implantation. (Main figure photo shows vitrectomy being performed after completion of posterior capsulectomy) (insert shows capsulectomy being enlarged in a circular fashion by the cutter in the vitrector handpiece).

option of later secondary implantation of a posterior chamber IOL. However, if a very small posterior chamber opening is made, the chances for closure and synechiae increase. The size of the PCCC is most important when attempting to capture the optic of the IOL. The optimum size (neither too small, which makes it difficult to capture the optic, nor too large, in which case the optic may not remain captured) is a prerequisite for ideal and stable capture.

Does No-Suture Vitrectomy Technology Have a Role?

Sutureless pars plana vitrectomy through self-sealing sclerotomies has been reported in the literature.[25–27] Kwok et al.[28] described the ultrabiomicroscopy of conventional and sutureless pars plana sclerotomies. They concluded that ultrabiomicroscopy showed no difference in the amount of visible vitreous incarceration in conventionally sutured versus sutureless sclerotomies. However, several complications have been reported with this technique, including wound leakage, extension, dehiscence, hemorrhage, vitreous and/or retinal incarceration, retinal tear, and retinal dialysis. Difficulty with passage of instruments has also been observed when tunnels are used. In addition, the scleral tunnel technique still requires conjuctival dissection, which often requires suturing. Fujii et al.[26] reported a 25-gauge vitrectomy system that allows for completely sutureless vitrectomy surgery, which can be performed without scleral or conjunctival suture.

Lam et al.[29] evaluated the safety and efficacy of sutureless pars plana anterior vitrectomy through self-sealing sclerotomies in children with thick posterior pseudophakic membranes (secondary capsulectomy and vitrectomy).

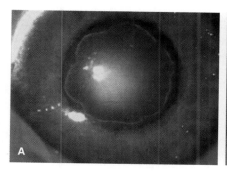
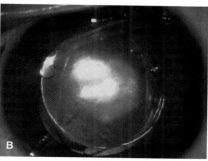

FIGURE 16-9. In the presence of a dense plaque **A,** it is better to perform the posterior capsulectomy and vitrectomy after IOL placement **B.**

They commented that although the scleral rigidity in children is lower, the self-sealing effect of this technique is good, with the integrity of the eyes well maintained. The authors concluded that the sutureless sclerotomy approach appears to be safe and effective and can be considered in selected cases.

Are Special Aids or Techniques for Visualization Needed?

Use of dye for posterior capsulorhexis has been described in the literature.[30–32] Details of this technique are given in Chapter 17. Dyes have been used less frequently for the posterior than for the anterior capsule.

Kenalog injection into the anterior chamber provides the anterior segment surgeon a means for localizing and identifying vitreous gel.[33] Clear visualization of the vitreous gel allows thorough removal of the prolapsed vitreous and alerts surgeons to residual strands of vitreous that might have gone unnoticed. It also allows surgeons to observe vitreous behavior so that they can avoid maneuvers that increase vitreous traction or prolapse.

How Is the End Point of the Vitrectomy Defined? How Much Vitreous Should Be Removed?

These questions have not been answered in a scientific manner. Sufficient vitreous should be removed centrally so that the lens epithelial cells cannot use the vitreous face as a scaffolding to create VAO. Any vitreous that tracks forward past the plane of the posterior capsulotomy needs to be removed. VAO after primary posterior

capsulotomy and anterior vitrectomy is often blamed on an inadequate posterior capsule opening or an inadequate vitrectomy. These assertions have not been verified scientifically. Most surgeons advise a "generous" anterior vitrectomy without placing the vitrector so deep that visualization would require a posterior vitrectomy viewing attachment to the operating microscope. As mentioned before, Kenalog can be injected into the anterior chamber to aid in visualization and thorough removal. Swiping the iris repositor can help to identify vitreous in the wound.[4–6]

TECHNIQUE

Posterior Capsulotomy

The technique of PCCC has been well described in the literature. After aspiration of the lens matter with two-port automated irrigation/aspiration, the capsule bag and anterior chamber are filled with high-viscosity sodium hyaluronate (Healon-GV or Healon-5) and posterior capsulorhexis is initiated. The central posterior capsule is thinnest. Grasp of the capsule is difficult at the initial stage. Therefore, initiation of the puncture and flap is better done with the help of the vertical element of the cystitome. The 26-gauge cystitome needle descends on the capsule at a slant. It engages the central capsule, lifts it up toward the surgeon, and, at the same time, initiates the puncture. A small flap is created by pushing the margin of the puncture inferiorly. High-viscosity sodium hyaluronate is injected through the puncture between the capsule and the vitreous face. This should be done slowly. Forceful injection through the tear can extend it toward the periphery. Then additional viscoelastic should be placed over the posterior

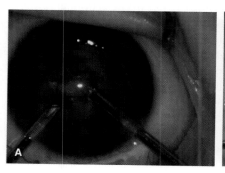
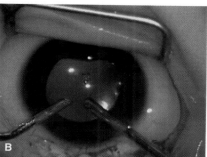

FIGURE 16-10. Vascularized plaque in an eye with persistent fetal vasculature (**A**). In this case, the IOL was placed in the ciliary sulcus with the optic captured in the anterior capsulotomy since most of the posterior capsule had to be removed to clear the plaque. Bleeding from the fetal vessels cleared spontaneously in the first postoperative week (**B**).

▶ TABLE 16-2 Limbal Versus Pars Plana Posterior Capsulectomy and Vitrectomy

	Limbal	Pars Plana
Cauterization	Can be avoided	Required
Size	Adequate size may not be obtained since IOL yet to be implanted (usually)	Larger opening is possible since IOL already in place
IOL implantation	Relatively difficult. It is common practice to perform limbal vitrectomy before IOL implantation. It is sometimes difficult to implant in soft vitrectomized eyes of young infants.	Relatively easy to implant in nonvitrectomized eye with posterior capsule still intact, as these are generally performed after IOL implantation when using this technique
Surgeon comfort and familiarity	Most anterior segment surgeons more accustomed to limbal approach	Most anterior segment surgeons not routinely accustomed to pars plana approach
Viscoelastic removal	More difficult since it is done after the posterior capsule is open	Easier since the removal is usually done after IOL insertion and before posterior capsulotomy
Posterior capsule plaque	Easy but posterior opening may need to be large and this would complicate in-the-bag insertion of IOL	Easy to insert IOL with plaque still present and remove posterior capsule through the pars plana—plaque makes posterior capsule easy to see under the IOL and opening can be safely made larger
Traction of vitreous base	If a vitreous strand remains attached to anterior wound, traction on retina is increased	Less likely to result in vitreous attached to anterior wound

capsule surrounding the puncture. This flattens the central posterior capsule and reduces potential peripheral extension. The flap is then held with capsulorhexis forceps and posterior capsulorhexis is accomplished. Frequent grasping and viscomanipulation of the flap becomes necessary. Posterior capsulorhexis can also be performed after placement of an IOL. This ensures IOL fixation in the desired plane. However, performing PCCC and anterior vitrectomy become more difficult with this method.

Vitrectomy

Machemer et al.[34] developed the vitreous infusion suction cutter in the early 1970s. The advent of the vitrectomy machine reduced the rate of retinal detachment as a late

▶ TABLE 16-3 Posterior Capsulotomy Before or After IOL Implantation?

Before IOL Implantation	After IOL Implantation
■ If capsulotomy extends during procedure, it may hamper achieving successful in-the-bag fixation.	■ Stable IOL fixation can be achieved.
■ IOL implantation becomes difficult in soft nonvitrectomized eyes.	■ IOL implantation is relatively easy.
■ Posterior capsulectomy and vitrectomy can be achieved under better visibility.	■ Visibility may be poor.
■ Generally aimed at a smaller opening to facilitate IOL implantation.	■ A wide posterior capsule opening can be achieved.

complication of pediatric cataract surgery. Similar to an anterior vitrectorhexis, a Venturi pump system is recommended, as it cuts the capsule more easily than a peristaltic pump. We recommend that readers follow the instruction manual of the manufacturer for using a specific machine and setting.

The unique surgical anatomy of infant eyes requires modification of standard vitreous surgery techniques. In addition to its small size, the infant eye differs from that of the adult with respect to the spatial relationship of various ocular structures. A major anatomic constraint is imposed by the relative size of the pars plana. In the newborn eye, the pars plana region is incompletely developed so that the anterior retina lies just behind the pars plicata. To avoid iatrogenic retinal breaks, entry incisions for vitreoretinal surgery, therefore, are made through or anterior to the region of the pars plicata.[35]

Aiello et al.[36] noted that the temporal ciliary body is longer than the nasal ciliary body in the pediatric age groups as well as in adults. These authors noted that the pars plana was 2.2 and 2.5 for the nasal and temporal aspect at <6 months of age, 2.7 and 3 at 6–12 months, 3.0 and 3.1 at 1–2 years of age, and 3.2 and 3.8 at 2–6 years of age. They estimated that the dimensions of the ciliary body in the vertical meridian fall between the measurements of the nasal and the temporal ciliary body, as observed in adults.

Good success has been reported with two-port phakic vitrectomies in infants when the sclerotomies were made 0.5 mm posterior to the limbus.[35] The most rapid phase of pars plana growth occurs at between 26 and 35 weeks of gestation. At full term, the mean pars plana width is 1.87 mm (range, 0.9 to 2.8 mm). Not until 62 weeks after conception does the pars plana attain a width >3 mm. Therefore, anatomically, it may be that a pars plana vitrectomy can be safely performed only after 62 weeks postconception.

Reporting the outcome of vitrectomy for infantile vitreous hemorrhage, Ferrone and de Juan[37] noted that two eyes had a retinal dialysis. The authors hypothesized that a potential reason for these dialyses was that the sclerotomies were 2 mm posterior to the limbus. This may be too far posterior in these young, developing eyes. In very young patients, it may also be that the pars plana is not wide enough to perform a pars plana vitrectomy safely. The two patients with dialyses in this series were only 44 and 47 weeks postconceptional. Hairston et al.[38] reported that the dimension of the pars plana is correlated closely with axial length and postconceptional age. A linear relationship between pars plana width and axial length existed once the axial length reached 12 mm. In cataractous eyes, the axial length may be even shorter, so we can assume that the pars plana is shorter also.

Considering the above, our current approach is to enter ≤2 mm (depending on the axial length of the eye) posterior to the limbus in patients <1 year old, 2.5 mm posterior in patients 1 to 4 years old, and 3 mm posterior in patients >4 years old. The entry angles should be toward the center of the vitreous when entering at 3 mm, however, it must be adjusted toward the optic disc when a more anterior entry site is used to avoid the equator of the capsular bag. Meier et al.[39] have recommended distances of 1.5, 2.0, and 2.5 mm at <3, 3–6, and >6 months of age, respectively.

As stated above, in the eye of the mature neonate, the pars plicata of the ciliary body is almost fully developed, whereas the pars plana is hardly established. *In the absence of the pars plana, ideally we should use the term* pars plicata posterior capsulectomy and anterior vitrectomy *in infants instead of the so-called pars plana* posterior capsulectomy and anterior vitrectomy *as used in recent literature.*

While performing vitrectomy during pediatric cataract surgery, the aim is to remove the central anterior vitreous without attempting to remove all of the peripheral or posterior vitreous. For this limited vitrectomy, we perform the procedure through two ports. Separating the irrigation from the cutting and aspiration reduces hydration of the vitreous. With an ocutome system (ATIOP) the reported desirable machine settings are a cut rate of 350 cuts/min, an aspiration flow rate of 20 mL/min, and a vacuum of 100 mm Hg.[5,6] Modern vitrectors have higher cut rates, and most now recommend that the vitreous be cut at a rate of at least 500 cuts/min. On the Accurus machine, we use an irrigation rate of ≤30 and a cutting rate of ≥500. At the end of the procedure, an iris spatula may be swiped from each port to rule out the possibility of vitreous strands entering the incisions. Buckley et al.[21] have mentioned a preplaced 8-0 Vicryl suture passed across the sclerotomy site to facilitate closure after vitreous removal.

Posterior Capsule Plaque

It is not uncommon to observe a plaque on the posterior capsule. This may be peeled free with a cystotome under sodium hyaluronate. It is also possible to do a large PCCC to encompass the plaque or to do a mechanized capsulotomy and vitrectomy large enough to fully remove the plaque. Other pathology associated with the posterior capsule such as a preexisting defect or persistent fetal vasculature (see Fig. 16-10) is discussed in other chapters. In the case of a preexisting defect, an attempt should be made to convert the preexisting opening into a primary PCCC with a Utrata forceps under high-viscosity sodium hyaluronate.

Secondary Surgical Posterior Capsulotomy

Removal of the center of the posterior capsule does not guarantee that secondary cataracts will not regrow, especially in young infants. When this occurs, an irrigation cannula is usually placed into the anterior chamber through a paracentesis incision. The posterior capsulectomy and vitrectomy are usually done through a pars plana entry if an IOL is present and is within the capsular bag. Sometimes the opacification can be easily reached from the limbal position by placing the vitrector posterior to the edge of the anterior capsulorhexis and then posterior to the IOL optic. Occasionally, a combined approach (anterior and posterior) may be needed to remove reproliferated cortex from both sides of the IOL.

CONCLUSION

To summarize, posterior capsulectomy and vitrectomy are an essential surgical step in the management of pediatric cataract surgery. Treatment of the posterior capsule determines the ultimate outcome of pediatric cataract surgery. Various alternatives have been suggested in the literature to achieve this goal. We need to choose the way in which the posterior capsule is managed for each patient based on the multiple factors discussed in this chapter.

REFERENCES

1. Parks MM. Management of the posterior capsule in congenital cataracts. *J Pediatr Ophthalmol Strabismus* 1984;21:114–117.
2. Alexandrakis G, Peterseim MM, Wilson ME. Clinical outcomes of pars plana capsulotomy with anterior vitrectomy in pediatric cataract surgery. *J AAPOS* 2002;6:163–167.
3. BenEzra D, Cohen E. Posterior capsulectomy in pediatric cataract surgery: the necessity of a choice. *Ophthalmology* 1997;104:2168–2174.
4. Vasavada A, Desai J. Primary posterior capsulorhexis with and without anterior vitrectomy in congenital cataracts. *J Cataract Refract Surg* 1997;23 (Suppl) 1:645–651.

5. Vasavada AR, Trivedi RH. Role of optic capture in congenital cataract and intraocular lens surgery in children. *J Cataract Refract Surg* 2000;26:824–831.

6. Vasavada AR, Trivedi RH, Singh R. Necessity of vitrectomy when optic capture is performed in children older than 5 years. *J Cataract Refract Surg* 2001;27:1185–1193.

7. Parks MM. Posterior lens capsulectomy during primary cataract surgery in children. *Ophthalmology* 1983;90:344–345.

8. Peyman GA, Sanders DR, Rose M, Korey M. Vitrophage in management of congenital cataracts. *Albrecht Von Graefes Arch Klin Exp Ophthalmol* 1977;202:305–308.

9. Peyman GA, Raichand M, Goldberg MF. Surgery of congenital and juvenile cataracts: a pars plicata approach with the vitrophage. *Br J Ophthalmol* 1978;62:780–783.

10. Peyman GA, Raichand M, Oesterle C, Goldberg MF. Pars plicata lensectomy and vitrectomy in the management of congenital cataracts. *Ophthalmology* 1981;88:437–439.

11. Maltzman BA, Caputo AR, Wagner RS, Celebre LJ. Neodymium:YAG laser capsulotomy of secondary membranes in the pediatric population. *J Am Intra-Oc Implant Soc* 1985;11:572–573.

12. Atkinson CS, Hiles DA. Treatment of secondary posterior capsular membranes with the Nd:YAG laser in a pediatric population. *Am J Ophthalmol* 1994;118:496–501.

13. Hutcheson KA, Drack AV, Ellish NJ, Lambert SR. Anterior hyaloid face opacification after pediatric Nd:YAG laser capsulotomy. *J AAPOS* 1999;3:303–307.

14. Stager DR Jr, Weakley DR Jr, Hunter JS. Long-term rates of PCO following small incision foldable acrylic intraocular lens implantation in children. *J Pediatr Ophthalmol Strabismus* 2002;39:73–76.

15. Koch DD, Kohnen T. A retrospective comparison of techniques to prevent secondary cataract formation following posterior chamber intraocular lens implantation in infants and children. *Trans Am Ophthalmol Soc* 1997;95:351–360, discussion 361–365.

16. Krag S, Andreassen TT. Mechanical properties of the human posterior lens capsule. *Invest Ophthalmol Vis Sci* 2003;44:691–696.

17. Comer RM, Abdulla N, O'Keefe M. Radiofrequency diathermy capsulorhexis of the anterior and posterior capsules in pediatric cataract surgery: preliminary results. *J Cataract Refract Surg* 1997;1:641–644.

18. Calhoun JH, Harley RD. The roto-extractor in pediatric ophthalmology. *Trans Am Ophthalmol Soc* 1975;73:292–305.

19. Green BF, Morin JD, Brent HP. Pars plicata lensectomy/vitrectomy for developmental cataract extraction: surgical results. *J Pediatr Ophthalmol & Strabismus* 1990;27:229–232.

20. Ahmadieh H, Javadi MA, Ahmady M, Karimian F, Einollahi B, Zare M, et al. Primary capsulectomy, anterior vitrectomy, lensectomy, and posterior chamber lens implantation in children: limbal versus pars plana. *J Cataract Refrac Surg* 1999;25:768–775.

21. Buckley EG, Klombers LA, Seaber JH, Scalise-Gordy A, Minzter R. Management of the posterior capsule during pediatric intraocular lens implantation. *Am J Ophthalmol* 1993;115:722–728.

22. Mackool RJ, Chhatiawala H. Pediatric cataract surgery and intraocular lens implantation: a new technique for preventing or excising postoperative secondary membranes. *J Cataract Refract Surg* 1991;17:62–66.

23. Squire C. Cited in Kwitko ML. *The Infant Eye.*

24. Caputo AR, Guo S, Wagner RS, Constad WH. A modified extracapsular cataract extraction for pediatric cataracts. *Ophthal Surg* 1990;21:396–400.

25. Fujii GY, de Juan E Jr, Humayun MS, et al. Initial experience using the transconjunctival sutureless vitrectomy system for vitreoretinal surgery. *Ophthalmology* 2002;109:1814–1820.

26. Fujii GY, de Juan E Jr, Humayun MS, et al. A new 25-gauge instrument system for transconjunctival sutureless vitrectomy surgery. *Ophthalmology* 2002;109:1807–1812, discussion 1813.

27. Chen JC. Sutureless pars plana vitrectomy through self-sealing sclerotomies. *Arch Ophthalmol* 1996;114:1273–1275.

28. Kwok AK, Tham CC, Loo AV, Fan DS, Lam DS. Ultrasound biomicroscopy of conventional and sutureless pars plana sclerotomies: a comparative and longitudinal study. *Am J Ophthalmol* 2001;132:172–177.

29. Lam DS, Chua JK, Leung AT, Fan DS, Ng JS, Rao SK. Sutureless pars plana anterior vitrectomy through self-sealing sclerotomies in children. *Arch Ophthalmol* 2000;118:850–851.

30. Pandey SK, Werner L, Escobar-Gomez M, Werner LP, Apple DJ. Dye-enhanced cataract surgery. Part 3: posterior capsule staining to learn posterior continuous curvilinear capsulorhexis. *J Cataract Refract Surg* 2000;26:1066–1071.

31. Wakabayashi T, Yamamoto N. Posterior capsule staining and posterior continuous curvilinear capsulorhexis in congenital cataract. *J Cataract Refract Surg* 2002;28:2042–2044.

32. Saini JS, Jain AK, Sukhija J, Gupta P, Saroha V. Anterior and posterior capsulorhexis in pediatric cataract surgery with or without trypan blue dye: randomized prospective clinical study. *J Cataract Refract Surg* 2003;29:1733–1737.

33. Burk SE, Da Mata AP, Synder ME, Schneider S, Osher RH, Cionni RJ. Visualizing vitreous using Kenalog suspension. *J Cataract Refract Surg* 2003;29:645–651.

34. Machemer R, Parel JM, Buettner H. A new concept for vitreous surgery. I. Instrumentation. *Am J Ophthalmol.* 1972;73:1–7.

35. Maguire AM, Trese MT. Lens-sparing vitreoretinal surgery in infants. *Arch Ophthalmol* 1992;110:284–286.

36. Aiello AL, Tran VT, Rao NA. Postnatal development of the ciliary body and pars plana. A morphometric study in childhood. *Arch Ophthalmol* 1992;110:802–805.

37. Ferrone PJ, de Juan E Jr. Vitreous hemorrhage in infants. *Arch Ophthalmol* 1994;112:1185–1189.

38. Hairston RJ, Maguire AM, Vitale S, Green WR. Morphometric analysis of pars plana development in humans. *Retina* 1997;17:135–138.

39. Meier P, Sterker I, Wiedemann P. Pars plana lentectomy for treatment of congenital cataract. *Graefes Arch Clin Exp Ophthalmol* 2001;239:649–655.

Dye-Enhanced Pediatric Cataract Surgery

Suresh K. Pandey

During the past few years there has been enormous interest in the use of vital dyes to enhance visualization during various steps of ophthalmic surgeries. In this chapter, we present applications of the two most commonly used dyes, trypan blue and indocyanine green (ICG), for anterior and posterior capsulorhexis in pediatric cataract surgery. We have also provided guidelines and recommendations for ophthalmic surgeons, based on the published experimental and clinical studies.

Use of 0.5% ICG and 0.1% trypan blue dye for anterior capsule staining was reported by Horiguchi et al.[1] and Melles et al.[2] A clinical study comparing both dyes was first reported by Chang.[3] Pandey and associates[4–7] extensively studied three types of capsular dyes—fluorescein sodium, ICG, and trypan blue—for anterior and posterior capsule staining. These experimental studies demonstrated that 0.5% ICG and 0.1% trypan blue dyes can be successfully used to stain the posterior lens capsule to enhance visualization while learning and performing posterior capsulorhexis, a technically challenging procedure (Figs. 17-1 and 17-2).[5] According to recently published reports, ophthalmic dyes are increasingly being used to facilitate anterior and posterior capsulorhexis during pediatric cataract surgery.[8–10] Intraoperative use of trypan blue to stain lens epithelial cell during pediatric cataract surgery has also been recently reported.[11]

Experimental studies using 0.5% ICG and 0.1% trypan blue for staining the posterior capsule, while performing posterior continuous curvilinear capsulorhexis (PCCC) in pediatric eyes, demonstrated that dye-enhanced visualization may help make this difficult maneuver safer (Fig. 17-2).[5] Posterior capsule staining also helps identify the presence of a posterior capsule tear as shown in Figure 17-2B.

PREPARATION OF THE DYES

Trypan blue is commercially available and ready for injection, requiring no dilution. Preparation of the ICG for capsule staining can be accomplished at the beginning of the surgical day. ICG can be prepared as described by Horiguchi and associates.[1] In brief, 0.5 mL of the provided diluent is mixed with the dry ICG powder, then 4.5 mL of balanced salt solution is added and the solution is mixed. This can be used for multiple cases throughout the surgical day.

AVAILABILITY AND COST OF THE DYES

Trypan blue has been recently approved by the U.S. Food and Drug Administration for anterior capsular staining. ICG dye is available in the United States, being approved for choroidal angiography. However, labeling issues prevent packaging of the ICG dye in a smaller, more cost-effective quantity. A 0.1% solution of trypan blue is commercially available under the trade name VisionBlue (Dutch Ophthalmic Research Company, the Netherlands). The 0.1% Vision Blue solution is ready for injection, requiring no dilution. At the time of this writing, the cost of 0.5-mL ampoule of VisionBlue is $5, compared to $90 for a 25-mg ampoule of ICG powder.

SURGICAL TECHNIQUE

A 0.5% solution of ICG and a 0.1% solution of trypan blue are commonly used to stain anterior or posterior lens capsules. For anterior capsulorhexis, ICG or trypan blue may be used under an air bubble. Posterior capsule staining can be done by instilling 1 drop of the dye solution into the capsular bag, after cortical cleanup. After 60–90 sec, the excessive dye is washed out. After the capsular bag is filled with viscoelastics (Healon; AMO Inc., Santa Ana, California), PCCC can be initiated using a 26-gauge needle cystotome. PCCC is completed using a Utrata's forceps. Optic capture of a posterior chamber intraocular lens (IOL), as well as anterior vitrectomy, can also be performed, if required.

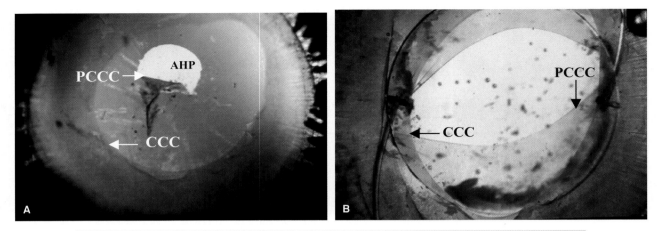

FIGURE 17-1. Gross photographs of a human eye obtained postmortem showing posterior continuous curvilinear capsulorhexis (PCCC) after staining of the capsular bag with indocyanine green. Cornea and iris were excised to allow better visualization. **A.** Anterior (surgeon's) view of the cleaned and stained capsular bag showing initiation of the PCCC. Note that it is easier to visualize the stained posterior capsule flap against the transparent (nonstained) anterior hyaloid face of the vitreous. **B.** Posterior capture of the intraocular lens (IOL) optic. Both IOL haptics are present in the capsular bag and the IOL optic is captured behind the posterior capsule.

Our experimental studies revealed that posterior capsule staining using ICG or trypan blue is very helpful when performing the PCCC procedure in children.[5] Recent clinical reports from other centers confirmed the experimental findings using these dyes to stain the posterior capsule when performing PCCC.[8,9] Wakabayashi and Yamamoto[8] reported using ICG staining for the anterior and posterior capsules combined in congenital cataracts. In their case of congenital cataract in a 6-month-old child, the visibility of both the anterior and the posterior capsules was poor without staining because of the corneal opacity. After cataract removal, ICG staining was used to better visualize the posterior capsule. PCCC was successfully completed because of the better visualization of the stained posterior capsule flap against the transparent anterior hyaloid face of the vitreous. Clear visual axes have been maintained post-operatively.

Learning and perfecting the anterior and posterior capsulorhexis procedure during pediatric cataract surgery, and achieving a consistent size of the anterior and posterior capsule opening for performing optic capture, can be difficult for the beginning surgeon due to the thin and transparent nature of the capsules. This is especially important in infantile eyes, which are particularly associated with a thin sclera and a positive vitreous pressure, thus making anterior and posterior capsulorhexis even

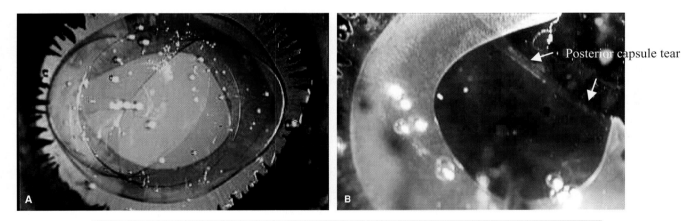

FIGURE 17-2. Dye-enhanced pediatric cataract surgery. Photographs of a pediatric eye obtained postmortem, taken from the anterior (surgeon's) view, illustrating the use of the capsular dye to enhance visualization during the pediatric cataract surgery. **A.** Posterior capsulorhexis and optic capture of a foldable intraocular lens after staining of the capsular bag with trypan blue. **B.** Visualization of a posterior capsule tear after staining of the capsular bag with indocyanine green.

more difficult than in older children or adults. It is relatively easy to perform a PCCC with IOL optic capture after staining the posterior capsule (Fig. 17-2).[5] Vitreous loss can also be identified by the formation of colored localized clumps, depending on the type of dye used. Even when utilizing the vitrector to open the posterior capsule, visualization of the capsulotomy edge can be difficult and would be enhanced by use of a dye. Also, IOL insertion into a soft pediatric eye after CCC and PCCC can be very difficult. Adequate visualization of the remaining capsule and of the capsulotomy edges is paramount to avoid inadvertent sulcus placement, asymmetric bag–sulcus fixation, or dislocation of the IOL through the PCCC.

SAFETY AND EFFICACY

Several laboratory, animal, and clinical studies have evaluated capsular dyes and capsule staining techniques for safety and efficacy during adult cataract surgery. Horiguchi et al.[1] reported the technique of staining the anterior capsule using a 2% solution of ICG in patients with mature cataracts. They compared the results of phacoemulsification and IOL implantation in two groups of 10 eyes. In the first group, the anterior capsule was stained with ICG before CCC, and in the second, no dye was used. No statistically significant difference was found between the two groups concerning specular microscopy endothelial cell counting or laser flare-cell photometry, thus the staining procedure was considered to be safe.

Clinical experience with ICG and trypan blue for anterior capsule staining in mature white or brunescent cataracts was first reported by David Chang[3] in two consecutive, nonrandomized series of mature or brunescent cataracts. The technique of dye injection under an air bubble was utilized. ICG dye was used in the first series, and trypan blue in the subsequent series. According to the author, both dyes provided consistently excellent visualization and clinical results, without any adverse effects. However, trypan blue created a more intense and persistent staining and provided superior visualization compared with ICG, according to this first clinical study.[3]

We emphasize using care when performing anterior capsule staining in vitrectomized patients during pediatric cataract surgery. Inadvertent staining of the posterior lens capsule may occur secondary to diffusion of dye into the vitreous cavity, thereby obscuring the red reflex.[12] However, the trypan blue molecule is large and, under normal circumstances, does not appear to cross the intact zonula ciliaris (ciliary zonules). It is likely that an intact anterior hyaloid face would prevent bulk flow of dye into the vitreous cavity. The surgeon should avoid using any ophthalmic dyes in pediatric cataract surgery combined with implantation of hydrophilic acrylic lenses having a high water content (>70%), as this can lead to permanent staining (discoloration) of the IOL by some ophthalmic dyes.[13] This discoloration may become associated with a decrease or alteration in the best-corrected visual acuity and, eventually, require IOL explantation/exchange.[13]

In an ongoing study, Tehrani and associates found that the anterior lens capsule stained using trypan blue was actually weaker, and less force was required to begin the tear at the capsule edge (M. Tehrani, personal communication, November 2003). These authors performed special elasticity tests using fresh lens capsules, which were removed during routine cataract surgery in human eyes. One half of the excised capsule was dyed with VisionBlue; the other half (nonstained) was used as a control. Analysis of 15 capsules suggested that capsules that stayed in contact with the trypan blue were actually weaker, in that only half the strength was necessary to tear the capsule. The precise mechanism is not clear at present and requires further investigation. However, this phenomenon seems to be related to the presence of preservative in the trypan blue solution.

GUIDELINES AND RECOMMENDATIONS FOR SURGEONS

We would like to offer some recommendations and guidelines for ophthalmic surgeons regarding suitable ophthalmic dyes and anterior and posterior capsule staining technique in pediatric cataract surgery. These are based on our experience in postmortem human eyes, used in patients at our institution, as well as clinical reports published by several other surgeons. Both ICG and trypan blue are currently preferred over fluorescein sodium dye, because of their better staining of the anterior capsule and the absence of vitreous leakage (owing to their high molecular weight).[5] Both of these dyes provide excellent visualization of the anterior capsule flap during CCC, without causing any toxic effects to the corneal endothelium. Trypan blue has the advantage of being less costly than ICG; to the best of our knowledge, the cost of a 0.5-mL ampoule of VisionBlue is $5, compared to $90 for a 25-mg ampoule of ICG powder. Currently, 0.1% trypan blue is the concentration used by most surgeons. Further studies may be helpful to determine the lowest concentration of trypan blue dye (e.g., 0.05, 0.025, or 0.01%) that can be used to stain the anterior lens capsule to perform CCC.

Staining using the air bubble technique is safer and therefore recommended for cataract patients presenting with a high intralenticular pressure and a fragile anterior lens capsule (e.g., pediatric traumatic cataract). When injecting under air, the dye should be injected after paracentesis but prior to creating the main incision, to help with anterior chamber stability. Viscoelastic solutions can be used to viscoseal the incision site to prevent escape of the air bubble and to minimize any anterior chamber fluctuations. Alternatively, mixing the dye with a viscoelastic solution may also provide better anterior capsule staining and limit contact with adjacent ocular tissues.

Use of nontoxic ophthalmic dyes for anterior capsule staining in advanced, white pediatric cataracts allows the performance of a safe and successful CCC.[5,9,10] The dyes can also be helpful when training residents in the techniques of CCC and when performing CCC in cases presenting with nebular and/or macular corneal opacity. Anterior capsule staining can also be useful when converting from a can-opener technique to CCC. Surgeons who only rarely operate on children may also find anterior and posterior capsule staining useful as an aid to dealing with the elastic nature of the capsule and the increased tendency for runaway rhexis. Even when the cataract is not completely white, the learning curve when beginning CCC in unfamiliar territory (such as infantile cataract cases) can be shortened by enhanced visualization of the capsular edge. These dyes may be useful for surgery in adult and pediatric cataract cases with poor or no red reflex, or for the surgeon who is learning, or in developing world settings in which inexpensive surgical microscopes with imperfect coaxial light may be a necessity.

In summary, capsular dyes can be successfully used in pediatric cataract surgery for performing anterior and posterior capsulorhexis. Posterior capsulorhexis, a technically challenging procedure, is relatively easy to perform after staining of the otherwise transparent posterior capsule, as demonstrated for the first time in our experimental study (Figs. 17-1 and 17-2)[5] and confirmed by clinical studies.[8,9] Posterior capsule staining may be especially useful for posterior capsulorhexis procedures performed in younger children with poor visualization. In addition to anterior and posterior capsulorhexis, staining of the lens epithelial cells using trypan blue dye, to facilitate intraoperative

removal during pediatric cataract surgery, has also been suggested recently.[11]

REFERENCES

1. Horiguchi M, Miyake K, Ohta I, Ito Y. Staining of the lens capsule for circular continuous capsulorhexis in eyes with white cataract. *Arch Ophthalmol* 1998;116:535–537.
2. Melles GRJ, Waard PWT, Pameyer JH, Beekhuis WH. Trypan blue capsule staining in cataract surgery. *J Cataract Refract Surg* 1999;24:7–9.
3. Chang DF. Capsule staining and mature cataracts: a comparison of indocyanine green and trypan blue dyes. *Br J Ophthalmol* (video report), July 2000.
4. Pandey SK, Werner L, Escobar-Gomez M, Roig-Melo EA, Apple DJ. Dye-enhanced cataract surgery. Part 1: Anterior capsule staining for capsulorhexis in advanced/white cataract. *J Cataract Refract Surg* 2000;26:1052–1059.
5. Pandey SK, Werner L, Escobar-Gomez M, Werner LP, Apple DJ. Dye-enhanced cataract surgery. Part 3: Posterior capsule staining to learn posterior continuous curvilinear capsulorhexis. *J Cataract Refract Surg* 2000;26:1066–1071.
6. Pandey SK, Werner L, Apple DJ, Wilson ME. Dye-enhanced adult and pediatric cataract surgery. In: Buratto L, Werner L, Zanini M, Apple DJ, eds. *Phacoemulsification: Principles and Techniques.* Thorofare, NJ: Slack, 2002:chap 41.
7. Pandey SK, Werner L, Wilson ME, et al. Anterior capsule staining: current techniques, guidelines and recommendations. *Indian J Ophthalmol* 2002;50:157–159.
8. Wakabayashi T, Yamamoto N. Posterior capsule staining and posterior continuous curvilinear capsulorhexis in congenital cataract. *J Cataract Refract Surg* 2002;28:2042–2044.
9. Saini JS, Jain AK, Sukhija J, Gupta P, Saroha V. Anterior and posterior capsulorhexis in pediatric cataract surgery with or without trypan blue dye: randomized prospective clinical study. *J Cataract Refract Surg* 2003;29:1733–1737.
10. Guo S, Caputo A, Wagner R, DeRespinis P. Enhanced visualization of capsulorhexis with indocyanine green staining in pediatric white cataracts. *J Pediatr Ophthalmol Strabismus* 2003;40:268–271.
11. Kiel AW, Butler T, Gregson R. A novel use for trypan blue to minimize epithelial cell proliferation in pediatric cataract surgery. *J Pediatr Ophthalmol Strabismus* 2003;40:96–97.
12. Birchall W, Raynor MK, Turner GS. Inadvertent staining of the posterior lens capsule with trypan blue dye during phacoemulsification. *Arch Ophthalmol* 2001;119:1082–1083.
13. Werner L, Apple DJ, Crema AS, et al. Permanent blue discoloration of a hydrogel intraocular lens caused by intraoperative use of trypan blue. *J Cataract Refract Surg* 2002;28:1279–1286.

Applications of the Fugo Blade

Daljit Singh and Ravi Shankar Jit Singh

The Fugo Blade is a unique cutting instrument that employs plasma, the fourth state of matter, for ablating incision paths in tissue in a manner similar to the Excimer laser and is approved for intraocular use by the U.S. Food and Drug Administration (FDA).[1–4]

This unit is referred to as the *Fugo Blade* (after its inventor, Dr. Richard Fugo) in the United States. It is also known as the *Plasma Blade* in many other parts of the world, since it ablates with plasma energy. The instrument consists of a console, a handpiece with a disposable tip. Three rechargeable battery cells provide the energy. The power generated is about 1 W, and little energy is needed to energize the cutting tip. One charge lasts for about an hour of cutting time. But the plasma that is generated on the 100-μm filament of the disposable tip is phenomenal from many points of view. It is visible under high magnification, looking like bees on a honeycomb. This plasma ablates in such a fashion that it creates a smooth wall along the ablation/incision path. The secret is that the electromagnetic waves are brought to a sharp focus by the electronics in the console and in the handle, onto the tip of the incising filament. The electromagnetic oscillations knock out electrons from their orbits in the atoms of the tissue. Thus plasma, the fourth state of matter, consisting of charged atoms and electrons, is produced. This plasma cloud at the activated tip–tissue junction is actually visible to the naked eye.

When viewed under a high-power microscope, the plasma cloud is visible as a 25- to 50-μm-wide pulsating yellow cloud on the activated tip. Around the plasma cloud, there is a much wider reddish photon cloud. The cutting power resides in the plasma cloud. The plasma sustains itself as long as the electromagnetic oscillations from the activated tip keep interacting with the tissue, which is ablated in the truest sense. The plasma cloud oscillations instantly shatter the macromolecules of the tissue into small fragments. The micromolecules thus produced mix with water vapor and are thrown out at great speed as a plume; just as is seen with the Excimer laser. The oscillation is not apparent inside the anterior chamber since the fluid inside retards it. Here it manifests in another way. The molecular oscillation produces cavitations that result in phase transformation of the water into vapor, which presents as small bubbles along the ablation path. Recent changes in electronic tuning have greatly reduced bubble formation while retaining the awesome cutting power. During extraocular procedures such as touching a bleeding area, the molecular oscillation throws the particles millimeters away. This produces a process called "autostasis" wherein these small particles plug the top of small vessels, thereby producing a noncauterizing hemostasis. The plasma energy at the tip is at a very high temperature. However, the heated field does not extend beyond 25 μm of the plasma, thus meaning that little or no heat is generated. Therefore, it does not burn or cauterize. The Fugo Blade has this important function of producing noncauterizing hemostasis in cut tissue. It does this in two ways—ablation of the vessels is the cutting path and particle oscillation tends to plug small bleeding vessels. Finally, it should be made clear that the Fugo Blade is completely different from a diathermy unit. The Fugo Blade uses minute amounts of energy yet cuts more sharply than a diamond, whereas diathermy uses large amounts of energy yet cuts poorly. Scanning electron micrographs show that the Fugo Blade creates a smooth, clean capsulotomy rim, whereas diathermy produces a blistered, burned appearance.

HOW IS THE FUGO BLADE USED?

The Fugo Blade is used in the presence of a well-formed anterior chamber, be it filled with saline, methylcellulose, or sodium hyaluronate. An empty anterior chamber invites injury to the tissues, especially the corneal endothelium. The chamber may be filled completely before the Fugo Blade is used. The moment the anterior chamber appears to shallow, the tip is withdrawn and the chamber refilled. The authors, however, prefer to have the assistant push the viscoelastic from the sideport and complete the procedure with relative calm and at a leisurely pace. This not only maintains the chamber but also helps to clear any cavitation bubbles that may form, hence maintaining a clear view of the capsulotomy.

HOW DOES THE FUGO BLADE HELP IN PEDIATRIC CATARACT SURGERY?

The Fugo Blade is capable of rapidly ablating any pediatric cataract, which can then simply be washed out. However, the device has a far greater utility in the following ways.

Anterior Capsulotomy

Pediatric capsulotomy is notorious for its erratic behavior, especially if the capsule is stretched by its contents. Low scleral rigidity along with vitreous upthrust makes the pediatric capsule prone to radial tearing. A capsular rent extending toward the equator is a perfect recipe for an impending vitreous problem, but a Fugo Blade incision ahead of the rent will stop its further progress. M. E. Wilson, R. H. Trivedi, and G. Lal of the Storm Eye Institute (USA) provided a creative analysis of the repair of a tear in a capsule. Therefore, Dr. Richard Fugo and his colleagues refer to the technique of repairing a capsule tear with the Fugo Blade as a "Wilson seal." The Fugo Blade helps make a perfectly controlled anterior capsulotomy of any size, without a risk of radial tear. The peculiar structure of the cut edge ensures that even if a deliberate Fugo Blade radial cut is made in the capsulotomy, it will not spontaneously extend toward the equator (Fig. 18-1).

Large Capsulotomy

Having the capability to make a very large anterior capsulotomy helps in many ways. It is easy to take out all the lens matter from the fornices, and it is easy to implant an in-the-bag intraocular lens. Such a case will not suffer capsular contraction and phimosis, vaulting, or decentration of the optic from fibrotic lens bag contraction. Secondary cataract formation is reduced in frequency and density.

Moreover, a primary posterior capsulotomy can now easily and quickly be performed with the Fugo Blade.

Anterior capsulotomy in pediatric cataract surgery is perhaps the most critical step. The perfect control over the capsulotomy with the Fugo Blade takes the variability out of the surgery. This translates into a shorter surgical time, which is of paramount importance for the busy cataract surgeon and also exposes the patient to lower doses of anesthetic gases.

Anterior capsulotomy is performed by tracing a path with the activated Fugo Blade tip on the surface of the capsule. The cutting is resistance-free and without tactile sensation to the surgeon. A beginner can start by making a small capsulotomy in the center. It can be followed by making one or more larger capsulotomies around the previous ones. This capsulotomy around another capsulotomy may sound peculiar but it underscores the ease and simplicity of the Fugo Blade capsulotomy. The capsulotomy may be made in one attempt or in many attempts, the result being the same—a strong capsular rim size of the surgeon's choice. Dr. David Apple has shown the Fugo Blade to have a postage stamp configuration along the capsulotomy rim, which makes it stronger than a capsulorhexis.

Managing Posterior Capsule Problems

Making a Fugo Blade incision around a tear in the posterior capsule can stop it. A deliberate round posterior capsulotomy can be fashioned for optic capture of the implanted posterior chamber lens. To avoid damaging the anterior vitreous face there the following two steps are taken: first, sodium hyaluronate is injected underneath the posterior capsule to push the vitreous away; second, the Fugo Blade tip, which normally is about 0.7 mm, is pared to about 0.2 mm (have it modified beforehand), so that ablation of the posterior capsule does not damage the vitreous.

Posterior Capsular Plaque

Posterior capsular plaque can be removed by performing a posterior capsulotomy around the plaque as described. Another way is to use the Fugo Blade as an "eraser." A video

FIGURE 18-1. A Fugo Blade anterior capsulotomy being done counterclockwise. The tip is introduced straight in. The capsulotomy starts at 12 o'clock. As the tip moves to the right, the Fugo Blade handle is moved to the left. When the capsulotomy reaches 6 o'clock, the handle is made straight once again. When cutting on the left, the handle is moved to the right. Initially a conscious effort is needed to change the position of the handle as the capsulotomy proceeds, but soon it becomes automatic.

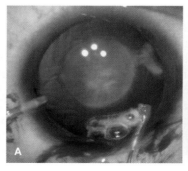
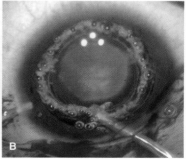

of this was shown at the 2003 ASCRS meeting, and the authors have performed many such cases. For this technique, the Fugo Blade tip is removed and the last 0.7 mm of the undersurface is denuded of its Teflon cover. The naked steel tip acts as an admirable eraser at medium settings. The plaque can be erased without damaging the vitreous face. Another approach is to make the plaque thin enough to be manageable by Nd:YAG laser later; however, a primary Fugo Blade posterior capsulotomy is easily performed.

Cutting Fibrovascular Membranes

Thick fibrous or fibrovascular membranes are encountered as congenital or acquired conditions. The latter category includes the sequeal of perforation, which leads to varying severity of adherent leukoma and the formation of adhesions between iris–lens, lens–iris–cornea, or vitreous–lens–iris. The blood vessels from the uvea invade the injured tissues. The injured lens assumes various appearances depending on the duration of the injury, amount of absorption, changes in the anterior and posterior capsule, and extent of vascular invasion. For cutting the various membranes and complexes, individual strategies have to be planned such as the site of incision, position of the sideport, and angle and size of the cutting tip. The disposable soft Fugo Blade tip can be easily modified with a needle holder. Fibrous or fibrovascular membranes may be seen on the posterior surface of any type of implanted intraocular lens. The Fugo Blade tip can be wriggled under the optic of any design of intraocular lens and the necessary membranectomy done. Sometimes, however, a posterior approach is unavoidable. In such cases a track is made through the pars plana with a micro vitreoretinal knife. The Fugo Blade tip is shaped to be directed anteriorly. Any thick membrane under the optic is cut with the greatest ease with the plasma of the Fugo Blade. Even though the tip touches the optic, the optic is not harmed.

Iridotomy

In some complicated cases, bleeding from the iris may be feared with a manual iridectomy. In pars plana vitrectomized cases, the blood may start trickling into the vitreous and cause immense problems in recovery. In these cases a bloodless iridotomy is done by simply rubbing the tip of the Fugo Blade across the iris and moving the tip in a circular fashion, to obtain a round hole of a desirable size. Iridotomy is also needed in cases of iris bombe. Wherever the limbal incision is placed, the Fugo Blade tip can reach any part of the anterior chamber to perform the task of iridotomy. It combines three functions in one tool—those of forceps, scissors, and noncauterizing hemostasis.

Pupilloplasty

Pupilloplasty may be needed in many patients undergoing surgery for traumatic cataract and for many more such patients needing a secondary implant. It may be performed before or after lens implantation. Needless to say, the Fugo Blade has revolutionized this procedure. With the Fugo Blade, the procedure is easy, is bloodless, and lacks a postoperative reaction as a result of plasma blade surgery. Pupilloplasty is also needed in many cases of a small fibrotic pupil adherent to a dense secondary cataract. The membrane and the iris are ablated as one unit. In darkbrown and black eyes with a microcornea, it is good to extend the ablation process beyond the edge of the optic, to make an additional passage for the aqueous.

Capsulotomy in a Subluxated Lens

The Fugo Blade instantly ablates any tissue that it touches. Thus, it is a simple matter to perform a free capsulotomy even on a subluxated lens, be it a case of Marfan, trauma, or something else. This allows one to dry-aspirate the lens contents without damage to the remaining zonules and the vitreous.

Anterior Vitrectomy

The Fugo plasma blade ablates any tissue that it touches, vitreous being no exception. The vitreous tags and mushroom in the anterior chamber, and under the iris-fixated lens, can easily be ablated. The main problem has been visual verification of what has been done. This has been facilitated in the past by injecting air into the anterior chamber. And recently it has been done by injecting opaque triamcinolone into the prolapsed vitreous and doing plasma ablation under visual control.

Making a Filtration Track

A patient with traumatic dislocation, with or without vitreous disturbance and hemorrhage in the anterior chamber, posterior chamber, or both, may have a high intraocular pressure, medically uncontrolled. The Fugo Blade can be used to perform a 1-min transconjunctival 100-μm filtration track into the anterior chamber for a smooth ocular decompression, making the eye fit for any procedure that is needed.[5,6] The filtration track remains functional for many days or weeks. As these eyes settle down from the consequences of trauma, many remain free of glaucoma.

CONCLUSION

It is obvious that the Fugo Blade has enormously important applications in the field of ophthalmic surgery. It certainly presents us with a new paradigm in pediatric cataract surgery and its importance has been underscored by its approval by the FDA for intraocular use.

REFERENCES

1. Fugo RJ, DelCampo DM. The Fugo Blade™: the next step aftercapsulorhexis. *Ann Ophthalmol* 2001;33(1):12–20.
2. Fugo RJ, Singh D, Fine IH. Automated Fugo Blade capsulotomy: a new technique and a new instrument. *Eyeworld* 2002;7(9); 49–54.
3. Singh SK. Fugo Blade capsulotomy: A new high tech cutting technology. *Trop Ophthalmol* 2001;1(1):14–16.
4. Singh D. Use of the Fugo Blade in complicated cases. *J Cataract Refract Surg* 2002;28(4):573–574.
5. Singh D. Singh micro-filtration for glaucoma; a new technique. *Trop Ophthalmol* 2001;1(6):7–11.
6. Singh D, Singh K. Transciliary filtration using the Fugo Blade. *Ann Ophthalmol* 2002;34(3):183–187.

Lensectomy and Anterior Vitrectomy When an Intraocular Lens Is Not Being Implanted

M. Edward Wilson, Jr. and Suresh K. Pandey

Intraocular lens (IOL) implantation at the time of cataract surgery is commonplace in older children. However, infants are often left aphakic. Optical rehabilitation is accomplished with contact lenses or aphakic glasses during the rapid years of eye growth. Later in childhood, secondary IOL implantation is usually performed. For infants, there are some significant advantages to the lensectomy and vitrectomy procedure compared to the lensectomy, vitrectomy, and IOL implantation procedure.

(1) Lensectomy and vitrectomy can be performed through two small corneal stab incisions, ≤20 gauge. This causes less surgical trauma for the baby eye compared to when an IOL is inserted. The avoidance of a larger incision makes a patch and shield unnecessary. We usually place a contact lens on the eye at the conclusion of surgery and leave the eye unpatched. Postoperative drops can be started immediately instead of waiting until the patch and shield are removed the day after surgery. Having the baby return after surgery with no eye bandage is a great psychological boost for the parents. The baby can "start seeing" right away.

(2) The risk of recurrent visual axis opacification after infant surgery is much lower when an IOL is not placed primarily. The anterior and posterior capsule remnants seal to each other more securely when an IOL is not placed between them. If a Soemmering's ring forms, it is more likely to remain peripheral to the visual axis. In contrast, infants with an IOL placed primarily are at higher risk of visual axis opacification from cortex that escapes the Soemmering's ring and reaches the visual axis.

(3) Aphakic contact lenses can be changed whenever the eye grows, allowing precise optical rehabilitation. When an IOL is placed in infancy, glasses must be worn for the residual hyperopia. Later in childhood, myopic glasses are often needed. Some parents find that contact lens wear (especially with the easy-to-handle extended-wear silicone contact lenses designed especially for infants) is easier to manage than glasses, at least in infancy. Later, if contact lens wear becomes more difficult, the eye has grown enough that the glasses (as an adjunct to an IOL) are less thick and less necessary for prevention or treatment of amblyopia.

The disadvantages of aphakia in infancy with optical replacement using contact lenses include worsening amblyopia whenever a contact lens is lost and the risk of corneal ulcers owing to the extended wear of the lenses during the day and night. These issues are also covered in other chapters in this book.

SURGICAL APPROACHES FOR LENSECTOMY AND ANTERIOR VITRECTOMY

Two main approaches exist for lensectomy and anterior vitrectomy in children: the pars plana/pars plicata approach and the limbal/corneal approach.[1-8]

The Pars Plana Approach for Lensectomy and Anterior Vitrectomy

The pars plana/pars plicata approach is not commonly used today for primary removal of a congenital cataract unless vitreoretinal pathology is also being addressed. When retina surgeons perform a lensectomy combined with a posterior vitrectomy and retinal repair in an infant, a pars plana approach is often preferred. Pediatric anterior segment surgeons are more likely to prefer a limbal approach. Pars plana posterior capsulotomy after limbal-approach lensectomy and IOL placement is covered elsewhere in this book.

Surgical Technique

Pars plana/pars plicata lensectomy requires a guillotine-type vitrectome. Epinephrine (adrenaline), 1:500,000, is mixed in balanced salt solution (BSS; Alcon Laboratories, Fort Worth, TX) to avoid intraoperative miosis. Conjunctiva is opened at the 10 o'clock and 2 o'clock positions to expose the sclera at the level of the pars plana. Two scleral perforations are made using a micro vitreoretinal (MVR) knife or a 20-gauge Stiletto knife (DORC, the Netherlands) at the pars plana/pars plicata level: one for the vitrectomy probe and the second for the infusion cannula. Stab incision placement recommendations are as follows: 2 mm posterior to the limbus in an infant, 2.5 mm in a toddler, and 3 mm in a school-aged child. A lensectomy–anterior vitrectomy is completed, sparing a peripheral rim of the capsular sac including the anterior, equatorial, and posterior capsule. These capsule remnants are used to create a shelf to support a posterior chamber IOL that may be implanted later in life. It is important to avoid vitreous incarceration in the wounds by turning off the infusion before withdrawing the vitrectome from the eye. This precaution reduces the chances of inducing retinal traction and retinal detachment later in life. The pars plana/pars plicata scleral incisions are closed with 8-0 synthetic absorbable suture. Recently, sutureless pars plana anterior vitrectomy through self-sealing sclerotomies in children has also been reported.[9]

Advantages and Disadvantages of the Pars Plana Approach

This approach minimizes the possibility of surgical trauma to the iris and the corneal endothelium because fewer maneuvers occur in the anterior chamber. However, there is a greater likelihood that inadequate capsule will remain for support of a secondary sulcus-fixated IOL using this approach.

The Limbal Approach for Lensectomy and Anterior Vitrectomy

The limbal/corneal approach is used most often by pediatric surgeons when operating on infants. Most use a bimanual technique but some use a single incision with an infusion sleeve attached to the vitrector handpiece.

Surgical Technique

Figure 19-1 illustrates our technique for pediatric cataract surgery with the limbal/corneal approach to lensectomy and anterior vitrectomy. Under general anesthesia, two

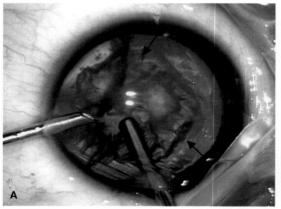
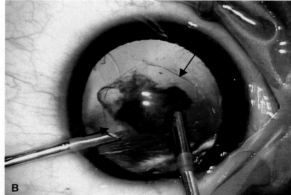
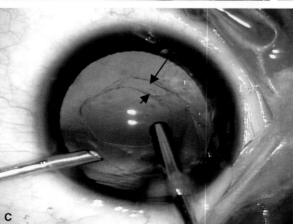

FIGURE 19-1. Techniques for pediatric cataract surgery using the limbal approach for lensectomy and anterior vitrectomy. **A** and **B.** Photographs showing the mechanized anterior capsulotomy (*vitrectorhexis*) technique and aspiration of the lens substance using an automated Venturi pump–driven vitrectomy machine. The arrow indicates the edge of vitrectorhexis. **C.** Photograph illustrating a mechanized posterior capsulectomy and anterior vitrectomy. The arrow indicates the edge of vitrectorhexis; the arrowhead indicates the posterior capsulotomy.

corneal stab incisions are recommended, using a 20-gauge MVR knife at the 10 o'clock and 2 o'clock positions: one for an irrigation cannula (connected to a BSS) and the other one for an aspiration/cutting handpiece. The stab incisions should be located at the terminal end of the limbal blood vessels as they reach the clear cornea. Care should be taken when making the incisions to assure a tight fit with the instruments to be inserted into the anterior chamber. The MVR knife is initially aimed posteriorly but is flattened out into the iris plane after the tip enters the anterior chamber. This maneuver will produce a tunneled incision about 1 mm wide and about 1 mm long. With the soft eyes (low tissue rigidity) of babies, an iris plane incision from the point of entry will result in a longer tunnel than expected. The anterior chamber will be entered closer to the visual axis than intended. Maneuvering the instruments will also be more difficult with this long tunnel due to the "oar locking" phenomenon. Also, the MVR knife needs to be backed out precisely along the path of entry. Beginning surgeons have a tendency to retract the knife along a slightly different path than the entry. This causes the soft corneal tissue of the infant to slice open wider than the blade width. Leakage around the instruments will result during surgery, leading to anterior chamber instability. Finally, the nondominant-side incision should be made first (left-hand incision for a right-handed surgeon). Usually, the incision can be made without resulting in a flat anterior chamber. In that circumstance, the second incision can be made without placing an ophthalmic viscosurgical device (OVD) into the eye. If the chamber flattens after the nondominant incision, the irrigating cannula can be placed in the eye through the initial opening and the second incision can be made with a fluid-filled chamber. No OVD is needed when an IOL is not being implanted.

Our preferred instruments are a 20-gauge blunt-tip, angled, beveled irrigating cannula (Nichamin cannula, Storz or Grieshaber 170.01, Alcon) and a 20-gauge vitrectomy (aspirating and cutting) handpiece (Accurus; Alcon). It is important that these instruments be equal in size. Subincisional cortex removal may require that the right- and left-hand instruments be switched. If the incisions and the instruments are of identical size, the tight fit can be maintained, which will keep the anterior chamber depth stable. Epinephrine (1:500,000) is usually added in the BSS to maintain the pupillary mydriasis. Although Ringer's lactate solution works well for irrigation associated with adult extracapsular cataract surgery, temporary corneal clouding can occur when it is used in the high-flow pediatric cataract surgery described here.

The anterior chamber is entered first (with the surgeon's nondominant hand using the nondominant-side incision) with the irrigating cannula. Care is taken to place the beveled tip in along the plane of the tunneled incision. A slight swirling motion often facilitates entry. The vitrectomy handpiece is more difficult to place because it is not beveled. Twirling movements aid entry. Take care not to aim too superficially within the incision. This will result in the instrument's missing the internal lip of the wound and tracking into the soft infantile corneal stroma. If this happens, back the instrument out and reenter with more posterior pressure on the tip of the instrument as it enters the wound. Occasionally, it will be necessary to have an assistant lift up on the incision outer lip to facilitate entry. Resist the temptation to enlarge the wound. Operating on very young infants requires a stable anterior chamber and a leaking wound will not facilitate chamber stability.

With both instruments in the anterior chamber, the vitrectorhexis can be performed. Our preferred settings on the Accurus machine are a fluid pressure of 50, aspiration of 200, and a cutting rate of 150. The vitrector is placed just anterior to the center of the anterior capsule, with the cutting port facing directly posterior. The aspiration foot pedal is depressed until the anterior capsule enters the cutting port and is opened. The surgeon should stay slightly anterior to the plane of the anterior capsule and let the capsule come to the cutter rather than chasing the capsule with the cutter and inadvertently reaching the posterior capsule prematurely. The anterior capsulotomy should be enlarged to the desired size using a gentle spiraling movement from the center outward. If the instrument slips posterior to the capsule edge, it should be pulled back anterior to the capsule where the cutter can be redirected. Care should be taken to avoid creating right-angled edges in the capsulotomy. The ideal size is 4.5 to 5 mm.

Without removing the instruments from the eye, the cutter is then turned off, leaving the instrument in the aspiration-only mode. The vitrector tip (now functioning as an aspiration handpiece) is directed under the anterior capsulotomy into the equator of the lens, with the port facing the equator of the lens and turned toward the surgeon. Peripheral cortex is aspirated first. Rather than pulling the instrument toward the center of the capsule, the aspiration foot pedal should be depressed (increasing the aspiration toward the maximum setting of 200) while the instrument is still near the lens equator. As the lens cortex begins to disappear into the aspiration port, some stripping toward the center is appropriate, but not to the degree usually used in adult surgery. The center of the lens is often aspirated last. This keeps the posterior capsule back until the equatorial cortex has been removed.

When the capsular bag has been cleaned of all lens material, the cutter is again turned on and the cutting port is positioned centrally, just anterior to the posterior capsule. The surgeon then aspirates the capsule up into the cutting port. Often, the posterior capsule is engaged with this technique without simultaneously engaging the vitreous face. Nonetheless, the cutter speed is increased to 500 cuts/min and the irrigation is decreased to 30, in case vitreous is encountered. As with the anterior capsule, enlargement of the posterior capsulotomy is done in a slow, spiraling manner. A central vitrectomy is performed after completion of the posterior vitrectorhexis. The irrigation cannula should be placed so as to direct fluid away from the vitrector tip.

At the end of the vitrectomy, the instruments are removed from the eye at nearly the same time. The irrigation cannula should exit just before (and not after) the removal of the vitrector tip. If a vitreous strand to either of the exit wounds is suspected, a miotic can be irrigated into the anterior chamber to constrict the pupil. If peaking of the pupil is seen, the vitrector is placed back into the anterior chamber until removal is complete. Rarely, an OVD will be needed along with a sweep of a vitreous strand from the wound using an iris spatula. Amazingly, vitreous rarely comes to the wound using this technique with infants. The formed vitreous of the baby combined with a generous central anterior vitrectomy results in an anterior segment devoid of vitreous nearly every time. The stab incisions are closed with one interrupted 10.0 vicryl suture each. A drop of 5% povidone iodine along with atropine and steroid/antibiotic drops is placed on the eye at the end of the surgery. An appropriate Silsoft aphakic contact lens (usually a 7.5-base curve, 29- or 32-diopter power for neonates) is place on the eye as well. The child is then awakened and recovered.

Advantages and Disadvantages of the Limbal/Corneal Approach

The limbal/corneal approach is more familiar to the anterior segment surgeon than the pars plana/pars plicata approach. The conjunctiva need not be disturbed and an adequate (for secondary IOL implantation later) capsular rim is more likely to remain when this approach is used. However, there is a greater risk of iris manipulation or iris damage by the cutting port when this approach is used. To avoid inadvertent iris cutting, the surgeon should take care to keep the vitrector cutting port facing away from the iris. If not, a sudden shallowing of the anterior chamber

from fluid leaking around the instruments can result in iris entering the cutting port.

SUMMARY

Lensectomy and anterior vitrectomy without an IOL constitute a widely used surgical technique for the removal of visually significant congenital cataracts in the first year of life. The technique, as described here, allows the anterior capsulotomy, lens aspiration, posterior capsulotomy, and anterior vitrectomy all to be done without ever having to take the instruments out of the eye. The procedure is fast and efficient, and it induces a minimal amount of surgical trauma. No conjunctival incision is needed. Closure is with two interrupted 10.0 synthetic absorbable sutures. The aphakic contact lens can be placed on the eye at the conclusion of surgery. No bandage or shield is necessary.

REFERENCES

1. Pandey SK, Wilson ME, Trivedi RH, et al. Pediatric cataract surgery and intraocular lens implantation: current techniques, complications and management. *Int Ophthalmol Clin* 2001;41:175–196.
2. Ram J, Pandey SK. Infantile cataract surgery: Current techniques, complications and their management. In: Dutta LC, ed. *Modern Ophthalmology.* New Delhi, India: Jaypee Brothers, 2000:378–384.
3. Wilson ME, Pandey SK, Thakur J. Pediatric cataract surgery in the developing world. *Br J Ophthalmol* 2003;87:14–19.
4. Basti S, Ravishankar V, Gupta S. Results of a prospective evaluation of three methods of management of pediatric cataracts. *Ophthalmology* 1996;103:713–720.
5. Parks MM. Posterior lens capsulotomy during primary cataract surgery in children. *Ophthalmology* 1983;90:344–345.
6. Taylor DSI. Choice of surgical technique in the management of congenital cataract. *Trans Ophthalmol Soc UK* 1981;101:114–117.
7. Meier P, Sterker I, Wiedemann P. Pars plana lentectomy for treatment of congenital cataract. *Graefes Arch Clin Exp Ophthalmol* 2001;239:649–655.
8. Ahmadieh H, Javadi MA, Ahmady M, et al. Primary capsulectomy, anterior vitrectomy, lensectomy, and posterior chamber lens implantation in children: limbal versus pars plana. *J Cataract Refract Surg* 1999;25:768–775.
9. Lam DS, Chua JK, Leung AT, et al. Sutureless pars plana anterior vitrectomy through self-sealing sclerotomies in children. *Arch Ophthalmol* 2000;118:850–851.

Chapter 20

Postoperative Medications and Follow-up

Hamid Ahmadieh and M. R. Ja'farinasab

Regular postoperative examinations and appropriate medical treatment are crucial for a successful outcome in all surgical interventions. There are certain aspects in pediatric cataract surgery that make the issue of follow-up more important. Children, especially infants, are unable to express complaints and depend on their parents or a caretaker for the use of medications; furthermore, ophthalmologic examinations including assessment of visual acuity, slit-lamp examination, and intraocular pressure measurement are tedious or impossible in some cases. Certain postoperative complications such as inflammation, glaucoma, and posterior capsular opacification are encountered more frequently in pediatric cataract surgery. Cataract surgery in a child is also different in the sense that the operation aims to provide lifelong useful vision in an individual whom amblyopia threatens a successful outcome.

The key to a successful outcome in pediatric cataract surgery lies in continuous and periodic reevaluation with the meticulous attention of the surgeon, a pediatric ophthalmologist, and the parents or caretaker. An uneventful operation is simply the first step toward achieving the main goals; only by careful observation for expected conditions, and also the unexpected, does one reach the ultimate objectives. The surgeon should inform the parents of the need for continuous follow-up prior to undertaking surgery and stress the importance of effort and dedication for the long period of observation. The postoperative care of pediatric cataract surgery consists of medical treatment and periodic examinations.

POSTOPERATIVE MEDICATIONS

Medical treatment is of prime importance following pediatric cataract surgery. The bases for postoperative medical therapy in children are studies performed on adults' and surgeons' experience. Although guidelines are often stated, the postoperative regimen should be tailored individually. There are certain points to be considered in small children.

Due to their lower body weight, one main consideration in the application of eye drops in children, especially infants and toddlers, is the possibility of systemic absorption and related side effects. Most postoperative medications for pediatric cataract surgery are prescribed for the first time, therefore attention to systemic side effects is mandatory. Measures to decrease systemic absorption, such as digital punctal occlusion and eyelid closure, are therefore more important in children.

Medications prescribed in the postoperative care of pediatric cataract surgery fall into two main categories. First are medications routinely prescribed in uncomplicated cases and, second, drugs used under certain circumstances and for specific indications. This chapter focuses on the first group of medications, which includes antibiotics, steroids, nonsteroidal anti-inflammatory drugs (NSAIDs), cycloplegics, mydriatics, and topical anesthetics.

Antibiotics

The use of perioperative antibiotics for prevention of infections and postoperative endophthalmitis remains a controversial issue. Postoperative endophthalmitis following pediatric cataract surgery is very uncommon and the overall incidence has been reported to be 7 per 10,000 operations.[1] Due to the severity of the condition and the potential of visual loss, surgeons generally take preventive measures to reduce its incidence; however, the efficacy of many of these measures remains unclear both theoretically and practically. Nevertheless, prophylactic use of antibiotics or antiseptics seems justified regarding ethical and medicolegal issues.

Povidone–iodine preparations are widely used for conjunctival antisepsis presurgically.[2] Injection of cefuroxime, 1 mg in 0.1 mL normal saline, into the anterior chamber at the end of surgery seems to be a safe measure; in newborns, 0.5 mg may suffice.[3] Gentamicin, 10 to 20 mg, or cephazolin, 50 to 100 mg, are among the more common antibiotics injected subconjunctively at the conclusion of surgery.[4–10] The addition of vancomycin to the irrigation bottle during surgery is not recommended due to the increased risk of cystoid macular edema and the possibility of causing bacterial resistance.[3]

Another preventive measure against endophthalmitis and wound infections is the use of perioperative topical antibiotics including gentamicin, neomycin, tobramycin, and polymyxin B.[6,11–13] Fluoroquinolones are another group of antibiotics used for this purpose. Certain characteristics make them attractive for prophylactic use. Fluoroquinolones exhibit good activity against gram-negative and gram-positive organisms that are the main causative agents of postoperative endophthalmitis. These drugs have minimal epithelial toxicity and when used frequently can attain effective concentrations in the corneal stroma and the anterior chamber. However, none of the fluoroquinolones can penetrate intact corneal epithelium very well, therefore drug levels may be inconsistent with prophylactic use. Among the three available topical fluoroquinolones, ofloxacin has the best transepithelial penetration. Ciprofloxacin is another suitable alternative since it is effective against the major organisms producing wound infections or endophthalmitis and also shows good coverage for gram-negative microorganisms. Ciprofloxacin has less epithelial toxicity compared to other fluoroquinolones. Perioperative use of both ciprofloxacin and ofloxacin reduces colony counts of external ocular flora. Norfloxacin is less suitable for prophylactic use in ophthalmic practice since it is less effective against gram-positive organisms and penetrates the epithelium less readily.[14]

One regimen for prophylactic use of fluoroquinolones is frequent preoperative instillation (every 5 to 15 min, 1 to 1.5 hr before surgery) and postoperative use every 6 hr for 5 to 7 days.[14] However, a study by Ta et al.[15] indicated that preoperative ofloxacin started 3 days prior to surgery was more effective than instillation 1 hr before the operation in reducing colony counts. All available fluoroquinolones are well tolerated, however, ciprofloxacin seems to be best tolerated by the corneal epithelium. Ciprofloxacin has minimal adverse systemic effects. Fluoroquinolones may cause damage to cartilage and arthropathy, therefore systemic administration should be avoided in children. Topical use in children entails no risk of arthropathy.[14]

Fourth-Generation Fluoroquinolones

Fourth-generation fluoroquinolones (such as gatifloxacin and moxifloxacin) offer a broader spectrum of coverage than previous generations of fluoroquinolones. These potent topical bactericidal agents promise to have greater antibacterial properties against gram-positive organisms and atypical mycobacteria. While fluoroquinolones were introduced for the treatment of corneal and conjunctival infections, ophthalmic surgeons now use them prophy-

lactically before intraocular surgery to prevent bacterial endophthalmitis. The drugs play a significant role in presurgical prophylaxis for pediatric cataract surgery to minimize the incidence of infectious endophthalmitis.

Two topical fourth-generation fluoroquinolones, *gatifloxacin* (Allergan Inc., Irvine, CA) and *moxifloxacin* (Alcon Laboratories, Fort Worth, TX), can be used for presurgical prophylaxis for pediatric cataract surgery. Preliminary studies suggest encouraging results with moxifloxacin, as it appears to be capable of reaching therapeutic levels against the offending microbes in the anterior chamber. Both gatifloxacin and moxifloxacin have recently been approved by U.S. Food and Drug Administration (FDA) and are currently available in the United States.

Steroids

The inflammatory response following cataract surgery is more intense in children, which increases the risk of some postoperative complications such as fibrinous membrane formation, pupillary block, pigmentary and cellular deposits on the intraocular lens (IOL), posterior synechiae, IOL capture, posterior capsule opacity, and cystoid macular edema. Frequent administration of topical and sometimes systemic steroids is needed to reduce the risk of these complications.

Corticosteroids

Corticosteroids are relatively potent anti-inflammatory agents with multimodal mechanisms of action. Despite the efficacy of steroids in reducing postoperative inflammation, their long-term use is associated with multiple adverse systemic and ocular effects. Systemic complications of long-term steroid use in children include growth retardation, affective disorders, Cushing syndrome, skin atrophy, hirsutism, acne, osteoporosis, femoral head avascular necrosis, myopathy, water and electrolyte imbalance, hypertension, duodenal ulcer, immunosuppression, and delayed wound healing. Intracranial hypertension (pseudotumor cerebri) has also been associated with discontinuation of steroids.[16] Ocular complications of long-term steroid use are ocular hypertension, glaucoma, predisposition to infections, and initiation or progression of cataract in the fellow eye.[16] Ocular side effects are related to the potency of the steroid and individual susceptibility. Generally speaking, in the pediatric age group, dexamethasone is considered the most potent and hazardous steroid; on the contrary, fluorometholone is the safest.

Following pediatric cataract surgery corticosteroids may be administered either regionally or systemically. Regional steroids may be used topically or locally in the form of eye drops, ointments, and subconjunctival or subtenon injections. Common steroids for sunconjunctival use include betamethasone and dexamethasone, 2 to 4 mg, injected into the inferior bulbar conjunctiva at the conclusion of surgery.[4,5,8,9,13,17,18] The authors usually inject betamethasone, 2 mg in patients under the age of 1 year and 4 mg in older patients. Steroids used for subtenon injection include methylprednisolone acetate and triamcinolone acetonide, 20 to 40 mg, depending on the age of the patient.[17,19] This form of periocular steroid has been associated with precipitous elevations of intraocular pressure.[20]

Steroid eye drops are generally prescribed from the first postoperative day. Steroid drops are an easy, safe, effective, and inexpensive method of drug delivery and usually do not entail systemic effects. Children are usually defensive against eye drop instillation, so one must take time and be patient. Topical steroid eye drops used in the postoperative care of pediatric cataract surgery include prednisolone acetate, betamethasone, and dexamethasone. Most authors recommend 1% prednisolone acetate eye drops for routine use[4,11,13,21–24]; our experience has shown 0.1% betamethasone to be an acceptable alternative.[19] The frequency of instillation is every 1 to 6 hr, depending on the clinical situation. In uncomplicated cases with minimal postoperative inflammation, 1% prednisolone acetate administered every 4 to 6 hr should suffice. With more severe inflammation, sterile uveitis, or preexisting intraocular inflammation, more frequent dosage (e.g., every 1–2 hr) may be required. The duration of topical steroid therapy is 4 to 12 weeks, depending on the clinical course. Steroid ointments are limited to bedtime use and are not recommended during waking hours because of the possibility of blurred vision.

Systemic steroid use is uncommon in adult cataract surgery. However, owing to the more severe inflammatory response, more extensive surgical manipulation (removal of the posterior capsule, anterior vitrectomy), and lack of adequate cooperation for eye drop instillation, systemic steroids may be needed for pediatric cataract surgery. The usual dose is 1 to 2 mg/kg oral prednisolone for 1 week, which is tapered and discontinued by 1–2 weeks.[4,11,17,18]

Nonsteroidal Anti-inflammatory Drugs

This class of medications reduces inflammation through inhibition of prostaglandin synthesis. The possible advantage of these medications is the potential for reduction of steroid-related complications such as increased intraocular pressure, risk of infections, and delayed wound healing. Investigations by slit-lamp biomicroscopy and fluorophotometry have proven the anti-inflammatory effect of NSAIDs including 1% indocin, 0.03% flurbiprofen, 0.5% ketorolac, and 0.1% diclofenac. Randomized double-blind clinical trials have shown the anti-inflammatory effect of 0.5% ketorolac and 0.01, 0.1, and 0.5% diclofenac to be equal to that of 0.1% dexamethasone and 1% prednisolone, respectively.[25] When used, NSAIDs are usually administered three or four times daily for 4 to 6 weeks following cataract surgery. These medications may cause ocular

irritation and, by interfering with platelet function, predispose to hemorrhage from the surgical wound. Therefore NSAIDs should be used with caution in patients receiving systemic anticoagulants or with hemorrhagic predisposition. Another contraindication for the use of topical NSAIDs is herpes simplex keratitis, however, experimental evidence suggests that flurbiprofen may be beneficial in some instances.[16] The above-mentioned studies have been performed in adults; at present, clinical experience with NSAID use after pediatric cataract surgery is rather limited.[8,12,18,26,27] However, no specific side effects have been reported in children.[16]

Cycloplegics and Mydriatics

Mydriatics and cycloplegics diminish ciliary spasm, stabilize the blood–aqueous barrier, and dilate the pupil, thereby reducing pain, inflammation, and the risk of pupillary block caused by synechiae or fibrinous membranes. The pupil dilating effect of these medications may remain for a few hours to a few days, depending on the drug potency and individual susceptibility. The latter depends on iris pigmentation (i.e., melanin content); dark irides tend to respond more slowly to these drugs and return to normal much sooner.[28] Commonly available cycloplegic eye drops include atropine, homatropine, cyclopentolate, and tropicamide.

Phenylephrine hydrochloride (PEH) is a potent mydriatic with no effect on accommodation and may be used separately or in combination with cycloplegics. PEH is available at 1, 2.5, 5, and 10% concentrations. The 10% solution should be avoided in children because of possible cardiovascular side effects.[29] PEH at 2.5% is preferred in children, however, neonates and premature infants should receive the 1% solution.[29]

There is no uniformity in the postoperative use of cycloplegics in pediatric cataract surgery; some surgeons prescribe these medications routinely for all patients one to three times daily for 1 to 4 weeks.[8,13,22,27,30,31]; others avoid the routine use of these drugs altogether.[11,12,21] Use of cycloplegics, especially long-acting ones, in cases where the posterior capsule is intact and anterior vitrectomy is not performed may predispose to IOL pupillary capture if the IOL has been implanted in the ciliary sulcus. However, when a continuous curvilinear capsulorhexis has been performed and the implant is well positioned in the capsular bag and when primary posterior capsulotomy with anterior vitrectomy has been done, the risk of pupillary capture is minimal.

Due to the insidious onset of pupillary capture of IOL, in our practice we refrain from routine prescription of cycloplegics when the pupillary reflex is fair and insignificant postoperative inflammation is present. We prefer in-the-office instillation of cycloplegics only when postoperative examination reveals an unresponsive pupil or a pupillary membrane in formation. After instillation of a single drop of 0.5% proparacaine, we use one drop of 2.5% phenylephrine followed by one drop of cyclopentolate or tropicamide. The patient is reexamined after 30 min, and if visible signs of drug effect are not noted, we repeat the preceding routine one time.

Topical Anesthetics

Topical ocular anesthetics commonly used in pediatric patients are 0.5% proparacaine and 0.5% tetracaine. Proparacaine hydrochloride causes anesthesia in a few seconds; however, the anesthesia wears off after 11 min.[32] Many ophthalmologists routinely administer 0.5% proparacaine hydrochloride with cycloplegics and mydriatics; the epithelial changes induced by proparacaine facilitate intracorneal penetration of cycloplegics and mydriatics, thereby enhancing their effect.[32] Additionally, the corneal and conjunctival anesthesia provided by proparacaine reduces reflex tearing upon instillation of the other drops, increasing patient comfort and promoting more effective contact of the medication with the ocular surface. Adverse effects of proparacaine include contact dermatitis, epithelial keratitis, pupillary dilation, and seizures.[32] Tetracaine is not as well tolerated as proparacaine; it is more irritating and the duration of its effect is shorter (<10 min).[32]

FOLLOW-UP

As previously stated, lifelong follow-up of children undergoing cataract surgery with or without IOL implantation is crucial for a successful outcome. Young children are unable to report symptoms; therefore regular follow-up and detailed examination are mandatory for early recognition of complications and to initiate timely treatment. The first postoperative month and the first week, in particular, are the period when complications such as wound problems, endophthalmitis, and sterile uveitis may occur. Furthermore, due to continuous growth of the globe, the refractive status of the eye undergoes constant change requiring regular refraction and necessary changes in correction to obtain optimal vision. Prevention and treatment of amblyopia by timely occlusion is another vital issue in the postoperative course. Such extensive efforts call for cooperation among the surgeon, pediatric ophthalmologist, and parents.

Perioperative Considerations

The overall atmosphere in the hospital, particularly in the operating room, causes uneasiness or frank fear in most children. Therefore it is preferable not to admit children if at all possible. Children are intolerant of being kept hungry and thirsty, therefore the operation time should be scheduled precisely to avoid undue expectation or delay. The parents, in particular, undergo a considerable amount of

stress and anxiety and are generally easily irritated by signs of inattention.

Postoperative visits should be scheduled well in advance so that both child and parents can be prepared for full cooperation. These examinations are best scheduled for the early hours of clinic or office activity, when the examiner can deal with the child with more energy and patience. One should avoid disrupting the child's sleeping schedule and avoid unnecessary delay. Taking a few moments before starting the examination to establish rapport or communication, either verbal or physical, will facilitate the process. It is better to start the examination with less invasive or frightening procedures such as evaluation of the red reflex; more invasive or painful procedures such as instillation of topical anesthetics and intraocular pressure measurement should be performed toward the end.

All surgeons routinely visit the patient on the first postoperative day, however, subsequent visits are scheduled depending on the patient's age, the presence of complications and condition of the operated eye at the first postoperative visit, and the surgeon's experience. Some authors recommend visits on day 1, week 1, and months 1, 3, and 6, followed by examinations every 6 months thereafter.[13] Others have suggested monthly visits for 1 year, with subsequent visits at 3- to 6-month intervals. Our routine for postoperative visits in uncomplicated cases is daily examinations for the first 3 days, weekly examinations for a month, and monthly visits for 3 months, followed by examinations every 3 months for 1 year and every 6 months thereafter.

At each postoperative visit, visual acuity, slit-lamp examination, and intraocular pressure (if feasible) should be assessed. Dilated fundus examination should be performed in the first week after the operation and repeated at 3 months and then every 6 months in uncomplicated cases. On slit-lamp examination, attention must be paid to corneal clarity, wound stability and sutures, anterior chamber reaction, iris, pupil reaction, and IOL position, including centration and distance from the pupil margin. In cases where slit-lamp examination is impossible and handheld slit lamps are not available, penlight-assisted examination may be adequate. In these cases, a detailed examination under anesthesia 1 to 2 months after the operation is mandatory. If the penlight examination causes suspicion of any complication, a detailed examination under sedation or anesthesia becomes necessary. Examination under sedation is another alternative in uncooperative children. Miyahara et al.[33] have reported the use of oral triclofos sodium, 8 mg/kg, for intraocular pressure measurement in children younger than 3 years.

Suture Removal

Wound healing occurs more rapidly in children, therefore sutures may become loose sooner than in adults. In addition to causing irritation and discomfort, loose sutures predispose to suture abscess and possible intraocular infection. Removal of loose sutures is necessary at the slit-lamp examination; if that procedure is not possible, suture removal under anesthesia in the operating room must be considered.

Surgically induced or preexisting astigmatism can be managed by suture removal. Postoperative corneal astigmatism may be assessed by keratometry or topography in cooperative children; in other cases retinoscopy may be a rough guide to corneal astigmatism. As a rule of thumb, with more than 3 and 1.5 diopters of suture-induced astigmatism 1 and 2 months after surgery, respectively, suture removal should be considered. Selective suture removal may be considered for patients able to cooperate for slit-lamp removal; otherwise, complete suture removal under anesthesia becomes necessary for significant postoperative astigmatism. Factors such as the type (corneal versus scleral), size, and location of the incision, patient's age, degree of scar formation, and required steroid dose affect the timing for suture removal.

Restrictions

Eye protection is of major concern for prevention of trauma to the operated eye, especially in the trauma-prone period of childhood. Eye shields or protective glasses may be used for waking hours and a shield may be applied during the nighttime. Owing to the rapid wound healing in childhood, use of eye protection is required for only 3 weeks during waking hours and 1 to 2 weeks during sleep. Because of the potential for amblyopia, protective glasses are preferred over eye shields during periods of activity. Strenuous physical activity including gym classes, contact sports, and swimming should be avoided for 3 weeks.[6,7]

Correction of Refractive Errors

An excellent surgical outcome and clear optical media are only prerequisites for useful vision after pediatric cataract surgery. Achievement of a successful visual outcome depends on timely correction of residual refractive errors, particularly aphakia. Bilateral and unilateral refractive errors, whether aphakic or pseudophakic, should be corrected at the first possible opportunity. Another important point is periodic recheck of refractive errors, especially during the first few years of life, when globe growth causes a myopic shift. Some studies have shown a mean decrease of 9 diopters in contact lens power during the first 4 years of life.[34] Options for postoperative correction of refractive errors include spectacles or contact lens use. Epikeratophakia for correction of aphakia, which was introduced in the early 1980s, is outdated due to related complications and the widespread implantation of IOLs in pediatric cataracts. Factors influencing the choice of correction include aphakia versus pseudophakia, unilaterality versus

bilaterality, socioeconomic status, access to eye care, and patient/parent compliance and devotion. The best method of correction in unilateral aphakia is contact lens use. Details on options for correction of aphakia are described in Chapter 49. Aphakic glasses are the next alternative, especially for bilateral aphakia or when contact lens use is not possible in unilateral aphakia. The rate of ulcerative keratitis increases six to eight times with overnight use of contact lenses,[34] parents should be warned of this serious complication. The compliance rate for contact lens use in unilateral aphakia was 44% in one study.[34] Neumann et al.[35] reported the rate of contact lens loss to be four times in the first year of use and twice in the second year; these figures may depend on the type of contact lens and the child's behavior. IOL implantation has become more popular in the past years, however, due to problems of IOL power calculation in children and changes in corneal curvature and axial length, postoperative refractive errors are common in pseudophakic eyes. Hiles[36] reported an overall rate of 66% for spectacle correction after pediatric cataract surgery with IOL implantation; this figure includes prescriptions for both spherocylindrical errors and near-vision correction. The corresponding figure in infants was reported to be 78%. To compensate for the naturally occurring myopic shift, there is a tendency to undercorrect the power of implanted IOLs in children <8 years, therefore postoperative hyperopia is the rule. Hyperopia probably causes amblyopia since neither far nor near objects are clearly focused on the retina. This fact calls for prompt correction of any residual refractive error. Moreover, the refractive status of the eye undergoes constant change in the first few years of life; reexaminations every 2 to 3 months in the first year of life and every 3 to 6 months thereafter are necessary to detect any significant change and corresponding need for a new prescription.

An aphakic or pseudophakic eye lacks effective accommodation. Bifocals are not properly used in toddlers; furthermore, in children <2 to 3 years of age most activities are within the range of 0.3 to 0.6 m. Therefore, a single prescription (contact lens or aphakic glasses) suitable for this distance is desirable. However, older children have a wider range of visual tasks; in this age group bifocal glasses with a near add of +2.5 are recommended.[6]

Amblyopia Therapy

Amblyopia and its treatment are one of the formidable obstacles in the postoperative course of pediatric cataract surgery, particularly in unilateral cases. Eyes with unilateral cataracts requiring surgery are amblyopic to varying degrees unless operated on by 6 weeks of age.[34] Furthermore, the ensuing unilateral aphakic or pseudophakic eye, even with appropriate correction, can never compete with the normal fellow eye with natural accommodation. Bilateral cases are less prone to develop amblyopia, however, one should always bear this possibility in mind. Amblyopia therapy should be considered in bilateral cases when fixation preference is present in one eye or when discrepancy in visual acuity between the eyes exceeds two Snellen lines.[5,13,22,36]

One of the cornerstones of successful amblyopia therapy is acceptance and compliance by the patient and family. The vital importance of proper correction and adherence to the amblyopia therapy schedule should be clearly explained to the parents. Zwaan et al.[37] described the effect of patient acceptance on visual outcomes of amblyopia therapy. According to their study only half of their operated patients were compliant with the regimen. Of children accepting treatment, 70% achieved a visual acuity of 20/80 or better, while the corresponding figure for those with poor compliance was only 38%. Conditions related to amblyopia and low vision include strabismus and nystagmus; the management of these conditions requires collaboration with a pediatric ophthalmologist.

SUMMARY

Postoperative care, including follow-up examinations and medical treatment, following cataract surgery is a delicate and sophisticated issue in children compared to adults. The follow-up schedule should be individualized as dictated by the clinical course. However, closely spaced examinations in the early postoperative period and lifelong observation are mandatory for all children undergoing cataract extraction.

Attention to postoperative inflammation and its control are of utmost importance. Topical steroids, NSAIDs, and cycloplegics are the cornerstones of treatment, however, systemic steroids may be required in certain cases. Periodic reassessment of the operated eye is necessary to detect media opacification, glaucoma, or any other complication.

One should always bear in mind that performing an uncomplicated pediatric cataract extraction with or without IOL implantation is only the first step toward visual rehabilitation. Timely correction of refractive errors and amblyopia therapy and early recognition of other complications are critical for a succesful outcome. Intimate cooperation among the surgeon, a pediatric ophthalmologis, and the parents is critical in achieving this goal.

REFERENCES

1. Aasuri MK, Gupta S. Management of pediatric cataract: current perspectives. In: Agarwal S, ed. *Phacoemulsification, Laser Cataract Surgery and Foldable IOLs*. New Dehli, India: Jaypee Brothers, 2000:389–998.
2. Rajpal RK, Glaser SR. Antiseptics and disinfectants. In: Zimmerman TG, ed. *Textbook of Ocular Pharmacology*. New York, Philadelphia: Lippincott–Raven, 1997:661–665.
3. Zetterstrom C. Cataract surgery in pediatric eye. In: Buratto L, Osher R, Masket S, eds. *Cataract Surgery in Complicated Cases*. Fabiano–Milano: Slack, 2000:1–14.
4. Devaro JM, Buckley EG, Awner S, Seaber J. Secondary posterior chamber intraocular lens implantation in pediatric patients. *Am J Ophthalmol* 1997;123:24–30.
5. Argento C, Badoza D, Ugrin C. Optic capture of the acrysof intraocular lens in pediatric cataract surgery. *J Cataract Refract Surg* 2001;27:1638–1642.
6. Cheng KP, Biglan AW. Pediatric cataract surgery. *Clin Ophthalmol* 6:1–24.
7. Biglan AW. Pediatric cataract surgery. In: Albert DM, ed. *Ophthalmic Surgery: Principles and Techniques*. Cambridge, MA: Blackwell, 1999:970–1014.
8. Pavlovic S, Jacobi FK, Graef M, Jacobi KW. Silicone intraocular lens implantation in children: preliminary results. *J Cataract Refract Surg* 2000;26:88–95.
9. Onol M, Ozdek SC, Koksal M, Hasanreisoglu B. Pars plana lensectomy with double-capsule-supported intraocular lens implantation in children. *J Cataract Refract Surg* 2000;26:486–490.
10. Behki R, Noel LP, Clarke WN. Limbal lensectomy in the management of ectopia lentis in children. *Arch Ophthalmol* 1990;108:809–811.
11. Awner S, Buckley EG, DeVaro JM, Seaber JH. Unilateral pseudophakia in children under 4 years. *J Pediatr Ophthalmol Strabismus* 1996;33:230–236.
12. Vasavada AR, Trivedi RH, Singh R. Necessity of vitrectomy when optic capture is performed in children older than 5 years. *J Cataract Refract Surg* 2001;27:1185–1193.
13. Alexandrakis G, Peterseim MM, Wilson ME. Clinical outcomes of pars plana capsulotomy with anterior vitrectomy in pediatric cataract surgery. *J AAPOS* 2002;6:163–167.
14. Ogawa GSH, Hyndiuk RA. Fluoroquinolones. In: Zimmerman TJ, ed. *Textbook of Ocular Pharmacology*. Philadelphia, New York: Lippincott–Raven, 1997:537–548.
15. Ta CN, Egbert PR, Singh K, Shiver EM, Blumenkranz MS, de Kaspar HM. Prospective randomized comparison of 3-day versus 1-hour preoperative ofloxacin prophylaxis for cataract surgery. *Ophthalmology* 2002;109:2036–2041.
16. Ellis FD. Ocular antinflammatory agents. In: Zimmerman TJ, ed. *Textbook of Ocular Pharmacology*. Philadelphia, New York: Lippincott–Raven, 1997:801–804.
17. Raina UK, Gupta V, Arora R, Mehta DK. Posterior continuous curvilinear capsulorhexis with and without optic capture of the posterior chamber intraocular lens in the absence of vitrectomy. *J Pediatr Ophthalmol Strabismus* 2002;39:278–287.
18. Pandey SK, Ram J, Werner L, Brar GS, Jain AK, Gupta A, Apple DJ. Visual results and postoperative complications of capsular bag and ciliary sulcus fixation of posterior chamber intraocular lenses in children with traumatic cataracts. *J Cataract Refract Surg* 1999;25:1576–1584.
19. Ahmadieh H, Javadi MA, Ahmady M, et al. Primary capsulectomy, anterior vitrectomy, lensectomy, and posterior chamber lens implantation in children: limbal versus pars plana. *J Cataract Refract Surg* 1999;25:768–775.
20. Stamper RL, Lieberman MF, Drake MV. *Diagnosis and Therapy of the Glaucomas*. Philadelphia, New York: Lippincott–Raven, 1999:317–355.
21. Jensen AA, Basti S, Greenwald MJ, Mets MB. When may the posterior capsule be preserved in pediatric intraocular lens Surgery? *Ophthalmology* 2002;109:324–328.
22. Crouch ER, Crouch JR, Pressman SH. Prospective analysis of pediatric pseudophakia: myopic shift and postoperative outcomes. *J AAPOS* 2002;6:277–282.
23. Cavallaro BE, Madigan WP, O'Hara MA, Kramer KK, Bauman WC. Posterior chamber intraocular lens use in children. *J Pediatr Ophthalmol Strabismus* 1998;35:254–263.
24. Plager DA, Lipsky SN, Snyder SK, Sprunger DT, Ellis FD, Sondhi N. Capsular management and refractive error in pediatric intraocular lenses. *Ophthalmology* 1997;104:600–607.
25. Vitale A, Foster CS. Nonsteroidal anti-inflammatory drugs. In: Zimmerman TG, ed. *Textbook of Ocular Pharmacology*. New York, Philadelphia: Lippincott–Raven, 1997:713–722.

26. Shepard D, Christiansen SP, Jacobi KW, Wright KW, Soheilian M. Consultation section: pediatric cataract. *Ann Ophthalmol* 1999;31:212–215.

27. Eidenbick AM, Amon M, Moser E, et al. Morphological and functional results of acrysof intraocular lens implantation in children prospective randomized study of age-related surgical management. *J Cataract Refract Surg* 2003;29:285–293.

28. Ellis FD. Cycloplegic agents. In: Zimmerman TG, ed. *Textbook of Ocular Pharmacology*. Philadelphia, New York: Lippincott–Raven, 1997:787–789.

29. Ellis FD. Topical ophthalmic preparations used for infants and children. In: Zimmerman TG, ed. *Textbook of Ocular Pharmacology*. Philadelphia, New York: Lippincott–Raven, 1997:783–786.

30. BenEzra D, Cohen E. Cataract surgery in children with chronic uveitis. *Ophthalmology* 2000;107:1255–1260.

31. Gimbel HV, Ferensowicz M, Raanan M, DeLuca M. Implantation in children. *J Pediatr Ophthalmol Strabismus* 1993;30:69–79.

32. Ellis FD. Topical and local anesthetic agents. In: Zimmerman TG, ed. *Textbook of Ocular Pharmacology*. Philadelphia, New York: Lippincott–Raven, 1997:791–793.

33. Miyahara S, Amino K, Tanihara H. Glaucoma secondary to pars plana lensectomy for congenital cataract. *Grafes Arch Clin Exp Ophthalmol* 2002;240:176–179.

34. Lambert SR, Drack AV. Major review: Infantile cataract. *Surv Ophthalmol* 1996;40:427–458.

35. Neumann D, Weissman BA, Isenberg SJ, Rosenbaum AL, Bateman JB. The effectiveness of daily wear contact lenses for the correction of infantile aphakia. *Arch Ophthalmol* 1993;111:927–930.

36. Hiles DA. Intraocular lens implantation in children with monocular cataracts. *Ophthalmology* 1984;91:1231–1237.

37. Zwaan J, Mullaney PB, Awad A, Al-Mesfer S, Wheeler DT. Pediatric intraocular lens implantation. *Ophthalmology* 1998;105:112–119.

Lens Implantation in Children

Chapter 21

Posterior Chamber Lens Implants: *Currently Available Lens Designs and Future Application*

Suresh K. Pandey and Randall J. Olson

Owing to the advent of small-incision cataract surgery made possible by phacoemulsification, age-related cataract surgery has been transformed from a major surgical procedure requiring several days of hospitalization to an outpatient procedure with an almost-immediate return to active life. Pediatric cataract–intraocular lens (IOL) surgery underwent significant advancement concurrent with adult cataract–IOL surgery. While the results of pediatric cataract surgery–IOL implantation have been improved, improvements in IOL power calculation and refraction precision are still needed. Comprehensive details on rigid and foldable implant biomaterials, designs, and visual results as well as complications related to the use of these devices in adult and pediatric cataract surgery have been reviewed in several recent publications.[1–13] In this chapter, we attempt to provide the relevant details on commonly implanted rigid and foldable biomaterials and designs and also to include brief details on newly available lenses that are not yet approved by the U.S. Food and Drug Administration (FDA). However, it is almost impossible to provide comprehensive details on each and every rigid/foldable IOL manufactured/implanted today. Since experience with newly available implants in children is very limited, a significant amount of the information

provided in this chapter (text and figures) on the various designs/biomaterials is derived from cataract–IOL surgery in adults.

RIGID AND SOFT IMPLANTS: TERMINOLOGY, BIOCOMPATIBILITY, AND MECHANICAL PROPERTIES

It may be pertinent for readers to be familiar with some of the specific terminology that is used to describe the properties of IOL biomaterials. All IOLs are made of polymers, each of which is made up of about 5,000 monomers cross-linked by a process called polymerization. These cross-linkages can form a polymer with a linear or a three-dimensional structure. In addition, all modern IOL optics contain integrated ultraviolet (UV) absorbing agents, which are incorporated to protect the retina from UV radiation in the 300- to 400-nm range. Normally this protection is provided by the human crystalline lens. Benzophenone and benzotriazole are two classes of UV absorbing chromophores used for manufacturing the artificial implant. Some new technology implants also now include blue light filtering agents, which may protect the retina from hazardous blue light (>400 nm).

Implant Biocompatibility

Lens material biocompatibility is an often-misunderstood term. Biocompatibility is defined as the capability of a prosthesis implanted in the body to exist in harmony with the tissue without causing deleterious changes (*International Dictionary of Medicine and Biology*, 1986). Biocompatibility of IOLs can be discussed in terms of the host cell response to trauma (cataract surgery) and foreign body reaction to the IOL. Uveal biocompatibility describes the level of the foreign body reaction to the IOL biomaterial. Capsular biocompatibility describes the level of biomaterial–lens epithelial cell (LEC) interaction, resulting in various levels of LEC outgrowth, anterior capsule opacification, posterior capsule opacification (PCO), and capsular contraction.

Refractive Index

The refractive index describes the ability of a biomaterial to bend light. Each lens biomaterial has a refractive index that, to a large degree, determines the lens thickness. The higher the refractive index of a lens material (e.g., 1.55 for AcrySof hydrophobic acrylic biomaterial, compared to 1.46 for IOLs manufactured from silicone), the thinner the IOL optic will be for the same dioptric power, all else being equal.

Mechanical Properties

The mechanical properties of a polymer are described by its tensile strength and tensile elongation. The ultimate tensile strength is the ability of a biomaterial to resist breaking under stress. Tensile elongation of a biomaterial is the percentage increase in length that occurs before it breaks under tension. These parameters are important for the resistance of the biomaterial to manipulation, such as folding.

Polymethylmethacrylate (PMMA) exhibits a high tensile strength with a low tensile elongation percentage, meaning that is it very resistant to tensile stress and, when breaking, does so without much deformation. This can be affected by various types of manufacturing processes, such as lathe cut, cast molding, and injection molding. The foldable IOL materials exhibit in general a lower tensile strength with higher percentages of elongation at their breaking points compared to PMMA.

Glass Transition Temperature

The mechanical properties of polymers are affected by temperature. The glass transition temperature (T_g) can be understood as the temperature at which a polymer will change its properties. At temperatures above T_g linear polymers will display viscous flow, whereas a cross-linked polymer will be rubbery or elastic. Below T_g polymers will be hard and glassy. The transition range is approximately 10°C.

Surface Energy

The surface energy describes the wetting capability of a biomaterial. It depends on the liquid, the biomaterial, and their surroundings. For example, if the adhesive forces of the liquid are weaker than their attraction to the solid surface, wetting occurs. Surface energy can be quantified by measurement of the contact angle of a drop of liquid placed on a solid surface. High surface energy means a low water-drop contact angle and a high wetting capability (hydrophilic materials). Low surface energy means a high water-drop contact angle and a low wetting capability (hydrophobic materials).[14]

BIOMATERIALS FOR RIGID AND SOFT IMPLANTS

IOLs are manufactured from acrylic or silicone biomaterials. Acrylic lenses can be further classified as rigid lenses manufactured from PMMA and soft or foldable lenses manufactured from hydrogels (hydrophilic acrylic) or hydrophobic acrylic biomaterial. We have provided a brief overview of IOL biomaterials. Interested readers may consult other comprehensive sources to become familiar with this subject.[15]

Pediatric Cataract Surgery and Rigid Polymethylmethacrylate Implants

Trends and Overview

The 2001 pediatric cataract surgery and IOL survey of ASCRS and AAPOS members, by Wilson and associates,[16] reports that rigid PMMA IOLs were preferred by 23.6 and 24.5% of the responders, respectively. PMMA is a polymer of methylmethacrylate (MMA), which means that it is an acrylic biomaterial made from only one type of monomer. IOLs made from PMMA have a T_g of approximately 110°C, making them rigid at room temperature. PMMA is flexible only when thinner than 0.12 mm. PMMA has a refractive index of 1.49, higher than that of silicone but lower than that of some acrylic copolymers. PMMA seems to have less uveal biocompatibility than silicone or hydrogel IOLs. Surface treating of PMMA lenses (e.g., heparin surface modification) significantly reduces postoperative inflammation, cell adhesion, and corneal endothelial cell damage. The lower incidence of inflammatory cell deposit formation in eyes with heparin surface-modified PMMA IOLs suggests that these IOLs have a greater bicompatibility than unmodified PMMA IOLs in pediatric cataract surgery.[17]

Pediatric Cataract Surgery and Foldable Silicone Implants

Trends and Overview

The 2001 pediatric cataract surgery and IOL survey of American Society of Cataract and Refractive Surgery (ASCRS) and American Association for Pediatric Ophthalmology and Strabismus (AAPOS) members, by Wilson and associates,[16] reports that silicone IOLs were preferred by 6.8 and 1.7% of the responders, respectively. Most silicone IOLs are low molecular weight polymers of oxygen and silicone (polysiloxanes) that are extensively cross-linked. The silicone–oxygen molecular backbone confers mechanical flexibility. The appendant organic groups, e.g., vinyl, methyl, and phenyl, determine the strength, clarity and

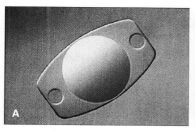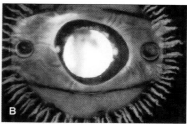

FIGURE 21-1. Large-hole silicone plate IOL (Elastic Lens) manufactured by Staar Surgical. **A.** Photograph of this currently available IOL. The diameter of the two holes in this IOL design has been increased from the original 0.3 mm to 1.15 mm for secure fixation in the capsular bag in adult cataract–IOL surgery. The role of the fixation hole has been confirmed in animal studies, however, further clinical studies are needed to confirm that the larger positioning holes help with fixation in the bag. **B.** Gross posterior photograph (Miyake–Apple technique) showing a large-hole silicone plate IOL implanted in a pseudophakic human eye obtained postmortem. Note the fibrosis of the anterior capsule with anterior capsular folds. (Courtesy of David J. Apple, MD, Salt Lake City, UT.)

refractive index. Newer generations of silicone have a higher refractive index (1.46 versus 1.41; still lower than that of PMMA) and, thus, thinner optics, resulting in a smaller wound size over a range of dioptric power. Silicone lenses have a T_g of approximately $-100°C$, making them very flexible at room temperature.

Silicone's angle of water contact is 99°, which makes it more hydrophobic than hydrophobic acrylic, which has an angle of water contact of 73°.[14] Newer silicone IOLs are known for their high uveal and capsular biocompatibility.[18,19] Once implanted, silicone IOLs may stimulate a varying degree of anterior capsule fibrosis, as reported in postmortem human eyes implanted with various IOLs.[20,21] The silicone IOL polymer had the lowest threshold for laser-induced damage and a greater linear extension of damage than the PMMA and acrylic IOL polymers.[22]

Currently Available Silicone Lens Designs

There are several designs of silicone IOLs available in the United States. The spherical types of the one-piece plate design are manufactured by Staar Surgical (Elastic Lens; Monrovia, CA) (Fig. 21-1) and Bausch and Lomb Surgical (Rocheseter, NY). Standard posterior chamber IOLs have only spherical refractive correction. A new Staar toric IOL (Fig. 21-2) may be useful in correcting preoperative astigmatism in pediatric cataract surgery. It has had limited follow-up but shows promising results in correcting preoperative astigmatism as reported for adult cataract surgery.[23,24] It is a single-piece silicone plate haptic that corrects 1.5 to 3.5 diopters of astigmatism. While spherical IOLs can be placed in and rotated into any position, a toric IOL must be placed in the correct axis to be effective. Researchers have reported good results implanting the Staar toric IOL and maintaining its orientation after adult cataract surgery. These IOLs have complications similar to those of the one-piece plate silicone lenses. However, owing to their cylindrical refractive correction, decentration or dislocation of these lenses has a more profound effect on the patient's visual acuity. These lenses are not recommended when a primary posterior capsulectomy and anterior vitrectomy are being performed. Plate silicone IOLs create the most capsular fibrosis of any IOL type and can dislocate posteriorly after Nd:YAG laser posterior capsulotomy.

Three-piece monofocal silicone lenses are very popular and well tolerated. These IOL designs include three-piece

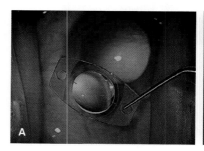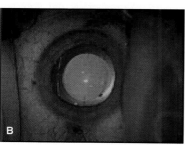

FIGURE 21-2. A current large-hole silicone plate IOL, the Staar Surgical model AA-4203TF toric IOL. **A** and **B.** Clinical photographs showing its implantation in a patient undergoing surgery for age-related cataract. (Courtesy of David F. Chang, MD, Los Altos, CA.)

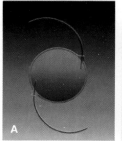
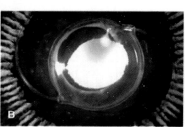

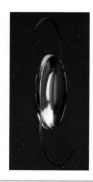

FIGURE 21-3. Advanced Medical Optics (AMO Inc.; formerly Allergan) was the first successful manufacturer of foldable three-piece silicone IOL designs, beginning with the prototype SI9 and SI13 designs in the early 1980s and continuing today with the successful SI30 and SI40 models. **A.** Photograph of the three-piece silicone SI40 IOL design. **B.** Miyake–Apple posterior view of an eye obtained postmortem containing the AMO SI40 foldable silicone IOL shows good centration and clarity. (B: Courtesy of David J. Apple, Salt Lake City, UT.)

FIGURE 21-5. Photograph showing the Clariflex IOL (AMO Inc.), with its modified truncated edge designed to minimize dysphotopsia.

monofocal silicone IOLs (SI30 and SI40), which have a rounded-edge optic profile (Fig. 21-3). The CeeOn Edge 911 (AMO Inc., Santa Ana, CA; formerly Pfizer Ophthalmics, New York) (Fig. 21-4) and AMO Clariflex IOL (AMO; Santa Ana, CA; formerly Allergan) (Fig. 21-5) have a sharp posterior edge, a design modification that is helpful in reducing PCO. Bausch & Lomb also has a new edge design for its SoFlex silicone IOL. The new SoFlex SE IOL also features a squared-off posterior edge to facilitate complete capsular contact and reduce LEC migration and the incidence of PCO.

Implantation of the Silicone Lens Designs

Recently, injectable devices have been designed to allow for remarkably safe, facile, and reproducible placement of IOLs in the capsular bag. A brief summary of the available injectors and injection methods for foldable implants is included in this chapter. Owing to the lack of published studies in the pediatric age group, interested readers may refer to the brochure/manual published by the manufacturer to become familiar with the comprehensive details of the individual IOL delivery system, suggested insertion techniques, incision size, etc.

One-piece silicone plate haptic IOLs have the advantage of insertion through a very small incision wound. Structurally, silicone has a "slippery" surface that makes it difficult to manipulate, especially if wet, and also makes it less adherent to ocular tissue. Both threaded- and syringe-style injectors exist for one-piece plate haptic silicone IOLs and allow for placement through incision sizes of ≤2.8 mm. The first of the injectable devices designed for three-piece silicone lenses was the Unfolder Sapphire Implantation System (AMO Inc., Santa Ana, CA; formely Allergan). The Silver Series is used to deliver three-piece silicone lenses SI30, SI40, and SA40N Array multifocal implants through unenlarged standard phacoemulsification incisions in adult cataract–IOL surgery. The Gold

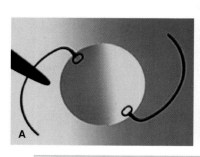
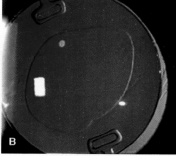
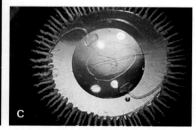

FIGURE 21-4. A foldable IOL in the AMO Inc. CeeOn 900 series: the CeeOn 911 Edge design lens. It has a silicone optic, a truncated edge, and polyvinylidene fluoride haptics. **A.** photograph showing the characteristic capsular C-shaped haptic configuration. **B.** Clinical photograph showing a well-centered CeeOn Edge 911 IOL implanted in an adult eye. Note that the lens is recognizable owing to the oval-rectangular configuration of the haptic tips at the site where they enter the peripheral optic. **C.** Gross photograph of a human eye obtained postmortem implanted with the CeeOn 911 Edge design, showing good centration of the lens within the capsular bag.

Series handpiece and cartridge are similar and are used for the 5.5-mm-optic three-piece silicone lenses (e.g., SI55). These metal-threaded injectors incorporate a soft, silicone-tipped plunger, which advances the optic and allows for placement of the trailing haptic. These injectors require partial rotation along their long axis during delivery for consistent and properly oriented implant placement within the capsular bag. Upon IOL insertion into the capsular bag, silicone IOLs may have a rapid unfolding action, depending on the insertion system, which can lead to uncontrolled insertion and intraocular damage. The metal threads have recently been enlarged, increasing the speed of delivery of the IOL. The M-port is a plastic syringe-style device that allows for one-handed delivery without rotation of the device. It is manufactured by Bausch & Lomb Surgical (Claremont, CA) and is used to deliver the three-piece silicone implant (model LI61U).

Pediatric Cataract Surgery and Hydrophilic Acrylic (Hydrogel) Implants

Trends and Overview

The 2001 pediatric cataract surgery and IOL survey of ASCRS and AAPOS members, by Wilson and associates,[16] reported that hydrogel IOLs were preferred by 2.4 and 1% of the responders, respectively. Hydrophilic acrylic IOLs are composed of a mixture of a hydroxyethylmethacrylate (poly-HEMA) backbone and a hydrophilic acrylic monomer. There are multiple types of hydrophilic acrylic IOLs, with varying water contents and copolymers. The amount of water absorbed, expressed as a percentage of the weight of the hydrated gel, is known as the equilibrium water content, which usually varies between 18 and 38%. These IOLs are soft and have an excellent biocompatibility because of their relatively hydrophilic lens surface. There have been reports that these IOLs show little or no surface alterations or damage from folding with insertion, most likely because of their soft flexible surface.[25]

Their low surface energy and thus hydrophilicity are a major reason for their uveal biocompatibility, as well as their low damage potential when touching the corneal endothelial cells. However, hydrogels seem to have a lower capsular biocompatibility than other biomaterials, resulting in more LEC outgrowth, anterior capsule contracture, and PCO formation after adult cataract surgery.[26] Fortunately, if a Nd:YAG capsulotomy is necessary, these lenses have a high threshold for Nd:YAG laser damage.[27] Also, the hydrophilic properties include a low surface energy, and in patients requiring vitreoretinal surgery, these IOLs have minimal adherence to silicone oil.[28]

Currently Available Hydrophilic Lens Designs and Their Implantation

There are several types of hydrophilic acrylic IOLs, described below.

The Hydroview

The Hydroview (Bausch & Lomb, Rochester, NY) (Fig. 21-6) is a three-piece lens made of a poly-HEMA mixture with a relatively low water content. This IOL has a high refractive index and a thin optic. The Hydroview IOL is currently being marketed internationally in conjunction with the Surefold delivery system. Interested readers may refer to the brochure/manual published by Bausch & Lomb for the details of the Surefold delivery system and insertion techniques.

The MemoryLens

The MemoryLens (IOLTECH Laboratories, Cedex 9, France) (Fig. 21-7) is a poly-HEMA–acrylic (MMA) mixture with a moderate water content and polypropylene loops. The CV 232 SRE from Ciba Vision is a modification of the unique MemoryLens design, which uses thermoplastic material. The CV 232 SRE's posterior edge is squared off to help prevent PCO; the rounded anterior edge is

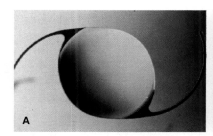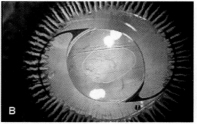

FIGURE 21-6. Bausch & Lomb Surgical, Inc. hydrophilic hydrogel design, the Hydroview H55S and H60M series, which was approved by the FDA in mid-1999. This IOL (formerly Storz Surgical) is a one-piece design with PMMA haptics fused to an 18% water content hydrogel polymer optic material. **A.** Photograph of the Hydroview model H60M. **B.** Photograph of a postmortem human eye from the posterior view implanted with a Hydroview IOL. Centration of the lens within the capsular bag is excellent.

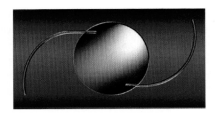

FIGURE 21-7. The MemoryLens (IOLTECH Laboratories, Cedex 9, France) is a poly-HEMA–acrylic (MMA) mixture with a moderate water content and polypropylene loops. Manufacturer's illustration of the IOL.

designed to give good optical quality. Unfortunately, there have been reports of delayed-onset acute, sterile, toxic anterior segment syndrome with the MemoryLens among adult cataract cases.[29] These patients present postoperatively with unexplained inflammation in the anterior segment. Most patients with toxic anterior segment syndrome improved with intensive topical steroids. It is unclear whether this inflammation is caused by the IOL itself or another factor. The manufacturers have blamed this problem on residual polishing compound. The lens was removed from the market and rereleased with the assurance that the issues have been resolved. However, we must carefully monitor hydrophilic acrylic biomaterials for outbreaks of inflammation and concern about refractive stability. Hopefully, manufacturers will eliminate these problems with time.

The MemoryLens is available prerolled from the manufacturer, obviating the need to fold the implant. It is simply removed from its package and inserted directly into the incision using a round-bodied forceps. Specifically designed instruments may be used to help minimize the incision size and improve the holding power on the grasped optic. As the leading haptic is being placed, care must be taken to angle it in a clockwise direction so that the broad C-shaped haptics are properly positioned under the anterior capsular leaflet. The trailing haptic is placed in a conventional manner. As the IOL slowly warms to the eye's temperature,

the optic unrolls, and the haptics move into position within the capsular bag.

The Centerflex IOL

The Centerflex IOL (Rayner Intraocular Lenses, East Sussex, UK) (Fig. 21-8) is another single–piece hydrophilic acrylic IOL with broad haptics. The round, tapered edge of the classic one-piece hydrophilic acylic IOL designs at the optic–haptic junction represents a theoretical *"Achilles' heel"* where ingrowing LECs may bypass the desired barrier. This may be important in pediatric cataract surgery owing to the high rate of PCO after cataract–IOL surgery in this population. The manufacturer has now introduced an IOL with an "enhanced square edge," as this profile provides a square edge (barrier, ridge, wall) for 360° around the lens optic, eliminating the potential defect. The Centerflex IOL can be inserted through an injector, and clinical investigation of the C-*flex* injectable IOL system is in progress.

Delayed Postoperative Opacification of Hydrophilic Acrylic Lens Designs

The issue of hydrophilicity now involves other concerns that have recently been reported. Probably the most disconcerting effect to date has been the calcification of these lenses. Although several hundred cases of calcification of Hydroview IOLs (Bausch & Lomb, Claremont, CA) in adult cataract surgery have been reported, this represents only a small percentage of all hydrophilic acrylic lenses implanted.[30–36] Other hydrophilic acrylic lenses with reported dystrophic calcification include the MDR SC60BOUV, AquaSense, Memory Lens, Morcher, and IOLTech.[37,38] Dystrophic calcification in pediatric implantations has been reported recently as well.[53]

Calcification tends to progress slowly and can be significant in some patients, even to the extent that the lens must be removed. Although there is no definitive explanation, the manufacturers have suggested that a breakdown in the blood–iris barrier caused by silicone particles from

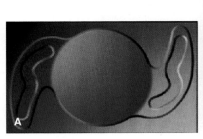 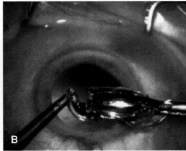 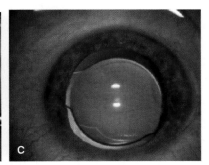

FIGURE 21-8. The Centerflex IOL (Rayner Inc., East Sussex, UK) is a single-piece hydrophilic acrylic IOL with a broad optic–haptic junction. **A.** Manufacturer's illustration. **B** and **C.** Clinical photographs showing implantation of the Centerflex IOL. Note the well-centered IOL in the capsular bag.

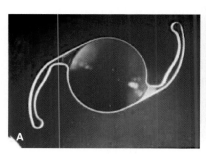
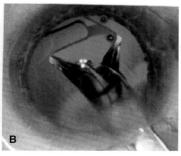

FIGURE 21-9. Single-piece hydrophobic acrylic (Alcon AcrySof) lens. **A.** Gross photograph. **B.** Photograph showing insertion of the lens.

the packaging may be the culprit. In vitro studies done by the manufacturer revealed a migration of silicone from a gasket in the SureFold packaging system. In addition to silicone, the presence of fatty acids also contributed to attracting calcium on the lens surface. Modifications in the IOL packaging were carried out by the manufacturer, and to the best of our knowledge, no cases of calcification have been reported since then. However, we should keep a careful eye on hydrophilic acrylic lenses with regard to this calcification issue. A more pertinent question is whether calcification is a potential problem with all hydrophilic materials.

Pediatric Cataract Surgery and Hydrophobic Acrylic Implants

Trends and Overview

The 2001 pediatric cataract surgery and IOL survey of ASCRS and AAPOS members, by Wilson and associates,[16] reported that hydrophobic acrylic IOLs were most commonly implanted in children, being preferred by 66.8 and 71.7% of the responders, respectively. Hydrophobic acrylic lenses are made of copolymers of acrylate and methacrylate, which makes them flexible and durable. Hydrophobic acrylic lenses are lightweight and relatively inert. The T_g of some hydrophobic acrylic (such as AcrySof) IOLs is 13°C, making them flexible at room temperature. Hydrophobic acrylic usually has a higher refractive index (1.44–1.55) than silicone (1.41–1.46) and PMMA (1.49), therefore the lenses are usually thinner. Owing to their thinness, hydrophobic acrylic lenses have also been implanted in a piggyback manner for correcting the refractive power after infantile cataract surgery. Interested readers should refer to Chapters 23 and 24 for details.

Currently Available Hydrophobic Lens Designs

These include the three-piece AcrySof single-piece AcrySof (Fig. 21-9), Sensar (Fig. 21-10), and Hoya (Fig. 21-11) IOLs. Hydrophobic acrylic lenses are known to have a high capsular biocompatibility, provoking less capsular bag opaci-

fication. The low rate of PCO/capsular bag opacification has been attributed, in part, to the sharp-edge optic design of lenses made from three-piece hydrophobic acrylic (AcrySof) biomaterial, but also in part to the adhesive properties of the biomaterial itself. One possible mechanism is that hydrophobic acrylic has a higher binding capacity to fibronectin, which mediates adherence to the lens capsule, thus impeding LEC migration.[39–41]

Blue Filtration Hydrophobic IOL–AcrySof Natural IOL Design

Prolonged exposure to visible blue light rays is widely considered to be a causative factor for damage to the retina and macula and is believed to be a possible contributor to age-related macular degeneration. A variation of the hydrophobic lens known as AcrySof Natural (Alcon Inc., Fort Worth, TX) has been approved by the FDA for age-related cataract surgery. This IOL contains a proprietary, integrated polymer dye designed to filter both invisible UV rays and visible blue rays of light. While traditional UV lenses provide light filtration from 200 to 400 nm, the AcrySof Natural lens provides filtration properties that approximate the crystalline lens of a 20-year-old. This means that the light transmission is gradually reduced from 500 to 400 nm, and at 500 nm and above the data overlap those for the average human crystalline lens of a 20-year-old. Improved contrast sensitivity, a decrease in central glare after IOL implantation, and restoration of normal, adult, precataract color vision (as traditional UV filters may result in

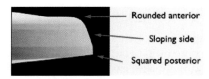

FIGURE 21-10. Three-piece hydrophobic acrylic Sensar lens (AMO Inc.) with OptiEdge technology. Scanning electron micrograph. Note the rounded anterior edge that scatters the light, thus reducing internal reflections. The sloping side edge minimizes the potential for edge glare and the square posterior edge facilitates a 360° capsular seal.

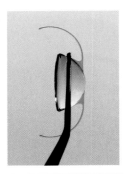

FIGURE 21-11. Three-piece hydrophobic acrylic lens (Hoya Inc.). This IOL filters out some blue light.

excessive unnatural blue color vision for the patient) are among the other theoretical advantages of the AcrySof Natural IOL design. Nevertheless, loss of scotopic vision is a potential negative of blue filtration IOLs and requires further study.[42]

Implantation of the Hydrophobic Lens Designs

Hydrophobic acrylic copolymers allow for a slower unfolding action, which some feel provides more controlled insertion and manipulation. However, the softer nature of this acrylic copolymer makes it fragile and more susceptible to cracks, dents, and scratches. Foldable one-piece and three-piece ArcySof IOLs can be inserted through the Monarch injector delivery system manufactured by Alcon. This system permits excellent visualization of the folding process and implant delivery in the capsular bag. The three-piece Sensar hydrophobic acrylic IOL may be delivered through the Sapphire injector, specifically designed by AMO Inc. for this implant. Owing to the lack of published studies on insertion techniques and incision size after pediatric cataract surgery, interested readers may refer to the brochure/manual published by the manufacturer for the details of the IOL delivery system, insertion techniques, and incision size.

NEWLY INTRODUCED IMPLANT DESIGNS

Globally, contemporary cataract surgeons have witnessed great advancements in cataract surgery, foldable IOLs, and surgical technology, with easier and safer cataract removal using a smaller incision. We provide, below, brief details of newly available IOL designs for adult cataract surgery. These include multifocal, ultrasmall-incision lenses, accommodative IOLs, and light-adjustable and aspherical lenses. Most of these IOLs have been used in adult cataract

surgery, and as we gain experience, they can be implanted in children after cataract surgery.

Pediatric Cataract Surgery and Multifocal Implants

The IOLs commonly in use are monofocal. It is not possible to see near and distant objects clearly with the same lens without correction and thus patients are at least potentially dependent on spectacles. Over the past decade, a variety of multifocal IOLs has been introduced and has enjoyed widespread clinical use. Both refractive and diffractive models have been shown to be effective in allowing each eye to achieve quality, uncorrected distance and near visual acuity after cataract surgery. The major concerns with the use of these lenses are the loss of contrast sensitivity and the inducement of glare and halos from light sources during night vision, which occurs more commonly with refractive designs. All multifocal lenses require careful attention to IOL power calculations and minimal refractive error after cataract surgery.

The only multifocal IOL currently approved for general use in the United States is the Array (AMO, Advanced Medical Optics, Santa Ana, Ca). The AMO Array SA40N multifocal IOL is a lens designed with a 2.1-mm central zone and five zones of near and distance powers on the anterior surface of the optic (Fig. 21-12). These power rings allow greater flexibility with different pupil sizes. The Array is considered a "distance dominant" lens and provides near acuities without correction in the J-3 range or better, offering good midrange and near acuity for most tasks. Some patients still require a near correction for finer print and under some low and high light conditions. The AMO Array is available in a foldable silicone biomaterial with PMMA haptics.

In a prospective, noncomparative, interventional case series, Jacobi and associates[43] reported the outcomes of multifocal IOL implantation in pediatric cataract surgery.

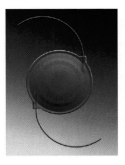

FIGURE 21-12. Photograph of the AMO Array multifocal lens, which is a three-piece silicone optic–PMMA haptic design.

Thirty-five eyes of 26 pediatric patients aged 2 to 14 years with multifocal IOL implantation with more than 1 year of follow-up were included. All eyes underwent a standard surgical procedure and implantation of a multifocal IOL (SA40-N; Allergan, Irvine, CA). At last follow-up, 71% of eyes were documented to have a visual acuity of 20/40 or better and 31% of eyes had a visual acuity of 20/25 or better. In the nine bilateral cases, spectacle dependency was moderate, with only two children (22%) reporting the permanent use of an additional near correction. Stereopsis also improved significantly after multifocal IOL implantation and the authors concluded that multifocal IOL implantation is a viable alternative to monofocal pseudophakia in the pediatric age group. However, in the same study, postoperative complications such as IOL decentration were noted (6 of 35 eyes), requiring explantation/exchange of the multifocal IOL with a monofocal lens. Posterior synechie was another postoperative complication, seen in as many as 54% of eyes. Based on some of these concerns, Hunter[44] cautioned against the widespread use of multifocal IOLs in children, who are especially at risk of amblyopia, and also in traumatic cataract patients. Traumatic cataract cases have more risk of implant decentration or postsurgical pupillary abnormalities, thus minimizing the potential advantages of multifocal lens designs.

The AcrySof ReSTOR Pseudoaccommodative Implant

The AcrySof ReSTOR pseudoaccommodative IOL design (MA60D3 or SA60D3), with its apodized diffractive optic, was found (in FDA trials) to provide patients with excellent near visual acuity without compromising distance vision. Good functional intermediate vision has also been demonstrated in ongoing early clinical studies. No significant reduction in contrast sensitivity was found and the incidence of severe visual disturbances was not increased compared to that in monofocal controls. This IOL has an anterior conventional refractive surface that provides distant viewing power and a posterior concentric diffractive plate that provides additional near viewing power ranging from 2.5 to 4.5 diopters.

Ultrasmall-Incision Implants and Their Application in Pediatric Cataract Surgery

Owing to the soft nature of pediatric cataracts, phacoemulsification is not needed, and the lens cortex and nucleus can be aspirated with an irrigation/aspiration or vitrectomy handpiece through a small to ultrasmall incision. Ultrasmall incisions are being evaluated in adult eyes at present, however, with time they will be used in children. The first ultrasmall-incision IOL available for im-

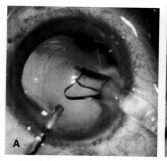
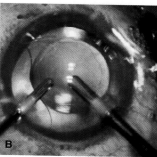

FIGURE 21-13. Acri.Tec Acry.Smart lens. **A** and **B.** Clinical photographs showing insertion of the Acry.Smart lens (model H44-IC-1) through a sub-2-mm incision. (Courtesy of Amar Agarwal, MD, Chennai, India.)

plantation in sub-2-mm incisions is the Acri.Smart (model H44-IC-1; Acri.Tec GmbH, Berlin, Germany).[45] This is a hydrophilic acrylic (25% water content) lens with a hydrophobic coating. The overall design is that of a plate haptic lens with square edges, which is loaded into the injector in a hydrated state so that unfolding is faster. It has an optical diameter of 6 mm and a total length of 12.3 mm. A folded +19-diopter lens has a width of about 1.2 to 1.3 mm. Following implantation, the Acri.Smart unfolds gradually in the capsular bag, being completely unfolded within 30 min (Fig. 21-13). Acri.Smart lenses (model 48S, with a 5.5-mm optic, and model 46S, with a 6.0-mm optic) have been developed for implantation with a specially designed injector through a 1.5-mm incision.

Another lens available for insertion through a sub-2.0-mm incision is the Ultrachoice (ThinOptX, Abingdon, VA).[46] The ThinOptX IOL is manufactured from off-the-shelf hydrophilic acrylic materials. The dioptric powers of this IOL range from −25 to +30, and the lens thickness ranges from 30 up to 350 μm. The ultrathin properties of the lens are attributable to its design, based on the Fresnel principle. Other unique properties of the ThinOptX IOL include its flexibility and ability to retain original memory. The manufacturer is now preparing to start clinical trials of the ThinOptX IOL in Europe and the United States.

For implantation of the ThinOptX IOL, the lens is taken from the container and gently held with a McPherson forceps (Fig. 21-14). The lens is then placed in a bowl of balanced salt solution (BSS; Alcon Inc., Fort Worth, TX) that is approximately body temperature. This is done to ensure that the IOL is pliable and to facilitate the rolling process. Once the lens is pliable, it is carefully taken with the gloved hand, holding it between the index finger and the thumb. The lens is then rolled in a rubbing motion by the surgeon. It is preferable to do this in the bowl of BSS so that the lens remains well rolled. An insertion system is

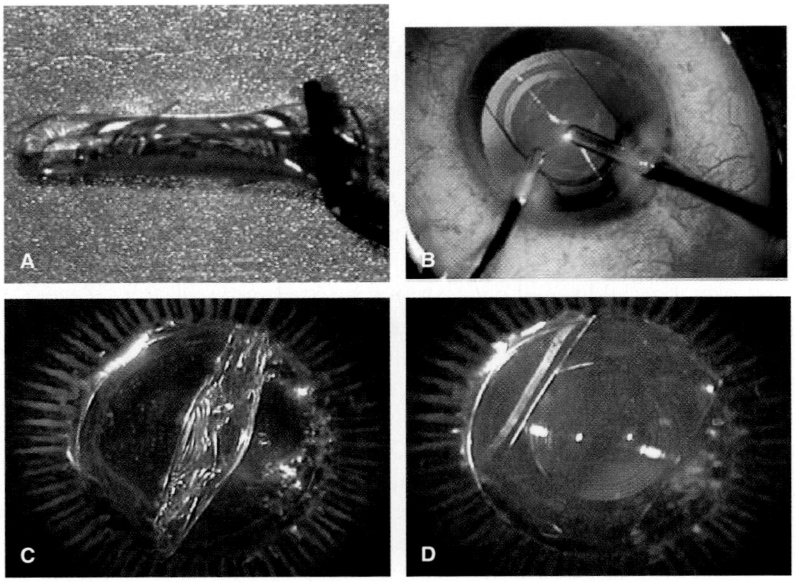

FIGURE 21-14. ThinOptX rollable IOL. **A.** Photograph of the IOL. **B.** Clinical photograph showing insertion of the ThinOptX IOL through a sub-2-mm incision. **C.** The ThinOptX IOL is unfolding inside the capsular bag upon reaching normal body temperature. **D.** Note the well-centered ThinOptX IOL in the capsular bag. (A, C, D: Courtesy of Nick Mamalis, MD, Salt Lake City, UT. B: Courtesy of Amar Agarwal, MD, Chennai, India.)

now available that can be used to roll the IOL. The lens is then carefully inserted through the sub-1.4-mm incision. The tip of the haptic should have a pointed shape to allow the lens to penetrate the clear corneal incision. The lens is then carefully implanted into the capsular bag after using a viscoelastic solution (Healon-GV; AMO Inc., Santa Ana, CA). To assure proper placement of the lens, the teardrop on the haptic should point in a clockwise direction. The smooth optic lenticular surface will be facing posteriorly. After implantation, the natural temperature of the eye causes the lens to open gradually within the capsular bag (Fig. 21-14C).

The third ultrasmall-incision IOL in the experimental, preclinical phase is the SmartIOL (Medennium, Inc., Irvine, CA). This is made of a thermodynamic hydrophobic acrylic gel polymer that can be formed to any size and shape with any dioptric power imprinted on it. At room temperature, the material is formed into a rod approximately 30 mm long and 2 mm wide. Therefore, it can be implanted into the patient's eye through a small incision. Inside the eye, the IOL slowly converts to its original size and shape as it reaches body temperature. It fills the entire capsular bag. This process takes about 30 sec and results in a lens about 9.5 mm wide and 2 to 4 mm thick (averaging about 3.5 mm) at the center, depending on the dioptric power. According to the Helmholtz theory, the loss of accommodation is caused by loss of flexibility in the mature, hard lens. Because of the entire filling of the capsular bag, the SmartIOL may theoretically restore accommodation. Due to its high refractive index, small changes in shape will result in significant changes in lens power. Even though the SmartIOL has not yet been implanted clinically, the hydrophobic acrylic biomaterial is expected to adhere to the capsule once in its contact, potentially re-

ducing PCO formation. Furthermore, a lens that has the dimensions of a natural lens will not cause problems with decentration and edge glare and will possibly overcome the spherical aberration induced by other artificial lens designs.

Laboratory studies performed by Nick Mamalis and associates using the Miyake–Apple posterior video technique and close-system technique demonstrated that both one-piece (Figs. 21-15A–C) and three-piece (Figs. 21-15D–F) SmartIOL designs can be inserted through sub-3-mm incisions with optimum filling of the capsular bag.[54]

Accommodating Implants and Their Application in Pediatric Cataract Surgery

The excellent results of modern small-incision cataract–IOL surgery have provided motivation to cataract surgeons to restore accommodation. Several manufacturers, ophthalmologists, and vision research scientists are in the process of designing and evaluating accommodative IOLs for placement in the capsular bag of patients to assess restoration of functional accommodation (as opposed to the pseudoaccommodation provided by multifocal IOLs) after cataract surgery. Another possible approach that has been experimentally explored in animals is the injection of a polymer lens into the capsular bag through a small capsulorhexis after phacoemulsification.

Accommodative implants have tremendous application in pediatric cataract surgery, as there is almost-total loss of accommodation after cataract surgery in this young age group. Most of the accommodative lens designs are currently being evaluated in adults and therefore most of

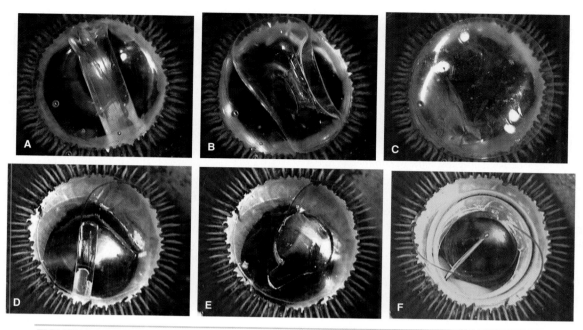

FIGURE 21-15. Experimental studies on the SmartIOL. **A–C.** Photographs showing the unfolding of the one-piece SmartIOL within the capsular bag of a postmortem human eye after injection of body-temperature BSS. **D–F.** Photographs showing the unfolding of the three-piece SmartIOL within the capsular bag of a postmortem human eye after injection of body-temperature BSS. (Courtesy of Nick Mamalis, MD, Salt Lake City, UT.)

the information summarized in the chapter is based on implantation of accommodative lenses in adult cataract surgery. Two of the accommodative lens designs undergoing clinical trials in adult cataract surgery are the *Crysta-Lens* AT-45 (Eyeonics, Aliso Viejo, CA, USA; now approved by the FDA) (Fig. 21-16), which is a modified plate haptic lens with a 4.5-mm optic, and the *Akkomodative* 1CU (HumanOptics, Erlangen, Germany) (Fig. 21-17), which is a hydrophilic acrylic IOL with a 5.5-mm optic. Both of these IOLs use the anterior movement of the optic to improve near vision.[47] Issues needing further study include dysphotopsia with these small optics, correlation of objective with subjective results, whether the aging eye loses pseudophakic accommodative amplitude, and the diminished result expected with low–dioptric power IOLs, as well as issues related to postoperative opacification of the capsular bag.

One manufacturer, Visiogen, Inc. (Irvine, CA) has developed a dual-optic, silicone, single-piece, foldable, accommodating lens called Synchrony (Fig. 21-18). This IOL features two optics connected by haptics that have a springlike action.[48,55] The optical power of the anterior optic is 30.00 to 35.00 diopters, and the posterior optic is assigned a variable diverging power to produce emmetropia for a given eye. The *Synchrony* accommodating IOL system is designed to work in the capsular bag, according to the traditional Helmholtz theory of accommodation. The distance between the two optics is minimal in the unaccommodated state and maximum in the accommodated state. Minimal movement results in large refractive changes owing to the dual-lens design. Early clinical results are promising but only time will tell if capsular contraction decreases accommodation amplitude over time.

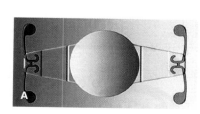

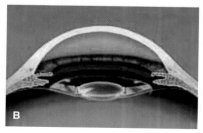

FIGURE 21-16. An accommodative lens. **A.** The CrystaLens. **B.** Schematic illustration of this IOL in the eye.

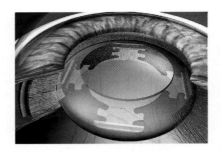

FIGURE 21-17. Schematic drawing of the Akkommodative 1CU lens in the capsular bag.

The Light Adjustable Lens and Its Application in Pediatric Cataract Surgery

It is well known that the majority of the eye's axial growth occurs during the first 2 years of life. This rapid eye growth makes selection of an IOL power for an infant difficult. Owing to its ability to provide changes in IOL power, the Light Adjustable Lens (LAL; Calhoun Vision, Pasadena, CA) has the potential to become a lens of choice after infantile cataract surgery. The major growth of the human eye occurs in the first 2 years of life, therefore IOL power calculation and adjustment are difficult. The LAL can theoretically adjust the IOL power commensurate with the growth of eyes in infancy. The LAL is currently undergoing in vivo study in rabbit eyes as well as preliminary clinical study in human eyes.

The LAL consists of a silicone matrix into which smaller, photosensitive molecules are embedded (Fig. 21-19).[49] Shining a low-level UV light onto the center of the lens polymerizes the photosensitive molecules, which creates a concentration gradient between the irradiated region where the photosensitive silicone molecules are polymer-

ized and the rest of the optic. Over a 12-hr period, the photosensitive molecules migrate from the untreated areas, down the concentration gradient, and into the irradiated region until there is no concentration gradient. This movement causes the irradiated region to swell and, thereby, increases the lens power. If, instead, the edges of the lens are treated, the photosensitive molecules will migrate outward from the central, untreated region, which will flatten the center of the lens and reduce its dioptric power. Treatment may also be directed along a specific meridian or region of the lens to correct astigmatic errors and high-order aberrations.

The amount of energy applied to the LAL determines the degree to which the lens power changes. This dose response is highly reproducible, and in vitro studies demonstrated power adjustments accurate to within less than 0.25 diopter. One day after the power adjustment, the patient returns so that the lens has the desired power. If satisfactory results are obtained, the entire lens is irradiated, which polymerizes all of the remaining photosensitive silicone molecules and locks the lens. After this lock-in step, the LAL is essentially a standard silicone IOL. Before lock-in, the LAL can be readjusted, a fact that will make it possible for the patient to try monovision or multifocality and then have that modality removed if it proves undesirable. Theoretically, lock-in may be avoided and the lens adjusted over time as changes in refractive precision occur, which would be perfect for pediatric cases (Fig. 21-19).

The Aspherical (Negative-Spherical) Implant

The Tecnis Z9000 IOL (AMO Inc., Santa Ana, CA) is an IOL designed to reduce spherical aberration. Investigators have demonstrated an improvement on the optical

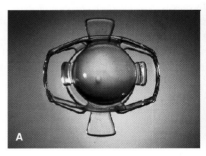
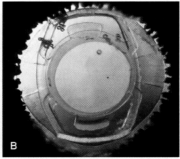
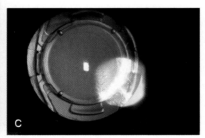

FIGURE 21-18. Dual-optic intraocular accommodating system: the Synchrony IOL, manufactured by Visiogen Inc. **A.** Gross photograph of the IOL. **B.** Gross photograph (anterior view) with retroillumination showing an experimental implantation of the Synchrony IOL in a human eye obtained postmortem (Miyake–Apple posterior video technique). The capsular bag was stained with trypan blue to enhance visualization. (A & B. Courtesy of Liliana Werner, MD, PhD, Salt Lake City, UT. C. Courtesy of Gerd U. Affarth, Heidelberg, Germany)

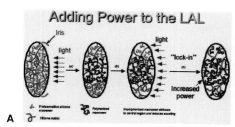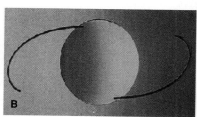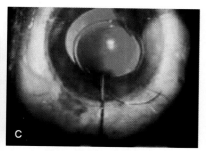

FIGURE 21-19. Light adjustable lens (LAL; Calhoun Vision). **A.** Manufacturer's illustration showing the principle of refractive adjustment. **B.** Photograph showing that this IOL is a typical three-piece silicone design. **C.** Clinical photograph showing implantation of the LAL. (Courtesy of A. Chayet, MD, Mexico.)

bench in contrast sensitivity under mesopic and photopic conditions with this technology. Recent advances in wavefront measurement of total ocular aberrations and corneal aberrations have demonstrated that the asphericity of the cornea remains constant throughout life, while the refractive gradient of the lens changes and produces increasing spherical aberration.

The Tecnis IOL is designed to reproduce the compensatory negative spherical aberration of the youthful crystalline lens and increase pseudophakic contrast sensitivity. Clinical trials have shown that this modified prolate IOL improves functional vision in most scenarios, however, decentration >0.5 mm will decrease the functional vision compared to that with spherical IOLs.[50–52]

The Tecnis Z9000 shares basic design features with the CeeOn Edge 911A (AMO Inc.), including a 6-mm, biconvex, square-edge silicone optic and angulated, cap C polyvinylidene fluoride haptics (Fig. 21-20). The implantation technique for the Tecnis Z9000 IOL is identical to that for the CeeOn Edge 911A. For the FDA-monitored study, the IOL is easily folded and implanted with forceps through a 3.5-mm incision. The Tecnis Z9000

IOL was recently approved by the FDA for use in adult eyes.

SUMMARY

Pediatric cataract surgery is constantly evolving and improving in terms of implant biomaterial and design. The stellar success and excellent results of current small-incision cataract–IOL surgery have provided motivation to cataract surgeons to restore accommodation, which is indeed very important in children. Ophthalmologists, vision scientists, and manufacturers are working together to obtain better refractive correction with a smaller wound size and a decreased host cell response to limit inflammation and maintain transparency of the capsular bag after cataract–IOL surgery.

REFERENCES

1. Olson RJ. Foldable IOL biomaterial and design. In: Chang DF, ed. *Ophthalmic Hyperguide.* Thorofare, NJ: Slack, 2001.
2. Chehade M, Elder MJ. Intraocular lens materials and styles: A review. *Aust NZ J Ophthalmol* 1997;25:255–263.
3. Doan KT, Olson RJ, Mamalis N. Survey of intraocular lens material and design. *Curr Opin Ophthalmol* 2002;13:24–29.
4. Apple DJ, Auffarth GA, Peng Q, Visessook N. *Foldable Intraocular Lenses: Evolution, Clinicopathologic Correlations, and Complications.* Thorofare, NJ: Slack, 2000.
5. Azar DT. Intraocular lenses in cataract and refractive surgery. Philadelphia: W. B. Saunders, 2001.
6. Wilson ME, Apple DJ, Bluestein EC, Wang XH. Intraocular lenses for pediatric implantation: biomaterials, designs and sizing. *J Cataract Refract Surg* 1994;20:584–591.
7. Wilson ME, Elliott L, Johnson B, et al. AcrySof acrylic intraocular lens implantation in children: clinical indications of biocompatibility. *J AAPOS* 2001;5:377–380.
8. Pavlovic S, Jacobi FK, Graef M, Jacobi KW. Silicone intraocular lens implantation in children: preliminary results. *J Cataract Refract Surg* 2000;26:88–95.
9. Pandey SK, Wilson ME, Trivedi RH, et al. Pediatric cataract surgery and intraocular lens implantation: current techniques, complications and management. *Int Ophthalmol Clin* 2001;41:175–196.

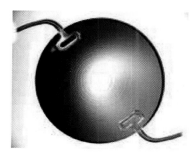

FIGURE 21-20. Manufacturer's illustration showing the Tecnis Z9000 aspheric IOL (AMO Inc.; formerly Pfizer Ophthalmics, New York).

10. Kuchle M, Lausen B, Gusek-Schneider GC. Results and complications of hydrophobic acrylic vs PMMA posterior chamber lenses in children under 17 years of age. *Graefes Arch Clin Exp Ophthalmol* 2003;241:637–641.

11. Trivedi RH, Wilson ME Jr. Single-piece acrylic intraocular lens implantation in children. *J Cataract Refract Surg* 2003;29:1738–1743.

12. Rowe NA, Biswas S, Lloyd IC. Primary IOL implantation in children: a risk analysis of foldable acrylic v PMMA lenses. *Br J Ophthalmol* 2004;88:481–485.

13. Vasavada AR, Trivedi RH, Nath VC. Visual axis opacification after AcrySof intraocular lens implantation in children. *J Cataract Refract Surg* 2004;30:1073–1081.

14. Cunanan CM, Ghazizadeh M, Buchen SY, Knight PM. Contact-angle analysis of intraocular lenses. *J Cataract Refract Surg* 1998;24:341–351.

15. Christ FR. Buchen SY, Deacon J, et al. Biomaterials used for intraocular lenses. In: Wise DL, Trantolo DJ, Altobelli DE, et al., eds. *Enclyopedic Handbook of Biomaterials and Bioengineering.* Part B: Applications, Vol. 2. New York: Mercel Dekker, 1995:1261–1313.

16. Wilson ME Jr, Bartholomew LR, Trivedi RH. Pediatric cataract surgery and intraocular lens implantation: practice styles and preferences of the 2001 ASCRS and AAPOS memberships. *J Cataract Refract Surg* 2003;29:1811–1820.

17. Basti S, Aasuri MK, Reddy MK, et al. Heparin-surface-modified intraocular lenses in pediatric cataract surgery: prospective randomized study. *J Cataract Refract Surg* 1999;25:782–787.

18. Abela-Formanek C, Amon M, Schild G, et al. Uveal and capsular biocompatibility of hydrophilic acrylic, hydrophobic acrylic, and silicone intraocular lenses. *J Cataract Refract Surg* 2002;28:50–61.

19. Abela-Formanek C, Amon M, Schauerberger J, et al. Results of hydrophilic acrylic, hydrophobic acrylic, and silicone intraocular lenses in uveitic eyes with cataract. *J Cataract Refract Surg* 2002;28:1141–1152.

20. Werner L, Pandey SK, Escobar-Gomez M, et al. Anterior capsule opacification: A histopathological study comparing different IOL styles. *Ophthalmology* 2000;107:463–471.

21. Werner L, Pandey SK, Apple DJ, et al. Anterior capsule opacification: correlation of pathologic findings with clinical sequelae. *Ophthalmology* 2001;108:1675–1681.

22. Newland TJ, McDermott ML, Eliott D, et al. Experimental neodymium:YAG laser damage to acrylic, poly(methyl methacrylate), and silicone intraocular lens materials. *J Cataract Refract Surg* 1999;25:72–76.

23. Chang DF. Early rotational stability of the longer Staar toric intraocular lens: fifty consecutive cases. *J Cataract Refract Surg* 2003;29:935–940.

24. Leyland M, Zinicola E, Bloom P, et al. Prospective evaluation of a plate haptic toric intraocular lens. *Eye* 2001;15:202–205.

25. Kohnen T, Magdowski G, Koch DD. Scanning electrom microscopic analysis of foldable acrylic and hydrogel intraocular lenses. *J Cataract Refract Surg* 1996;22:1342–1350.

26. Hollick EJ, Spalton DJ, Ursell PG. Surface cytologic features on intraocular lenses: Can increased biocompatibility have disadvantages? *Arch Ophthalmol* 1999;117:872–878.

27. Trinavarat A, Atchaneeyasakul L, Udompunturak S. Neodymium:YAG laser damage threshold of foldable intraocular lenses. *J Cataract Refract Surg* 2001;27:775–780.

28. Arthur SN, Peng Q, Apple DJ, et al. Effect of heparin surface modification in reducing silicone oil adherence to various intraocular lenses. *J Cataract Refract Surg* 2001;27:1662–1669.

29. Jehan FS, Mamalis N, Spencer TS, et al. Postoperative sterile endophthalmitis (TASS) associated with MemoryLens. *J Cataract Refract Surg* 2000;26:1773–1777.

30. Werner L, Apple DJ, Escobar Gomez M, et al. Postoperative deposition of calcium on the surfaces of a hydrogel intraocular lens. *Ophthalmology* 2000;107:2179–2185.

31. Fernando GT, Crayford BB. Visually significant calcification of hydrogel intraocular lenses necessitating explantation. *Clin Experiment Ophthalmol* 2000;28:280–286.

32. Izak AM, Werner L, Pandey SK, et al. Calcification on the surface of the Bausch & Lomb Hydroview intraocular lens. *Int Ophthalmol Clin* 2001;41:63–77.

33. Yu AK, Shek TW. Hydroxyapatite formation on implanted hydrogel intraocular lenses. *Arch Ophthalmol* 2001;119:611–614.

34. Izak AM, Werner L, Pandey SK, Apple DJ. Calcification of modern foldable hydrogel intraocular lens designs. *Eye* 2003;17:393–406.

35. Dorey MW, Brownstein S, Hill VE, et al. Proposed pathogenesis for the delayed postoperative opacification of the Hydroview hydrogel intraocular lens. *Am J Ophthalmol* 2003;135:591–598.

36. Pandey SK, Werner L, Apple DJ, Gravel JP. Calcium precipitation on the optical surfaces of a foldable intraocular lens: a clinicopathological correlation. *Arch Ophthalmol* 2002;120:391–393.

37. Werner L, Apple DJ, Kaskaloglu M, Pandey SK. Dense opacification of the optical component of a hydrophilic acrylic intraocular lens: a clinicopathological analysis of 9 explants. *J Cataract Refract Surg* 2001;27:1485–1492.

38. Pandey SK, Werner L, Apple DJ, Kaskaloglu M. Hydrophilic acrylic intraocular lens optic and haptics opacification in a diabetic patient: bilateral case report and clinicopathological correlation. *Ophthalmology* 2002;109:2042–2051.

39. Linnola R. Sandwich theory: bioactivity-based explanation for posterior capsule opacification. *J Cataract Refract Surg* 1997;23:1539–1542.

40. Linnola RJ, Werner L, Pandey SK, et al. Adhesion of fibronectin, vitronectin, laminin, and collagen type IV to intraocular lens materials in pseudophakic human autopsy eyes. Part 1: Histological sections. *J Cataract Refract Surg* 2000;26:1792–1806.

41. Linnola RJ, Werner L, Pandey SK, et al. Adhesion of fibronectin, vitronectin, laminin, and collagen type IV to intraocular lens materials in pseudophakic human autopsy eyes. Part 2: Explanted intraocular lenses. *J Cataract Refract Surg* 2000;26:1807–1818.

42. Mainster MA, Sparrow JR. How much blue light should an IOL transmit? *Br J Ophthalmol* 2003;87:1523–1529.

43. Jacobi PC, Dietlein TS, Konen W. Multifocal intraocular lens implantation in pediatric cataract surgery. *Ophthalmology* 2001;108:1375–1380.

44. Hunter DG. Multifocal intraocular lenses in children. *Ophthalmology* 2001;108:1373–1374.

45. Agarwal A, Agarwal S, Agarwal A. Phakonit with an AcriTec IOL. *J Cataract Refract Surg* 2003;29:854–855.

46. Pandey SK, Werner L, Agarwal A, et al. Phakonit: cataract removal through a sub-1.0 mm incision and implantation of the ThinOptX rollable intraocular lens. *J Cataract Refract Surg* 2002;28:1710–1713.

47. Kuchle M, Seitz B, Langenbucher A, et al. Erlangen Accommodative Intraocular Lens Study Group. Stability of refraction, accommodation, and lens position after implantation of the 1CU accommodating posterior chamber intraocular lens. *J Cataract Refract Surg* 2003;29:2324–2329.

48. McLeod SD, Portney V, Ting A. A dual optic accommodating foldable intraocular lens. *Br J Ophthalmol* 2003;87:1083–1085.

49. Schwartz DM. Light-adjustable lens. *Trans Am Ophthalmol Soc* 2003;101:417–436.

50. Kershner RM. Retinal image contrast and functional visual performance with aspheric, silicone, and acrylic intraocular lenses. *J Cataract Refract Surg* 2003;29:1684–1694.

51. Packer M, Fine IH, Hoffman RS, Piers PA. Prospective randomized trial of an anterior surface modified prolate intraocular lens. *J Refract Surg* 2002;18:692–696.

52. Mester U, Dillinger P, Anterist N. Impact of a modified optic design on visual function: clinical comparative study. *J Cataract Refract Surg* 2003;29:652–660.

53. Kleinmann G, Werner L, Pandey SK, et al. Opacification on the surface of hydrophilic acrylic lenses in children. Presented at the ASCRS Symposium on Cataract, IOL, and Refractive Surgery, San Diego, CA, 2004.

54. Pandey SK, Werner L, Mamalis N, et al. Evaluation of ultra-small incision intraocular lenses using Miyake–Apple posterior video technique. Poster presented at the ASCSR Symposium, San Diego, CA, 2004.

55. Pandey SK, Werner L, Apple DJ, et al. Evaluation of an accommodative silicone IOL in human eyes obtained postmortem. Presented at the ASCRS Symposium on Cataract, IOL, and Refractive Surgery, Philadelphia, 2002.

Intraocular Lens Types and Sizes for Pediatric Cataract Surgery

Suresh K. Pandey and M. Edward Wilson, Jr.

Intraocular lens (IOL) implantation at the time of cataract surgery has become the most common means of optical correction for children beyond infancy. A growing number of case series and a survey of practice styles and preferences of American Society of Cataract and Refractive Surgery (ASCRS) and American Association for Pediatric Ophthalmology and Strabismus (AAPOS) members have now been published supporting the safety and effectiveness of IOLs for children.[1-8] An IOL can provide a full-time correction with optics that closely simulate those of the crystalline lens. However, some concern still remains about the unknown risks of an IOL over the long lifespan of a child. In addition, predicting the refractive change of even older children is difficult since individual variation is common.

The major advantage of an IOL is that it provides permanent continuous correction of the aphakia. This may be important in preventing amblyopia and encouraging normal visual development. Although glasses are usually necessary to obtain the best vision, uncorrected pseudophakic vision is probably better than uncorrected aphakic vision.

IOL IMPLANTATION IN PEDIATRIC CATARACT SURGERY

Intraocular lenses manufactured from various rigid and foldable biomaterials have been used for pediatric cataract surgery. Interested readers should refer to Chapter 21 for details concerning IOL biomaterials, newly available IOL designs, and insertion techniques. Rigid implants manufactured from polymethylmethacrylate (PMMA) have been implanted since 1949. An IOL implanted in a child's eye must stay there for several decades without biodegrading. PMMA has the longest safety record in both adults and children.

Visual rehabilitation in children in the industrialized world is now being revolutionized by the IOL. The three most important reasons for increased use of IOLs in children are as follows.

(1) Appropriately sized (11.5- to 12.0-mm), more flexible implants made are now available and can be inserted much more easily into the capsular bag of the child. Despite their increased flexibility, newer lens designs retain enough "memory" to resist the intense equatorial capsular fibrosis seen in children after implantation. In addition, PMMA as an implant material now has a tract record of biocompatibility that extends to 50 years or more. Heparin surface modification of PMMA has increased its biocompatibility even more. Also, copolymerization of different acrylate and methacrylate acids has resulted in foldable lenses with many of the same biocompatibility features as PMMA. As an example, foldable hydrophobic acrylic lenses, such as the AcrySof (Alcon, Inc., Forth Worth, TX, USA), are being implanted in children's eyes with greater frequency. The biocompatibility of the hydrophobic acrylic lenses may equal or exceed that of the tried PMMA lenses. The foldable hydrophobic acrylic lenses are easier to insert in a small eye, and the squared edge of the AcrySof IOL optic design may result in delayed posterior capsule opacification in young eyes. Pavlovic and coworkers[5] reported that foldable silicone IOL implantation in children is also a safe procedure with stable short-term anatomic results.

(2) Refined surgical techniques can more predictably ensure capsular fixation of the IOL. Surgeons have gained more confidence in the safety of "in-the-bag" implantation even over the extended lifespan of a child. Capsular fixation provides sequestration of the implant away from vascularized tissues. Although ciliary sulcus fixation of the IOL may also be safe, uveal contact for a lifetime is not as desirable. In addition, complications such as pupillary capture and IOL decentration are more common with ciliary sulcus

fixation. The preference for capsular fixation over ciliary sulcus placement has resulted in more IOLs being implanted in children at the time of cataract extraction (rather than secondary implantation in the ciliary sulcus later), even at very young ages.

(3) Finally, customized management of the anterior and posterior capsules for pediatric eyes at the time of implantation has improved outcomes and decreased complications. These improvements have provided for long-term centration of the IOL and a reduction in opacification of the visual axis after implantation.

IOL SIZING FOR PEDIATRIC CATARACT SURGERY

The mean axial length of a newborn's eye is 17.0 mm, compared to 23 to 24 mm in an adult. The pediatric eye, especially in the first 1 to 3 years of life, is significantly smaller than the adult eye.[9] This has led to concerns about implantation of adult-sized IOLs in these patients. In an effort to determine the size of the pediatric lens, Bluestein et al.[9] examined 50 fresh, nonpreserved autopsy eyes from patients ranging in age from 1 day to 16 years. A variety of measurements was made, including the anterior–posterior, vertical, and horizontal lengths of the globe, corneal diameter, lens diameter, and diameter of the zonular free zone. The most rapid growth of the globe, the lens (Fig. 22-1), and the capsular bag occurred from birth to 2 years of age.

Currently available adult-sized IOLs are slightly oversized in relation to capsular bag measurements but may actually fit into eyes in the first 2 years of life, although possibly not into very small infantile eyes. The small capsular bag may become misshaped into an oval with these adult-sized IOLs. The ovality may vary from minimal to severe, depending on the design, type, and overall diameter of the implanted IOL (Fig. 22-2). There are several possible consequences of implantation of adult-sized IOLs into the relatively small capsular bag of infants and young children. First, in contrast to adult cataract surgery, dialing of the IOL haptics into the capsular bag can be difficult in infants and children. The combination of a small soft eye with vitreous upthrust and an oversized IOL will increase the risk of asymmetric (bag–sulcus) IOL fixation, which can lead to decentration of the IOL. Second, implantation of an oversized IOL in the capsular bag of a child may cause marked capsular bag stretching, resulting in posterior capsular folds and striae. The lens epithelial cells may migrate toward the visual axis, through the capsular folds, leading to opacification of the posterior capsule. Third, implantation of an oversized IOL in the capsular bag of a small child may cause zonular stress in the direction parallel to the IOL haptics. The long-term sequalae of the capsular bag stretching (and also the zonular stress) on the axial growth of the globe remains to be further investigated.

In a nonrandomized comparative trial, Pandey and associates[10] compared the amount of capsulorhexis ovaling and capsular bag stretch produced by various rigid and foldable IOLs when implanted into pediatric human eyes obtained postmortem. In this study, 16 pediatric human eyes obtained postmortem were divided into two groups: Eight eyes were obtained from children <2 years of age (group A) and eight eyes were obtained from children >2 years of age (group B). All eyes were prepared according to the Miyake–Apple posterior video technique.[11,12]

Six IOL types (listed below), manufactured from rigid and foldable biomaterials, were implanted to determine the IOL design best suited for implantation in pediatric eyes.

1. Single-piece hydrophobic acrylic IOL (AcrySof, SA30AL; 5.5-mm optic, 12.5-mm overall diameter; Alcon Inc. Fort Worth, TX).
2. Three-piece hydrophobic acrylic optic–PMMA haptic (AcrySof, MA60BM; 6-mm optic, 13-mm overall diameter; Alcon Inc.)
3. Three-piece silicone optic–PMMA haptic (SI40NB; 6-mm optic, 13-mm overall diameter; AMO Inc., Santa Ana, CA).
4. Three-piece silicone optic–polyimide haptic (elastimide; 6-mm optic, 12.5-mm overall diameter; Staar Surgical Co., Monrovia, CA).

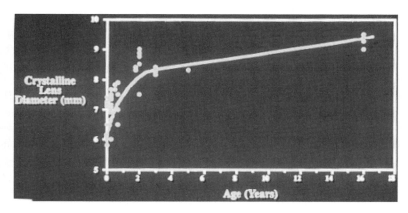

FIGURE 22-1. Graph showing the growth of the crystalline lens. The most rapid growth occurs from birth to 2 years of age and the growth of the crystalline lens is almost completed by the age of 2 years. (Reprinted with permission from Bluestein EC, Wilson ME, Wang XH, et al. Dimensions of the pediatric crystalline lens: Implications for intraocular lenses in children. *J Pediatr Ophthalmol Strabismus* 1996;33:18–20.)

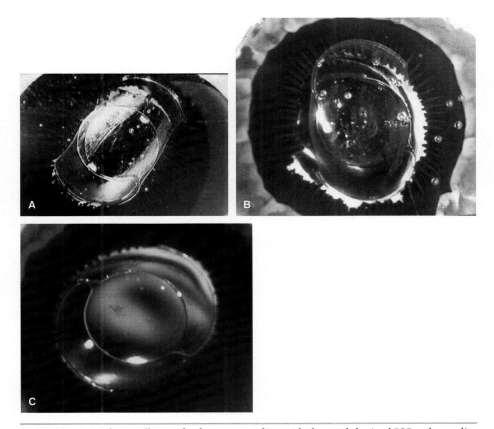

FIGURE 22-2. The small capsular bag may ovalize with these adult-sized IOLs; the ovality may vary from minimal to severe, depending on the design, type, and overall diameter of the implanted IOL. **A.** Miyake–Apple view after in-the-bag implantation of a one-piece, flexible open-loop, all-PMMA IOL, 13.75 mm in overall length, into an eye obtained postmortem from a 2-year-old child. Note the severe capsular bag stretch and ovaling between 1 o'clock and 7 o'clock. These indicate marked oversizing of the IOL in relation to the size of the capsular bag. **B.** Miyake–Apple view after in-the-bag implantation of a one-piece PMMA, flexible open-loop, modified C-loop capsular IOL, 12.5 mm in diameter, into an eye obtained postmortem from a 5-year-old child. Note the marked ovaling and elongation of the bag between 12 o'clock and 6 o'clock, indicating the slightly oversized IOL. **C.** Miyake–Apple posterior photographic view showing a one-piece, all-PMMA, 12.0-mm-diameter, modified C-loop IOL experimentally placed into the capsular bag in a cadaver eye of a 2-year-old child. Note the very optimum "fit" of the implanted IOL. (Reprinted with the permission from Wilson ME, Bluestein EC, Wang XH. Current trends in the use of intraocular lenses in children. *J Cataract Refract Surg* 1994;20:579–583.)

5. One-piece silicone plate IOL (AA-4203VF; 6-mm optic, 10.5-mm overall diameter; Staar Surgical Co.).
6. One-piece PMMA optic–PMMA haptic (809 P; 5-mm optic, 12-mm overall diameter; Pfizer Ophthalmics [formerly Pharmacia Inc.], New York).

The capsulorhexis opening and the capsular bag diameters were measured before IOL implantation and subsequently after in-the-bag IOL fixation with the haptics (or the main axis) of the lens at the 3–9 o'clock meridian. The percentage ovaling of the capsulorhexis opening was calculated by noting the difference in its horizontal diameter before and after IOL implantation. The percentage capsular bag stretch was also calculated by noting the difference

in the horizontal capsular bag diameter before and after IOL implantation.

All of the IOLs produced ovaling of the capsulorhexis opening, and stretching of the capsular bag, parallel to the IOL haptics. Figures 22-3 and 22-4 illustrate ovaling of the capsulorhexis opening and capsular bag stretch after implantation of rigid and foldable lenses in postmortem human eyes obtained from both group A and group B. Comparison of all six lens types within each group of eyes revealed significant differences in capsulorhexis ovaling and capsular bag stretch ($P < 0.001$, analysis of variance). However, the postcomparison difference was found to be significant only between the single-piece hydrophobic acrylic (AcrySof) lens and the other lenses. The single-piece

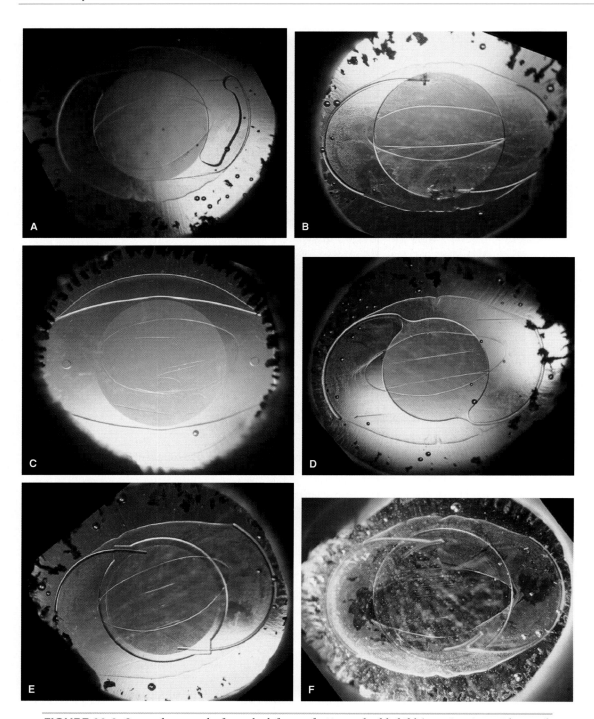

FIGURE 22-3. Gross photographs from the left eye of a 5-month-old child (anterior view with retroillumination). Note the variable degree of capsulorhexis ovaling and capsular bag stretch after implantation of the following rigid and foldable lens designs. Minimal capsulorhexis ovaling and capsular bag stretch were documented after implantation of a single-piece hydrophobic acrylic lens design. **A.** Single-piece hydrophobic acrylic (AcrySof) IOL. **B.** Three-piece hydrophobic acrylic optic–PMMA haptic IOL. **C.** One-piece silicone plate IOL. **D.** One-piece PMMA optic–PMMA haptic IOL. **E.** Three-piece silicone optic–PMMA haptic IOL. **F.** Three-piece silicone optic–polyimide haptic IOL.

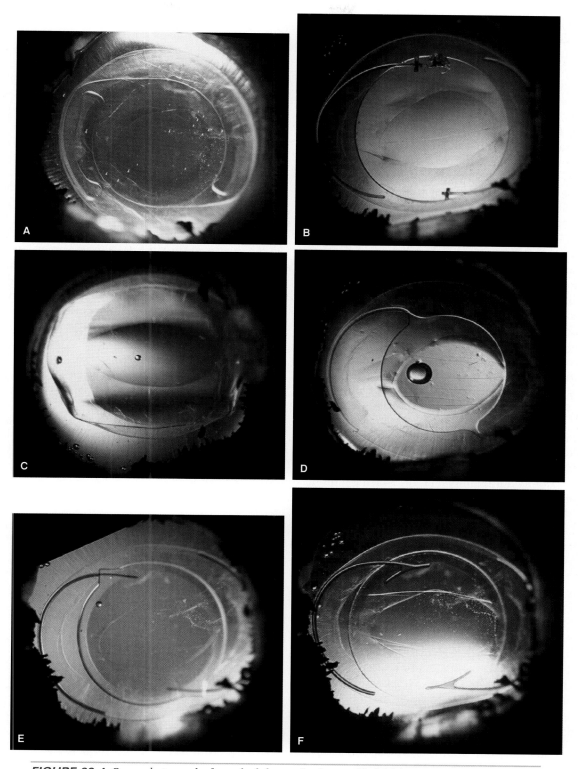

FIGURE 22-4. Gross photographs from the left eye of a 4-year-old child (anterior view with retroillumination). Note the variable degree of capsulorhexis ovaling and capsular bag stretch after implantation of the following rigid and foldable lens designs. Minimal capsulorhexis ovaling and capsular bag stretch were documented after implantation of a single-piece hydrophobic acrylic lens design. **A.** Single-piece hydrophobic acrylic (AcrySof) IOL. **B.** Three-piece hydrophobic acrylic optic–PMMA haptic IOL. **C.** One-piece silicone plate IOL. **D.** One-piece PMMA optic–PMMA haptic IOL. **E.** Three-piece silicone optic–PMMA haptic IOL. **F.** Three-piece silicone optic–polyimide haptic IOL.

hydrophobic acrylic lens was associated with significantly less capsulorhexis ovaling and capsular bag stretch in both group A and group B (12.06 ± 0.59 and 7.6 ± 1.47%, respectively).

Our study using postmortem human eyes suggests that modern rigid and foldable IOLs, designed for the adult population, can be implanted in the capsular bag of infants and children. However, a variable degree of ovaling of the capsulorhexis opening and capsular bag stretch was seen after implantation of the adult-sized rigid and foldable IOLs. Miyake–Apple posterior video technique confirmed the well-maintained configuration of the capsular bag (with minimal ovaling) after implantation of the single-piece hydrophobic acrylic lens in both groups due to its flexible haptic design.

The reason for this minimal ovaling of the capsulorhexis opening and capsular bag stretch is probably the result of the unique optic/haptic design. The memory and flexibility of the hydrophobic acrylic biomaterial allow the haptics of the single-piece design to bend and twist during entry and then conform to any size of capsular bag to a much greater degree than the other lenses tested. The modified "L"-loop haptics are described as Stable-Force haptics and are made of the same hydrophobic acrylic biomaterial used for the optic of the lens.[13] The loop memory of the Stable-Force haptics has not been addressed in the previous laboratory studies.[14,15] However, these haptics appear to have very good memory (reexpansion) characteristics despite being more flexible than PMMA or prolene haptics. The single-piece AcrySof seems to have an ideal combination of softness and flexibility during implantation, causing minimal ovaling of the capsule, and enough memory to resist the equatorial fibrosis of the capsular bag known to occur in children. Our clinical follow-up has verified this fact. We have not seen any examples of the soft single-piece AcrySof haptics being compressed over the optic by the equatorial capsular fibrosis. Besides the IOL haptic design and memory, the stickiness of the hydrophobic acrylic biomaterial may also play some role in reducing the extent of capsulorhexis and capsular bag distortion in young eyes.

Wilson and coworkers[16] conducted an experimental IOL implantation study in 50 pediatric eyes obtained postmortem to determine the biomaterials, designs, and sizes that may be appropriate for pediatric implantation. Based on this study, using the Miyake–Apple posterior video technique, these researchers recommended clinical trials of capsular IOLs, downsized to approximately 10.0-mm diameter, for children <2 years of age. Capsular IOLs were defined as flexible open-loop, one-piece, all-PMMA, modified C-loop designs made especially for in-the-bag placement. Since that report was published, the AcrySof single-piece IOL has been introduced and the most common material for pediatric implantation has changed from PMMA to hydrophobic acrylic. These advances have eliminated the need for downsized IOLs, even in infancy.

In summary, visual rehabilitation in children in the industrialized world is now being revolutionized by the implantation of the IOL. Highly refined and perfected microsurgical techniques have now propelled the cataract–IOL procedure in adults toward being one of the most successful surgical techniques in history. Application of this procedure to children is now improving the treatment of pediatric cataract. Surgeons are now applying the best tried and true techniques perfected over the years for adult cataract surgery. They are modifying these to meet the specific characteristics of the infantile eye.

Several reports indicate that IOL implantation is technically feasible in even the youngest children. To date, IOLs have been found to be efficacious in providing good short- to intermediate-term results after implantation over a wide range of ages at the time of cataract surgery for congenital, developmental, and traumatic cataracts. Long-term results are needed and are now beginning to appear in the literature, giving the surgeon even more confidence in the lifelong safety of these implanted devices.

REFERENCES

1. Wilson ME Jr, Bartholomew LR, Trivedi RH. Pediatric cataract surgery and intraocular lens implantation: practice styles and preferences of the 2001 ASCRS and AAPOS memberships. *J Cataract Refract Surg* 2003;29:1811–1820.
2. Mullner-Eidenbock A, Amon M, Moser E, et al. Morphological and functional results of AcrySof intraocular lens implantation in children: prospective randomized study of age-related surgical management. *J Cataract Refract Surg* 2003;29:285–293.
3. Trivedi RH, Wilson ME Jr. Single-piece acrylic intraocular lens implantation in children. *J Cataract Refract Surg* 2003;29:1738–1743.
4. Ram J, Brar GS, Kaushik S, Gupta A, Gupta A. Role of posterior capsulotomy with vitrectomy and intraocular lens design and material in reducing posterior capsule opacification after pediatric cataract surgery. *J Cataract Refract Surg* 2003;29:1579–1584.
5. Pavlovic S, Jacobi FK, Graef M, Jacobi KW. Silicone intraocular lens implantation in children: Preliminary results. *J Cataract Refract Surg* 2000;26:88–95.
6. Basti S, Aasuri MK, Reddy MK, et al. Heparin-surface-modified intraocular lenses in pediatric cataract surgery: prospective randomized study. *J Cataract Refract Surg* 1999;25:782–787.
7. Pandey SK, Ram J, Werner L, et al. Visual results and postoperative complications of capsular bag versus ciliary sulcus fixation of posterior chamber intraocular lenses for traumatic cataract in children. *J Cataract Refract Surg* 1999;25:1576–1584.
8. Wilson ME. Intraocular lens implantation: Has it become the standard of care for children? (Editorial). *Ophthalmology* 1996;103:1719–1720.
9. Bluestein EC, Wilson ME, Wang XH, et al. Dimensions of the pediatric crystalline lens: implications for intraocular lenses in children. *J Pediatr Ophthalmol Strabismus* 1996;33:18–20.
10. Pandey SK, Werner L, Wilson ME, et al. Capsulorhexis ovaling and capsular bag stretch after rigid and foldable intraocular lens implantation: an experimental study in pediatric human eyes. *J Cataract Refract Surg* 2004;30:2183–2191.
11. Miyake K, Miyake C. Intraoperative posterior chamber lens haptic fixation in the human cadaver eye. *Ophthalm Surg* 1985;16:230–236.
12. Apple D, Lim E, Morgan R, et al. Preparation and study of human eyes obtained postmortem with the Miyake posterior photographic technique. *Ophthalmology* 1990;97:810–816.

13. Caporossi A, Casprini F, Tosi GM, Baiocchi S. Preliminary results of cataract extraction with implantation of a single-piece Acrysof intraocular lens. *J Cataract Refract Surg* 2002;28:652–655.
14. Assia EI, Legler UFC, Castaneda VE, Apple DJ. Loop memory of posterior chamber intraocular lenses of various sizes, designs, and loop materials. *J Cataract Refract Surg* 1992;18:541–546.
15. Izak AM, Werner L, Apple DJ, et al. Loop memory of different haptic materials used in the manufacture of posterior chamber intraocular lenses. *J Cataract Refract Surg* 2002;28:1229–1235.
16. Wilson ME, Bluestein EC, Wang XH. Current trends in the use of intraocular lenses in children. *J Cataract Refract Surg* 1994;20:579–583.

Primary Intraocular Lens Implantation in Infantile Cataract Surgery

Rupal H. Trivedi and M. Edward Wilson, Jr.

The functional outcome of infantile cataract surgery has been greatly influenced by several factors such as amblyopia, compliance, and need for parental care. The capability of the intraocular lens (IOL) to provide *constant visual input* is an important advantage for the functional outcome of infantile cataract surgery. Because of the advantages it offers, primary IOL implantation has slowly gained acceptance for the management of infantile cataracts. However, as of 2004, it remains a controversial issue.[1–9] Table 23-1 describes the arguments for and against primary IOL implantation in infantile cataract surgery.

The main concerns about *IOL implantation* are the poor predictability of IOL power, postoperative complications, inflammation, and the technical difficulty of the surgery.[10] In addition to the smaller eyes, decreased scleral rigidity makes IOL implantation more challenging in infants compared to older children. Also, infantile cataracts are often associated with microphthalmos and anterior segment anomalies. Frequent secondary complications due to the lens material and design and enhanced inflammatory response in these small eyes have been issues of concern in the past. Studies on the anatomical outcome of IOL implantation have revealed that such eyes are at high risk for reoperations for visual axis opacification (VAO).[1,2,5,11]

The main concerns with contact lens correction are poor compliance, high lens loss rate, high cost, and keratitis (Fig. 23-1).[10] For these reasons, contact lenses are not practically applicable in all cases, especially in most parts of the developing world. Although it is possible for an eye undergoing infantile cataract surgery followed by contact lens correction to achieve an excellent visual outcome, this has continued to be the exception rather than the rule, especially in eyes with unilateral cataracts.

Despite all these controversies, IOLs are being implanted in infants at a gradually increasing frequency. In 2001, we surveyed the ASCRS and AAPOS communities for trends in pediatric cataract surgery. Our survey data noted that 15.9 to 31.8% (unilateral cataract, 31.8 and 30.0%; bilateral cataract, 19.8 and 15.9%; ASCRS and AAPOS, respectively) of the respondents performed or advised IOL implantation in the first year of life.[9] In 2003, Lambert and coworkers published an update of perceptions of AAPOS members and of parents. For AAPOS surgeons, reporting on a scale from 1 to 10, with 1 strongly favoring an IOL implant and 10 strongly favoring a contact lens, the median score was 7.5. The authors concluded that although most AAPOS members still favor contact lens correction after cataract surgery for a unilateral congenital cataract, five times more surgeons had implanted an IOL in an infant in 2001 than in 1997 (21 versus 4%). Parents were almost equally divided in their preference for IOL implant versus contact lens correction.[10]

Our current strategy for selecting one modality over another depends on several factors. When a child presents in infancy with a visually significant cataract, we spend time explaining the options for correcting the aphakia to the parents. Although we do not have any absolute contraindication for primary implantation in infants, a corneal diameter <9 mm is a relative contraindication for us. We also must not forget that very microphthalmic eyes or eyes with poorly formed anterior segment structures are not good candidates for primary IOL implantation. With that said, mild to moderate microphthalmos does not necessarily preclude IOL placement at the time of cataract surgery.

In unilateral cases we more often choose an implantation. This is especially true in families in which contact lens care would be difficult. In our state, Medicaid does not pay for contact lenses even when we write letters stating that the contact lenses are medically necessary. We prefer silicone SilSoft contact lenses because they are relatively well tolerated, are easy to fit, and can be worn for a month at a

▶ **TABLE 23-1** Arguments For and Against Primary IOL Implantation in Infantile Cataract Surgery

Proponents of Contact Lens	Proponents of IOL Implantation
1. The power of a contact lens can be easily changed to compensate for the rapid myopic shift that occurs during the first 2 years of life. An IOL can be implanted in these eyes when these children are older and their refractive errors have stabilized.	1. Compliance with contact lens wear is a major concern. Noncompliance may result in dense amblyopia by the time their refractive error stabilizes.
2. Implanting an adult-size IOL in the small capsular bag of an infant is techically difficult.	2. With the availability of foldable IOLs and injectors, the success of implanting in-the-bag is relatively high.
3. IOLs in infantile eyes lead to a high rate of reoperations for visual axis opacification.	3. Eyes with aphakia more often need other surgery, e.g., strabismus or secondary IOL. If we consider total reoperations, the incidences may be similar.
4. A good visual outcome is possible if a child is compliant with contact lens wear and occlusion therapy.	4. Compliance to contact lens wear is a major hurdle. The available data suggest that a good visual outcome can be obtained more consistently in infants with unilateral congenital cataracts who undergo IOL implantation at the time of surgery.
5. The long-term safely of an artificial lens is not known.	5. Contact lens wear, long-term, can lead to corneal vascularization, and a risk for corneal ulceration and scarring.

time between cleanings (we recommend weekly cleaning). However, these lenses are more than $100 U.S. each and are often lost or in need of frequent replacement. Many poor families will not be able to afford this expense. In these families, IOL implantation with glasses for residual hyperopia is the only viable option when the cataract is unilateral.

On the other hand, for parents who are more experienced with contact lens care and are willing and able to buy contact lenses whenever they are needed, we are likely to leave a neonatal eye aphakic. In the later months of infancy (beyond 6 months) IOLs are more often implanted in all eyes. Piggyback IOL implantation (temporary polypseudophakia) is also a good option for eyes >6 months of age but <2 years. This is discussed in Chapter 27. Bilateral IOL implantation may also be favored in mentally retarded children whose behavior makes them poor candidates for glasses or contact lens use.

Before moving forward with implantation, it is important to discuss the major pros and cons of the available options with the parents/legal guardians. They should be made aware that the IOLs are market approved by the U.S. Food and Drug Administration (FDA) for adults and that no formal FDA testing has been done for children. Parents of children receiving implants should also be made aware that glasses will likely still be needed postoperatively.

Ophthalmologists who perform IOL implantation in very young children have had to approximate the IOL power considering the age of the child and other factors and need to develop a predictor of how the eye will grow.[3] This is one of the most important reasons why physicians are reluctant to implant in infants. The eye grows rapidly in the first 2 years of life. Opponents of IOLs argue that waiting for implantation until at least 2 years of age allows the IOL power to be calculated more precisely and the future growth to be predicted more accurately. Proponents of infantile IOL implantation argue that many of these children are noncompliant with contact lens wear, resulting in dense amblyopia by the time their refractive errors are stabilized (Table 23-1).

IOL power calculation is discussed in detail in Chapter 7. We prefer the Holladay formula to calculate IOL power. The target postoperative refraction is based on the patient's age and the fellow eye status. In general, we recommend a target refraction of +12 D (diopters) in the first month of life, +8 to +10 D in the second to third month, +6 D in the fourth to sixth month, and +4 D in the sixth to twelfth month. Our preferred IOL is a single-piece AcrySof (Alcon Laboratories; Fort Worth, TX) for infantile eyes. In a microphthalmic eye, the target postoperative refraction was not always attainable with the +30-D lens, which was the highest-power lens available until recently. IOLs with powers up to +40 D are now available if needed for these very small eyes.

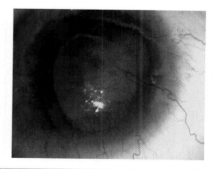

FIGURE 23-1. A healed corneal ulcer in an eye followed by the use of contact lens correction for pediatric aphakia. Note the corneal vascularization.

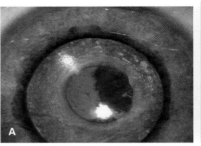
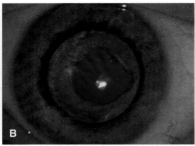

FIGURE 23-2. **A.** Cortex proliferation and anterior capsule fibrosis. **B.** After removal of opacification. Proliferated cortex was easy to wash out, however, dense anterior capsule fibrosis was difficult to remove.

SURGICAL TECHNIQUE

General principles described in this book should be followed. Specific points to remember when operating on infantile eyes are as follows.

1. Conjuctival peritomy and scleral tunnel: For infant eyes we have converted back to a scleral tunnel instead of the corneal tunnel used in eyes beyond infancy. Corneal tunnels in infants often heal with a noticeable opaque scar. Scleral tunnels in infants are more likely to be invisible after healing;

2. Vitrectorhexis is recommended in infants instead of a manual continuous curvilinear capsulorhexis;

3. Bimanual irrigation–aspiration;

4. IOL implantation: The single-piece AcrySof IOL (SA and SN series acrylic lenses; Alcon Laboratories, Fort Worth, TX) can be inserted into even the smallest of capsular bags using the Monarch II injector. In-the-bag fixation is the best available position for IOL placement and all efforts should be made to achieve it. We prefer to implant an IOL before performing posterior capsulectomy and vitrectomy via the pars plana route in infantile eyes. This avoids some of the difficulties of implanting an IOL in a soft vitrectomized eye;

5. Pars plana posterior capsulectomy and vitrectomy (2 to 2.5 mm away from the limbus, depending on the age of the child and size of an eye;)

6. Suturing of the incision with 10/0 vicryl. Pars plana entry sites are closed with 8/0 vicryl.

OUTCOME OF INTRAOCULAR LENS IMPLANTATION IN INFANTILE EYES

Visual Axis Opacification

VAO requiring secondary intervention is the most common complication of infantile cataract and IOL implantation surgery (Figs. 23-2 and 23-3). Despite the performance of a primary posterior capsulectomy and vitrectomy, secondary surgery was required in as many as 80% of the eyes operated in the first 6 months of age.[5]

It is unclear why IOL implantation leads to a higher rate of VAO in infants. Without an IOL in place, perhaps the capsular edges of Soemmering's ring seal better, making it difficult for any proliferated cortex to reach the visual axis. In eyes with an IOL, the capsule may not seal as well to the IOL as it can to itself. This may allow some of the new lens cortex to reach the central visual axis. Also, it has been hypothesized that the IOL may act as scaffolding to which fibrous tissue can attach. In our experience, VAO in infants does not involve attachment of cells or membranes to the IOL itself.

■ *Age at surgery.* We have reported that the relative risk of eyes needing secondary surgery for VAO is 2.7 if the cataract surgery is performed on or before 6 months of age, compared to after 6 months of age. Eyes operated

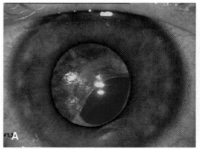
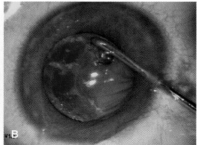
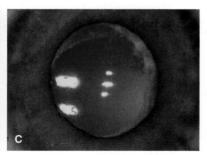

FIGURE 23-3. **A.** Fibrous opacification of visual axis in an eye operated on for cataract at 7 months of age. **B.** Kloti radiofrequency diathermy was used to remove the fibrous opacification. **C.** After removal of opacification.

in the first 6 months of age are at higher risk than eyes operated at 6 to 12 months of age. In our recent series, 50% of eyes (9/18) operated at or before 6 months of age were opacified, while 18.2% (2/11) of eyes operated after 6 months of age were opacified ($P = .09$). Eyes with associated ocular anomalies were found to have a higher VAO rate (see below), and these cases are often initially operated on early in life.

- *Ocular anomalies.* In our series, eyes with associated ocular anomalies (e.g., anterior segment dysgenesis, Peters anomaly, persistent fetal vasculature, iris hypoplasia) were 8.6 times more likely to need secondary surgery for VAO than eyes without ocular anomalies.[11]

- *Ethnicity.* In our series, all 11 eyes requiring reoperation for VAO were of Caucasian ethnicity.[11] However, these Caucasian patients were more often associated with ocular anomalies compared to our African-American study patients.

- *Kaplan–Meier survival time.* The first 6 months postoperative period is a very high-risk period for development of VAO. Frequent postoperative follow-up visits are needed for pediatric cataract surgery patients operated on during the first year of life, especially during the first 6 months following cataract surgery, to ensure the early detection of VAO. Figure 23-4 shows a Kaplan–Meier curve representing the secondary surgery-free survival of eyes following primary cataract surgery. Excellent maintenance of visual axis clarity after 6 postoperative months is shown in the survival analysis.

- *Type of opacification.* Cortex proliferation is the most common type of opacification, followed by fibrous changes and Elschnig pearls. Many times a mixed type of opacification is observed in such eyes. Proliferation of the cortex occurs more often in eyes with bag-fixated haptics. In sulcus-fixated eyes, fibrous opacification is the most common form. Opacification can be in front of and/or behind the optic of the IOL. Cortex proliferation is easy to remove, however, fibrous opacification, especially when dense, can be difficult to remove. It is advisable to remove fibrous VAO soon after it develops. As time elapses, the fibrotic material may become more densely fibrotic and more difficult to remove.

Literature Search

A multicenter pilot study in the United States reported 11 infants implanted with either an acrylic or a PMMA IOL at a mean age of 10 weeks. With an average 13 months of follow-up, 8 of the 11 patients needed one or more reoperations and 2 patients developed glaucoma.[1] Plager et al.[5] reported that 12 (80%) of 15 eyes operated on in the first 6 months of life required secondary surgery to clear recurrent VAO. Two of these 12 eyes required a third surgery. We have reported that a secondary surgical procedure to clear postoperative VAO was required in 37.9% of eyes (11/29) at a median of 4.8 months after initial cataract surgery. In 1988, Tablante et al.[12] reported the outcome of nine eyes operated on in the first 2 years of life. All eyes with an intact posterior capsule required intervention as early as 2 weeks after the initial surgery ($n = 5$). Four eyes with epilenticular posterior chamber IOL implantation followed by pars plana endocapsular lensectomy did not opacify (follow-up ranged from 6 to 25 months). Vasavada and Chauhan[7] reported a series of eyes with IOL implantation in the first year of life. All 17 of the eyes that did not receive a primary posterior capsulectomy required secondary surgery at an average of 4 months following primary cataract surgery. O'Keefe et al.[4] reported that 10 (90.9%) of 11 eyes with an intact posterior capsule opacified.

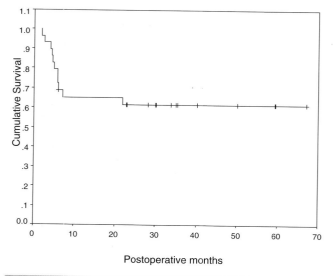

FIGURE 23-4. Kaplan–Meier curve representing the secondary surgery-free survival of eyes without visual axis opacification following primary cataract surgery at <1 year of age and showing excellent maintenance of visual axis clarity after 6 postoperative months. (Reprinted with permission from Trivedi RH, Wilson ME Jr, Bartholomew LR, Lal G, Peterseim MM. Opacification of the visual axis after cataract surgery and single acrylic intraocular lens implantation in the first year-of-life. *J AAPOS* 2004;8: 156–164.)

Rate of Reoperations in Aphakic and Pseudophakic Eyes

A nonrandomized pilot study performed in anticipation of a planned randomized clinical trial found a higher rate of reoperation in infants receiving IOLs compared with infants left aphakic.[2] Plager et al.[5] reported that 4 (12.1%) of 33 aphakic eyes required a secondary procedure for VAO, compared to 12 (80.0%) of 15 eyes in their pseudophakic group. We reviewed 27 consecutive aphakic eyes (cataract surgery also in the first year of life) that underwent lens aspiration without IOL implantation at our institution between 1997 and 2002.[11] The number of eyes that required secondary surgery for VAO in the aphakic group was 3 of 27 (11.1%), compared to 11 of 29 (37.9%) eyes in the pseudophakic population. The number of reoperations due to other ocular causes was 10 in the aphakic group (3 secondary IOL, 3 strabismus, 4 glaucoma), representing 10 of 27 (37.0%) eyes, compared to 3 in our pseudophakic study population, all involving a single eye that required three glaucoma operations (1 of 29 eyes [3.4%]).

Posterior Synechiae

The incidence of posterior synechia formation is higher when an IOL is implanted early in life compared to in older children. We have reported synechiae in 31.0% of eyes (9/29).[11] For three-piece AcrySof IOLs, synechiae have been reported in 35.1% of eyes implanted in the first 13 months of life and 1.7% in eyes implanted at between 2 and 16 years of age.[13]

Glaucoma

Eyes operated on early in life are at high risk for development of glaucoma. A recent report[14] concluded that chronic glaucoma is common after cataract surgery performed at or before, but not after, a certain age in childhood. The data suggest that this age threshold is 9 months. Continued follow-up will be necessary to determine the impact of an IOL implantation in pseudophakic eyes.

Functional Outcome and Parental Stress

Lambert et al.[2] noted that correcting aphakia after unilateral congenital cataract surgery with primary IOL implantation results in an improved visual outcome. Also, the incidence of strabismus was 75% in the IOL group compared with 23% in the contact lens group. Drews et al.[15] noted a higher stress level in parents with children who had unilateral congenital cataracts and did not receive IOLs—particularly stress related to their child's reaction to sensory stimulation and mood—compared with parents of pseudophakic children.

In summary, despite posterior capsulectomy and vitrectomy, the occurrence of VAO is very high. This is especially true in eyes associated with other ocular anomalies. It is prudent to caution families preoperatively about the likelihood of requiring secondary surgery for VAO during the first 6 months after surgery. IOL implantation has the benefit of providing at least a partial optical correction at all times and a potentially improved functional outcome, but this gain must be balanced against the high reoperation rate for VAO. For children with unilateral cataracts presenting in the first 6 months of life, we are truly in equipoise

about whether (in the best of circumstances) the visual outcome will be better with primary IOL and glasses or with aphakia and contact lens. The IATS (Infant Aphakia Treatment Study) will give us this answer by randomizing these eyes to a primary IOL or aphakia with a contact lens. The National Eye Institute (NEI) has now funded this multicenter clinical trial. We urge surgeons throughout the United States to refer eligible infants to the study center nearest to the parents' home. The IATS is an important study because it not only will compare two treatment options for infantile cataracts, but also will give us valuable data on parental stress and patching compliance. The field of pediatric cataract surgery has been devoid of well-designed NEI-sponsored randomized multicenter clinical trials. Adequate recruitment for the IATS is a prerequisite for additional important clinical trials in the field of pediatric cataract surgery.

REFERENCES

1. Lambert SR, Buckley EG, Plager DA, Medow NB, Wilson ME. Unilateral intraocular lens implantation during the first six months of life. *J AAPOS* 1999;3:344–349.
2. Lambert SR, Lynn M, Drews-Botsch C, et al. A comparison of grating visual acuity, strabismus, and reoperation outcomes among children with aphakia and pseudophakia after unilateral cataract surgery during the first six months of life. *J AAPOS* 2001;5:70–75.
3. Lloyd IC. Intraocular lens implantation in infants. *Clin Exp Ophthalmol* 2000;28:338–340.
4. O'Keefe M, Fenton S, Lanigan B. Visual outcomes and complications of posterior chamber intraocular lens implantation in the first year of life. *J Cataract Refract Surg* 2001;27:2006–2011.
5. Plager DA, Yang S, Neely D, Sprunger D, Sondhi N. Complications in the first year following cataract surgery with and without IOL in infants and older children. *J AAPOS* 2002;6:9–14.
6. Buckley E, Lambert SR, Wilson ME. IOLs in the first year of life. *J Pediatr Ophthalmol Strabismus* 1999;36:281–286.
7. Vasavada A, Chauhan H. Intraocular lens implantation in infants with congenital cataracts. *J Cataract Refract Surg* 1994;20:592–598.
8. Wilson ME, Peterseim MW, Englert JA, Lall-Trail JK, Elliott LA. Pseudophakia and polypseudophakia in the first year of life. *J AAPOS* 2001;5:238–245.
9. Wilson ME Jr, Bartholomew LR, Trivedi RH. Pediatric cataract surgery and intraocular lens implantation: Practice preferences of the 2001 ASCRS and AAPOS memberships. *J Cataract Refract Surg* 2003;29:1811–1820.
10. Lambert SR, Lynn M, Drews-Botsch C, et al. Intraocular lens implantation during infancy: perceptions of parents and the American Association for Pediatric Ophthalmology and Strabismus members. *J AAPOS* 2003;7:400–405.
11. Trivedi RH, Wilson Jr ME, Bartholomew LR, Lal G, Peterseim MM. Opacification of the visual axis after cataract surgery and single acrylic intraocular lens implantation in the first year-of-life. *J AAPOS* 2004;8:156–164.
12. Tablante RT, Lapus JV, Cruz ED, Santos AM. A new technique of congenital cataract surgery with primary posterior chamber intraocular lens implantation. *J Cataract Refract Surg* 1988;14:149–157.
13. Vasavada AR, Trivedi RH, Nath V. AcrySof Intraocular lens implantation in children. *J Cataract Refract Surg* 2004;30:1073–1081.
14. Rabiah PK. Frequency and predictors of glaucoma after pediatric cataract surgery. *Am J Ophthalmol* 2004;137:30–37.
15. Drews C, Celano M, Plager DA, Lambert SR. Parenting stress among caregivers of children with congenital cataracts. *J AAPOS* 2003;7:244–250.

AcrySof® Intraocular Lens Implantation in Eyes with Pediatric Cataracts

Rupal H. Trivedi and M. Edward Wilson, Jr.

Following Sir Harold Ridley's invention of the intraocular lens (IOL) in 1949, Dr. Edward Epstein implanted an IOL in the eye of a child in 1952 (cited in Ref. 1). However, many earlier attempts at IOL implantation in children resulted in frequent complications secondary to poor lens design and the increased inflammatory response that occurs in a child's eye after intraocular surgery. As a result, the use of an IOL in pediatric cataract surgery was slow to catch on and did not become common practice until the 1990s. Newer and more refined surgical techniques and technologies have resulted in a remarkable reduction in the postsurgical inflammatory response even in the highly reactive eyes of children. Advancement in IOL material is one of the most important contributing factors in this regard.

Polymethylmethacrylate (PMMA) IOLs, although time tested, are associated with a higher rate of complications.[2] The AcrySof® IOLs (Alcon, Ft. Worth, TX, USA) are made of hydrophobic acrylic and have become a favorite for implantation in children. Soon after its introduction in 1994, the AcrySof® IOL assumed a prominent role in adult cataract surgery. Pediatric surgeons, however, continued to implant PMMA IOLs, almost exclusively. Slowly, in the later half of the 1990s, more and more pediatric surgeons began implanting AcrySof® IOLs in children. In 2001, we surveyed surgeons worldwide and found that 66.8% of ASCRS respondees and 71.7% of AAPOS respondees preferred hydrophobic acrylic IOLs for implanting in children.[3] Although not specifically asked, many of the respondees in our 2001 survey wrote that the newer single-piece AcrySof® IOL was even better suited to pediatric implantation than the three-piece AcrySof® had been (unpublished data). The trend away from PMMA and in favor of the AcrySof® lens for childhood implantation has been driven by a desire for a biocompatible material that can be inserted via a smaller incision.[4] AcrySof® IOLs exhibit a high capsular biocompatibility. In addition, compared to PMMA IOLs, AcrySof® IOLs are associated with fewer posterior synechiae and fewer lens deposits when implanted in children.[5] Since visual axis opacification (VAO) is one of the most frequent and severe complications in pediatric cataract surgery, reports that the AcrySof® IOL decreased the incidence of capsule opacification after adult cataract surgery prompted many pediatric cataract surgeons to use this lens for pediatric cataract surgery also (Figs. 24-1 and 24-2).

Recent reports have documented outcomes of implantation of the three-piece as well as the newer single-piece AcrySof® acrylic IOLs in children.[4-18] More than 624 primary AcrySof® IOL implantations have now been reported in the literature. Herein we review the literature with regard to AcrySof® IOL implantation in eyes with pediatric cataracts. First, we report the intraoperative performance of the AcrySof® IOL in pediatric eyes. Afterward, we review articles related to postoperative outcome in children when AcrySof® IOLs are used.

When comparing literature, a cautionary note should be kept in mind. Results from different studies are difficult to compare because of common inconsistencies including variations in age at surgery, surgical technique, and associated ocular pathology. Major factors to keep in mind when interpreting these results are as follows.

1. *Age at surgery.* Children who are the youngest at the time of cataract surgery may also be the ones most prone to subsequent complications regardless of which IOL is used. Some studies include only older children, while others have a predominance of infants.

2. *Associated ocular anomalies.* Eyes with associated ocular anomalies (such as "complex microphthalmia") are at high risk for subsequent VAO regardless of the IOL used, even when a posterior capsulotomy is performed.[16]

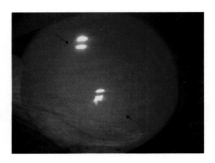

FIGURE 24-1. Single-piece AcrySof® (SA60AT; 22.5 diopters) in an eye operated on for cataract at the age of 44 months. Note the edge of the anterior capsulotomy (long arrow) and posterior capsulotomy (short arrow).

3. *Etiology of cataracts.* In general, eyes with traumatic cataracts develop a more severe inflammatory response after IOL implantation than eyes of similar-aged children with nontraumatic cataracts.

4. *Posterior capsule and anterior vitreous management.* Posterior capsule and anterior vitreous management greatly influences the ultimate maintenance of visual axis clarity and ultimate visual outcome in children (see Chapter 16).

5. *Follow-up.* Studies with longer follow-ups will have high rates of opacification. Eyes with an intact posterior capsule tend to opacify between 18 months and 3 years after surgery. Studies that include eyes with <3 years of postsurgical follow-up probably underestimate the incidence of VAO in the study population. In contrast, Trivedi et al.[16] have reported that eyes that undergo cataract removal in infancy and receive a primary posterior capsulectomy and vitrectomy (and AcrySof® IOL implantation) tend to be at risk for recurrent opacification mainly during the first 6 months after surgery.[16] Therefore, studies of this population will predict long-term VAO accurately as long as 6 months of postsurgical follow-up is included.[16]

With this background, we focus first on the intraoperative performance and then on the postoperative outcome of AcrySof® IOL implantation in children.

INTRAOPERATIVE PERFORMANCE

Historically, one of the most commonly cited reasons for surgeons' lack of enthusiasm about using IOLs in children was that the surgical trauma related to the difficulty of implanting an IOL into a small eye could potentially cause harm. When foldable IOLs made of acrylic materials became available, pediatric surgeons finally had biocompatible implants that could be inserted into small eyes less traumatically and through a smaller incision. In our experience, in addition to their superior biocompatibility, other important benefits of AcrySof® IOLs relate to their intraoperative performance in pediatric eyes.

We at the Storm Eye Institute, Medical University of South Carolina, were the first to actively advocate the use of AcrySof® IOLs for children. We have been implanting these IOLs in children since November 1995. We reported our initial series of 110 pediatric eyes implanted with AcrySof® IOLs and compared them with 120 pediatric eyes implanted with PMMA IOLs.[5] Rowe and coworkers[15] recently reported that primary implantation of foldable AcrySof® IOLs in pediatric eyes is associated with fewer perioperative complications than implantation of rigid PMMA IOLs (P <0.05).

Single-piece AcrySof® SA series IOLs are ideal for children based on the implantation characteristics as of 2004.[4] They can be inserted more easily into even the smallest of capsular bags. Extremely flexible haptics, combined with excellent memory, make this lens both easy to implant and not prone to deformation. The haptics unfold very slowly and adapt to any size capsular bag, yet retain enough memory after placement to resist equatorial lens capsule fibrosis. In our series, we did not find a single lens to be compressed (haptic deformation or bending of the haptic behind the optic) by capsular fibrosis.[4] This compression was a common finding in the 1980s and early 1990s when PMMA IOLs with Prolene haptics were implanted in children. These intraoperative advantages of AcrySof® SA lenses also apply to AcrySof® SN "natural" IOLs. The single-piece AcrySof® IOL is the lens of choice for the Infant Aphakic Treatment Trial, a multicenter clinical trial recently funded by the National Eye Institute to compare primary IOL implantation to primary aphakia with

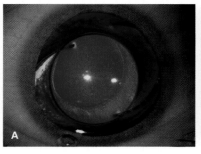
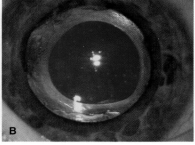

FIGURE 24-2. Postoperative follow-up showing a clear visual axis. **(A)** Note haptic distortion peripheral capsular changes. **(B)** Note well centered IOL and anterior capsule opacification.

secondary IOL implantation at a later age in infants having cataract surgery at age <7 months.

Laboratory investigations at the Storm Eye Institute have shown that the flexible haptic design of the single-piece acrylic AcrySof® IOL appears to minimize the ovaling of the rhexis opening and capsule bag in children compared to the other IOL designs tested.[19] Pandey and associates[19] compared the amount of capsulorhexis ovaling and capsular bag stretch produced by various rigid and foldable IOLs when implanted into pediatric human eyes obtained postmortem. Six types of IOLs manufactured from rigid and foldable biomaterials were implanted to determine which IOL design was best suited for implantation in pediatric eyes. All of the IOLs produced ovaling of the capsulorhexis opening, and stretching of the capsular bag, parallel to the IOL haptics. However, the single-piece hydrophobic acrylic AcrySof® lens was associated with significantly less capsulorhexis ovaling and capsular bag stretch.

POSTOPERATIVE OUTCOME

Visual Axis Opacification

VAO is rapid and virtually inevitable in the very young child after pediatric cataract surgery when adult-style surgery, leaving the posterior capsule intact, is performed. The incidence of VAO is a common outcome measure of pediatric cataract surgery. A review of the literature on the incidence and characteristics of VAO is presented in Table 24-1.

In aggregate, the literature on VAO in children suggests that when the posterior capsule is left intact, pediatric patients show a similar VAO rate when implanted with an AcrySof® IOL or a PMMA IOL. However, VAO after AcrySof® implantation with an intact posterior capsule is more "proliferative," as opposed to the "fibrous" reaction commonly seen in conjunction with PMMA IOLs. The proliferative VAO may progress more slowly, be less visually significant, and require secondary intervention less often. After a primary posterior capsulotomy and an anterior vitrectomy, VAO is rare regardless of whether an AcrySof® or a PMMA IOL is inserted. When it does occur, it is usually in a baby operated on in the first year of life. This form of VAO tends to occur within the first 6 months after cataract and implant surgery if it is going to occur at all. Finally, the AcrySof® IOL has been documented to stimulate what has been called an "anterior vitreous reticular response" when exposed to the vitreous face after pediatric cataract surgery and posterior capsulotomy but no vitrectomy.[13] This finding on the anterior vitreous face was usually not visually significant. The authors recommended AcrySof® IOL implantation combined with a posterior capsulotomy and an anterior vitrectomy from infancy until age 5 years.[13,17] For children between 5 and 8 years of age, a primary posterior capsulotomy was performed without an anterior vitrec-

tomy.[17] After age 8, the authors recommended implanting an AcrySof® IOL and leaving the posterior capsule intact.[17]

The published investigations into the issue of VAO after AcrySof® are listed and discussed below in chronologic order from the oldest (2001) to the most recent (2004).

Wilson et al.[5] reported on 110 eyes receiving an AcrySof® implantation at an average age of 60.4 months, with an average follow-up of 14.9 months. In comparison, 120 eyes had a PMMA lens inserted at an average age of 71.9 months, with an average postoperative follow-up of 31.5 months. Twenty-two AcrySof®-implanted eyes and 28 PMMA-implanted eyes had an intact posterior capsule. The YAG laser caspulotomy rate was similar in the two groups: 45.4% for AcrySof® and 50% for PMMA. The average time from surgery to YAG posterior capsulotomy was 18.6 months for an AcrySof® lens and 18.3 months for a PMMA lens. None of the patients with AcrySof® IOLs have needed more than one YAG capsulotomy. Five of the patients with PMMA IOLs have needed multiple YAG laser treatments for recurrent opacification ($P \leq 0.05$).

Argento and coworkers[6] published the results of AcrySof® IOL optic capture in children with cataracts. Eight children were included, with a mean follow-up of 28.9 ± 5.3 months (age at cataract surgery, 2 to 8 years). The visual axis remained clear in all cases. No case required a secondary procedure. The article by Argento et al.[6] does not make clear whether the advantage was provided by optic capture or by the AcrySof® material. The study did not have a control group (AcrySof® implantation with no optic capture).

Kugelberg and Zetterstrom[7] evaluated aftercataract formation in children undergoing cataract surgery with or without anterior vitrectomy. This was a retrospective study comprised of 85 eyes (age, birth to 15 years) who had cataract surgery with or without anterior vitrectomy after the implantation of an IOL. All patients had primary posterior capsulorhexis but no optic capture. Thirty-five patients received a heparin-surface-modified (HSM) PMMA IOL (809C; Pharmacia & Upjohn), and 50 patients a foldable acrylic IOL (AcrySof®; Alcon). In children older than 7 years in the AcrySof® IOL group, there was no difference in the frequency of aftercataract surgery for the vitrectomy versus the no-vitrectomy group ($P > 0.05$). In children younger than 7 years with an AcrySof® IOL, the rate of aftercataract surgery was significantly lower in those who had an anterior vitrectomy at the time of cataract surgery compared to those who did not ($P < 0.05$). Interestingly, in this series, some patients with an HSM PMMA IOL developed aftercataracts even though surgery was performed with an anterior vitrectomy, in contrast to the AcrySof® group, in which all eyes with vitrectomy remained clear. Of the children with an AcrySof® IOL, none who had an anterior vitrectomy developed aftercataracts, whereas 8 of 31 patients who did not have an anterior vitrectomy developed

▶ TABLE 24-1 Literature Review of Outcome of Primary AcrySof® IOL Implantation in Children

Authors (Ref. No.)	Year	Age (yr)[a]	N	Follow-up (yr)[a]	IOL	Posterior Capsule Management	Secondary Intervention (%)
Wilson et al. (5)	2001	5	110	1.2	MA60BM, MA30BA	Intact PC = 22; Rest: PC + V	45.4
Argento et al. (6)	2001	3.4 ± 1.9 (2–8)	8	2.4	MA60BM, MA30BA	PC ± V (IOL optic capture)	0
Kugelberg & Zetterstrom C (7)	2002	5.7 (median)	50	1.6	MA30BA	PC: 31 / PC + V: 19	26 / 0
Plager et al. (8)	2002	<0.5	15	ND	MA30BA	PC + V	80
		0.8–5.0	16	ND	MA30BA	PC + V	0
Stager et al. (9)	2002	8.3 ± 3.7	26	2.7	MA30BA	Intact PC	50
Mullner-Eidenbock et al. (10)	2003	2–16	50	1.7	MA60BM	2–6 yr: PC + V (n = 12)	8
						PC + V + OC (n = 8)	0
						6–16 yr: PC (n = 8)	0
						PC + OC (n = 7)	0
						Intact PC (n = 15)	13.3
Ram et al. (11)	2003	0.3–12	64	Min 2	MA30BA	PC + V (n = 16)	12.5
						Intact PC (n = 16)	75
Kuchle et al. (12)	2003	8.4 ± 4.6	10	1.0 ± 0.7	MA60BM	PC ± V (n = 4)	0
						Intact PC	16.7
Trivedi & Wilson (4)	2003	2.8 (0.04–9.1)	42	1.0 (0.1–2.3)	SA30AL, SA60AT	PC + V	16.7
Vasavada et al. (14)	2004	1.8	24	1.5	MA30BA	PC + V	0
Rowe et al. (15)	2004	0.1–15	35	2	MA30BA, MA60BM	PC (n = 8), intact PC (n = 26)	45.7
Trivedi et al. (16)	2004	0.4	29	2.7	MA30BA, MA60BM, SA30AL, SA60AT	PC + V	37.9
Vasavada et al. (17)	2004	5.2 ± 5.0	103	2.3 ± 0.9	MA30BA	<2 yr: PC + V	8.1
						>2 yr: Intact PC	27.7
						PC + V	0
						PC – V	7
Raina et al. (18)	2004	6.5	42	1.1	MA30BA, MA60MB	Intact PC	16
						PC ± V	0

PC, posterior capsulotomy; V, vitrectomy.
[a]Mean unless specified otherwise.

aftercataracts. In the HSM IOL group, 6 of 31 patients who had an anterior vitrectomy needed surgery for aftercataracts, whereas 3 of 4 eyes that did not have an anterior vitrectomy developed aftercataracts.

Plager and colleagues[8] reported on the role of IOLs in infants and older children. The authors noted that 12 of 15 (80.0%) eyes operated in the first 6 months of life required secondary surgery to clear the visual axis. None of the eyes operated on between 10 months and 5 years required intervention for VAO.

Stager et al.[9] reported rates of posterior capsule opacification (PCO) following foldable acrylic IOL implantation in children. With a mean age at surgery of 8.25 years and a mean follow-up of 2.75 years, 13 of 26 eyes (50%) developed visually significant PCO requiring intervention. In the group of children <4 years of age, 100% of the eyes with an intact posterior capsule developed opacification of the visual axis and required a secondary intervention. In children between 4 and 14 years old, 38% (8/21) of eyes developed opacification. Four of 26 eyes (15%) required two procedures (either repeat Nd–YAG laser capsulotomy or pars plana secondary membrane removal) to clear the visual axis. The authors further noted that three of five (60%) eyes developed recurrent opacification following Nd–YAG laser in the younger age group (<4 years), which suggested that surgical capsulotomy combined with anterior vitrectomy, rather than YAG laser capsulotomy, may be needed in these young children to keep the visual axis clear.

Mullner-Eidenbock et al.[10] reported the results of a prospective, randomized study comprised of 50 eyes of 34 children between 2 and 16 years of age. Eyes of children between 2 and 5.9 years were consecutively randomized to Group 1a (primary posterior capsulotomy and anterior vitrectomy) or Group 1b (optic capture in addition). Eyes of children between 6 and 16 years old were consecutively randomized to Group 2a (primary posterior capsulotomy without anterior vitrectomy), Group 2b (optic capture in addition), or Group 2c (in-the-bag IOL implantation without opening of the posterior capsule). The visual axis was clear at the last follow-up in all eyes in Groups 1a, 1b, 2a, and 2b except for one eye in Group 1a (8.33%). In the eye of a healthy boy with a unilateral cataract, severe PCO occurred. The eye developed fibrosis and phimosis of the posterior capsulorhexis 6 months postoperatively, causing significant decentration of the capsulorhexis. The patient required a second operation 12 months postoperatively. Nine of 15 eyes (60.0%) in Group 2c (with an intact posterior capsule) developed PCO, which was mild in 7 eyes (77.8%). The first signs of mild PCO developed a mean of 6.2 months postoperatively (range, 0.5 to 13.0 months); however, treatment was not necessary as of the last follow-up. One eye had moderate PCO, with the first signs developing 2 months postoperatively. This eye had a YAG laser capsulotomy at 24 months. One eye of a 10-year-old boy who developed severe anterior uveitis 1 month postoper-

atively that required a reoperation 6 months later had severe PCO. His left eye, also in Group 2c but without signs of postoperative uveitis, had a clear visual axis at the last examination.

Ram and coworkers[11] evaluated the effect of a primary posterior capsulotomy with anterior vitrectomy and various IOL materials on the development of PCO after pediatric cataract surgery. Sixty-four eyes of 52 children, ranging in age from 3 months to 12 years, who had cataract extraction with IOL implantation were prospectively evaluated for a minimum postoperative period of 2 years. Thirty-two eyes received a AcrySof® acrylic IOL, and 32 a single-piece PMMA IOL. Sixteen eyes in each IOL group had posterior capsulectomy and vitrectomy; in the remaining 16 eyes in each group, the posterior capsule was left intact. Postoperatively, 25 eyes in the intact capsule group and 5 in the other group developed PCO; the difference between groups was significant (*P* <0.05). Of eyes with an intact capsule, 12 with an AcrySof® acrylic IOL and 13 with a PMMA IOL developed PCO (*P* >0.05). In the vitrectomy group, two eyes with an acrylic IOL and three with a PMMA IOL developed PCO (P >0.05). Overall, 14 eyes with an acrylic lens and 16 eyes with a PMMA lens developed PCO (*P* >0.05). After surgery, there was a significant short-term delay in the development of PCO in the acrylic group (14 eyes; mean, 6.66 ± 1.57 months) compared to the PMMA group (16 eyes; mean, 3.16 ± 0.83 months; *P* <0.05). For eyes with an intact capsule, 10 of 13 with a PMMA IOL developed a fibrotic membrane and 12 of 12 eyes in the AcrySof® acrylic group developed Elschnig pearl opacification (*P* <0.05). Development of PCO in the postoperative period was delayed with a AcrySof® acrylic IOL compared to a PMMA lens, but ultimately the PCO rate was similar for the lenses studied.

Kuchle et al.[12] analyzed and reported the results of cataract surgery and posterior chamber IOL implantation in 30 eyes of 30 patients aged 1 to 16 years. In 10 eyes AcrySof® acrylic IOLs, and in 20 eyes single-piece PMMA PCIOLs, were implanted. Mean patient age at surgery was 8.6 (3 to 16) years for the AcrySof® acrylic group and 6.3 (1 to 16) years for the PMMA group. Mean follow-up was 1 year for the AcrySof® acrylic and 1.8 years for the PMMA group. Primary anterior vitrectomy was performed in seven eyes in the PMMA group and in three eyes in the AcrySof® acrylic group. Evaluating all complications together (at least one complication versus no complications), there were significantly fewer complications in the AcrySof® acrylic group (2 of 10 versus 15 of 20; *P* = 0.007). The rate of PCO requiring YAG capsulotomy was 1 of 6 in the AcrySof® acrylic group without posterior capsulorhexis, versus 7 of 12 in the PMMA group without posterior capsulorhexis. The postoperative time for YAG capsulotomy was 21 months in the AcrySof® acrylic group and 19 months in the PMMA group. In this series none of the eyes with posterior capsulorhexis developed PCO, in either the AcrySof® acrylic or the PMMA group.

Trivedi and Wilson[4] reported outcomes of single-piece AcrySof® IOL implantation in children. Their retrospective case review comprised 42 consecutive implantations of single-piece hydrophobic acrylic IOLs: AcrySof® SA30AL (5.5-mm optic, 12.5-mm overall size) or AcrySof® SA60AT (6.0-mm optic, 13.0-mm overall size). Forty-two eyes with posterior capsulectomy and vitrectomy were analyzed. Eyes with traumatic cataracts and secondary IOLs were excluded. The mean age was 33.5 ± 28.9 (SD) months (range, 0.5 to 110 months), and the mean follow-up, 12.0 ± 8.2 months (range, 1.0 to 27.5 months). Postoperative VAO occurred in seven eyes (16.7%). Secondary surgical procedures were required in five eyes (11.9%). The mean age at surgery was 7.9 ± 6.6 months in patients who required a secondary procedure and 37.0 ± 29.0 months in those who did not (*P* = 0.0001). Five of 17 eyes (29.4%) operated before 18 months of age required a second surgery to clear the visual axis; none of the 25 eyes operated at or after 18 months of age required a second surgery. The secondary procedures were required a mean of 10.7 months (range, 4.4 to 21.9 months) after cataract surgery. One patient had SA30AL IOL implantation at the ages of 10.6 and 10.8 months, respectively. The right-eye surgery was uneventful. In the left eye, a tear was noted in the anterior capsule during IOL manipulation. At the 22.1- and 21.9-month follow-ups, respectively, the right eye had a clear visual axis, with the anterior capsule completely covering the optic. The left eye had VAO caused by Elschnig pearls. This opacification was visually significant and required a second procedure. In this eye, the anterior capsule edge no longer completely covered the optic for 360°, which exposed the IOL edge for 1 clock hour at the 3 o'clock position. The relationship of the anterior capsule to the IOL optic may have led to the need for the second procedure by allowing Elschnig pearls to migrate into the visual axis. Although one case is not sufficient to draw a conclusion, this possible explanation concurs with a report in the literature on adult cataract surgery.[20] We concluded that single-piece acrylic lenses are well suited for implantation in the small capsular bags of children. The IOL can be placed in the eye through a 3.0-mm incision with good control using the Monarch II injector, even in very soft eyes. Although long-term clinical experience with these newer IOLs is necessary to draw firm conclusions regarding the biocompatibility of this material in pediatric eyes, our preliminary data suggest that the single-piece acrylic IOL can be safely implanted in the pediatric eye.

Vasavada and associates[14] recently reported on the management of congenital cataract with a preexisting posterior capsule defect. The mean age was 21.9 (SD, 33.3) months. Twenty eyes had an AcrySof® MA30BA IOL in the bag and four eyes (14.81%) had the same IOL placed in the ciliary sulcus. The visual axis remained clear in all eyes, with a mean follow-up of 17.9 months (range, 6–67 months).

Rowe and colleagues[15] recently reported that YAG laser rates in their children were similar for PMMA versus AcrySof® acrylic IOLs (*P* >0.05). Mean times until intervention for PMMA and acrylic IOLs were 30.1 months (95% CI, 22 to 38 months) and 19.8 months (95% CI, 12 to 27 months), respectively (log rank test statistic, 1.53; *P* = 0.22). Fifteen of 25 PMMA cases, and 16 of 35 eyes implanted with AcrySof® acrylic IOLs, underwent at least one subsequent laser or surgical capsulotomy during a total of 594 months of total at-risk follow-up for PMMA and 392 total months of at-risk follow-up for AcrySof® acrylic. At 12 months post–implant surgery, 76% (95% CI, 59 to 93%) of PMMA cases and 54% (95% CI, 35 to 72%) of acrylic cases had not required intervention for PCO; these proportions fell to 55% (95% CI, 35 to 75%) and 38% (95% CI, 14 to 61%) for PMMA and acrylic cases, respectively, at 2 years postsurgery. After adjustment for age at surgery, primary posterior caspulorhexis, and perioperative complications, the relative risk of intervention after acrylic IOL implantation was 1.6 (95% CI, 0.66–3.9; *P* = 0.29). However, we should interpret the results carefully since 32% (8/25) of eyes in the PMMA group had an intact posterior capsule, but 76% (26/34) of eyes in the AcrySof® acrylic group had an intact posterior capsule.

Trivedi and colleagues[16] reported the incidence and risk factors for secondary surgical intervention to treat VAO after cataract surgery and AcrySof® acrylic IOL implantation during the first year of life. We concluded that 11 of 29 (37.9%) eyes developed VAO requiring secondary surgical intervention at a median of 4.8 months (95% CI, 3.4 to 6.2 months). The relative risk of subsequent VAO surgery was 2.7 times for primary surgery performed at or before 6 months of age. Opacification was significantly related to eyes with associated ocular anomalies (e.g., anterior segment dysgenesis, iris hypoplasia, or PFV), with a relative risk of 8.6. When secondary surgery was required, it occurred primarily (i.e., 9 of 11 eyes) during the first 6 months after the initial surgery. The median survival period was 4.8 months in Kaplan–Meier survival analysis. For comparison, we reviewed an age-matched group of 27 consecutive aphakic eyes (cataract surgery also in the first year of life) that underwent lens aspiration without IOL implantation at our institute (Storm Eye Institution). The number of eyes that required secondary surgery for VAO in the aphakic group was 3 of 27 (11.1%), compared with 11 of 29 (37.9%) eyes in the pseudophakic group. However, the number of reoperations to treat other ocular problems was 10 in the aphakic group (3 secondary IOL, 3 strabismus, and 4 glaucoma), versus 1 in the pseudophakic study population.

Vasavada et al.[17] published a study evaluating VAO and the need for a secondary procedure after AcrySof® IOL implantation in pediatric eyes. This prospective randomized study evaluated 103 consecutive eyes of 72 children with pediatric cataracts. In contrast to most other published series, the authors excluded eyes with associated ocular anomalies. Two groups were formed based on age at surgery: Group 1, younger than 2 years; and Group 2, older than 2 years. All eyes in Group 1 ($n = 37$) had primary posterior continuous curvilinear capsulorhexis (PCCC) with anterior vitrectomy. In Group 2 ($n = 66$), management of the posterior capsule was assigned randomly to no PCCC (Group 2A; $N = 37$) or PCCC (Group 2B; $N = 29$). The PCCC group was further randomized into two subgroups: no vitrectomy (Group 2BN; $N = 14$) or vitrectomy (Group 2BV; $N = 15$). The primary outcome measures were VAO and the resulting need for a secondary procedure. The mean age of the patients was 5.2 ± 5.0 years (range, 0.2 to 16.0 years) and the mean follow-up was 2.3 ± 0.9 years (range, 1.0 to 4.0 years). Overall, 41 eyes (39.8%) developed VAO and 14 (13.6%) required secondary intervention.

- In Group 1, four eyes (10.8%) developed VAO and three (8.1%) had a secondary pars plana vitrectomy.
- In Group 2A, 31 eyes (83.8%) developed PCO and 10 eyes (27.7%) had secondary intervention. The incidence of PCO was highest between 2 and 3 years postoperatively. The mean age was 11.3 ± 5.3 years for those who did not develop PCO and 7.2 ± 3.6 years for those who did ($P = 0.02$). For eyes with an intact posterior capsule, PCO occurred in 10 of 15 whose age at surgery was >8 years and 21 of 22 whose age at surgery was 2 to 8 years ($P = 0.01$). Of 31 eyes with opacification, 21 (67.7%) had proliferative PCO, 9 (29.0%) had mixed PCO, and 1 (3.2%) had fibrous PCO. The mean age of those developing proliferative PCO was significantly higher than that of those developing mixed PCO (proliferative and fibrous) (8.2 ± 3.6 versus 5.2 ± 3.0 years, respectively; $P = 0.03$). Ten eyes required a secondary procedure; four had surgery and six had an Nd:YAG laser capsulotomy to clear the visual axis. The secondary procedures were done a mean of 2.0 ± 0.6 years (range, 1.1 to 3.0 years) after the initial cataract surgery. Opacification recurred in two eyes; one had an Nd:YAG capsulotomy and one had surgery to clear the visual axis. An increased incidence of PCO in eyes with an intact capsule is expected. The need for primary posterior capsulotomy was evident in children younger than 8 years. Besides its frequent occurrence, PCO is a greater concern in children younger than 8 years because of the increased risk that patients will be noncompliant during Nd:YAG laser capsulotomy and because of the risks associated with anesthesia in a secondary procedure. Other factors such as the availability of an Nd:YAG laser, condition of the posterior capsule (e.g., plaque, defect), and type of PCO (proliferative or fibrous) also influence the choice of posterior capsule management. The

proliferative type of PCO is probably less amblyogenic than the fibrous type. This explains the low rate of secondary procedures. The authors noted that in their experience with PMMA IOLs, PCO was predominantly fibrous. They believe that the type of PCO is dependent on the IOL material and that the PCO with AcrySof® IOLs is proliferative.

- In Group 2BN five eyes (37.5%) had opacification of the anterior vitreous face, one of which required a secondary procedure 2.7 years after cataract surgery. Of these, 60% (three of five) had a fine meshworklike reticular response, termed the anterior vitreous reticular response; 20% (one of five) had a scaffold response and 20% had a mixed response at the last follow-up. The mean age of eyes developing anterior vitreous face changes was 5.1 ± 3.4 years. All eyes of patients ≤5 years and one eye of children >5 years developed an anterior vitreous reticular response ($P = 0.0015$). Based on the results in this group, the authors believe that one can avoid vitrectomy in children >5 years old. When the AcrySof® IOL came in contact with the anterior vitreous face, a fine, reticular meshwork change on the anterior vitreous face was noted and was termed "the anterior vitreous reticular response."[13] Further study of this group revealed that this response did not have a significant effect on visual acuity. There was no significant difference in visual acuity before versus after the development of the anterior vitreous reticular response ($P = 0.072$). In a previously published study Vasavada et al.[21] noted that the visual axis opacified as a result of anterior vitreous fibrosis in 70% of eyes when vitrectomy was not performed.
- In Group 2BV, 1 (6.7%) of 15 eyes had VAO with a fibrous band across the visual axis in front of the IOL, which did not require a secondary procedure as of the last follow-up. In this eye, the anterior continuous curvilinear capsulorhexis (ACCC) was incomplete and a posterior capsule plaque was present, which was converted to a PCCC. No eye in this group needed a secondary procedure. In the eyes with and without primary management of the posterior capsule (Groups 2B and 2A), children ≥2 years old had a relative risk for a secondary procedure of 7.9. It is not surprising that in this group, almost all eyes had a clear visual axis, as the group comprised relatively older children who had a PCCC and vitrectomy.

The authors concluded that AcrySof® IOL implantation with appropriate management of the posterior capsule maintained a clear visual axis in 60.2% of eyes. Of the 39.8% of eyes with VAO, 13.6% had visually significant opacification and required a secondary procedure.

Raina and associates[18] evaluated outcomes of in-the-bag implantation of acrylic IOLs at the time of pediatric cataract surgery. Forty-two eyes of 25 children were included in this prospective study. All of them had in-the-bag implantation of an AcrySof® IOL. Twenty-five eyes had an intact posterior capsule (Group A). Seventeen eyes had PCCC (Group B), four had anterior vitrectomy combined with PCCC (Group C), and six had PCCC with IOL optic capture through the PCCC (Group D). Secondary opacification of the visual axis, visual acuity, and possible complications were observed and analyzed. The mean age of the patients was 78 months (range, 36 to 144 months). The mean follow-up was 13 months (range, 6 to 18 months). Patients were relatively older in Group A in this series. The average age in the group with no PCCC was 92 months. However, Groups B, C, and D had an average age of 68, 66, and 66 months, respectively. Four eyes (16%) in Group A developed visually significant PCO involving the central visual axis and required secondary capsulotomy. All eyes in Groups B, C, and D had a clear visual axis at the last follow-up and did not require a secondary procedure. The authors concluded that an optimal-sized ACCC followed by in-the-bag implantation of a foldable acrylic IOL helped maintain a clear visual axis by delaying the onset of PCO and leading to milder PCO. The benefits of a foldable acrylic IOL in pediatric cataract surgery can be increased by combining it with PCCC, with or without anterior vitrectomy, or with optic capture of the IOL. Raina et al.[18] noted that in Group A (ACCC alone), 15 eyes (60.0%) had visually insignificant (grade 0 to 1+) PCO at the 3-month follow-up. At 6 months, eight eyes (32.0%) had grade 2+ PCO and one eye had grade 3+ PCO. Of these, two eyes (one with grade 2+ and one with grade 3+) required secondary capsulotomy. Two other eyes (one with grade 2+ and one with grade 3+) required a secondary capsulotomy at 1 year. Thus, four eyes (16.0%) in this group required secondary capsulotomy (two surgical and two Nd:YAG). No eye had reopacification of the visual axis until the last follow-up. In Group B (ACCC with PCCC), four eyes (57.1%) had mild opacification of the paracentral or peripheral posterior capsule at the last follow-up. In one of these eyes (14.2%), mild haze of the anterior vitreous face (grade 1+ PCO) was noticed at 1 year; however, the haze did not affect visual acuity. In Group C (PCCC with anterior vitrectomy), two cases (50.0%) had mild peripheral PCO at the last follow-up. No eye developed VAO. Authors further noted that the PCO was pearl-type and mild in most cases and fibrous in only two cases.

Other Outcomes

Fibrin

Fibrinous uveitis due to increased tissue reactivity is a common complication during the early postoperative period in eyes undergoing pediatric cataract surgery. Kuchle and colleagues[12] reported that postoperative fibrin formation was less frequent in eyes with an AcrySof® IOL compared to eyes with a PMMA IOL (1 of 10 in the acrylic group versus 9 of 20 in the PMMA group).

Pigment Deposits

Deposits on the surface of an IOL optic are often seen during the postoperative period in children. Assessment of type and amount of deposits helps us to understand uveal biocompatibility. Wilson et al.[5] noted that IOL deposits were seen in 6.4% (7/110) of AcrySof® lenses (6.4%), compared with 21.7% (26/120) of PMMA lenses. Several other series have reported the incidence of deposits as 25%,[10] 35.9%,[17] and 24.1%.[16] The incidence of deposits was significantly higher in younger age groups (age at surgery, <2 years) than in the older groups ($P < 0.04$)[17].

Synechiae

Younger age at the time of cataract surgery increases the risk for synechiae formation. Wilson et al.[5] noted posterior synechiae in 5 of 110 AcrySof® lenses (4.5%), compared with 23 of 120 PMMA lenses (19.2%). Evaluating single-piece IOLs in children, Trivedi et al.[4] noted that synechiae were seen in five eyes (11.9%). None produced enough corectopia to cause a noticeable cosmetic deformity. In most cases, the synechiae were pinpoint adhesions of the iris to the anterior capsulotomy edge. No adhesions were seen between the iris and the IOL. Kuchle et al.[12] noted formation of posterior synechiae in none of 10 eyes in the AcrySof® acrylic group versus 6 of 20 eyes in the PMMA group. Vasavada et al.[17] noted posterior synechiae in 14 eyes (13.6%). The incidence of synechia formation was significantly higher in Group 1 (age at surgery, <2 years) than in the other groups ($P < 0.001$). In Group 1, 35.1% developed posterior synechiae. Trivedi et al.[16] noted that synechiae were seen in 31% of eyes in the first year of life.

Glistening

Mullner-Eidenbock et al.[10] noted glistening in both eyes of one patient 1 week postoperatively. The glistenings increased during the first 2 postoperative years to a degree of 3+ and then remained stable until the last follow-up at 40 months.

Centration of IOL

Excessive capsular fibrosis and asymmetric IOL fixation are the most common causes leading to decentration of an IOL. Trivedi et al. noted that all eyes maintained a clinically centered IOL in a series of single-piece AcrySof® IOL implantations in children.[4] Vasavada et al.[17] noted that all eyes in all groups had well-centered AcrySof® IOLs. Trivedi et al.[16] noted mild, clinically nonsignificant decentration of an AcrySof® IOL in 2 of 29 (6.9%) eyes operated on for cataracts during the first year of life.

Cystoid Macular Edema

Pediatric cataract surgery using modern techniques and technologies does not predispose the child to an increased risk of cystoid macular edema. Two articles report that fundus examination did not reveal cystoid macular edema in any eye after pediatric cataract surgery and AcrySof® IOL implantation.[7,14]

Retinal Detachment

The incidence of retinal detachment after pediatric cataract surgery is very low. Kugelberg et al.[7] noted that retinal detachment was not observed in any eyes with AcrySof® IOL implantation in children.

Ocular Hypertension and Glaucoma

Asrani and coworkers[22] noted a low incidence of glaucoma in postcataract patients who had received an IOL. This study did not specifically include only eyes with AcrySof® IOLs. This may represents a selection bias since the more severely maldeveloped and microphthalmic eyes are the ones least likely to be implanted with an IOL.

Vasavada et al.[17] noted that the mean postoperative intraocular pressure after AcrySof® implantation was 15.8 ± 3.8 mm Hg. Five eyes (4.8%) developed an intraocular pressure of ≥ 21 mm Hg. Trivedi et al.[16] noted that both eyes of one patient developed glaucoma, one of which required glaucoma surgery. This patient had anterior segment dysgenesis in both eyes.

Visual Acuity

Wilson et al.[5] reported the Snellen visual acuity recorded for 67 eyes implanted with an AcrySof® IOL. Of those, 48 (72%) had 20/40 or better best corrected visual acuity (BCVA) at the last follow-up and 63 eyes (94%) had 20/100 or better visual acuity. Argento et al.[6] noted that the mean preoperative BCVA in the pediatric cataract patients in their series was 0.06 ± 0.06. Postoperatively, after AcrySof® IOL implantation, the mean BCVA was 0.88 ± 0.11. Mullner-Eidenbock et al.[10] reported that after AcrySof® IOL implantation, a BCVA of 20/25 was achieved in 78% of eyes with bilateral cataracts operated on at 2 to 6 years of age, 45% of eyes with unilateral cataracts operated on at 2 to 6 years of age, and 61% of eyes with bilateral cataracts operated on at between 6 and 16 years of age.

SPECIAL SITUATIONS

Sutured IOLs

Packer et al.[23] reported the case of a 5-year-old boy with severe ectopia lentis who had bilateral lensectomy and suture fixation of a foldable acrylic IOL. The patient experienced an uncorrected visual acuity of 20/40 in both eyes. The conjunctiva was quiet and well healed over the scleral flaps. The corneas were clear and the chambers deep and quiet. The IOLs were positioned centrally in the posterior chambers. The authors concluded that the unique design characteristics of the single-piece AcrySof® IOL make possible the suture fixation of a foldable posterior chamber IOL. However, longer follow-up is needed to ascertain the stability of this suture-fixated IOL over time.

Secondary IOL Implantation

Despite widespread acceptance of the use of primary IOL implantation in children, surgery for infantile cataracts often leaves behind aphakia. Difficulty in determining IOL power, intraoperative difficulties, and higher rates of reoperation are reasons why some surgeons are not very enthusiastic about IOL implantation in neonates and infants with congenital cataracts. In 2001, we surveyed the ASCRS and AAPOS communities for the trend in pediatric cataract surgery. The majority of respondees (unilateral cataract, 68.2 and 70.0%; bilateral cataract, 80.2 and 84.1%; ASCRS and AAPOS, respectively) in both societies choose aphakia as the initial management strategy when cataract surgery is performed in the first year of life.[3,16] It is likely that many of these aphakic patients will later need or desire secondary IOL implantation. Secondary implantation of an IOL is generally recommended when traditional spectacle or contact lens correction of aphakia has become unsuccessful. The technical success of secondary implantation depends mainly on how much capsular support is left behind at the time of primary cataract surgery. At the time of secondary IOL implantation, the surgeon faces two important decisions: what type of lens material to use and where in the eye to implant.

Crnic and associates[24] recently reported the use of AcrySof® acrylic foldable IOLs for secondary implantation in children. Fifty-five eyes, with a mean age at surgery of 7.4 years and a mean follow-up of 28 months, were included in the series. Complications noted were IOL decentration in three eyes (5%), wound leak in three eyes (5%), secondary membrane formation in five eyes (9%), and pupillary block glaucoma in one eye (2%). The authors concluded that an AcrySof® IOL in the ciliary sulcus is a safe and effective method to correct aphakia in pediatric patients with adequate capsular support.

Recently we analyzed the data from our cases of secondary IOL implantation in pediatric aphakia.[25] We excluded eyes with traumatic cataract and eyes with <6 months of follow-up. Seventy-seven eyes were identified with an average age at secondary implantation of 7.8 ± 5.0 years. Age at primary cataract surgery was 1.5 ± 2.6 years. Average follow-up after secondary implantation was 2.7 ± 1.9 years. Thirty eyes received AcrySof® IOLs, while 47 eyes received rigid PMMA IOLs. Complications included clinically significant decentration (5.2%), VAO (5.2%), dislocation of the IOL (2.6%), and pupillary capture required repositioning of the IOL (1.3%). Clinically significant decentration requiring surgical intervention was noted exclusively in eyes with sulcus-fixed AcrySof® IOLs (28.6%; 4/14). None of the 29 eyes with sulcus-fixed PMMA IOLs developed decentration. All of the decentrations were in an inferior direction and all occurred in male eyes. Eyes with an axial length >23 mm were four times more likely to develop decentration when implanted with a sulcus-fixed foldable IOL compared to eyes measuring <23 mm.[25] Postoperative geometric BCVA was significantly better than preoperative acuity (P <0.001). In our series, in-the-bag fixation of AcrySof® IOLs was associated with a low rate of complications. More and more, we strive for secondary in-the-bag implantation of an AcrySof® IOL using a technique we reported previously.[26] However, sulcus-fixed AcrySof® lenses appear to have a higher rate of decentration than PMMA lenses. Myopic males may be at a higher risk for lens decentration. For secondary IOLs we recommend using an AcrySof® IOL if the capsular bag can be reopened but a PMMA IOL if the ciliary sulcus will be the site of implantation. Exceptions to that rule are made for microphthalmic eyes of young children undergoing secondary IOL implantation into the ciliary sulcus especially if optic capture through the anterior and posterior capsulotomy can be achieved. In these small eyes, a three-piece AcrySof® IOL is used without fear of decentration. As mentioned above, decentration occurred only in eyes >23 mm in axial length.

CONCLUSION

The findings of this chapter can be summarized as follows.

1. AcrySof® IOLs have improved the intraoperative performance of pediatric cataract surgery. These hydrophobic acrylic IOLs not only allow easier and safer implantation in small (even microphthalmic) pediatric eyes, but also help the surgeon to consistently achieve the desired in-the-bag fixation in these eyes.

2. In eyes with an intact posterior capsule, PCO is inevitable in children, even with AcrySof® IOLs. However, some studies have documented a delay of the PCO with use of AcrySof® compared to PMMA lenses. This delay may allow children to reach an age at which they can cooperate for a YAG laser capsulotomy in the office. Also, at the amblyopic ages, any delay in the onset or progression of PCO may be beneficial. Proliferative PCO is more common with AcrySof® IOLs, whereas fibrous PCO is more common with PMMA IOLs.

3. In children beyond infancy, combined posterior capsulectomy, vitrectomy, and AcrySof® IOL implantation

eliminates the need for a secondary intervention in most eyes.

4. In infant eyes, VAO is much more common than primary aphakia when an IOL of any type is implanted, even when a posterior capsulotomy and an anterior vitrectomy are performed. Pilot studies suggest, however, that the visual outcome may be better when an IOL is implanted in infancy rather than relying on aphakic contact lenses. The Infant Aphakic Treatment Study, a multicenter randomized clinical trial now under way, will investigate whether an IOL or aphakia will produce the better outcome after unilateral cataract surgery in the first 6 months of life. AcrySof® IOLs will be utilized in the National Eye Institute–funded study under an Investigational Device Exemption (IDE) from the FDA.

With all that said, we must still remember that an IOL implanted in a child's eye must stay there for several decades, perhaps 70 years or more, without biodegrading. To date, AcrySof® IOLs have been found to be efficacious in providing good short- to intermediate-term results after implantation in congenital, juvenile, and traumatic cataract surgery. Long-term outcome will remain an open question for the years to come.

REFERENCES

1. Letocha CE, Pavlin CJ. Follow-up of 3 patients with Ridley intraocular lens implantation. *J Cataract Refract Surg* 1999;25:587–591.
2. Hollick EJ, Spalton DJ, Ursell PG, Pande MV, Barman SA, Boyce JF, et al. The effect of polymethylmethacrylate, silicone, and polyacrylic intraocular lenses on posterior capsular opacification 3 years after cataract surgery. *Ophthalmology* 1999;106:49–54.
3. Wilson Jr ME, Bartholomew LR, Trivedi RH. Pediatric cataract surgery and intraocular lens implantation: Practice preferences of the 2001 ASCRS and AAPOS memberships. *J Cataract Refract Surg* 2003;29:1811–1820.
4. Trivedi RH, Wilson ME Jr. Single-piece acrylic intraocular lens implantation in children. *J Cataract Refract Surg* 2003;29:1738–1743.
5. Wilson ME, Elliott L, Johnson B, Peterseim MM, Rah S, Werner L, et al. AcrySof acrylic intraocular lens implantation in children: clinical indications of biocompatibility. *J AAPOS* 2001;5:377–380.
6. Argento C, Badoza D, Ugrin C. Optic capture of the AcrySof intraocular lens in pediatric cataract surgery. *J Cataract Refract Surg* 2001;27:1638–1642.
7. Kugelberg M, Zetterstrom C. Pediatric cataract surgery with or without anterior vitrectomy. *J Cataract Refract Surg* 2002;28:1770–1773.
8. Plager DA, Yang S, Neely D, Sprunger D, Sondhi N. Complications in the first year following cataract surgery with and without IOL in infants and older children. *J AAPOS* 2002;6:9–14.
9. Stager DR Jr, Weakley DR Jr, Hunter JS. Long-term rates of PCO following small incision foldable acrylic intraocular lens implantation in children. *J Pediatr Ophthalmol Strabismus* 2002;39:73–76.
10. Mullner-Eidenbock A, Amon M, Moser E, Kruger A, Abela C, Schlemmer Y, et al. Morphological and functional results of AcrySof intraocular lens implantation in children: prospective randomized study of age-related surgical management. *J Cataract Refract Surg* 2003;29:285–293.
11. Ram J, Brar GS, Kaushik S, Gupta A. Role of posterior capsulotomy with vitrectomy and intraocular lens design and material in reducing posterior capsule opacification after pediatric cataract surgery. *J Cataract Refract Surg* 2003;29:1579–1584.

12. Kuchle M, Lausen B, Gusek-Schneider GC. Results and complications of hydrophobic acrylic vs PMMA posterior chamber lenses in children under 17 years of age. *Graefes Arch Clin Exp Ophthalmol* 2003;241:637–641.

13. Vasavada AR, Nath VC, Trivedi RH. Anterior vitreous face behavior with AcrySof in pediatric cataract surgery. *J AAPOS* 2003;7:384–388.

14. Vasavada AR, Praveen MR, Nath V, Dave K. Diagnosis and management of congenital cataract with preexisting posterior capsule defect. *J Cataract Refract Surg* 2004;30:403–408.

15. Rowe NA, Biswas S, Lloyd IC. Primary IOL implantation in children: a risk analysis of foldable acrylic v PMMA lenses. 2004;88:481–485.

16. Trivedi RH, Wilson ME, Bartholomew LR, Lal G, Peterseim MM. Opacification of the visual axis after cataract surgery and single acrylic intraocular lens implantation in the first year of life. *J AAPOS* 2004;8:156–164.

17. Vasavada AR, Trivedi RH, Nath V. Visual axis opacification after AcrySof intraocular lens implantation in children. *J Cataract Refract Surg* 2004;30:1073–1081.

18. Raina UK, Mehta DK, Monga S, Arora R. Functional outcomes of acrylic intraocular lenses in pediatric cataract surgery. *J Cataract Refract Surg* 2004;30:1082–1091.

19. Pandey SK, Werner L, Wilson ME et al. Capsulorhexis ovaling and capsular bag stretch after rigid and foldable intraocular lens implantation: experimental study in pediatric human eyes. *J Cataract Refract Surg* 2004;30:2183–2191.

20. Hollick EJ, Spalton DJ, Meacock WR. The effect of capsulorhexis size on posterior capsular opacification: one-year results of a randomized prospective trial. *Am J Ophthalmol* 1999;128:271–279.

21. Vasavada AR, Trivedi RH, Singh R. Necessity of vitrectomy when optic capture is performed in children older than 5 years. *J Cataract Refract Surg* 2001;27:1185–1193.

22. Asrani S, Freedman S, Hasselblad V, Buckley EG, Egbert J, Dahan E, et al. Does primary intraocular lens implantation prevent "aphakic" glaucoma in children? *J AAPOS* 2000;4:33–39.

23. Packer M, Fine IH, Hoffman RS. Suture fixation of a foldable acrylic intraocular lens for ectopia lentis. *J Cataract Refract Surg* 2002;28:182–185.

24. Crnic T, Weakley DR, Stager D, Felius J. Use of AcrySof acrylic foldable intraocular lens for secondary implantation in children. *J AAPOS* 2004;8:151–155.

25. Trivedi RH, Wilson ME, Facciani J. Secondary intraocular lens implantation for pediatric aphakia (submitted for publication to *J AAPOS*).

26. Wilson ME, Jr., Englert JA, Greenwald MJ. In-the-bag secondary intraocular lens implantation in children. *J AAPOS* 1999;3:350–355.

The Iris-Claw (Artisan) Lens

Daljit Singh, Kiranjit Singh, Arun Verma, and Ravi Shankar Jit Singh

The iris-claw (artisan) lens is the culmination of Jan Worst's research into iris fixation of an intraocular lens (IOL).[1–6] Proceeding from nylon fixation in 1970 through steel wire fixation, he eventually redesigned a pair of haptics that captured or grasped the iris, the so-called "claw." The iris-claw lens was first used by Jan Worst in 1978. Since then, over 300,000 of them have been used worldwide. We have been using them for pediatric patients since 1980 (see Figs. 25-1 and 25-2). Dr. Worst is fond of telling the story of the history of the acceptance of his lens. The lens was named after him (i.e., the "Worst lens"). Dr. Worst states that this was a marketing disaster in English-speaking countries. When physicians told patients that they were going to implant the "Worst" lens, the patient reaction was uniform. They did not want the "worst" lens; they wanted the "best" lens. For this reason, the lens was eventually renamed the iris-claw lens and, later, the artisan lens. The details of ophtec *pediatric artisan aphakia lenses* can be viewed at www.ophtec.com.

The iris-claw lens is now a one-plane polymethylmethacrylate (PMMA) lens, whereas originally it was a two-plane lens, which had loops behind the iris and the optic in the anterior chamber. The lens is oval in construction, with the center being the optic and the two wings being the haptics. Each PMMA haptics is shaped like a round or oval ring, 0.17 mm thick and 0.25 mm wide. The haptics has a cut in it that provides the claw grasping mechanism. The iris is passed through the cut in the haptics (the "claw") to effect fixation of the lens. The optic is convexoplane for normal use and convexoconcave for use in phakic eyes. The size of the optic and the overall width of the lens vary, depending on the requirement. We have used optics from 3 to 5 mm in diameter. Our most commonly used optic diameter is 4.25 mm, the next most common size being 3.5 mm (for microcornea). Currently, the width of the lenses in our cases varies from 6 to 7.25 mm. In exceptional cases, it is 5.0 mm. The optic configuration most often used is convexoplane. Recently, our preference has been to use a vaulted lens with a convexoconcave optic, which is the hyperopic phakic lens. The reason is that this minimizes iris touch, except at the site of fixation. Thereby, the vaulted design is better tolerated than its convexoplane counterpart. The original Worst lens has the claw placed at 180°. The *Singh variation* has an eccentric claw opening, namely, positioned 45° upward. Also, the claw toward the surgeon is smaller and stiffer, while the one away from the surgeon is longer and more flexible.

ROLE IN PEDIATRIC CATARACTS

The iris-claw lens differs from all other lenses as follows. All other IOLs are larger than the space in which they were designed to be fixed. The lens is pushed into the space and the tissues bounding the space capture the lens. The iris claw is much smaller than the tissue space, therefore it must capture or grasp the tissue (the iris) in order to be fixed. The peculiar design of the IOL endows it with special characteristics, utilities, and advantages, as follows.

a. The iris-claw lens has universal application, provided that iris tissue is available for fixation. The presence or absence of the posterior capsule is immaterial. It is eminently suitable for pediatric use at any age, in congenital or traumatic cataract, for primary or secondary implantation.
b. The pupil may be fully dilated without fear of dislocation. A midperipheral fixation of the iris allows an hourglass dilation.
c. The lens is far away from the angle of the anterior chamber, therefore it eliminates the problems associated with anterior chamber angle–supported lenses.
d. It is far away from the corneal endothelium, if the correct size has been chosen and it is fixed properly.
e. Every part of the lens and the tissue in relation to it are always available for direct examination under the slit lamp.
f. A small iris-claw lens is used in the patients with microcornea.

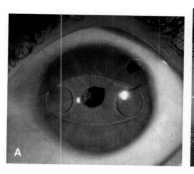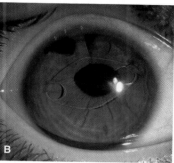

FIGURE 25-1. A. A 22-year-old patient operated on at age 1 year (using 1.5× magnification). Vision is 6/9. Specular endothelial microscopy with Topcon: 2005 cells/mm². The intraocular pressure is normal. The child's other eye, implanted with a similar lens, developed glaucoma and uveitis and became blind. **B.** Age 11 years: a case of perforating injury leading to traumatic cataract and pupil deformation. A vaulted artisan lens was implanted 3 years earlier. The BCVA is 6/9.

g. A standard lens is suitable for a case of megalocornea. What the eye needs is an optic on the pupil. The application of the iris-claw lens is unrelated to the large size of the cornea.

h. One or two sides of the lens can be fixed on the back of the iris in special circumstances of traumatic cataract or traumatic aphakia.

i. In the presence of a central corneal opacity, the iris-claw lens can be fixed in an eccentric position.

j. The iris-claw lens can be fixed across a large iris coloboma and it may actually help to reduce the size of the gap.

k. Phakic lenses are available for treating high myopia or hyperopia.

l. Iris-claw lenses for albinos can be used with or without refractive correction, in phakic or aphakic eyes.

m. Customized lenses can be designed for specific purposes, for example, a three-claw lens for a mydriatic pupil and a hybrid lens with loops and claws to adjust to the anatomy of the traumatized eye.

n. For a medical or refractive reason, the lens can be easily and safely explanted or exchanged.

o. It is an excellent lens for an aphakic or a traumatic cataract case undergoing keratoplasty.

p. Nd:YAG lasering for an opacified posterior capsule is easy. The capsule is situated far from the IOL, therefore pitting should not occur. The laser is focused directly on the capsule, therefore less energy is needed to open it. Accordingly, the vitreous face sus-

tains much less injury than with posterior chamber lenses.

q. Elschnig pearls can be easily aspirated or irrigated out from under the iris-claw lens.

r. A dense membrane formation in the pupillary area that is not amenable to Nd:YAG laser treatment can be easily managed by manual capsulotomy with one or two discission needles, with an erbium laser, or with the Fugo Blade.

FIXATION OF THE IRIS-CLAW LENS

Fixation should be done in such a way that:

a. The optic is centrally placed over the pupil.

b. An adequate amount of iris tissue is passed through the claws of the lens.

c. The iris root is not pulled in the process.

d. The sphincter muscle/pupil margin does not get drawn toward the claw.

e. There is no injury to the corneal endothelium either by the implant or by the instruments used to manipulate it.

The instruments used for claw-lens fixation are as follows.

a. A horizontally acting utility forceps is used to slip the lens inside the anterior chamber and to rotate it to the horizontal or any other desired position.

b. A thin iris forceps is used to hold and carry the iris through the claw.

c. A number of forceps designs can be used. A narrow forceps may be used to hold one side of the haptics close to the claw, while a wide forceps may be used to hold the lens by the optic.

d. A small, irrigating 26-gauge cannula is used to coax the iris into the claw, while it releases saline or viscoelastic material to keep the anterior chamber formed. For injecting viscoelastic material, the irrigating handle is connected by silicone tubing to a syringe that is held and operated by the assistant.

e. A 26-gauge needle, suitably bent at a distance of 4 to 6 mm from the tip, is used to engage, partially penetrate,

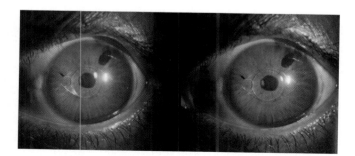

FIGURE 25-2. An artisan lens in an eye with megalocornea.

and lift the iris, then to carry it through the claw. The needle is used when the iris has a tendency to fall back, owing to the absence of vitreous support.

Iris-claw lens insertion and fixation require the presence of three incisions: two sideports and one main incision. The pupil is contracted by an intracameral miotic—acetylcholine, pilocarpine, or carbachol. The anterior chamber is deepened with viscoelastic. The iris-claw lens is inserted with the convex side facing up. It is then rotated to the desired meridian by a nudge from the irrigating cannula. If the lens happens to float toward the opposite limbus, the anterior chamber is filled with viscoelastic. As the lens holding forceps is introduced, positioned, and opened in the anterior chamber, the lens comes floating into the forceps's waiting jaws. The most important precaution is to keep the anterior chamber formed when a manipulation is done to fix the lens. The passage of the iris through the claw (enclavation) must be understood thoroughly. It is a bimanual procedure requiring simultaneous attention to many details; keeping the lens away from the endothelium, holding and centering the optic over the pupil, and passing the iris through the claw. These steps may seem difficult to perform if viscoelastic is lost from the eye. In this case, the lens holding and enclavation instruments must be withdrawn and the anterior chamber refilled. Then the claw fixation is reassessed and a fresh start made. With experience, the process becomes easy. However, there is a moderate learning curve.

The lens is held steady either at the optic or by the small side of the claw (as in the Singh variation). The iris is brought into the claw by any of the instruments for enclavation: a thin forceps, a cannula, or a needle. In the beginning, a small amount of iris, situated directly under the claw, is passed through the lens on one side. After it is clear that enclavation is at the right place, more iris tissue is added. It is important that the iris tissue be added by a movement of the iris tangential to the pupillary margin. If the iris is pulled peripherally, the pupil becomes oval. If the iris is pulled toward the pupil, the iris root can be torn, thereby causing bleeding. The Worst design has symmetrical claws. The enclaving instrument carries the iris tissue directly into the claw. The haptics is touching, in fact pressing, the iris when this is done. In the Singh variation, one side of the claw is small and rigid for all practical purposes. The lens is preferably held on this side. The long distal arm of the claw is flexible. The iris holding forceps lifts the long arm. As the rigid forceps passes through the claw, the claw mechanism shuts and grips the iris underneath the forceps. Our preferred method is to use one of the forceps tips to push iris tissue into the claw. On rare occasions, when the iris seems friable, a pinch of the iris tissue is held with a forceps and passed through the claw.

The second approach to lens fixation is to steadily hold the iris with thin iris forceps. While the lens claw is pressed on the iris by the force of the lens holding forceps, the thin forceps open the backward-moving claw and carry the iris into the lens. It is always advisable to first make a small enclavation. The optic must be centered; only then can the amount of the iris in the claw be increased.

There are special circumstances in which the iris-claw lens can be fixed to the back of the iris. An example of this is when the anterior chamber is very shallow, usually the result of trauma. Viscoelastic is injected under the iris to increase the distance between the iris and the posterior capsule or the vitreous. The iris-claw lens is held very carefully and steadily, especially if there is not posterior capsular support. The lens is then slipped under the iris and tilted by the haptics to raise the iris on one side. The iris tissue is pressed back with a needle or thin cannula at the proper place on the claw. The iris easily enters the gap, thereby causing one side of the lens to become fixated. The same thing is done on the other side. One can progressively increase the amount of the iris in the claw, but it is clumsy and more difficult to reduce the amount of iris in the claw and to explant the behind-the-iris fixed lens. In certain situations, one claw may be fixed under the iris and the other over the iris. In exceptional cases, for instance, in the absence of iris tissue, it may be possible to fix the claw to a fibrous band.

There is another important variation of claw fixation that can to be used in extremely difficult cases. In these cases, the surgeon will find a flat leathery iris that is difficult to gather in a forceps and pass through the claw. It is apparent that the lens may eventually dislocate. The solution to this problem is that a hole is produced in the iris tissue at the intended point of fixation and the claw of the lens is made to hold the iris through and through at the edge of the opening. Many trauma cases have a scarred and stretched iris, which is locally or widely adherent to the capsule underneath. Claw fixation in these situations carries a high risk of dislocation later or is nearly impossible. Manual separation of the iris from the underlying scar tissue leads to local bleeding from the pulled iris root. The way to deal with such a situation is to make holes in the thick iris–capsule complex with either the Fugo Blade or an erbium laser.[7] In our experience, both are effective. Cavitation bubbles from the tip of the Fugo Blade may actually split the iris from the scar tissue, thus allowing a full-thickness pure iris fixation. If separation does not occur and the hole formation involves both the iris and the capsular scar, the claw is made to hold both of them at the edge of the Fugo Blade– or erbium laser–produced hole.

When there is no posterior capsule support and the pupil is large, the use of a Sheets glide is mandatory. The Sheets glide is especially helpful in cases that have undergone pars plana vitrectomy and lensectomy for posterior chamber problems such as traumatic endophthalmitis. At the end of incision, the eye becomes so soft that an unsupported iris-claw lens is likely to sink into the saline-filled vitreous cavity. Unlike vitreous, saline does not provide support. Furthermore, the iris fixation can be successful if only the tip of a 26-gauge disposable irrigating needle is used to engage and lift the iris at the desired point for passage through the claw. Sometimes, bleeding from the site of the prick gravitates into the vitreous and delays visual recovery.

During the iris enclavation process, the iris tissue should be moved into the claw, either from directly under the claw or by an iris movement that is tangential to the pupillary margin. Pulling the iris tissue radially outward makes the pupil oval. Pulling the iris tissue toward the pupil may cause an iris root tear and bleeding.

How Much Iris in the Claw?

The idea is to catch the fibrous structures of the iris. In light-colored eyes, these structures are on the surface and easy to pick, then pass through the claw. The iris may be caught at a crypt. The case with brown and dark eyes is different in that the surface stroma containing pigment is quite thick, with few fibrous elements. The crypts are difficult to find. A superficial fixation runs the risk of late erosion of the tissue in the claw, leading to dislocation. Recall that children are more liable to ocular trauma in day-to-day life and therefore require healthy claw fixation. The most reliable fixation in any type of iris is to capture a fold of iris right up to the posterior pigment of the iris.

POSTOPERATIVE PROBLEMS

Early Problems

a. *Closure of peripheral iridectomy.* The iridectomy is occluded by adhesions with the underlying anterior or the posterior capsule, by the growth of Elschnig pearls, or by a natural repair process of the iris that may occlude the opening. The iridectomy may close with a surprising swiftness, even in days or weeks. To minimize the closure, we often choose to do a larger iridectomy involving the mid-iris and the pupillary margin. The iridotomy opening size decreases over a period of months. However, the longer it remains open, the greater is the chance for patency.
b. *Posterior synechia.* The pupillary margin may become adherent to the underlying posterior capsule. Wider adhesions can occur between the posterior surface of the iris and the posterior capsule. Thick, unbreakable bonds may be produced between them.
c. *Iris bombe.* This occurs if a and b co-occur. The pupil constricts and a thick membrane forms underneath.

These three problems are indicative of a pseudophakic pupillary block that must be dealt with urgently. Use of the Nd:YAG laser is more difficult in brown or dark eyes.

Adhesion formation and inflammation are usually seen together. Both are treated by providing a free passage to the aqueous. Originally, we treated them with pupilloplasty and membranectomy with a vitrector. Later, we successfully used an erbium laser for this purpose. The problem with both of these devices is that they often generate significant bleeding, which may sometimes trickle into the vitreous. In recent years we have shifted to the use of the Fugo Blade, which ablates without bleeding.

Late Problems

After a few months have elapsed postsurgery, the severity and the frequency of the above-noted problems are greatly reduced. Peripheral iridectomy closure and thin secondary cataract are managed easily with Nd:YAG. Surgical intervention is less often necessary.

a. *Dislocation of the lens.* Most often this is due to trauma, to which children are more prone. One claw opens and the lens hangs in the anterior chamber from the other claw. The condition is easy to handle. The old lens may be refixed or a new one may be fixed, if the refraction has changed over the years.
b. *Endothelial cell damage.* The main cause of endothelial cell damage is a neglected dislocated iris-claw lens rubbing against the endothelium for months or years. Unfortunately, this often happens in a third world situation. The treatment is corneal transplant. Endothelial damage is a rare problem now as lens design and manufacturing techniques have evolved over the years.
c. *Glaucoma.* Glaucoma may result from complications or as an independent entity. It is important to check the intraocular pressure at least once a year.

CONCLUSION

In 1980, we hoped that the iris-claw lens would be a safe solution for pediatric cataracts and aphakia. We can now say that time has proved this to be true. Whenever possible, we prefer to use the vaulted iris-claw lens.

REFERENCES

1. Singh D. Correspondence: Iris claw lens usage in India. *Eur J Implant Ref Surg* 1989;1:285–287.
2. Singh D, Singh IR, Singh R. Use of the Worst–Singh lobster claw intraocular lens in children. *Ophthalmic Pract* 1987;5:18–20.
3. Worst JGF. Iris-fixated lenses: evolution and application. In: Percival P, ed. *A Color Atlas of Lens Implantation*. London: Wolfe, 1991.
4. Pol BAE, van der Worst JGF. Iris claw intraocular lenses in children. *Documenta Ophthalmol* 1996;92:29–35.
5. Menezo JL, Martinez MC, Cisneros AL. Iris-fixated Worst claw versus sulcus-fixated posterior chamber lenses in the absence of capsular support. *Cataract Refract Surg* 1996;22:1476–1484.
6. Singh D, Worst J, Singh R, Singh IR. *Cataract and IOL*. New Delhi: Jaypee, 1993:82–97, 189–200.
7. Singh D. Use of the Fugo Blade in complicated cases. *J Cataract Refract Surg* 2002;28(4):573–574.

Role of Optic Capture in Pediatric Cataract–Intraocular Lens Surgery

Abhay R. Vasavada and Rupal H. Trivedi

The concept of capturing an intraocular lens (IOL) optic through an anterior capsulorhexis was first suggested in a case of posterior capsule tear in an adult. The haptics were placed in the ciliary sulcus, and the IOL optic was then placed through the anterior capsulorhexis to "capture" the IOL for stable optic fixation. Gimbel et al.[1–4] have used the concept to develop the technique of *posterior capsulorhexis with optic capture*. They believe that placing the optic behind the primary posterior continuous curvilinear capsulorhexis (PCCC) and fixating the haptics in the bag (optic capture through posterior capsulorhexis) minimize the risk of visual axis opacification (VAO) and may allow surgeons to avoid planned anterior vitrectomy. Optic capture fuses the anterior and posterior leaflets of the capsular bag for almost 360°, except at the haptic–optic junction. Theoretically, capsule fusion anterior to the IOL optic might reduce central lens epithelial cell migration or at least direct the cell movement anteriorly over the lens optic, which is presumably an unsuitable substrate for lens survival and thus may help to decrease VAO. To us, the main advantage of optic capture is its ability to achieve well centered IOL.[5]

The *optic capture* technique was subsequently utilized for various other indications and at various sites of fixation (see Fig. 26-1).[4–9]

Conventional (or posterior) optic capture techniques utilized the *posterior capture* technique. This can be achieved by capturing the optic through the anterior capsulorhexis (haptics in the ciliary sulcus), the posterior capsulorhexis (haptics in the bag), or both the rhexes (haptics in the ciliary sulcus). Optic capture with haptics in the ciliary sulcus can be helpful for both primary and secondary IOL implantation.[5,6] IOL decentration was the most common complication in eyes with secondary IOL implantation. Optic capture through fused anterior and posterior rhexes (haptics in the ciliary sulcus) helps to achieve well-centered IOLs.[6] As noted previously, optic capture through the pos-

terior capsulorhexis was proposed to avoid the step of anterior vitrectomy in pediatric cataract surgery.[1–4] Although it helps to achieve IOL centration, its role in maintaining a clear visual axis in pediatric IOL surgery, without the need for an anterior vitrectomy, is controversial.[1–5,7–15] The success of this technique may depend on the IOL haptic–optic junction design.[4]

Reversed optic capture (capturing from behind the IOL optic) has been described as capturing from the posterior to the anterior side[4] (see Fig. 26-1).

This chapter describes the technique of optic capture and reviews the literature related to the outcome of this technique in pediatric cataract–IOL surgery.

TECHNIQUE OF OPTIC CAPTURE

Posterior capture of the IOL optic is performed under a high-viscosity ophthalmic viscosurgical device. The capture process is achieved by gentle pressure on the IOL optic. The IOL optic is slid through the PCCC with an iris spatula and Lester hook until the entire optic is placed posterior to the capsulorhexis. Optic vaulting through the PCCC requires careful manipulation because of the thin posterior capsule. When the round opening is stretched into an elliptical one, this indicates complete capture (Fig. 26-2).

Optic capture is a technically challenging procedure. The key point is to achieve a "capturable" PCCC. The opening in the posterior capsule should not only be continuous but also well centered and of an optimum size. The optimum size (neither too small, which makes it difficult to capture the optic, nor too large, in which case the optic may not remain captured) is a prerequisite for ideal and stable capture. The diameter of the PCCC opening must be at least 1.0 mm smaller than the IOL optic. We achieved capturable PCCC in 96.4% eyes of older

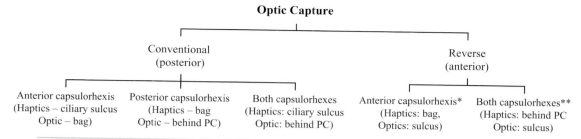

FIGURE 26-1. Schematic diagram showing different sites for capturing the IOL optic. *In the case of a large posterior capsule tear noticed after IOL implantation and in-the-bag fixation; not considered stable. **In the case of posterior dislocation (pars plana repositioning) of an IOL.

children and 64.5% eyes of younger children.[5,8] Total optic capture was achieved in 92.6% of eyes of older children and in 85% of eyes of younger children.[5,8] In addition to size, we believe that a centered capsulorhexis is also important to IOL centration. Koch and Kohnen[9,13] reported that a decentered PCCC can cause IOL decentration.

Of note, for optic capture the IOL power may need to be adjusted to 0.5 to 1 diopter higher than for bag-fixated IOL. In addition to difficulty with the optic capture technique, the following intraoperative problems may arise.

1. The main idea behind the use of this technique is to avoid the need for vitrectomy. However, occasionally the vitreous face is disturbed during the performance of PCCC, and it may require vitrectomy (unplanned). The vitreous face was disturbed in 12.2% of our study cases.

2. Removal of the ophthalmic viscosurgical device may sometimes cause the optic to vault forward. This vaulting can undo the optic capture.

POSTOPERATIVE OUTCOME

Spontaneous Release of Optic Capture

Spontaneous release of optic capture through the posterior capsulorhexis has been reported in the literature.[5] We

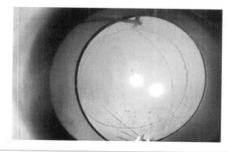

FIGURE 26-2. AcrySof IOL captured through posterior capsulorhexis (optic behind posterior capsule; haptics in the bag).

have noted that the optic did not remain captured in 4.9% of eyes in an older cohort and in 30.0% of eyes in a younger cohort.[5,8] This phenomenon is observed more frequently in eyes with a large posterior capsulorhexis. Too large a PCCC not only makes it difficult to achieve total optic capture but also can lead to spontaneous release of the optic capture in the postoperative period.

Visual Axis

a. Gimbel[3] reported that optic capture nearly eliminated posterior capsule opacification (PCO) in 16 patients (nonvitrectomized) with a mean age of 5.85 years.

b. Koch and Kohnen[13] reported that four of five eyes with optic capture and without anterior vitrectomy developed visually significant PCO by 2.5 years postoperatively.

c. Vasavada and Desai[7] noted that anterior vitrectomy is desirable in children <5 years old because capturing the optic through the posterior capsulorhexis without primary anterior vitrectomy does not always ensure a clear visual axis.

d. We evaluated the role of optic capture in anterior vitrectomy in eyes of younger children (age at surgery, <5 years) in a prospective, randomized, controlled clinical trial.[5] Note that all eyes received vitrectomy; however, optic capture was assigned randomly. All eyes in the *no-capture* group maintained a clear visual axis. One eye in the *optic capture* group developed a membrane in front of the IOL that required secondary surgical intervention. The anterior and posterior capsulorhexes in that eye were noted to be relatively small (3.0 and 3.2 mm, respectively). The central elliptical area of the captured optic, bracketed on both sides by capsule leaflets, was obliterated by a membrane. Koch and Kohnen[13] also reported this as a unique complication of anterior IOL surface opacification.

e. Dada et al.[11] studied the efficacy of using PCCC with optic capture in pediatric cataract surgery. The authors reported that all eyes in the PCCC and optic capture group remained clear, while 57% eyes in the no-PCCC group developed PCO. PCO can be because of an intact posterior capsule. In addition to optic capture, PCCC was another variable in this study.

f. In another study, we questioned whether vitrectomy is necessary when optic capture is performed in children between 5 and 12 years old.[8] In this prospective, randomized, controlled clinical trial, vitrectomy was assigned randomly. Note that all eyes in both groups received optic capture. All eyes in the vitrectomy group and 30% eyes in the no-vitrectomy group had a clear visual axis. The visual axis was obscured as a result of anterior vitreous fibrosis in 70% of eyes in the no-vitrectomy group. This fibrosis of the anterior vitreous face did not affect high-contrast visual acuity; however, it significantly decreased low-contrast sensitivity.

g. Argento and coworkers[10] published the results of AcrySof IOL optic capture in children with cataracts. Eight children were included, with a mean follow-up of 28.9 ± 5.3 months (age at cataract surgery, 2 to 8 years). The visual axis remained clear in all cases. No case required a secondary procedure. In the article by Argento and coauthors,[10] it was not clear whether the advantage was provided by optic capture or by the AcrySof material. The study did not have a control group (AcrySof implantation with no optic capture).

h. Raina and coauthors[15] reported a prospective randomized study of 34 eyes with a mean follow-up of 17.5 months. The authors concluded that PCCC with optic capture prevents PCO of the visual axis even in the absence of an anterior vitrectomy.

i. *Mullner-Eidenbock et al.*[14] concluded, in a prospective, randomized, clinical trial of AcrySof IOL, that optic capture was not necessary to ensure a clear visual axis.

j. Raina et al.[16] recently reported the outcome of Acrysof IOL use in pediatric cataract surgery. The authors noted that all six eyes with optic capture of an AcrySof IOL maintained a clear visual axis (age at surgery, 4 to 8 years).

Synechiae

The incidence of synechia formation was reported to be significantly high in the optic-capture group.[5] Both the capsules in front of an IOL may predispose the eye to synechia formation.[5]

Deposits on an IOL Optic

Cellular deposits were observed more frequently in the optic-capture group.[5,14] These deposits were closer to the posterior synechiae.

Centration of an IOL

In our opinion, the most important benefit of optic capture is that the continuous capsule margin locks the IOL optic and prevents it from decentering.[5]

IOL Exchange

Later IOL exchange, if necessary to manage anisometropia or a lens-related complication, may become difficult.[9]

CONCLUSION

To summarize, the role of optic capture in preventing VAO in the absence of vitrectomy is controversial. However, optic capture helps to achieve a well-centered IOL.

REFERENCES

1. Gimbel HV, DeBroff BM. Posterior capsulorhexis with optic capture: maintaining a clear visual axis after pediatric cataract surgery. *J Cataract Refract Surg* 1994;20:658–664.
2. Gimbel HV. Posterior capsulorhexis with optic capture in pediatric cataract and intraocular lens surgery. *Ophthalmology* 1996;103:1871–1875.
3. Gimbel HV. Posterior continuous curvilinear capsulorhexis and optic capture of the intraocular lens to prevent secondary opacification in pediatric cataract surgery. *J Cataract Refract Surg* 1997;23(Suppl 1):652–656.
4. Gimbel HV, DeBroff BM. Intraocular lens optic capture. *J Cataract Refract Surg* 2004;30:200–206.
5. Vasavada AR, Trivedi RH. Role of optic capture in congenital cataract and intraocular lens surgery in children. *J Cataract Refract Surg* 2000;26:824–831.
6. Trivedi RH, Wilson ME, Facciani J. Secondary intraocular lens implantation for pediatric aphakia (in press).
7. Vasavada A, Desai J. Primary posterior capsulorhexis with and without anterior vitrectomy in congenital cataracts. *J Cataract Refract Surg* 1997;23(Suppl 1):645–651.
8. Vasavada AR, Trivedi RH, Singh R. Necessity of vitrectomy when optic capture is performed in children older than 5 years. *J Cataract Refract Surg* 2001;27:1185–1193.
9. Koch DD, Kohnen T. Retrospective comparison of techniques to prevent secondary cataract formation after posterior chamber intraocular lens implantation in infants and children. *J Cataract Refract Surg* 1997;23(Suppl 1):657–663.
10. Argento C, Badoza D, Ugrin C. Optic capture of the AcrySof intraocular lens in pediatric cataract surgery. *J Cataract Refract Surg* 2001;27:1638–1642.
11. Dada T, Dada VK, Sharma N, Vajpayee RB. Primary posterior capsulorhexis with optic capture and intracameral heparin in paediatric cataract surgery. *Clin Exp Ophthalmol* 2000;28:361–363.
12. Dadeya S. Posterior continuous curvilinear capsulorhexis with and without optic capture of the posterior chamber intraocular lens in the absence of vitrectomy. *J Pediatr Ophthalmol Strabismus* 2003;40:130–131.
13. Koch DD, Kohnen T. A retrospective comparison of techniques to prevent secondary cataract formation following posterior chamber intraocular lens implantation in infants and children. *Trans Am Ophthalmol Soc* 1997;95:351–360, discussion 361–365.

14. Mullner-Eidenbock A, Amon M, Moser E, Kruger A, Abela C, Schlemmer Y, et al. Morphological and functional results of AcrySof intraocular lens implantation in children: prospective randomized study of age-related surgical management. *J Cataract Refract Surg* 2003;29:285–293.

15. Raina UK, Gupta V, Arora R, Mehta DK. Posterior continuous curvilinear capsulorhexis with and without optic capture of the posterior chamber intraocular lens in the absence of vitrectomy. *J Pediatr Ophthalmol Strabismus* 2002;39:278–287.

16. Raina UK, Mehta DK, Monga S, Arora R. Functional outcomes of acrylic intraocular lenses in pediatric cataract surgery. *J Cataract Refract Surg* 2004;30:1082–1091.

Polypseudophakia

M. Edward Wilson, Jr. and Rupal H. Trivedi

Implantation of multiple intraocular lenses (IOLs; polypseudophakia or piggyback IOLs) has been described as a solution to the problem of providing adequate IOL power to adult patients with microphthalmos and extreme hyperopia.[1–5] We have used this concept in children with nanophthalmos, implanting primary piggyback IOLs to achieve the required high IOL power. In addition, we have used piggyback secondary IOL implantation in aphakic patients who become contact lens intolerant and are nearly full-grown but still have microphthalmia and require a high IOL power. These are situations in which the piggyback IOLs are expected to remain in the eye from that point forward.

In contrast, we have also used the concept of piggybacking IOLs to develop the technique of *temporary polypseudophakia* for infantile eyes.[6] The posterior lens is implanted in the capsular bag (permanent) and the anterior lens is placed in the ciliary sulcus (temporary) (Fig. 27-1). This approach may help in the prevention and treatment of amblyopia by eliminating residual hyperopia in small children after IOL implantation. The combination of a permanent IOL sequestrated in the capsular bag and a temporary IOL placed in the ciliary sulcus—a location from which it can be easily removed later—makes this *temporary polypseudophakia* option attractive for the correction of aphakia in infancy, especially when compliance with glasses or contacts is expected to be poor.

Although uncorrected aphakia can be eliminated by implanting a single IOL in infancy, undercorrected aphakia may remain a frequent occurrence. Because the eye grows an average of 4.5 mm in axial length in the first 2 years of life, IOLs implanted in infancy are usually selected to produce a 20% or more undercorrection. This approach often produces from 6 to 18 D (diopters) of residual hyperopia. If compliance with glasses or contact lens is poor, an amblyogenic hyperopic refractive error will be present despite the implantation of an IOL. However, if the combined IOL power implanted could be enough for early emmetropia, the amblyopia risk from residual hyperopia could be

eliminated. If a single IOL is implanted early in life with enough power to achieve emmetropia, a high degree of myopia would undoubtedly occur later. In an effort to address this problem, we recommended piggyback IOL. A permanent IOL is placed in the capsular bag intended to be retained by the infant throughout life. An additional IOL is placed in a piggyback fashion in the ciliary sulcus.

As the eye grows, myopia develops and increases. Because it is well known that myopia is much less amblyogenic than hyperopia, we have hopes that ultimately the visual acuity will be improved and amblyopia more easily treated. After the myopia increased beyond 4 D, glasses should be prescribed. However, if compliance with glasses is poor, the child can still attain a sharp focus with the polypseudophakic eye during occlusion of the normal eye by holding the object of interest close.

It must be noted, however, that high myopia can also be amblyogenic, and a second *planned surgery* will be needed to remove the sulcus-fixated IOL. When needed due to refractive growth, the lens implanted in the ciliary sulcus is explanted/exchanged. In this way, a total IOL power sufficient for the infant to reach emmetropia in the early months of life can be implanted. IOLs placed in the ciliary sulcus do not scar in place and they can be easily rotated, exchanged, and removed even several years after implantation. This has been a consistent finding for us over many years.

When choosing *IOL power*, we must remember that using two or more lenses to achieve high dioptric powers is optically superior to using a single lens of the same total power. When implanting piggyback lenses in the first few weeks of life, we keep a target of +2 or +3 D because this mild hyperopia would likely disappear in the first 4 to 6 weeks. After 2 months of age, we keep the target postoperative refraction as plano or mild myopia. Glasses may not need to be prescribed if a low residual refractive error is present. The power of the temporary anteriormost IOL is chosen based on how much refractive change is anticipated during growth and development. This has

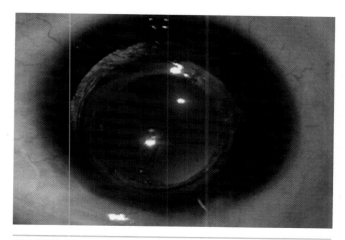

FIGURE 27-1. Postoperative appearance of an eye with piggyback IOL implantation (of two single-piece AcrySof IOLs—One IOL is in-the-bag, while another temporary IOL is in the ciliary sulcus.

often amounted to approximately one third of the total IOL power.

Our operative *technique* of piggyback IOL implantation is identical to that used for single IOL insertion except that an additional IOL is implanted in the ciliary sulcus immediately after the initial IOL is placed in the capsular bag. We prefer to use Alcon AcrySof lenses for both the permanent and the temporary IOL. The material's high refractive index (1.55) allows the lens to be thinner and flatter than PMMA (polymethyl methacrylate) or silicone lenses. The center thickness of a 24-D Alcon AcrySof MA30BA lens is 0.72 mm, versus 1.0 mm for the thinnest available silicone IOL (Allergan SI-30NB). A single-piece AcrySof IOL is used for placement within the capsular bag. For sulcus fixation, we use the three–piece AcrySof IOL. Interlenticular opacification (ILO), a recently reported complication of capsule-fixed piggyback IOLs in adults, is avoided in our patients because one of the IOLs is placed in the ciliary sulcus.[7-9] ILO seemed to be related to two posterior capsule IOLs being implanted in the capsular bag through a small capsulorhexis, with its margins overlapping the optic edge of the anterior IOL for 360°. Analyses of the above-described cases of ILO concluded that the opacification within the interlenticular space is derived from retained/regenerative cortex and pearls. This is similar to the pathogenesis of the pearl form of posterior capsule opacification (PCO).

Pupillary capture of an IOL optic was noted in one of our patients with a sulcus-fixed IOL 1 day after the procedure and required reoperation.[6] We now constrict the pupil with an intracameral miotic at the end of surgery.

Gayton et al.[10] have also noted pupillary capture of secondary piggyback IOL implantation.

Of note, we have also used the concept of polypseudophakia to treat pseudophakic refractive error, to avoid the risks associated with lens exchange. The additional manipulation required for the removal process of an IOL, particularly if the IOL is strongly fixed, increases the risk of complications. A second IOL can be implanted anteriorly to the primary IOL. The power of a secondary piggyback IOL implant is also more predictable than that of an IOL exchange.

To summarize, infants who are anticipated to have difficulty complying with contact lens wear and amblyopia therapy can be candidates for piggyback IOL implantation. It must be noted that not all infant eyes are suitable for piggyback lens placement; piggyback IOL implantation should be confined to eyes in which the benefit of this implantation exceeds the potential risks. With marked microphthalmia, we have sometimes elected not to place a second IOL because of insufficient space in the eye. To date, more than 30 infantile eyes have undergone this procedure successfully. Although we are waiting for long-term results in terms of the safety of this procedure and its impact on rapid myopization and visual outcome, it appears to be a useful option for addressing some of the questions associated with infantile IOL implantation.

REFERENCES

1. Gayton JL, Sanders VN. Implanting two posterior chamber intraocular lenses in a case of microphthalmos. *J Cataract Refract Surg* 1993;19:776–777.
2. Mittelviefhaus H. Piggyback intraocular lens with exchangeable optic. *J Cataract Refract Surg* 1996;22:676–681.
3. Masket S. Piggyback intraocular lens implantation. *J Cataract Refract Surg* 1998;24:569–570.
4. Holladay JT, Gills JP, Leidlein J, Cherchio M. Achieving emmetropia in extremely short eyes with two piggyback posterior chamber intraocular lenses. *Ophthalmology* 1996;103:1118–1123.
5. Fenzl RE, Gills JP 3rd, Gills JP. Piggyback intraocular lens implantation. *Curr Opin Ophthalmol* 2000;11:73–76.
6. Wilson ME, Peterseim MW, Englert JA, Lall-Trail JK, Elliott LA. Pseudophakia and polypseudophakia in the first year of life. *J AAPOS* 2001;5:238–245.
7. Werner L, Shugar JK, Apple DJ, Pandey SK, Escobar-Gomez M, Visessook N, et al. Opacification of piggyback IOLs associated with an amorphous material attached to interlenticular surfaces. *J Cataract Refract Surg* 2000;26:1612–1619.
8. Trivedi RH, Izak AM, Werner L, Macky TA, Pandey SK, Apple DJ. Interlenticular opacification of piggyback intraocular lenses. *Int Ophthalmol Clin* 2001;41:47–62.
9. Trivedi RH, Werner L, Apple DJ, Pandey SK, Izak AM. Post cataract-intraocular lens (IOL) surgery opacification. *Eye* 2002;16:217–241.
10. Gayton JL, Sanders V, Van Der Karr M. Pupillary capture of the optic in secondary piggyback implantation. *J Cataract Refract Surg* 2001;27:1514–1515.

Transscleral Suture Fixation of Posterior Chamber Intraocular Lenses

Suresh K. Pandey and M. Edward Wilson, Jr.

Optical rehabilitation of aphakia, especially when it is unilateral, in eyes with incomplete or absent capsular support is problematic in pediatric patients. If contact lens or spectacle correction is not viable, secondary placement of an intraocular lens (IOL) is the method of choice in these eyes. The choice of IOL mainly depends on the preoperative status of the eye (e.g., aphakia and amount of capsular rim remaining) and the selected location for the implant. Several IOL implantation approaches have been reported in the literature for pediatric cases without capsular support: using an angle-supported anterior chamber (AC-) IOL, an iris-claw IOL, and a transsclerally sutured posterior chamber (PC-) IOL.[1–8] A technique for placing a secondary IOL within the capsular bag in pediatric cases has also been suggested when a Soemmering's ring remains.[9] For secondary lens placement during adult cataract surgery, implantation of modern open-loop ACIOLs and iris-fixated claw ACIOLs has regained popularity and provides a valuable alternative to sutured PCIOLs. However, experience with the aforementioned IOL designs in children is limited, and at present, no consensus exists on the indications or on the relative safety and efficacy of these different options.

Transsclerally sutured PCIOLs may be suitable for certain pediatric cases in the absence of capsular support. Because of its anatomic location, the sutured PCIOL is more appropriate for eyes with compromised corneal endothelium, peripheral anterior synechiae, shallow anterior chamber, or glaucoma.[10,11] *In this chapter we focus on surgical techniques and visual outcome of transscleral suture fixation of PCIOLs in children. Interested readers should consult Chapters 25 and 29 to learn about other options for secondary IOL implantation such as ACIOLs and iris-claw lenses.*

TRANSSCLERALLY SUTURED POSTERIOR CHAMBER IMPLANTS

Preoperative Examination

Children who are being considered for secondary lens placement should undergo a complete ocular history and office examination. In addition, an examination under general anesthesia just prior to implant surgery may be helpful. If possible, as part of the ocular examination, a careful refraction and determination of the best corrected visual acuity should be undertaken in both operative and nonoperative eyes. A thorough anterior segment biomicroscopic examination should be performed, with particular attention paid to corneal clarity, the integrity of the hyaloid face and posterior capsule, the corneal endothelium, the anatomy of the iris, the presence or absence of capsular support, and the location of the vitreous. Examination of the anterior sclera should be performed to rule out scleral ectasia, especially in children who are highly myopic. In addition, gonioscopy and evaluation for glaucoma risk factors are important. The ocular examination should also include careful inspection of the posterior segment of the eye to rule out any posterior segment pathology.

Surgical Technique

Implantation of a sutured PCIOL is indicated in conditions in which capsule support for in-the-bag or ciliary sulcus IOL implantation is lacking and the anterior segment/angle structures are compromised (e.g., poor corneal endothelium cell count, peripheral anterior synechiae, shallow anterior chamber, or glaucoma) so that ACIOL placement may not be appropriate.

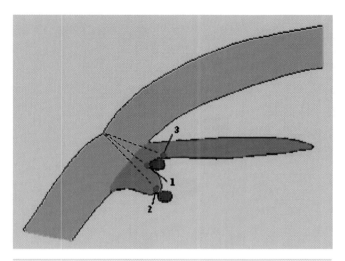

FIGURE 28-1. Schematic diagram showing that a correctly positioned (1) sulcus-fixated IOL haptic (blue) and its suture (red) should be placed directly into the ciliary sulcus. Complications may ensue when the haptic(s) and suture(s) are placed too far posteriorly (2), encroaching on the pars plicata, or even too far anteriorly (3), so the suture encroaches on the iris. Malposition of the haptics and suture is one of the cause of perioperative and postoperative complications (e.g., vitreous hemorrhage).

Proper placement of the sutures within the ciliary sulcus is very important for secured fixation of the sutured PCIOL haptics, as malposition of the haptics and suture is one of the causes of intrasurgical and postoperative hemorrhage (Fig. 28-1). Anatomical and histological studies have shown that the ciliary sulcus is 0.83 mm posterior to the limbus in the vertical meridian and only 0.46 mm posterior to the limbus in the horizontal meridian.[12,13] Duffey and coworkers[13] passed the needle perpendicular to the sclera 1, 2, and 3 mm posterior to the limbus and found that the needle exited internally at the ciliary sulcus, pars plicata, and pars plana, respectively. Based on these guidelines, the surgeon should pass the needles 1 mm posterior to the limbus and should avoid the 3 and 9 o'clock positions due to the presence of the long ciliary artery and nerves.[10] Fixation of sutured PCIOLs too anteriorly (iris) or too posteriorly (pars plicata) can lead to sight-threatening complications (Fig. 28-1).

A scleral-fixated PCIOL can be sutured by passing the needles from the outside of the eye inward (ab externo) or from the inside out (ab interno). The ab externo approach is usually preferred over the ab interno approach. Adequate anterior vitrectomy is mandatory before placement of sutures and the IOL to avoid complications related to the vitreous base.

Ab Interno Approach

Initially the ab interno technique was described for the scleral-fixated PCIOL. In this technique, two partial-thickness scleral flaps are made, 180° apart. Right-handed surgeons should create the superior flap toward 1 o'clock and the inferior flap toward 7 o'clock for ease of maneuverability. The Ethicon CIF-4 long tapered needle can be used to pass a polypropylene suture through the inferior scleral flap and the Ethicon TG 160-6 small curved needle can be used to pass a polypropylene suture through the superior scleral flap. The sutures can be looped through the eyelets of the haptics or tied to the haptic or a girth hitch suture can be used. These sutures can be used for two-point or four-point fixation of the IOL. After passing out the polypropylene sutures through the scleral flaps, the ends of the sutures are tied in a 3–1–1 knot. The ends of the knot are cut 1 mm long. The scleral flaps are tied with 6.0-mm vicryl. The corneoscleral wound is closed with 10-0 monofilament nylon or Vicryl and the overlying conjunctical wound is closed with 6-0 plain gut suture.

Ab Externo Approach

Some surgeons are not comfortable passing sutures below the iris through the sclera blindly using the ab interno method. The ideal location for IOL placement is with the haptics positioned in the ciliary sulcus. To ensure this placement, the ab externo approach was introduced. However, this outside-to-inside approach is more time-consuming than the inside-to-outside approach. For the ab externo approach the surgeon needs to have long straight needles, for example, Ethicon STC-6 or Alcon SC-5. After making partial-thickness flaps, the straight needle is passed approximately 0.75 posterior to the limbus through one side; on the other side a 25-, 27-, or 28-gauge hypodermic needle should be passed. The straight needle is then negotiated through the hollow hypodermic needle. The hypodermic needle should be withdrawn with the straight solid needle inside it. The AC is entered and the suture is taken out with a hook. The suture is cut and the end is tied to the eyelet of the IOL haptic. If the surgeon desires four-point fixation of the IOL, the above steps are repeated (Figs. 28-2 and 28-3). It should be noted that the main advantage of the ab externo approach is its greater precision in the location of scleral sutures.

The polypropylene suture knot should not be kept exposed because it may cause irritation and may increase the chances of endophthalmitis. Scleral flaps are recommended to cover it. If possible, the knot should be buried in the sclera. More recently, a four-point fixation technique with no scleral flaps has been introduced (Fig. 28-4), in which the knots are rotated and buried in the site where the hypodermic needle had been introduced, as discussed above. Alternatively, we have recently begun merely leaving the polypropylene suture ends long and tucking them under the conjunctiva toward the fornix. We reason that while the short ends of the suture tend to extrude, the long ends tend to lie down against the sclera and are well tolerated. The PCIOLs used for scleral fixation should ideally

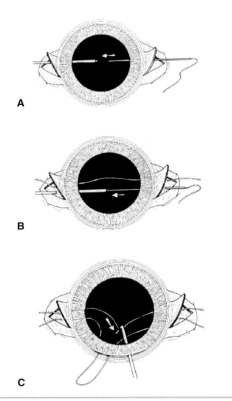

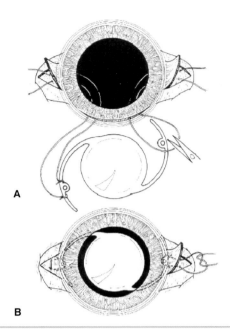

FIGURE 28-2. **A.** The double-suture variant of the Lewis ab externo technique begins similarly to the single-suture technique, except that the suture entry point under the scleral flap is displaced to one side. **B.** The second suture is passed parallel to the first, with 1 to 1.5 mm between the two sutures. **C.** Care must be taken to keep the sutures taut, to avoid crossing them or confusing which suture originates from each scleral site, while a Kuglen hook or similar instrument withdraws the suture loop through the previously prepared principal incision. (Reprinted with permission from Steinert RF, Arkin MS. Secondary intraocular lenses. In Steinert RF [ed], *Cataract Surgery: Techniques, Complications, Management.* Philadelphia: Saunders, 2004:429–441.)

FIGURE 28-3. **A.** To achieve four-point stable fixation, the cut sutures are tied to the haptic on either side of the eyelet. **B.** The IOL is placed in the posterior chamber, keeping the sutures taut to avoid enlargement. The ends are then tied under the scleral flaps, and the conjunctiva closed over the flaps. (Reprinted with permission from Steinert RF, Arkin MS. Secondary intraocular lenses: In Steinert RF [ed], *Cataract Surgery: Techniques, Complications, Management.* Philadelphia: Saunders, 2004:429–441.)

have large-diameter optics (6.5 to 7 mm) and the haptics should ideally have large and well-polished eyelets. Some of the scleral sutured IOLs available on the market are Alcon C270BD, and ORC Optical Radiation Corporation C540MC. When these IOLs are not available or not preferred, any standard IOL can be sutured in place by tying a polypropylene suture to the midportion of the haptic.

In cases in which partial capsular support is present for ciliary sulcus IOL fixation, we have sometimes sewn one haptic to the sclera in the area of least capsular support but left the other haptic unsutured. Often the area of missing capsular support is superior. If only 2 or 3 clock hours of support is missing, no suturing is needed. The IOL is merely oriented with the haptics at the 3 and 9 o'clock positions where an adequate capsular rim exists. In these situations, a large polymethylmethacrylate IOL is recom-

mended since softer foldable IOLs may rotate into the area of no support.

A method of suturing a three-piece AcrySof (Alcon Fort Worth, TX) IOL to the peripheral iris is also gaining popularity because it can be done through a small corneal incision. For soft pediatric eyes, this is an advantage. Advocates claim that suture fixation to the relatively nonmobile midperipheral iris does not lead to any increase in inflammation compared to scleral fixation or anteriorly placed IOLs.

The iris fixation technique begins with the application of a miotic into the AC to constrict the pupil. An AcrySof MA-60 IOL is placed through a corneal tunnel folder in a "mustache" fashion, with both haptics facing posteriorly. The haptics are delivered through the pupil and allowed to unfold. An iris spacula is used under the optic to promote a purposeful pupillary capture of the optic. The haptics are, therefore, in the PC but the optic is in the AC, captured in the pupil. A polypropylene suture is passed through the cornea, through the iris, under the haptic, and back out of the eye. The suture ends can then be pulled out of a paracentesis opening, tied, and placed back into the eye. In this manner, both haptics are tied to the peripheral iris using a single through-and-through iris knot. After the haptics are secured, the optic is placed through the pupil into the posterior segment.

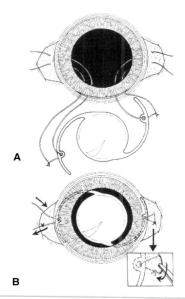

FIGURE 28-4. In this variant of the double-suture ab externo technique, the goal is to achieve a loop of suture where the knot can be rotated beneath the sclera, avoiding the necessity for a scleral flap and the potential for the late erosion of the knot or suture ends. **A.** Cut ends of each suture are passed through the haptic positioning hole and tied. **B.** As the IOL is positioned in the posterior chamber, one end of the suture on each side is pulled so that the knot passes through the sclera to the external eye, where it is cut off. The remaining suture ends are then tied together, and the knot is rotated beneath the sclera (*inset*), achieving the same results as illustrated in Fig. 28-3. (Reprinted with permission from Steinert RF, Arkin MS. Secondary intraocular lenses: In Steinert RF [ed], *Cataract Surgery: Techniques, Complications, Management*. Philadelphia: Saunders, 2004:429–441.)

Complications

There is a tendency toward an increased risk of serious complications with scleral sutured PCIOLs, especially in the hands of less experienced surgeons. These include retinal detachment, posterior dislocation of the IOL, suprachorodal, and vitreous hemorrhage. Glaucoma is one of the reported complications but it may not be related to the scleral-fixated PCIOL. Other reported complications include endophthalmitis, polypropylene knot erosion, corneal edema, lens tilt, refractive surprises, and risk of late failure of the polypropylene suture with subsequent decentration/displacement of the IOL posteriorly.[10,11] To obviate the risk of suture erosion, a partial-thickness scleral flap was recommended. To decrease the incidence further, some surgeons recommend burying the sutures in the sclera.

In order to avoid the complications associated with PCIOL scleral fixation in children, Beltrame and associates[1] have suggested securing the IOL at the ciliary sulcus by suturing the haptics to the sclera at three points (the 3, 5, and 9 o'clock positions). The authors used this technique for secondary IOL implantation in 21 aphakic eyes with a mean follow-up of 18 months. All eyes that underwent secondary IOL implantation had equal or better visual acuity postoperatively and none developed serious intra- or postoperative complications. No tilt or decentration of the IOL was observed postoperatively. According to the author, this technique was easy to perform and produced good visual outcomes with stable transscleral fixation of the IOL.

A few isolated antidotal cases of polypropylene breakage (early or late) have led some surgeons to change from 10.0 to 9.0 polypropylene suture. In addition, newer suture materials are being tested as substitutes for polypropylene.

Published Clinical Studies

Epley and associates[2] reported their experience with pediatric secondary lens implantation in the absence of capsular support. Postoperative results of 18 eyes with PCIOLs sutured to the ciliary sulcus and 10 eyes implanted with ACIOLs were reviewed. Visual outcomes were divided into two groups: onset of aphakia during the critical period of visual development (≤9 years) and onset after the critical period (>9 years). Visual outcomes and complications were recorded after an average follow-up of 10.3 months (in the PCIOL group) and 49.2 months (in the ACIOL group). In their series, eyes that became aphakic after the critical period of visual development achieved better overall final visual acuity than eyes that became aphakic during the critical period. Complications in the ACIOL group included corectopia, haptic migration through the operative wound requiring removal, and pigment deposits on the lens. There were no complications reported in the PCIOL group. The authors concluded that PCIOLs sutured to the ciliary sulcus offer a superior option to ACIOLs for correction of childhood aphakia in children lacking capsular support. ACIOLs had a high rate of serious complications (10%) in this small series. According to the authors, secondary implantation with transsclerally sutured PCIOLs should be considered in complicated cases when more conservative options have been exhausted.

Mittelviefhaus and associates[3] studied transscleral suture fixation of PCIOLs in three children <3 years of age with traumatic cataracts. Clinical outcome, visual acuity, and course of refraction were studied. Four eyes of three children with contact lens intolerance were also operated on. PCIOLs were sutured in the ciliary sulcus by transscleral sutures. To allow adjustment of refraction in situ without removing the primarily implanted and transsclerally fixed PCIOL, the authors used the piggyback IOL system for implantation. Results of the study suggest that visual acuity improved in all four eyes. The two children with traumatic cataracts achieved visual acuity of 0.7 and 1.0, respectively, and stereopsis. The authors observed no complications related to the technique of transscleral suture fixation of the PCIOL.

Buckley[4] reported the short-term results and complications of unilateral scleral-fixated PCIOLs in a pediatric population. All patients with scleral-fixated lenses <16 years old were retrospectively reviewed. Nine patients aged 12 months to 15 years underwent unilateral scleral-fixated PCIOL implantation using buried polypropylene fixation sutures. Postoperative visual acuity improved in all patients after an average follow-up of 2 years. Refractive goals were achieved in all but one patient. Complications included elevated intraocular pressure controlled with medications, anterior uveitis, and mild IOL decentration (one patient each). According to the author, short-term visual results appeared encouraging, but the scleral-fixated PCIOL procedure was technically more difficult and had an increased incidence of postoperative complications compared with secondary sulcus-fixated IOLs supported by capsular remnants. The author suggested caution when recommending this procedure for pediatric patients because the long-term risks are unknown.

In a retrospective study of 21 eyes of 13 children, Zetterstrom and associates[5] evaluated long-term follow-up in eyes of children who had sulcus fixation of an IOL without capsular support. Seven eyes had Marfan's syndrome, seven essential lens dislocation, two perforation with lens injury, and five spherophakia. The IOL implantation was primary in 16 eyes and secondary in 5 eyes. Lensectomy was performed via a limbal approach, and an IOL with fixation holes in the haptics was sutured in the ciliary sulcus, with the knots buried in the scleral bed. No complications occurred during surgery. In all cases, after IOL implantation, the best corrected visual acuity was equal to or better than that preoperatively. After a maximum follow-up of 33 months, posterior synechia formation occurred in four eyes, and four had cells on the IOL surface. In two eyes, the IOL optic subluxated into the AC, but both were successfully treated with 4% pilocarpine. Results of this study suggest that ciliary sulcus placement with scleral fixation of an IOL without capsular support is an option for correcting aphakia in children.

Sharpe et al.[6] reported their experience with scleral fixation of PCIOLs in children. Seven PCIOLs were sutured in the ciliary sulcus of children who could not wear contact lenses. In each eye, the lens capsule remnants were inadequate to provide sufficient support for the haptics of a PCIOL. Results of their study suggested that six of seven patients had improved visual acuity, with an average improvement of four lines. Complications related to scleral fixation included exposure of the scleral fixation suture in one eye, lens decentration in one eye, and lens tilt in one eye, after an average follow-up of 26 months.

CONCLUSION

To summarize, implantation of a scleral-fixated PCIOL offers an alternative to placement of an angle-supported ACIOL or an iris-claw implant for visual rehabilitation of aphakic children who are spectacle- and contact lens–intolerant and who lack capsular support. Further studies on these patients will help determine the long-term safety of this technique.

REFERENCES

1. Beltrame G, Driussi GB, Salvetat ML, et al. Original three-point fixation technique for sutured posterior chamber intraocular lens. *Eur J Ophthalmol* 2002;12:219–224.
2. Epley KD, Shainberg MJ, Lueder GT, Tychsen L. Pediatric secondary lens implantation in the absence of capsular support. *J AAPOS* 2001;5:301–306.
3. Mittelviefhaus H, Mittelviefhaus K, Gerling J. Transscleral suture fixation of posterior chamber intraocular lenses in children under 3 years. *Graefes Arch Clin Exp Ophthalmol* 2000;238:143–148.
4. Buckley EG. Scleral fixated (sutured) posterior chamber intraocular lens implantation in children. *J AAPOS* 1999;3:289–294.
5. Zetterstrom C, Lundvall A, Weeber H Jr, Jeeves M. Sulcus fixation without capsular support in children. *J Cataract Refract Surg* 1999;25:776–781.
6. Sharpe MR, Biglan AW, Gerontis CC. Scleral fixation of posterior chamber intraocular lenses in children. *Ophthal Surg Lasers* 1996;27:337–341.
7. van der Pol BA, Worst JG. Iris-claw intraocular lenses in children. *Doc Ophthalmol* 1996–97;92:29–35.
8. Biglan AW, Cheng KP, Davis JS, Gerontis CC. Secondary intraocular lens implantation after cataract surgery in children. *Am J Ophthalmol* 1997;123:224–234.
9. Wilson ME Jr, Englert JA, Greenwald MJ. In-the-bag secondary intraocular lens implantation in children. *J AAPOS* 1999;3:350–355.
10. Arkin MS, Steinert RF. Sutured posterior chamber intraocular lenses. *Int Ophthalmol Clin* 1994;34:67–85.
11. Hannush SB. Sutured posterior chamber intraocular lenses: indications and procedure. *Curr Opin Ophthalmol* 2000;11:233–240.
12. Lubniewski AJ, Holland EJ, Van Meter WS, et al. Histologic study of eyes with transclerally sutured posterior chamber intraocular lenses. *Am J Ophthalmol* 1990;110:237–243.
13. Duffey RJ, Holland EJ, Agapitos PJ, Lindstorm RL. Anatomic study of trans-sclerally sutured intraocular lens implantation. *Am J Ophthalmol* 1989;108:300–308.

Secondary Intraocular Lens Implantation in Children

Rupal H. Trivedi and M. Edward Wilson, Jr.

The use of primary intraocular lenses (IOLs) for pediatric aphakia has become increasingly common in recent years and is now a well-accepted approach for children beyond infancy. Nevertheless, the implantation of an IOL at the time of cataract surgery in children younger than 1 year remains controversial.[1-4] The main stumbling blocks are the IOL power calculation, IOL sizing, and reported higher rate of visual axis opacification. It is very likely that many of these patients will later require secondary IOL implantation.

To the best of our knowledge, the first IOL implantation in a child was performed as a secondary implantation in 1952. Dr. Edward Epstein performed this secondary IOL implantation for a traumatic cataract in a 12-year-old girl. A cruciate needling was performed on a cataractous lens on April 2, 1952. The lens became hydrated and much of the cortex was absorbed. The four quadrants of the anterior lens capsule (ALC) became adherent to the posterior iris. On June 26, 1952, the residual cortex was washed out and a Ridley IOL was inserted. Forty-six years later the best corrected visual acuity was 20/20 and the IOL remained centered and optically clear (cited in Ref. 5).

Secondary implantation of an IOL is generally recommended when traditional spectacle or contact lens correction of aphakia is unsuccessful. When deciding on secondary IOL implantation, surgeons face some important questions. Should I implant in this eye? If yes, what is the best site for fixation and what type of lens material should I use? This chapter addresses these questions.

Before the recommendation for secondary IOL implantation, a complete ophthalmic examination including visual acuity, slit-lamp biomicroscopy, and fundus examination after mydriasis should be performed. The technical success of secondary implantation depends mainly on how much capsular support was left behind at the time of primary cataract surgery. Three hundred sixty degree visibility of the fused edge of the posterior and anterior capsulectomy from the previous surgery increases the chances of achieving successful posterior segment implantation of an IOL. If the posterior capsule (PC) is not visible, a depression needs to be made posterior to the limbus using blunt-tipped forceps. Sometimes, examination by peripheral iridectomy (if present) is useful to look for capsular remnants. Presence of posterior synechiae, presence of vitreous in the anterior chamber (AC), and associated ocular anomalies should also be documented. In children who do not permit reliable examination, examination should be performed under general anesthesia. When inadequate capsular support is present for sulcus fixation in a child, implantation of an IOL is not recommended unless every contact lens and spectacle option has been fully explored.

SITE OF FIXATION

It sufficient capsular support is available, the most desirable position for the IOL is between the ALC and the PC, widely known as "in-the-bag" fixation. However, occasionally, fibrosis and scarring make the ALC and PC inseparable, and this option may not be feasible.[6] Ciliary sulcus fixation is possibly the best second alternative site for fixation of the IOL.[7] If capsular support is absent, the decision is more controversial. Sutured PCIOLs have become increasingly popular over the past decade (see Chapter 28), but an open-loop flexible ACIOL is used widely recently. An iris-claw lens can also be an option (see Chapter 25).

In the presence of available capsular support, secondary IOLs in children are relegated more commonly to the *ciliary sulcus*.[6,8-10] Several case series have been reported, indicating that a lens placed in the ciliary sulcus is reasonably safe and effective over the short term. Awad et al.[7] performed ultrabiomicroscopy on the ciliary sulcus in 10 eyes after secondary IOL implantation. No gross haptic erosion into the sclera, ciliary body, or sulcus was seen.

The structure of the sulcus in the implanted eye appeared similar to the sulcus in the contralateral normal eye.

However, *in-the-bag* implantation is the best position, as it sequestrates the IOL from the highly reactive uveal tissues and maintains optimum centration of the IOL. Ciliary sulcus-fixated IOLs are more prone to develop pupillary capture, pigment dispersion, ciliary body erosion, decentration, unstable loop fixation, and lens tilt than IOL with bag fixation.[11] Amino et al.[12] reported, in a study of adult eyes, that even more than 2 years after cataract surgery, AC flare counts in eyes with sulcus-to-sulcus IOL fixation were significantly higher than in eyes with in-the-bag fixation.

The technique of in-the-bag secondary IOL implantation in children was reported in 1999.[10] In young children, the process of equatorial epithelial cell proliferation produces a ring of cortex trapped between the lens equator and the fused anterior and posterior capsulectomy edges. Therefore, a potential space for in-the-bag placement of an IOL may be maintained between the ALC and the PC leaflets. In our experience, in-the-bag fixation is more consistently achieved in eyes made primarily aphakic during early infancy. Eyes operated in the first 6 months of life have much more exuberant cortex proliferation within the capsular bag remnant than children operated on at a later age. This material helps to maintain a potential space for lens implantation. In older children, the AC and PC leaflets often fuse together from the central opening far into the equator.

Optic capture through fused ALC and PC and haptics in the ciliary sulcus is another viable option in such cases. It helps to achieve centration of an IOL.

In the absence of sufficient lens capsule support, choosing the best site for the IOL is more difficult and controversial.[13–16] Several reports of *sutured IOL* outcomes in the pediatric population have appeared in the literature.[15–17] Various techniques have been suggested over the years for suturing an IOL.[18–20] Scleral fixation of PCIOLs in children have been well tolerated according to some recent studies, but complications such as pupillary capture, suture erosion, and refractive error from lens tilt or anterior/posterior displacement have been reported. Sutured IOLs are described in more depth in Chapter 28.

Modern, flexible open-loop *ACIOLs* seem to be well tolerated when the anterior segment is developmentally normal. ACIOLs are not usually recommended in eyes with preexisting glaucoma, peripheral anterior synechiae, a shallow AC, or iris defects. It is commonly stated that ACIOLs are easy to insert but difficult to insert correctly.[21] The three most common mistakes made during insertion are incorrect sizing, not taking sufficient steps to avoid iris tuck, and insufficient attention to location of iridectomies and the capacity of haptics to rotate through them.[21] Complications of AC lenses include corneal endothelial cell loss and subsequent corneal decompensation, iris sphincter erosion, glaucoma, and hyphema. We note that two of six ACIOL-implanted eyes in our series required a secondary surgical intervention—one for corectopia and the other for traumatic dislocation.

OUTCOME OF SECONDARY IOL IMPLANTATION

We recently presented our experience with and outcome of secondary IOL implantation in children (Trivedi et al., presented at AAPOS meeting, Washington, DC, 2004). Seventy-seven eyes with a minimum follow-up of 6 months were reported. The mean patient age at surgery was 7.8 ± 5.0 years (range, 0.5 to 18.9 years).

Secondary IOL implantation in our patients was performed most commonly during the 2 to 4 years of age time frame. This is an age when contact lens compliance can be difficult to achieve, yet there is still hope to reverse amblyopia. An additional smaller peak is seen in our group at 12 to 14 years of age. Most of these were bilaterally aphakic patients who requested IOL implantation for cosmetic purposes.

Complications included clinically significant decentration (5.2%), visual axis opacification (5.2%), dislocation of the IOL (2.6%), and pupillary capture necessitating IOL repositioning (1.3%).

Decentration of the IOL was the most common complication. Foldable IOLs in the sulcus are associated with a high rate of decentration or dislocation.[22] Decentration/dislocation was responsible for 21% of explanted three-piece hydrophobic acrylic IOLs in a 2001 survey.[23] In our series clinically significant decentration requiring surgical intervention was noted exclusively in eyes with sulcus-fixated foldable IOLs (28.6%; 4/14) (see Fig. 29-1). Perhaps the rigidity of polymethylmethacrylate (PMMA) IOLs helped to avoid decentration. All of the decentrations were in an inferior direction and all occurred in male eyes. Perhaps this is due to the higher incidence of trauma among males. Another possible reason is that male eyes have been noted to have a longer axial length than female eyes (Trivedi et al., Axial length and keratometry in eyes

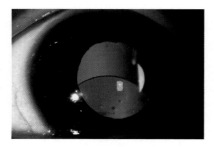

FIGURE 29-1. Decentration of AcrySof IOL 3 weeks postoperatively in a 13.8-year-old male.

with pediatric cataract. Poster presented at ASCRS, 2003). We hypothesized that longer eyes may also have a "wider" anterior segment. A wider sulcus-to-sulcus distance may promote IOL decentration. Eyes with an axial length >23 mm were four times more likely to develop decentration if implanted with a sulcus-fixated foldable IOL compared to eyes measuring <23 mm.

Another recent study has reported decentration in 6% of eyes after secondary placement of foldable AcrySof IOLs in the ciliary sulcus.[24] Jacobi and associates noted decentration of a scleral fixation of a secondary foldable monofocal or multifocal IOL implant in 19.2% of eyes of children and young adults.[25] We commonly use heparin-surface-modified (HSM) PMMA IOLs for the sulcus fixation of an IOL unless microphthalmia is present or optic capture can be achieved.

A higher incidence of *cystoid macular edema* with secondary IOL implantation in adults in whom vitreous loss occurred at the time of initial cataract surgery has been reported. Other studies, however, reported excellent results when a careful and controlled vitrectomy was performed with secondary IOL implantation. Although we did not perform angiography, we did not observe clinical significant cystoid macular edema after secondary implantation in pediatric eyes.

Some reports in the adult literature have reported a higher incidence of *endophthalmitis* in secondary IOL patients compared to primary cataract surgery with IOL placement[26] (cited in Ref. 27). We have witnessed one patient who underwent surgery for bilateral secondary IOL implantation and developed unilateral endophthalmitis.

Bilateral uveitis (possibly sympathetic ophthalmia) resulting in blindness in a child following secondary IOL implantation for unilateral congenital cataract has been reported.[28]

We have noted significant improvement in visual acuity outcome. The geometric mean visual acuity increased from 0.29 to 0.4. Another recent series reported that 42% of patients implanted with an IOL secondarily had a best corrected visual acuity of 20/40 or better, and 78%

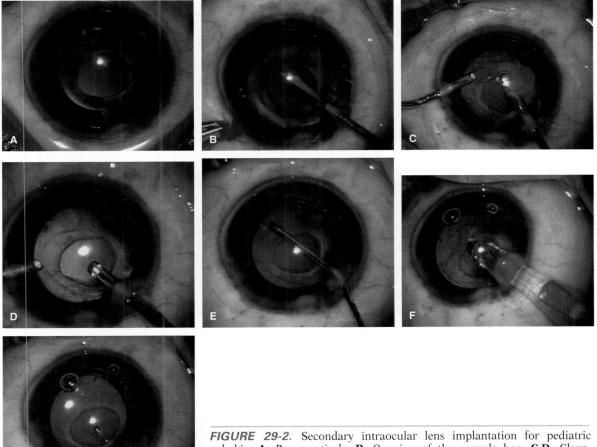

FIGURE 29-2. Secondary intraocular lens implantation for pediatric aphakia. **A.** Preoperatively. **B.** Opening of the capsule bag. **C,D.** Cleaning of the capsular bag. **E.** Viscoelastic injection between capsular leaflets. **F.** Implantation of a single-piece AcrySof IOL. **G.** Well-centered in-the-bag IOL.

better than 20/80.[7] In a 1984 series, Hiles reported that 10% of infantile cataract patients achieved best postoperative visual acuities of 20/40 or better. Twelve years later[6] another series reported that 27% of infantile cataract patients achieved a visual acuity of 20/40 or better.

LESSONS LEARNED

1. When performing infantile cataract surgery without primary IOL implantation, leave an adequate capsular rim for subsequent IOL placement. A 4.5-mm central posterior and anterior capsulectomy is usually adequate to prevent opacification of the visual axis but assures an adequate rim of support when secondary IOL implantation is elected.

2. In a patient with bilateral aphakia, it is sometimes a clever idea to choose the eye with the worst capsular support first. If it is not feasible to safely achieve implantation, bilateral aphakia can still be chosen. This approach can help avoid an IOL in one eye and aphakia in the other.

3. Scleral tunnel incision is preferable for secondary IOL implantation even if a foldable IOL is to be used. In our experience, scleral tunnels are easier to enlarge than corneal tunnels. After the posterior synechiae are severed, a change to a PMMA IOL may be warranted when capsular support is limited. This change can be accomplished more easily from a scleral incision.

4. Change of fixation site may require adjusting the *IOL power*.

5. Assess whether it is possible to reopen the capsular bag leaflets. Figure 29-2 describes the surgical steps for in-the-bag secondary IOL implantation. The key is to locate one area in which the anterior capsule edge is not strongly adherent to the PC.[21] Using the entry point, viscoelastic agents can be very useful in the separation of the capsular layers. If adhesions are very strong, alternative dissection (with iris reposition and/or a micro vitreoretinal knife) techniques must be used. Remove the Soemmering's ring by bimanual irrigation/aspiration and place a secondary IOL into the capsular bag whenever possible. A foldable lens is recommended for this location. In our experience, in-the-bag fixation is more consistently achieved with foldable IOLs—either three-piece or single-piece. The newer single-piece foldable AcrySof model is difficult to explant from the bag and should be avoided if future exchange/explantation is expected for refractive error changes.

6. When the ciliary sulcus is the intended placement site for a secondary IOL, our preferred lens is a HSM PMMA IOL. Perhaps the rigidity of this IOL helps prevent the decentration associated with the use of foldable IOLs. Foldable IOLs work well when microphthalmia is present or optic capture through the ALC and PC can be accomplished.

7. In the absence of available capsular support, sutured IOLs, iris-claw lenses, or ACIOLs can be used, depending on the surgeon's preference, ocular environment, and IOL availability. We will wait for long-term follow-up before commenting on the superiority of one over another.

REFERENCES

1. Lambert SR, Lynn M, Drews-Botsch C, Loupe D, Plager DA, Medow NB, et al. A comparison of grating visual acuity, strabismus, and re-operation outcomes among children with aphakia and pseudophakia after unilateral cataract surgery during the first six months of life. *J AAPOS* 2001;5:70–75.
2. Plager DA, Yang S, Neely D, Sprunger D, Sondhi N. Complications in the first year following cataract surgery with and without IOL in infants and older children. *J AAPOS* 2002;6:9–14.
3. Drews C, Celano M, Plager DA, Lambert SR. Parenting stress among caregivers of children with congenital cataracts. *J AAPOS* 2003;7:244–250.
4. Trivedi RH, Wilson ME Jr, Bartholomew LR, Lal G, Peterseim MM. Opacification of the visual axis after cataract surgery and single acrylic intraocular lens implantation in the first year-of-life. *J AAPOS* 2004;8:156–164.
5. Letocha CE, Pavlin CJ. Follow-up of 3 patients with Ridley intraocular lens implantation. *J Cataract Refract Surg* 1999;25:587–591.
6. DeVaro JM, Buckley EG, Awner S, Seaber J. Secondary posterior chamber intraocular lens implantation in pediatric patients. *Am J Ophthalmol* 1997;123:24–30.
7. Awad AH, Mullaney PB, Al-Hamad A, Wheeler D, Al-Mesfer S, Zwaan J. Secondary posterior chamber intraocular lens implantation in children. *J AAPOS* 1998;2:269–274.
8. Biglan AW, Cheng KP, Davis JS, Gerontis CC. Secondary intraocular lens implantation after cataract surgery in children. *Am J Ophthalmol* 1997;123:224–234.
9. Biglan AW, Cheng KP, Davis JS, Gerontis CC. Results following secondary intraocular lens implantation in children. *Trans Am Ophthalmol Soc* 1996;94:353–373, discussion 374–379.
10. Wilson ME, Jr., Englert JA, Greenwald MJ. In-the-bag secondary intraocular lens implantation in children. *J AAPOS* 1999;3:350–355.
11. Apple DJ, Mamalis N, Loftfield K, Googe JM, Novak LC, Kavka-Van Norman D, et al. Complications of intraocular lenses. A historical and histopathological review. *Surv Ophthalmol* 1984;29:1–54.
12. Amino K, Yamakawa R. Long-term results of out-of-the-bag intraocular lens implantation. *J Cataract Refract Surg* 2000;26:266–270.
13. Evereklioglu C, Er H, Bekir NA, Borazan M, Zorlu F. Comparison of secondary implantation of flexible open-loop anterior chamber and scleral-fixated posterior chamber intraocular lenses. *J Cataract Refract Surg* 2003;29:301–308.
14. Ozmen AT, Dogru M, Erturk H, Ozcetin H. Transsclerally fixated intraocular lenses in children. *Ophthalmic Surg Lasers* 2002;33:394–399.
15. Epley KD, Shainberg MJ, Lueder GT, Tychsen L. Pediatric secondary lens implantation in the absence of capsular support. *J AAPOS* 2001;5:301–306.
16. Zetterstrom C, Lundvall A, Weeber H Jr, Jeeves M. Sulcus fixation without capsular support in children. *J Cataract Refract Surg* 1999;25:776–781.
17. Buckley EG. Scleral fixated (sutured) posterior chamber intraocular lens implantation in children. *J AAPOS* 1999;3:289–294.
18. Malbran ES, Malbran E Jr, Negri I. Lens guide suture for transport and fixation in secondary IOL implantation after intracapsular extraction. *Int Ophthalmol* 1986;9:151–160.

19. Tomikawa S, Hara A. Simple approach to secondary posterior chamber intraocular lens implantation in patients without a complete posterior lens capsule support. *Ophthalmic Surg* 1995;26:160–163.

20. Stark WJ, Gottsch JD, Goodman DF, Goodman GL, Pratzer K. Posterior chamber intraocular lens implantation in the absence of capsular support. *Arch Ophthalmol* 1989;107:1078–1083.

21. Steinert RF, Arkin MS. *Secondary Intraocular Lenses*. Philadelphia: Saunders, 2004.

22. Mamalis N. Explantation of intraocular lenses. *Curr Opin Ophthalmol* 2000;11:289–295.

23. Mamalis N. Complications of foldable intraocular lenses requiring explantation or secondary intervention—2001 survey update. *J Cataract Refract Surg* 2002;28:2193–2201.

24. Crnic T, Weakley DR, Stager D, Felius J. Use of AcrySof acrylic foldable intraocular lens for secondary implantation in children. *J AAPOS* 2004;8:151–155.

25. Jacobi PC, Dietlein TS, Jacobi FK. Scleral fixation of secondary foldable multifocal intraocular lens implants in children and young adults. *Ophthalmology* 2002;109:2315–2324.

26. Kattan HM, Flynn HW Jr, Pflugfelder SC, Robertson C, Forster RK. Nosocomial endophthalmitis survey. Current incidence of infection after intraocular surgery. *Ophthalmology* 1991;98:227–238.

27. Scott IU, Flynn HW Jr, Feuer W. Endophthalmitis after secondary intraocular lens implantation. A case-report study. *Ophthalmology* 1995;102:1925–1931.

28. Wilson-Holt N, Hing S, Taylor DS. Bilateral blinding uveitis in a child after secondary intraocular lens implantation for unilateral congenital cataract. *J Pediatr Ophthalmol Strabismus* 1991;28:116–118.

Anatomical Anomalies That May Complicate Cataract Surgery

Chapter 30

Cataracts Associated with Type I Diabetes Mellitus

M. Edward Wilson, Jr. and
Rupal H. Trivedi

Cataract formation as a complication of Type I diabetes mellitus in young children and adolescents is rare.[1-8] Most information regarding this entity in the literature is found in the form of case reports. One large study, in which 600 cases of insulin-dependent diabetes mellitus (IDDM) were reviewed, found the incidence of related cataract to be only 1%.[1] Cataracts in patients with IDDM were first documented by John Rollo in 1798 (cited in Ref. 2). In 1934, O'Brien and Malsberry studied 126 cases of diabetic patients between 2 and 33 years of age and found cataracts in 16% (cited in Ref. 2).

Cataracts in younger patients with diabetes are usually bilateral (Fig. 30-1). However, patients may present with a unilateral cataract. These patients needs close follow-up since they are prone to develop a cataract in the fellow eye. Diabetic cataracts are unique to younger patients with diabetes who have a long duration of symptoms or history of poorly controlled disease. Acute cataracts, however, have been described in young people as a presenting feature of their diabetes. Thus, cataracts can be a presenting sign of diabetes. One study showed that good metabolic control did not protect against cataract formation.[1] However, most studies, including the one just mentioned,[1]

noted that metabolic control of these patients is generally poor.

These cataracts typically have a band of anterior or posterior subcapsular vacuoles or dense white cortical "snowflake" opacities.[1-3] The cataracts may arrest, partially regress, or progress with the appropriate treatment of diabetes. Early cataracts have been shown to resolve with metabolic control and normalization of fluid and electrolyte status but are permanent once lens protein coagulation occurs.[6]

The mechanism of cataract formation from diabetes appears to be multifactorial since all children with diabetes do not form cataracts.[3] Local factors, genetic predisposition, and nutritional status, combined with other potential known causes such as steroid use, may play a role in development of diabetic cataracts.[2] The osmotic hypothesis, with aldose reductase playing a key role in hyperglycemic-associated cataracts, has been supported by studies using cell cultures, galactose-fed rats, and aldose reductase inhibitors in rats.[9] Dog studies have shown a similar mechanism involving aldose reductase. Its activity in an adult dog lens is similar to that in a human.[10] The polyol pathway involves intracellular excess glucose being reduced to sorbitol by aldose reductase. Sorbitol is then reduced by sorbitol dehydrogenase to fructose, which can penetrate the cell membrane. The increase in intracellular sorbitol causes an osmotic gradient leading to swelling of lens fibers and subsequent alterations of membrane permeability. There is a resultant loss of potassium ions and amino acids, with a rise in sodium ions and a cessation of lens protein production. Continued lens hydration and electrolyte disturbances result in lenticular opacification.[9]

Ehrlich et al.[7] reported 10 cases of cataracts in children with IDDM in a 10-year period. IDDM in these patients had been diagnosed at age 3 weeks to 14 years, with the cataracts diagnosed at age 6 to 16 years. Metabolic control was considered average to poor in these 10 patients.

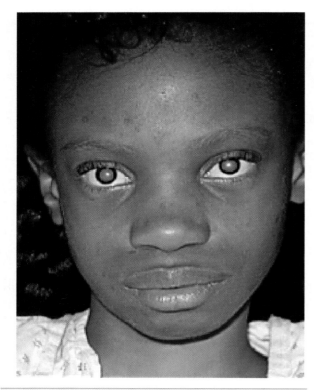

FIGURE 30-1. Bilateral total cataracts in a diabetic patient.

Montgomery and Batch[2] have reported nine cases of diabetic cataracts over 16 years. The average age of the diabetic cataract patient was 10.1 years. Two of nine patients had cataracts at the time of diagnosis of IDDM, one within 3 weeks of diagnosis, and the other six patients developed cataracts 1.7 to 13.0 years after diagnosis. The authors noted that metabolic control of the nine patients was generally poor, with only one patient achieving a satisfactory average hemoglobin A_{1C}.

Falck and Laatikainen[1] retrospectively analyzed the occurrence and possible predisposing factors of diabetic cataracts in a population-based series of some 600 children. Six patients (1%) needed cataract surgery. At the diagnosis of cataracts they were 9.1 to 17.5 years old, and the duration of diabetes was between 0 months and 3 years 11 months. The type of cataract was similar in all patients, characterized by bilateral snowflake-type cortical deposits and posterior subcapsular cataract. Four of the six patients had at least a 6-month history of diabetic symptoms before treatment was started, and five patients had ketoacidosis at initial admission to hospital. In 1 of the 11 operated eyes, diabetic retinopathy was observed immediately after surgery. Three patients developed proliferative retinopathy within 7 to 10 months after the operation, after 6.3 of 11.8 years of diabetes.

We have collected 11 cases (22 eyes) from the accumulated data of six pediatric ophthalmic practices from 1985 to 2000 in order to review this clinical entity as well as discuss its management. All patients <21 years of age with available data who carry the diagnosis of IDDM and cataract were included. The mean age at the time of diagnosis of diabetes was 9.6 years (range, 6 months to 14 years), while the mean age at the time of cataract diagnosis was 10.7 years (5.0 to 15.5 years). In two patients the diagnosis of cataract preceded the diagnosis of IDDM, while in three patients the diagnoses were simultaneous. In some patients the cataracts were bilateral at presentation and in others a unilateral cataract was present, with subsequent cataract development in the other eye. Various studies have reported a preponderance of girls.[2,3] Our results were similar, with 8 of 11 patients being female. The description of cataracts in our patients included posterior subcapsular, lamellar, flakelike opacities throughout the nucleus and cortex, and dense white milky cataracts. Nine of 11 patients (17 eyes) underwent cataract extraction, with a postoperative visual acuity 20/40 or better in 15 eyes. In 13 of these eyes an intraocular lens was implanted. In 6 eyes a primary posterior capsulotomy was performed, while in 11 the posterior capsule was left intact. The literature on adults has reported that diabetic patients developed significantly more posterior capsule opacification after cataract surgery than did nondiabetic patients.[11] Pediatric eyes are at high risk for posterior capsule opacification if the posterior capsule is left intact. Eyes with diabetic cataracts may be at higher risk. Eight of these 11 eyes eventually required Nd:YAG laser capsulotomy.

Two patients developed diabetic retinopathy postoperatively in our series. It has been reported in the literature that cataract surgery increases the risk of diabetic retinopathy.[12] However, to the best of our knowledge, an influence of primary posterior capsulectomy and vitrectomy on diabetic retinopathy has not been reported. Theoretically, these eyes may be at higher risk for diabetic retinopathy.

To summarize, since cataracts can be a presenting symptom of diabetes, children with acquired cataracts of unknown etiology should be questioned about classic symptoms of diabetes and evaluation for hyperglycemia should be performed. Early diagnosis and initiation of metabolic control are important since cataract formation may be influenced by the duration of symptoms prior to treatment. Early detection of cataracts, determination of etiology with subsequent glycemic control, and evaluation by an ophthalmologist for surgical removal are essential in the treatment of diabetic cataracts in children. Modern cataract surgery techniques can be performed safely when visual acuity is diminished provided that there is close observation to monitor the potential onset of diabetic retinopathy.

REFERENCES

1. Falck A, Laatikainen L. Diabetic cataract in children. *Acta Ophthalmol Scand* 1998;76:238–240.
2. Montgomery EL, Batch JA. Cataracts in insulin-dependent diabetes mellitus: sixteen years' experience in children and adolescents. *J Pediatr Child Health* 1998;34:179–182.
3. Datta V, Swift PG, Woodruff GH, Harris RF. Metabolic cataracts in newly diagnosed diabetes. *Arch Dis Child* 1997;76:118–120.
4. Scarpitta AM, Perrone P, Sinagra D. The diabetic cataract: an unusual presentation in a young subject: case report. *J Diabetes Complicat* 1997;11:259–260.
5. Datiles MB 3rd, Kador PF. Type I diabetic cataract. *Arch Ophthalmol* 1999;117:284–285.
6. Santiago AP, Rosenbaum AL, Masket S. Insulin-dependent diabetes mellitus appearing as bilateral mature diabetic cataracts in a child. *Arch Ophthalmol* 1997;115:422–423.
7. Ehrlich RM, Kirsch S, Daneman D. Cataracts in children with diabetes mellitus. *Diabetes Care* 1987;10:798–799.
8. Bilginturan AN, Jackson RL, Ide CH. Transitory cataracts in children with diabetes mellitus. *Pediatrics* 1977;60:106–109.
9. Kinoshita JH, Kador P, Catiles M. Aldose reductase in diabetic cataracts. *JAMA* 1981;246:257–261.
10. Sato S, Mori K, Wyman M, Kador PF. Dose-dependent prevention of sugar cataracts in galactose-fed dogs by the aldose reductase inhibitor M79175. *Exp Eye Res* 1998;66:217–222.
11. Hayashi K, Hayashi H, Nakao F, Hayashi F. Posterior capsule opacification after cataract surgery in patients with diabetes mellitus. *Am J Ophthalmol* 2002;134:10–16.
12. Chung J, Kim MY, Kim HS, Yoo JS, Lee YC. Effect of cataract surgery on the progression of diabetic retinopathy. *J Cataract Refract Surg* 2002;28:626–630.

Persistent Fetal Vasculature

Irene Anteby

Persistent fetal vasculature (PFV) is one of the most common congenital malformations of the human eye. It includes a complex spectrum of clinical manifestations, which develop due to the abnormal persistence of fetal vasculature. The term PFV, coined by Goldberg[1] in his 1997 Jackson Memorial Lecture, replaced the more commonly used persistent hyperplastic primary vitreous (PHPV).[2] The substitution of the term PFV reflects Goldberg's more accurate description of anatomic and pathologic features of this disease. In PFV some, or all, components of the fetal intraocular vasculature remain after birth. This malformation may affect the anterior, retrolental, and/or posterior parts of the infant eye. The extent of the vascular anomaly directly influences both the prognosis for and the therapeutic approach to the PFV eye.

CLINICAL MANIFESTATIONS

It is important to recognize the range of clinical manifestations in PFV. Knowledge of the embryological milestones responsible for the development of fetal vasculature is crucial for the understanding of the diversity of symptoms and signs appearing in PFV. During fetal development transient sets of proliferating blood vessels extend throughout the posterior and anterior poles of the eye. The vessels anastomose freely, creating a rich network by the equator and thus connecting all compartments of the eye. These fetal vessels start to grow during the first month of gestation, reach their maximum proliferative activity by the second to third month, and begin to involute at 4 months' gestation. Normally these fetal vessels disappear by birth.[1,3] In eyes with PFV, the process of fetal vascular regression is arrested. Persistence of some or all fetal vasculature may have profound morphological consequences. Although individual components of the fetal vasculature often persist in combination with others, any one of the vascular remnants either may predominate in such combinations or may occur alone. Therefore, PFV may cause any of several clinical variants.[1]

1. *Persistent pupillary membrane.* These threadlike vessels appearing in the pupil are the remnants of the anterior tunica vasculosa lentis. Occasionally the pupil is deformed by these vessels. Congenital ectropion or entropion uvea may also occur. Vision may be unaffected or reduced, depending on the extent of pupillary occlusion. The presence of a pupillary membrane may aid in the diagnosis of PFV in an eye with total cataract or whitish retrolental mass.

2. *Iridohyaloid blood vessels.* These fetal vessels appear as radial, short, and parallel vessels by the equator of the lens. They constitute a vascular connection between the posterior and the anterior tunica vasculosa lentis. When these vessels do not regress by the second trimester of gestation, they contribute to the appearance of radial superficial vessels in iris stroma. Often, white limbal connective tissue malformation may be seen in the same meridian. When the vessels reach the pupil they make hairpin loops, inducing a small pupillary notch.

3. *Persistence of the posterior fibrovascular sheath of the lens.* Persistence of the posterior tunica vasculosa lentis causes the appearance of a fibrovascular mass behind the lens. Reese[2] described this as the hallmark of PHPV syndrome. The retrolental membrane may be small or may cover the entire posterior capsule of the lens. It may be associated with a clear lens or cause variable degrees of lenticular opacification. Typically the retrolental membrane is white or pink in color, differentiating it from the yellow tissue seen in Coats' disease or the snow-white tissue typical of calcified retinoblastoma. Formation of a retrolental membrane in PFV is often accompanied by elongation of the ciliary processes, which may become visible as the pupil is dilated. Although prominent ciliary processes were once considered pathognomonic for PHPV, they are also seen in retinopathy of prematurity stage V, Norrie's disease, trisomy 13, and congenital subluxated lenses.[1]

4. *Mittendorf dot.* This small white dot on the posterior surface of the lens is typically found 0.5 mm to the nasal side of the center of the posterior pole and designates the point of incomplete regression of the hyaloid artery, where it attaches to the posterior surface of the lens. It is normally found in 0.7 to 2.0% of the population and rarely causes any visual disturbance.[3]

5. *Persistent hyaloid artery.* The fetal hyaloid artery lies within the Cloquet canal and normally loses perfusion around the seventh month of gestation. When this vessel persists, it may be seen stretching from the optic nerve to the lens.

6. *Bergmeister papilla.* This is often the benign remnant of the posterior part of the hyaloid artery and can be seen as an epipapillary vascular tissue. Its effect on vision depends on the presence of other associated optic nerve abnormalities.

7. *Congenital tent-shaped retinal detachment.* Congenitally detached retina is caused by traction from PFV on the retina. It typically has the shape of a traction retinal detachment and it adheres to the posterior surface of the lens, ciliary body, or both. The detachment may progress, and it has grave visual consequences.

8. *Macular abnormalities.* Various dysplastic and hypoplastic abnormalities of the macula may occur in PFV and these will inevitably affect vision.

9. *Optic nerve abnormalities.* Both primary and secondary abnormalities of the optic nerve, including optic disc hypoplasia, may be seen in PFV.

10. *Microphthalmos.* Retention of fetal vasculature may be accompanied by an arrest in the growth of the eye globe. Typically, eyes with severe forms of PFV have some degree of microphthalmos. Additional changes include a decreased corneal diameter and distortion of the configuration of globe wall, with colobomatous microphthalmos as a result.

ADJUNCTIVE TOOLS FOR DIAGNOSIS

Despite the wealth of clinical manifestations, diagnosing PFV may sometimes be challenging. Any child with a cataract, unilateral or bilateral, especially when associated with a microphthalmic globe, should be suspected of having PFV. When PFV is associated with cataract the differential diagnosis includes diseases causing leukocoria. When clinical signs are nonconclusive, adjunctive imaging may aid in making the correct diagnosis. The most helpful and noninvasive tool is echography. Both posterior segment echography and ultrasound biomicroscopy of the anterior segment[4] are valuable. Posterior segment echography typically shows a small globe with a retrolental membrane and a vitreous band extending from the

posterior lens capsule to the disc area.[5] It can also reveal whether a retinal detachment is present, which may influence the choice of surgical technique used to remove the cataract. High-frequency ultrasonography may demonstrate an anteriorly placed and swollen lens with a resultant shallow anterior chamber, centrally dragged ciliary processes, and thickened anterior vitreous face appearing as a double linear echo by the pars plana or pars plicata.[4] In addition, color Doppler imaging of the persistent hyaloid artery may detect blood flow within the stalk (Fig. 31-3). Computerized tomography and magnetic resonance imaging have also been reported as excellent adjunctive devices in the evaluation of PFV.[6–8] The demonstration of calcifications within the globe is suggestive of retinoblastoma, which is the most important differential diagnosis to rule out in eyes with leukocoria. The rare occurrence of retinoblastoma in an eye with PHPV has been reported.[9]

PFV AND ASSOCIATED ANOMALIES

Although PFV mostly appears as a single anomaly, sometimes it may be associated with other ocular abnormalities such as Peters' anomaly,[10] Riegers anomaly,[11] and morning glory syndrome.[12,13] Only 5 to 10% of children with PFV have binocular involvement. Bilaterality represents a more widespread degree of abnormal embryological development. Associated systemic anomalies may occur, especially neurological abnormalities.[14] Haddad et al.[15] reported systemic abnormalities including cleft palate and lip, polydactyly, and microcephaly in association with bilateral PHPV. Goldberg reported on the association of PFV with trisomy 13.[1] A few pedigrees with familial PFV have been described, suggesting the possibility of an autosomal recessive[16] or autosomal dominant[17] inheritance pattern in selected cases.

MANAGEMENT

Historically, eyes with PFV, especially when accompanied by dense cataracts hampering ocular stimuli during the critical period of visual development, were doomed to be blind.[18,19] Surgery was indicated only to avoid or treat complications such as angle-closure glaucoma, vitreous hemorrhage, progressive retinal detachment, and phthisis.[2] Many eyes eventually required enucleation, with a resultant poor cosmetic outcome.[20] Since the advent of closed-system vitrectomy instrumentation, removal of the cataract, retrolental mass, and persistent hyaloid stalk has been made possible. By surgical release of the traction on the ciliary body in eyes with PFV, the eye is allowed to grow and acceptable cosmetic improvement achieved.[21] Even though initial surgical goals in eyes with PFV were mainly to avoid the complications of the disease and improve cosmesis, reports of useful postoperative vision following microsurgical vitrectomy techniques began to appear in the 1980s.[22–25] Successful visual rehabilitation has been reported for the most part in PFV with anterior presentation, i.e., without disc or macular involvement.[26]

Today, the introduction of sophisticated microsurgical techniques, in combination with aggressive amblyopia therapy, has resulted in more favorable visual outcomes for eyes with PFV.[27–30] Therapeutic goals should therefore be expanded to include saving useful vision. Several surgical approaches removing the cataract and persistent vasculature in PFV have been described. During the past 15 years we have applied a modified surgical approach in the treatment of PFV, similar to that previously described for uncomplicated cataracts.[31,32]

Surgical Methods

Two techniques are described briefly: the pars plana (posterior) approach and the limbal (anterior) approach. In both, the cataract is removed by a lensectomy in combination with an anterior vitrectomy and removal of the persistent hyaloid system.

Posterior Approach

Using the posterior approach, a micro vitreoretinal (MVR) blade (20 gauge) is used to perform a sclerotomy at the 10 o'clock position 1.5 to 2.0 mm from the limbus. The MVR blade is then pierced through the lens by the equator, leaving an opening in the anterior capsule. A cannula with irrigation fluid is introduced through a similar sclerotomy site at the 2 o'clock position. A vitrectomy handpiece is then introduced through the sclerotomy site at 10 o'clock and inserted in the opened bag, and the lens material is aspirated within the bag. After removal of all lens material, the lens capsule and adjacent retrolental membranes are removed by the vitrector. When the retrolental membrane is too thick to be cut with a vitrector alone, intraocular scissors may help to segmentally cut the membrane into fragments small enough for the vitrector to remove.[33] An anterior vitrectomy with removal of the anterior part of the hyaloid stalk is then performed. Possible bleeding from the patent hyaloid artery can usually be controlled by raising the infusion set or by applying diathermy to the bleeding stump. Since all lens capsule material is removed when using this posterior approach, the eye remains aphakic. When posterior abnormalities are present, a complete posterior vitrectomy is suggested, with peeling of membranes to release retinal traction and folds. In some patients an air–fluid exchange may be indicated.

Anterior Approach

A second approach to cataract removal in PFV is the anterior (limbal) approach. The main advantage of this method is the feasibility of intraocular lens (IOL) implantation, enabling better visual rehabilitation and final cosmetic outcome.[27] In addition, the anterior approach facilitates surgery by avoiding the peripheral retina, which might be attached to the ciliary body or be drawn into the retrolental membrane.[15] Briefly, in the anterior approach an MVR blade is used to perform two openings by the limbus: superotemporally for the vitrector and inferotemporally for the anterior chamber maintainer (irrigation set). A mechanized anterior capsulotomy is performed. The lens is aspirated within the bag. A posterior capsulotomy and removal of retrolental membranes are performed using the vitrector. In cases where the membranes are thick and stiffened, scissors may be used to fragment the membrane before final removal with the vitrector. Through the opening in the posterior capsule, the anterior vitreous and anterior portions of the persistent hyaloid artery are removed using the vitrectomy-cutting instrument. An IOL can then be inserted either in the bag or in the sulcus, similarly to uncomplicated childhood cataract.

VISUAL OUTCOME

To achieve favorable vision in children with PFV, irrespective of surgical approach, early intervention followed by aggressive antiamblyopic patching therapy is indicated.[27–30] Anteby et al.[27] reported the visual outcome in 89 eyes with unilateral PFV, comparing 60 operated eyes (using the above-mentioned surgical techniques) to 29 nonoperated eyes. In this large series a final visual acuity of 20/200 or better in 25% of 60 operated eyes was achieved. Mittra et al.[30] reported even more encouraging results of 14 eyes managed by surgery and aggressive antiamblyopic therapy, with 66% achieving 20/100 or better vision. However, in this series no long-term follow-up was available and possible late complications affecting vision were not taken into account. Alexandrakis et al.,[28] in a study of 30 eyes managed by surgery, reported 47% of the operated eyes achieving 20/400 or better, compared to 12% in nonoperated eyes. Successful visual results have been reported after surgery with PFV of the anterior type.[20,26] More limited visual success is to be expected in PFV involving the posterior segment.[29]

Traditionally, operated PFV eyes remained aphakic. With an anterior surgical approach, the insertion of an IOL during the initial surgery is feasible. IOLs facilitate postoperative care by avoiding the need for contact lenses. Due to the microphthalmos often encountered in PFV, contact lenses need a high refractive power and can be difficult to fit on a small cornea. Recent reports have included attempts to rehabilitate vision in PFV eyes by IOL implantation. Anteby et al.[27] inserted IOLs in 30 eyes with unilateral PFV over the past 15 years. A good visual acuity, 20/50 or better, was seen in 20% of these eyes and a fair visual acuity, 20/200 or better, was obtained in 33.3%. Mittra et al.[30] reported on the use of IOL in two eyes with PFV with a resultant acceptable visual outcome.

POSTOPERATIVE COMPLICATIONS

The main postoperative complications in PFV eyes include glaucoma, secondary membrane formation, vitreous hemorrhage, retinal detachment, and strabismus. Dass et al.[29] reported a general reoperation rate of 32% in 27 eyes with PFV.

The rate of glaucoma in eyes with PFV varies from series to series. Anteby et al.[27] reported a 15% overall rate of glaucoma in 89 PFV eyes. Glaucoma developed twice as often in eyes with aphakia (22%) as in nonoperated eyes (11%). The rate of glaucoma in PFV eyes with pseudophakia was only 8%.[27] This suggests that IOL implantation in these eyes does not increase the risk for glaucoma, although eyes selected for IOL implantation may have less severe forms of PFV. Others reported glaucoma to occur in up to 30% of eyes operated for PFV.[34] Glaucoma is often diagnosed within the first year after lensectomy but may also develop several years after surgery.[34]

Despite the performance of a relatively large posterior capsulotomy in eyes with PFV, the rate of secondary cataract and membrane formation necessitating further surgery is high—up to 30%.[27,34] The rate seems unaffected by insertion of an IOL during the initial lensectomy.[27] Possibly this high rate of secondary cataract can be attributed to the microphthalmos itself, as typical postoperative complications have been found to be less common in PFV eyes that are myopic.[35]

COSMETIC OUTCOME

One of the major goals of surgical treatment of eyes with PFV should include the achievement of good cosmetic rehabilitation. If the PFV eye is not treated surgically, complications such as glaucoma, vitreous hemorrhage, corneal opacification, and phthisis may gravely disfigure the globe. In addition, as no significant vision is achieved, sensory strabismus develops, further blemishing the child (Fig. 31-1). The quality of life for children with PFV is severely affected by the development of phthisis and deformed eye or the need for a cosmetic shell or prosthesis. Anteby et al. reported 30% of PFV eyes developing a visible cosmetic blemish due to advanced microphthalmos, buphthalmos, extensive corneal leukoma, or total phthisis. Interestingly, 25% of aphakic eyes and 7.1% of nonoperated eyes needed a prosthesis or cosmetic shell during the years of follow-up, whereas none of the eyes with pseudophakia needed this type of rehabilitation.[27] Pollard[20] reported that only 2 of 83 eyes with PFV required cosmetic shell. None of the patients needed enucleation. In Scott and coworkers'[25] series the rate of enucleation was also low: 8% in nonoperated and 4% in aphakic PFV eyes.

CONCLUSION

The key to success in managing the child with PFV is early diagnosis of the disease. In eyes where vision is gravely impaired by optic axis occlusion owing to cataract and retrolental membranes, early surgery should be attempted to enable visual and cosmetic rehabilitation. During surgery, whether using an anterior or a posterior approach, lensectomy, anterior vitrectomy, release of ciliary body traction, and removal of the hyaloid stalk should be performed. The rehabilitation of vision may be further facilitated using an

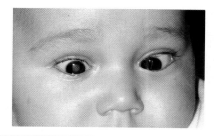

FIGURE 31-1. A 6-month-old boy with PFV in the right eye. Progressive swelling of the lens has induced shallowing of the anterior segment, with resultant angle-closure glaucoma. The boy suffers from marked epiphora from the microphthalmic and leukocoric eye. In addition, his increased irritability prompted his parents to bring him in for examination.

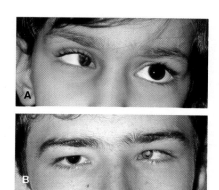

FIGURE 31-2. When left untreated, eyes with PFV become a cosmetic blemish. These young children have a microphthalmic PFV eye (**A & B**), with leukocoria (**B**), ectropion uvea (**B**), and large-angle esotropia (**A & B**).

IOL when technically possible. Final visual outcome depends not only on the extent of the disease, but also on the promptness of treatment, including aggressive antiamblyopic therapy after surgery (Fig. 31-2). Children with PFV need to be carefully monitored for years, for the possible development of common postoperative complications such as glaucoma and secondary cataract formation. To assure a good quality of life for children with PFV, the goals of therapy should include saving useful vision and achieving a good cosmetic outcome.

REFERENCES

1. Goldberg M. Persistent fetal vasculature (PFV): An integrated interpretation of signs and symptoms associated with persistent hyperplastic primary vitreous (PHPV). LIV Edward Jackson Memorial Lecture. *Am J Ophthalmol* 1997;124:587–626.
2. Reese AB. Persistent hyperplastic primary vitreous. *Am J Ophthalmol* 1955;40:317–331.
3. Wright KW, ed. Embryology. In: Cook CS, Sulik KK, Wright KW, eds. *Pediatric Ophthalmology and Strabismus*. St. Louis, MO: Mosby, 1995:1–43.
4. MacKeen LD, Nischal KK, Lam WC, Levin AV. High-frequency ultrasonography findings in persistent hyperplastic primary vitreous. *J AAPOS* 2000;4:217–224.
5. Frazier Byrne S, Green RL. Intraocular tumors. In: Fraziet Byrne S, Green RL, eds. *Ultrasound of the Eye and Orbit*. St. Louis, MO: Mosby, 1992:201–204.
6. Mafee MF, Goldberg MF. Persistent hyperplastic primary vitreous (PHPV): role of computed tomography and magnetic resonance. *Radiol Clin North Am* 1987;25:683–692.
7. Potter PD, Shields CL, Shields JA, Flanders AE. The role of magnetic resonance imaging in children with intraocular tumors and simulating lesions. *Ophthalmology* 1996;103:1774–1783.
8. Kuker W, Ramaekers V. Persistent hyperplastic primary vitreous: MRI. *Neuroradiology* 1999;41:520–522.
9. Irvine AR, Albert DM, Sang DN. Retinal neoplasia and dysplasia. II. Retinoblastoma occurring with persistence and hyperplasia of the primary vitreous. *Invest Ophthalmol Vis Sci* 1977;16:403–407.
10. Matsubara A, Ozeki H, Matsunaga N, et al. Histopathological examination of two cases of anterior staphyloma associated with Peters' anomaly and persistent hyperplastic vitreous. *Br J Ophthalmol* 2001;85:1421–1425.
11. Storimans CW, Van Schooneveld MJ. Riegers eye anomaly and persistent hyperplastic primary vitreous. *Ophthalm Paediatr Genet* 1989;10:257–262.
12. Brown GC, Gonder J, Levin A. Persistence of the primary vitreous in association with the morning glory disc anomaly. *J Pediatr Ophthalmol Strabismus* 1984;21:5–7.
13. Cennamo G, Liguori G, Pezone A, Iaccarino G. Morning glory syndrome associated with marked persistent hyperplastic primary vitreous and lens coloboma. *Br J Ophthalmol* 1989;73:684–686.
14. Marshman WE, Jan JE, Lyons CJ. Neurological abnormalities associated with persistent hyperplastic primary vitreous. *Can J Ophthalmol* 1999;34:17–22.
15. Haddad R, Font RL, Reeser F. Persistent hyperplastic primary vitreous. A clinicopathologic study of 62 cases and review of the literature. *Surv Ophthalmol* 1978;23:123–134.
16. Khaliq S, Hameed A, Ismail M, et al. Locus for autosomal recessive nonsyndromic persistent hyperplastic primary vitreous. *Invest Ophthalmol Vis Sci* 2001;42(10):2225–2228.
17. Lin AE, Biglan AW, Garver KL. Persistent hyperplastic primary vitreous with vertical transmission. *Ophthalm Paediatr Genet* 1990;11(2):121–122.
18. Jensen OA. Persistent hyperplastic primary vitreous. Cases in Denmark. *Acta Ophthalmol (Copenh)* 1968;46:418–429.
19. Olsen J, Moller PM. Persistent primary hyperplastic vitreous. *Acta Ophthalmol (Copenh)* 1968;46:412–417.
20. Pollard ZF. Persistent hyperplastic primary vitreous: diagnosis, treatment and results. *Trans Am Ophthalmol Soc* 1997;95:487–549.
21. Federman JL, Shields JA, Altman B, Koller H. The surgical and nonsurgical management of persistent hyperplastic primary vitreous. *Ophthalmology* 1982;89:20–24.
22. Stark WJ, Lindsey PS, Fagadau WR, Michels RG. Persistent hyperplastic primary vitreous. Surgical treatment. *Ophthalmology* 1983;90(5):452–457.
23. Pollard ZF. Treatment of persistent hyperplastic primary vitreous. *J Pediatr Ophthalmol Strabismus* 1985;22:180–183.
24. Karr DJ, Scott WE. Visual acuity results following treatment of persistent hyperplastic primary vitreous. *Arch Ophthalmol* 1986;104:662–667.
25. Scott WE, Drummond GT, Keech RV, Karr DJ. Management and visual acuity results of monocular congenital cataracts and persistent hyperplastic primary vitreous. *Aust NZ J Ophthalmol* 1989;17:143–152.
26. Pollard ZF. Results of treatment of persistent hyperplastic primary vitreous. *Ophthalm Surg* 1991;22:48–52.
27. Anteby I, Cohen E, Karshai I, BenEzra D. Unilateral persistent hyperplastic primary vitreous: course and outcome. *J AAPOS* 2002;6:92–99.
28. Alexandrakis G, Scott IU, Flynn HW Jr, et al. Visual acuity outcomes with and without surgery in patients with persistent fetal vasculature. *Ophthalmology* 2000;107:1068–1072.
29. Dass AB, Trese MT. Surgical results of persistent hyperplastic primary vitreous. *Ophthalmology* 1999;106:280–284.
30. Mittra RA, Huynh LT, Ruttum MS, et al. Visual outcomes following lensectomy and vitrectomy for combined anterior and posterior persistent hyperplastic primary vitreous. *Arch Ophthalmol* 1998;116:1190–1194.
31. BenEzra D. The surgical approaches to pediatric cataract. *Eur J Implant Refract Surg* 1990;2:241–244.
32. BenEzra D, Cohen E. Posterior capsulectomy in pediatric cataract surgery: The necessity of a choice. *Ophthalmology* 1997;104:2168–2174.
33. Paysse EA, McCreery KM, Coats DK. Surgical management of the lens and retrolental fibrotic membranes associated with persistent fetal vasculature. *J Cataract Refract Surg* 2002;28:816–820.
34. Johnson CP, Keech RV. Prevalence of glaucoma after surgery for PHPV and infantile cataracts. *J Pediatr Ophthalmol Strabismus* 1996;33:14–17.
35. Cheung JC, Summers CG, Young TL. Myopia predicts better outcome in persistent hyperplastic primary vitreous. *J Pediatr Ophthalmol Strabismus* 1997;34:170–176.

Cataract Surgery in Eyes with Retinopathy of Prematurity

Rupal H. Trivedi and M. Edward Wilson, Jr.

Retinopathy of prematurity (ROP) is a proliferative disease of premature infants in which peripheral retinal blood vessels fail to develop. ROP remains a leading cause of vision impairment in children in the United States. Prematurity per se and its associated low birth weight are the cause of most cases of ROP. Improvement in neonatal intensive care has increased the survival of premature newborns from 0 to 65% at some centers.[1] The Multicenter Trial of Cryotherapy for Retinopathy of Prematurity reported an incidence of ROP of 65.8% in 4,099 infants weighing <1250 g at birth.[2] A growing concern is the increasing incidence of ROP in middle-income countries. As living conditions and access to medical technology have improved in these countries, more premature infants are surviving.[3]

Cataract can be an associated ocular pathology in eyes with ROP, as low birth weight and prematurity are risk factors for both entities.[4,5] Alden et al.[6] reported transient lens opacities in 2.7% of low–birth weight infants. These opacities, which are reversible in nature, are characterized by clear fluid vacuoles just anterior to the posterior capsule of the lens. However, occurrence of secondary cataract (secondary to treatment of ROP) has been reported more frequently in the literature, and our focus in this chapter is to review that in detail.

During the past decade, laser photocoagulation has supplanted cryotherapy as the standard treatment for threshold ROP. Laser treatment is effective and easier to perform, patients are more comfortable after surgery, and better structural and functional outcomes can be achieved. Laser therapy in ROP patients can be applied with an argon laser or diode laser. The current trend for selecting an argon or a diode laser is based on laser availability and physician preferences. Compared with cryotherapy for ROP, laser treatment is associated with a lower rate of retinal detachment, less myopia, less postoperative lid edema, and conjuctival chemosis. Nevertheless, an iatrogenic cataract is a serious, potentially blinding complication that can occur as a result of transpupillary laser photocoagulation. Argon laser–treated eyes for ROP are at higher risk of developing secondary cataract; however, occurrence of cataract has also been reported in diode laser–treated eyes and with cryotherapy. A survey performed by Gold in 1995[7] reported 68 cataracts in association with ROP treatment. Sixty-two percent of these were associated with argon laser, 31% with diode laser, and 7% with cryotherapy.

TYPES OF CATARACTS

1. *Transient.* Focal opacities (either punctate or vacuolated) may occur at the capsular or subcapsular level. These are generally visually insignificant and often resolve spontaneously.[8]

2. *Progressive and visually significant.* Progressive lens opacification generally leads to total cataract and completely obstructs the visual axis.[9]

3. *Associated with retinal detachment.* A cataract develops frequently in eyes with stage 4 or 5 retinal detachments. These cataracts differ from the two types of cataracts described above in that their onset is later and they occur as a sequel of retinal detachment or of vitreoretinal surgery. Knight and associates[10] reported on the outcome of treatment for advanced cicatrical ROP. The authors found cataracts in 54.8% (17/31) of eyes.

DURATION

Cataract formation after argon laser photocoagulation has been noted immediately, during the laser treatment, to as long as 99 days after the laser treatment, with most occurring in the first few postoperative weeks. Lambert et al.[11] reported a median interval of 3 weeks for diagnosis of a cataract after laser photocoagulation.

ETIOPATHOGENESIS

1. *Tunica vasculosa lentis.* Premature infants have much of the tunica vasculosa lentis intact, which may allow for absorption of energy on the lens surface. Hazy vitreous and miosis in these infants also necessitate high-power settings.

2. *Anterior segment ischemia.* Associated clinical findings of anterior segment ischemia such as pupillary membranes, iris and ciliary process atrophy, pigment on the anterior lens surface, posterior synechiae, corneal edema, hyphema, and a shallow anterior chamber may be seen in association with cataracts.

3. *Thermal injury.* Paysse et al.[12] have reported that postlaser cataracts are more likely the result of thermal injury. This results from absorption of laser energy by lens proteins or hemoglobin in the blood circulating through a persistent anterior tunica vasculosa lentis, and they should, for the most part, occur in the first postoperative weeks after laser treatment. This hypothesis is further supported by the lower incidence of cataract formation with diode laser compare to argon laser, as this phenomenon of laser energy absorption is likely to be less frequent because of the reduced absorption of diode laser energy by hemoglobin.

4. *Uveal effusion.* Diode laser application in nanophthalmic eyes has been reported to cause uveal effusion that resulted in anterior rotation of the ciliary body and shallowing of the already narrow anterior chamber. The resulting corneolenticular apposition led to cataract formation in these eyes.[13]

5. *Vitreoretinal pathology.* Cataract may be associated with retinal detachment or may occur after vitreoretinal surgery.

6. *Rent in lens capsule.* Lambert et al.[11] have reported the detection of a rent in the posterior lens capsule at the time of cataract surgery. The authors noted lens material to be liquefied in some eyes. They also noted that, in addition to the above-mentioned findings, associated iridocyclitis supports this hypothesis. At times this occurs during vitreous surgery.

RISK FACTORS

1. *Prominent anterior tunica vasculosa lentis.* Sufficient laser energy may be absorbed by the persistent lens vasculature to cause thermal injury to the lens.

2. *Inadvertent burns placed on the iris.* Energy absorption caused by the iris pigment epithelium can cause heating of the anterior lens.

3. *Confluent laser therapy.* Extensive use of laser energy may add to the risk of lens injury.

4. *Vitreoretinal surgery.* Cataracts occur more commonly after intraocular surgery.

REVIEW OF THE LITERATURE

Argon Laser Therapy

1. *1992.* Drack et al.[8] reported transient punctate and comma-shaped opacities at the level of the anterior cortex/lens capsule, associated with a few posterior synechaie.

2. *1995.* Christiansen and Bradford[14] reported an incidence of 6% (6/100) visually significant cataracts and 1% (1/100) transient cataracts. Cataract was diagnosed between 19 and 99 days (median, 20 days) after treatment. All eyes with permanent cataract were noted to have permanent tunica vasculosa lentis at the time of treatment. After laser therapy these eyes developed hyphema, shallowing of the anterior chamber, corneal edema, and progressive opacification of the lens. The number of laser burns was higher (average, 1,320) in eyes developing a subsequent cataract compared to eyes that did not develop a cataract (average, 1,126).

3. *1997.* A survey conducted by Gold[7] revealed a total of 42 cataracts treated by argon laser—22 visually significant and 20 nonsignificant.

4. *1998.* O'Neil et al.[15] reported a total of 4 of 374 eyes (1%) with cataracts. In two of the four eyes it was judged that the cataract was related to the laser treatment. The incidence of cataract formation in eyes with persistent tunica vasculosa lentis was not significantly higher than in eyes without it ($P = 0.057$).

5. *2000.* Lambert et al.[11] reported five eyes developing visually significant cataract.

Diode Laser Therapy

1. *1994.* Capone and Drack[16] reported transient cavitary lenticular changes in two infants.

2. *1994.* Pogrebniak et al.[9] published a case report of a visually significant cataract.

3. *1995.* Seiberth et al.[17] noted that neither lenticular opacity nor cataract formation was observed in eyes with tunica vasculosa lentis. The number of burns was 1,556 ±315 in their series.

4. *1995.* Campolattaro and Lueder[13] reported development of a cataract in an eye with nanophthalmos; the fellow eye remained clear.

5. *1997.* A survey conducted by Gold[7] revealed a total of 21 cataracts in eyes treated by diode laser—9 were visually significant and 12 were not.

6. *1997.* Christiansen and Bradford[18] reported a case of bilateral visually significant cataracts that developed in a premature infant treated for threshold ROP in one eye with persistent tunica vasculosa lentis in both eyes. A total of 1,529 burns were delivered to the right eye, and 1,259 to the left eye.

7. *2000.* Lambert et al.[11] reported five eyes that developed visually significant cataracts a mean of 9.6 weeks after laser treatment.

8. *2002.* Fallaha et al.[19] reported the clinical outcome of confluent diode laser photoablation for ROP. The authors noticed postoperative cataracts in 4.9% of eyes (4/81). Two infants were noted to develop bilateral cataracts. One patient developed visually insignificant peripheral cortical lens opacities 6 months after laser treatment. The second infant developed dense central lens opacities 5 months after laser photoablation and underwent bilateral cataract surgery. This infant had received 1,500 laser burns in both eyes.

9. *2002.* Paysee et al.[12] reported a low incidence of acquired cataracts following transpupillary diode laser photocoagulation for threshold ROP in a large group of treated eyes. Only one eye (0.003%) developed small nonprogressive peripheral cortical lenticular opacities that were noted shortly after treatment. The advantage of diode over argon may be most visible in infants with significant persistent anterior tunica vasculosa lentis.

Cryotherapy

1. *1997.* A survey conducted by Gold[7] revealed a total of five cataracts in eyes treated with cryotherapy—three were visually significant and two were not.

2. *1998.* Repka et al.[5] reported that cataract surgery was required in 2% of eyes with threshold ROP and was

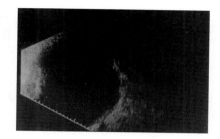

FIGURE 32-1. Preoperative B-scan in the left eye of a 44-month-old girl with a secondary cataract. Same child as described in the legend to Fig. 32-2.

performed equally often in treated (4/235) and control (3/231) eyes. An association with cryotherapy was not found, as control eyes were as likely as treated eyes to have cataracts develop of sufficient severity to warrant surgery.

3. *2001.* Shalev and associates[20] reported a randomized comparison of cryotherapy versus diode laser and reported no cataract in either group at 7 years of follow-up.

MANAGEMENT

Preventive

A near-confluent pattern of treatment may be equally effective at preventing retinal detachment (compared to confluent treatment) and less likely to result in the formation of a cataract for an infant with threshold ROP.[21] Also, use of longer-wavelength laser energy, such as the diode laser (810 nm), which is minimally absorbed by hemoglobin, could decrease the risk of cataract formation. This is especially true for eyes with persistent tunica vasculosa lentis.

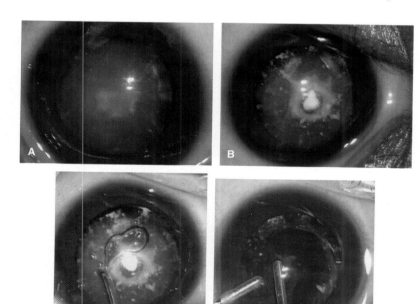

FIGURE 32-2. A 44-month-old girl with ROP had received laser treatment during infancy. Gradually she developed cataracts in both eyes. Associated findings include degenerative myopia (axial length, 26 mm OU) and strabismus. The right eye also has a macular scar. Right eye fundus examination 1 week postoperatively revealed chorioretinal scarring almost up to the border of zone 1. **A.** Right eye with total cataract. Note changes in anterior capsule. **B–D.** Left eye with total cataract. Note dense fibrous changes in anterior capsule (B). A Kloti radiofrequency diathermy unit was used to create capsulotomy (C). Note changes in anterior and posterior capsules.

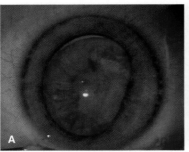
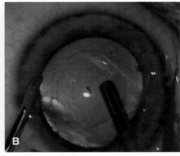
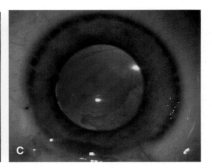

FIGURE 32-3. A 3.5-year-old girl who was born premature and developed ROP. The right eye developed inoperable retinal detachment and became phthisical. The left eye underwent laser therapy and developed cataract. Note fibrous changes in anterior capsule. This eye received a 14.5-diopter SA60 (Alcon AcrySof) intraocular lens implantation.

Therapeutic

A thorough retinal examination is necessary. If the retina cannot be visualized, a B-scan ultrasound is recommended (Fig. 32-1). Lambert et al. recommended to defer cataract surgery if there are objective signs of anterior segment ischemia, because cataract surgery may accelerate the process of these eyes becoming phthisical.[11] The general principles of pediatric cataract surgery described in this book should be applied to such eyes (Figs. 32-2A–D and 32-3A–C).

We have observed that these eyes are more often associated with fibrous changes in the anterior capsule (Figs. 32-2 and 32-3). When performing anterior capsulotomy in eyes with a fibrous capsule, we try to avoid the fibrous area if possible. If that is not possible, we have found a Kloti diathermy unit or Fugo unit useful to make an opening through a fibrous capsule. It is also important to remember that sometimes the posterior capsule may have been compromised during previous surgery.

OUTCOME

Nine of the 10 eyes described by Lambert et al.[11] progressed to phthisis bulbi after cataract surgery. A Medline search performed by Lambert et al. revealed clinical reports of 16 infants who developed a cataract(s) after transpupillary laser photoablation for threshold ROP. Cataracts were visually significant in six of these patients, and in three patients they resolved spontaneously. The remaining 10 patients had a total cataract(s) and underwent cataract surgery. Nine of these 16 patients developed bilateral cataract. Five of the eyes were reported to progress to inoperable retinal detachment, even though the retinas were reported to be attached in all but one patient at the time of cataract surgery. Some recent studies have reported an encouraging surgical outcome for posterior chamber intraocular lens implantation in premature infants with cataracts regardless of the presence of ROP,[22] and there are literature reports of favorable outcomes for cataract surgery in adult eyes with ROP.[23,24]

CONCLUSION

To summarize, cataracts rarely occur in eyes with ROP. Argon laser–treated eyes are at higher risk of developing secondary cataracts. Eyes with persistent fetal vasculature undergoing laser therapy are at higher risk for development of cataracts. Preventive measures play a significant role in minimizing the risk of cataract formation in eyes with ROP. For cataract surgery and intraocular lens implantation, general principles of pediatric cataract surgery should be followed.

REFERENCES

1. Ward RM, Beachy JC. Neonatal complications following preterm birth. *BJOG* 2003;110:8–16.
2. Palmer EA, Flynn JT, Hardy RJ, Phelps DL, Phillips CL, Schaffer DB, et al. Incidence and early course of retinopathy of prematurity. The Cryotherapy for Retinopathy of Prematurity Cooperative Group. *Ophthalmology* 1991;98:1628–1640.
3. Gilbert C, Rahi J, Eckstein M, O'Sullivan J, Foster A. Retinopathy of prematurity in middle-income countries. *Lancet* 1997;350:12–14.
4. SanGiovanni JP, Chew EY, Reed GF, Remaley NA, Bateman JB, Sugimoto TA, et al. Infantile cataract in the collaborative perinatal project: prevalence and risk factors. *Arch Ophthalmol* 2002;120:1559–1565.
5. Repka MX, Summers CG, Palmer EA, Dobson V, Tung B, Davis B. The incidence of ophthalmologic interventions in children with birth weights less than 1251 grams. Results through 5 1/2 years. Cryotherapy for Retinopathy of Prematurity Cooperative Group. *Ophthalmology* 1998;105:1621–1627.
6. Alden ER, Kalina RE, Hodson WA. Transient cataracts in low-birth-weight infants. *J Pediatr* 1973;82:314–318.
7. Gold RS. Cataracts associated with treatment for retinopathy of prematurity. *J Pediatr Ophthalmol Strabismus* 1997;34:123–124.
8. Drack AV, Burke JP, Pulido JS, Keech RV. Transient punctate lenticular opacities as a complication of argon laser photoablation in an infant with retinopathy of prematurity. *Am J Ophthalmol* 1992;113:583–584.

9. Pogrebniak AE, Bolling JP, Stewart MW. Argon laser-induced cataract in an infant with retinopathy of prematurity. *Am J Ophthalmol* 1994;117:261–262.
10. Knight-Nanan DM, Algawi K, Bowell R, O'Keefe M. Advanced cicatricial retinopathy of prematurity—Outcome and complications. *Br J Ophthalmol* 1996;80:343–345.
11. Lambert SR, Capone A Jr, Cingle KA, Drack AV. Cataract and phthisis bulbi after laser photoablation for threshold retinopathy of prematurity. *Am J Ophthalmol* 2000;129:585–591.
12. Paysse EA, Miller A, Brady McCreery KM, Coats DK. Acquired cataracts after diode laser photocoagulation for threshold retinopathy of prematurity. *Ophthalmology* 2002;109:1662–1665.
13. Campolattaro BN, Lueder GT. Cataract in infants treated with argon laser photocoagulation for threshold retinopathy of prematurity. *Am J Ophthalmol* 1995;120:264–266.
14. Christiansen SP, Bradford JD. Cataract in infants treated with argon laser photocoagulation for threshold retinopathy of prematurity. *Am J Ophthalmol* 1995;119:175–180.
15. O'Neil JW, Hutchinson AK, Saunders RA, Wilson ME. Acquired cataracts after argon laser photocoagulation for retinopathy of prematurity. *J AAPOS* 1998;2:48–51.
16. Capone A Jr, Drack AV. Transient lens changes after diode laser retinal photoablation for retinopathy of prematurity. *Am J Ophthalmol* 1994;118:533–535.
17. Seiberth V, Linderkamp O, Vardarli I, Knorz MC, Liesenhoff H. Diode laser photocoagulation for threshold retinopathy of prematurity in eyes with tunica vasculosa lentis. *Am J Ophthalmol* 1995;119:748–751.
18. Christiansen SP, Bradford JD. Cataract following diode laser photoablation for retinopathy of prematurity. *Arch Ophthalmol* 1997;115:275–276.
19. Fallaha N, Lynn MJ, Aaberg TM Jr, Lambert SR. Clinical outcome of confluent laser photoablation for retinopathy of prematurity. *J AAPOS* 2002;6:81–85.
20. Shalev B, Farr AK, Repka MX. Randomized comparison of diode laser photocoagulation versus cryotherapy for threshold retinopathy of prematurity: seven-year outcome. *Am J Ophthalmol* 2001;132:76–80.
21. Ferrone PJ, Banach MJ, Trese MT. Cataract and phthisis bulbi after laser photoablation for threshold retinopathy of prematurity. *Am J Ophthalmol* 2001;132:948–949.
22. Yu YS, Kim SJ, Chang BL. Cataract surgery in children with and without retinopathy of prematurity. *J Cataract Refract Surg* 2004;30:96–101.
23. Krolicki TJ, Tasman W. Cataract extraction in adults with retinopathy of prematurity. *Arch Ophthalmol* 1995;113:173–177.
24. Farr AK, Stark WJ, Haller JA. Cataract surgery by phacoemulsification in adults with retinopathy of prematurity. *Am J Ophthalmol* 2001;132:306–310.

Cataract Surgery in Eyes Treated for Retinoblastoma

Rupal H. Trivedi and M. Edward Wilson, Jr.

Retinoblastoma (RB) is the most common primary intraocular tumor in children[1–3] (Fig. 33-1). Several options are available for the treatment of RB, and the treatment selected depends on the size, extent, and laterality of the tumors, visual potential of the eye, and patient's systemic status. Treatments that are currently advocated include enucleation, chemoreduction, external beam radiotherapy (EBRT), scleral plaque irradiation, photocoagulation, cryotherapy, thermotherapy, and chemotherapy.[3–16] Although primary enucleation is still the preferred method for advanced unilateral cases, application of modern treatment techniques in the management of RB has resulted in a decrease in the frequency of enucleation. The direction in the management of less advanced cases of RB has now shifted toward conservative measures aimed at salvaging the eye and possibly preserving vision.[4,17] EBRT was the first commonly used therapeutic alternative to enucleation. It offers a better structural and functional outcome than enucleation. A recently reported approach has used chemoreduction (the use of chemotherapy to reduce the size of tumors) followed by local therapies to destroy any residual tumor (laser, cryotherapy, or plaque irradiation).[5–13,17]

Conservative modalities, however, can lead to various ocular complications.[3,18] The major ocular complication of EBRT and of episcleral plaque brachytherapy is radiation-induced cataracts. The crystalline lens is the most radiosensitive structure in the eye. Radiation-induced cataracts can be formed, as these rays penetrate the cornea and interact with the molecular components of the lens. The morphology of radiation-induced cataract was described by Cogan and Donaldson.[19] Following exposure of the lens to radiation, there is a latent period of variable length, depending largely on the radiation dose and the age of the patient. The initial changes are seen as vacuoles at the posterior pole, followed by involvement of the cortex. Posterior subcapsular cataract is the most common morphology seen in such eyes.

In a retrospective series, Amandola et al.[14] reported that 2 of 23 (8.7%) eyes developed cataracts after episcleral plaque therapy, 4 of 21 (19.0%) developed cataracts after EBRT, and 9 of 29 (31.0%) after combined episcleral plaque and EBRT therapy. Chemoreduction often leads to satisfactory RB control for Reese–Ellsworth (RE) stages I–IV, with treatment failures necessitating additional EBRT in only 10% of the eyes. In another series, eyes with RE stage V required EBRT in 47.0%.[5]

In one study, cataracts occurred in 87% of eyes treated with radiotherapy.[15] In 1939, Reese[20] reported on the examination of 112 eyes with radiation cataract. More recently, the incidence of radiation-induced cataracts has decreased dramatically because of lens-sparing radiotherapy techniques, and the growing popularity of chemotherapy rather than radiation. Cataract surgery after RB treatment was needed in 45 of 900 (5%) eyes in a recent series.[17]

The interval from EBRT to documentation of a radiation-induced cataract ranged from 9 to 48 months (median, 20 months).[21] Portellos and Buckley[22] performed surgery for cataract a mean of 54 months after EBRT. In a series by Honavar et al.,[17] the mean time interval for cataract surgery was 26 months after the final treatment for RB. As the average age at diagnosis of RB is 18 months, it is reasonable to assume that most of the eyes developing cataracts are still within the amblyogenic age range. Secondary cataract formation complicates the management of RB by precluding visualization of the tumor and may necessitate enucleation if there is suspicion of tumor recurrence. Intraocular surgery in these eyes raises genuine concerns about the patient's systemic outcome because of the risks for viable tumor seeding.[17,23,24] However, surgical intervention for cataracts is justified in certain clinical

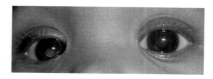

FIGURE 33-1. A 9-month-old boy with bilateral retinoblastoma. (Courtesy of Dr. O. Arambulo, Hospital Universitario de Maracaibo, Maracaibo, Venezuela.)

settings, especially if the tumor is judged to be clinically stable and in regression.[17]

Few case reports have documented simultaneous association of RB with cataract.[25–27] Our focus in this chapter is to review the literature and provide guidelines regarding management of secondary cataracts in eyes with RB (Figs. 33-2 and 33-3). In 1939, Reese[20] first reported operative treatment of radiation cataracts. Of the 112 eyes with cataracts, 25 eyes were operated on; intracapsular extraction was done on 16, extracapsular extraction on 6, and linear extraction on 3.[20] Reese[20] noted that

in cataract caused by irradiation there is a tendency toward a proliferation of the epithelium un-

der the anterior capsule into a metaplastic fibrous layer. This strengthens the anterior capsule and makes this type of cataract particularly suitable for intracapsular extraction. Extracapsular extraction in such cases is contraindicated because the lens epithelium remaining after the nucleus is extracted may continue to proliferate and form dense fibrous tissue, which tends to produce iridocyclitis and secondary glaucoma.

Since then, numerous other innovations in pediatric cataract surgery have evolved. During the past six-decades there have been several reports of successful and innovative surgical procedures in patients treated for RB.[16,21,22,28] In 2000, Honavar et al. published an article analyzing the results of intraocular surgery in patients treated for RB.[17] However, there is still concern regarding the safety of performing any intraocular surgery in such eyes, mainly because of the risk for tumor dissemination and systemic metastasis after open globe manipulation of eyes with RB.[17,23,24]

Following are some practical considerations one should keep in mind when treating such eyes.

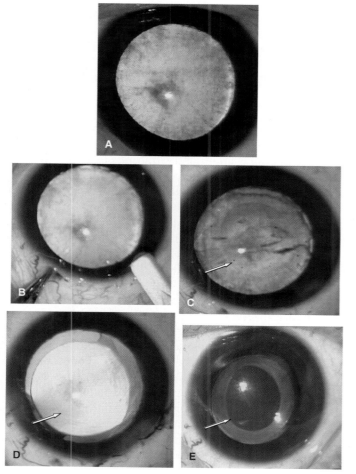

FIGURE 33-2. A. An eye with a radiation-induced cataract (OD) in a 4-year-old child. Retinoblastoma was treated with radiotherapy and chemotherapy. **B.** Corneal incision. **C.** Anterior capsulotomy (arrow shows the edge of the capsulotomy). **D.** AcrySof IOL implantation in-the-bag. Note the intact posterior capsule; the arrow shows the edge of the anterior capsule. **E.** Two months after cataract surgery. The arrow shows the edge of the anterior capsule.

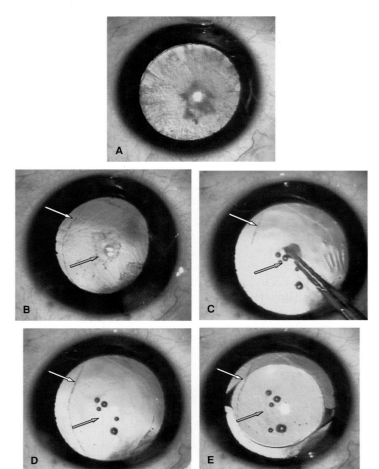

FIGURE 33-3. A. Left eye of the child described in the legend Fig. 33-2. **B.** A Fugo plasma blade was used to perform anterior capsulotomy. During hydrodissection, a radial tear developed. The white arrow shows the edge of the anterior capsule. Note posterior capsule plaque (black arrow). **C.** Manual posterior capsulorhexis was performed to remove the posterior capsule plaque. Care was taken to avoid disturbing the vitreous face. **D.** Posterior capsulorhexis. **E.** A single-piece Acyrsof IOL was implanted in the capsular bag. Haptics were positioned away from the areas of anterior capsule tear.

1. *Consultation with an experienced RB specialist* is prudent during preoperative and postoperative management of such eyes.

2. The *optimum interval* between completion of treatment of RB and intraocular surgery is not clearly established. Intraocular surgery should be withheld if the tumor is viable or if there is uncertainty about its activity. Even in patients with documented tumor regression, it may be worthwhile to allow observation for at least 6–12 months before attempting cataract removal.[17] Tumor status and risk of surgery must be assessed individually and discussed in detail with the family and physician treating RB before arriving at a decision about cataract removal.

3. Dissemination of RB cells through the cataract surgery *incision* has been reported.[21] The clear corneal incision may reduce the risk of inadvertent conjuctival implantation of viable tumor cells and may allow for direct inspection of the incision site for tumor recurrence (unlike the limbal or scleral incision, which may be obscured by the overlying conjuctival flap)[17] (Fig. 33-2B).

4. The presence of a *posterior capsule* opening theoretically increases the risk of dissemination of viable RB cells to the anterior chamber and extraocular extension through the incision site. In a multicenter trial published in 1990,[21] major complications occurred only in those eyes that underwent pars plana or pars plicata lensectomy. One eye that underwent pars plana lensectomy developed a retinal detachment. Authors recommended avoidance of posterior capsulotomy in eyes with persistent vitreous haze. If RB regression has been deemed stable for at least 6 to 12 months after cataract surgery, Nd:YAG laser posterior capsulotomy may be cautiously performed where required. However, Portellos and Buckley[22] later reported the safety of extracapsular cataract extraction and posterior chamber intraocular lens (IOL) implantation in combination with pars plana posterior capsulotomy and anterior vitrectomy in a series of eight patients (11 eyes) with radiation-induced cataracts after RB treatment. We prefer to avoid opening the posterior capsule if the posterior capsule is not associated with plaque and age limits permit (Fig. 33-2D). However, more often these eyes are associated with posterior capsule plaque (Fig. 33-3B) or defect. In this case, it may become necessary to perform posterior capsulotomy. However, we still try to achieve manual posterior capsulorhexis (with intake anterior vitreous face), to avoid vitreous face disturbance and subsequent vitrectomy (Figs. 33-3C and D).

5. Implantation of an *IOL* by itself may not increase the risk of recurrence of RB or systemic metastasis and can be considered for providing optimal visual rehabilitation after cataract surgery.[17] It is important to remember that these eyes are *poor candidates for contact lens wear due to dry eyes associated with decreased tear production from lacrimal gland irradiation.* Thus in unilateral cases IOL implantation is the only reasonable option for the correction of aphakia.

6. *Cytologic examination* of vitrectomy fluid can provide direct intraoperative evidence of viable RB. Prompt enucleation and adjuvant chemotherapy with or without orbital radiotherapy may be considered in such situations.

7. *Close long-term follow-up* is warranted, for several years, to detect possible tumor recurrence and systemic metastasis. Recurrence of RB after intraocular surgery is a potentially serious problem. Tumor recurrence has been reported to range from 0 to 45% after various intraocular procedures. One study[21] reported a recurrence of RB in three eyes (8%), necessitating enucleation of two eyes. Orbital exenteration was required in one case for subconjuctival RB recurrence that developed at the site of cataract incision. RB recurrence was confined primarily to eyes with persistent vitreous haze or vitreous hemorrhage at the time of surgery. There was no systemic metastasis. Use of the limbal approach and avoidance of primary posterior capsulotomy and scleral incision was recommended. Honavar et al.[17] reported recurrence of RB in 20.6% (7/34) of eyes undergoing cataract surgery, all of which underwent subsequent enucleation. None of the patients who underwent cataract surgery developed metastasis. Most recurrence occurred within the first year, with the longest interval being 19 months in that series. Patients needing a scleral buckling procedure or pars plana vitrectomy seemed to be at greater risk for RB recurrence compared with those needing cataract surgery.[17] RB continued to regress in 31 eyes (69%) after pars plana vitrectomy. A viable tumor was detected by cytologic examination of the vitrectomy fluid in two patients (4%) in whom vitreous hemorrhage had precluded visualization of the tumor immediately before intraocular surgery. Both of these patients underwent immediate enucleation.

Long-term follow-up of these eyes is helpful to see whether surgery in eyes harboring regressed RB allows for a reasonable visual outcome, as opposed to recurrence of RB necessitating enucleation or systemic metastasis. Even after a successful surgical outcome, the final *visual acuity* depends on several factors. In addition to clarity of the visual axis, other factors such as amblyopia, refractive error,

macular tumors,[29] radiation complications (keratopathy and/or retinopathy), optic atrophy, and chronic retinal detachment can affect visual outcome.

CONCLUSION

It is important to weigh the expected benefit of visual rehabilitation against the risk of tumor recurrence and metastasis and to discuss it with the family before proceeding to cataract surgery.[17] Current techniques for pediatric cataract and IOL surgery can be applicable for radiation-induced cataracts after complete regression of RB. However, considering the risk of tumor recurrence, it is advisable to take a cautious approach, including clear corneal incision and preservation of the posterior capsule if possible.

REFERENCES

1. Bhurgri Y, Bhurgri H, Usman A, Faridi N, Malik J, Puri R, et al. Epidemiology of ocular malignancies in Karachi. *Asian Pac J Cancer Prev* 2003;4:352–357.
2. Cheng CY, Hsu WM. Incidence of eye cancer in Taiwan: an 18-year review. *Eye* 2004;18:152–158.
3. Shields JA, Shields CL. Managment and prognosis of retinoblastoma. In: Shields JA, Shields CL, eds. *Intraocular Tumors: A Text and Atlas.* Philadelphia, PA: WB Saunders, 1992:377–392.
4. Sussman DA, Escalona-Benz E, Benz MS, Hayden BC, Feuer W, Cicciarelli N, et al. Comparison of retinoblastoma reduction for chemotherapy vs external beam radiotherapy. *Arch Ophthalmol* 2003;121:979–984.
5. Shields CL, Honavar SG, Meadows AT, Shields JA, Demirci H, Singh A, et al. Chemoreduction plus focal therapy for retinoblastoma: factors predictive of need for treatment with external beam radiotherapy or enucleation. *Am J Ophthalmol* 2002;133:657–664.
6. Simpson AE, Gilbert JA, Rudnick DE, Geroski DH, Aaberg TMJ, Edelhauser HF. Transscleral diffusion of carboplatin: an in vitro and in vivo study. *Arch Ophthalmol* 2002;120:1069–1074.
7. Shields CL, Shields JA. Recent developments in the management of retinoblastoma. *J Pediatr Ophthalmol Strabismus* 1999;36:8–18.
8. Sorbin L, Hayden BC, Murray TG, et al. External beam radiation "salvage" therapy in transgenic murine retinoblastoma. *Arch Ophthalmol* 2004;122:251–257.
9. Shields CL, Shields JA, Cater J, Othmane I, Singh AD, Micaily B. Plaque radiotherapy for retinoblastoma: long-term tumor control and treatment complications in 208 tumors. *Ophthalmology* 2001;108:2116–2121.
10. Hamel P, Heon E, Gallie BL, Budning AS. Focal therapy in the management of retinoblastoma: when to start and when to stop. *J AAPOS* 2000;4:334–337.
11. Scott IU, Murray TG, Feuer WJ, Van Quill K, Markoe AM, Ling S, et al. External beam radiotherapy in retinoblastoma: tumor control and comparison of 2 techniques. *Arch Ophthalmol* 1999;117:766–770.
12. Pradhan DG, Sandridge AL, Mullaney P, Abboud E, Karcioglu ZA, Kandil A, et al. Radiation therapy for retinoblastoma: a retrospective review of 120 patients. *Int J Radiat Oncol Biol Phys* 1997;39:3–13.
13. Blach LE, McCormick B, Abramson DH. External beam radiation therapy and retinoblastoma: long-term results in the comparison of two techniques. *Int J Radiat Oncol Biol Phys* 1996;35:45–51.
14. Amendola BE, Lamm FR, Markoe AM, Karlsson UL, Shields J, Shields CL, et al. Radiotherapy of retinoblastoma. A review of 63 children treated with different irradiation techniques. *Cancer* 1990;66:21–26.

15. Fontanesi J, Pratt CB, Hustu HO, Coffey D, Kun LE, Meyer D. Use of irradiation for therapy of retinoblastoma in children more than 1 year old: the St. Jude Children's Research Hospital experience and review of literature. *Med Pediatr Oncol* 1995;24:321–326.

16. Shields CL, Shields JA, De Potter P. New treatment modalities for retinoblastoma. *Curr Opin Ophthalmol* 1996;7:20–26.

17. Honavar SG, Shields CL, Shields JA, Demirci H, Naduvilath TJ. Intraocular surgery after treatment of retinoblastoma. *Arch Ophthalmol* 2001;119:1613–1621.

18. Merriam GR, Focht EF. A clinical study of radiation cataracts and their relationship to dose. *Am J Roentgenol Radiat Ther* 1957;77:759–785.

19. Cogan DG, Donaldson DD. Experimental radiation cataracts. I. Cataracts in the rabbit following single x-ray exposure. *Arch Ophthalmol* 1951;45:508.

20. Reese AB. Operative treatment of radiation cataracts. *Arch Ophthalmol* 1939;21:476–485.

21. Brooks HR Jr, Meyer D, Shields JA, Balas AG, Nelson LB, Fontanesi J. Removal of radiation-induced cataracts in patients treated for retinoblastoma. *Arch Ophthalmol* 1990;108:1701–1708.

22. Portellos M, Buckley EG. Cataract surgery and intraocular lens implantation in patients with retinoblastoma. *Arch Ophthalmol* 1998;116:449–452.

23. Shields CL, Honavar S, Shields JA, Demirci H, Meadows AT. Vitrectomy in eyes with unsuspected retinoblastoma. *Ophthalmology* 2000;107:2250–2255.

24. Stevenson KE, Hungerford J, Garner A. Local extraocular extension of retinoblastoma following intraocular surgery. *Br J Ophthalmol* 1989;73:739–742.

25. Friendly DS, Parks MM. Concurrence of hereditary congenital cataracts and hereditary retinoblastoma. *Arch Ophthalmol* 1970;84:525–527.

26. Brown GC, Shields JA, Oglesby RB. Anterior polar cataracts associated with bilateral retinoblastoma. *Am J Ophthalmol* 1979;87:276.

27. Hasan SJ, Brooks M, Ambati J, Kielar R, Stevens JL. Retinoblastoma with cataract and ectopia lentis. *J AAPOS* 2003;7:425–427.

28. Bhattacharjee H, Bhattacharjee K, Chakraborty D, Talukdar M, Das D. Cataract surgery and intraocular lens implantation in a retinoblastoma case treated by external-beam radiation therapy. *J Cataract Refract Surg* 2003;29:1837–1841.

29. Desjardins L, Chefchaouni MC, Lumbroso L, Levy C, Asselain B, Bours D, et al. Functional results after treatment of retinoblastoma. *J AAPOS* 2002;6:108–111.

Preexisting Posterior Capsule Defects

Daljit Singh, Seema K. Singh, and Kiranjit Singh

We have been observing and puzzling over preexisting posterior capsular defects (PPCD) since 1981. In 1992, the noted Indian anatomist and embryologist, Professor Indarjit Dewan, explained that it is possible for any membrane, including a part of the posterior capsule membrane, to disappear at any time during the course of embryonic development. We encounter PPCD in about 10% of pediatric cataract cases (Fig. 34-1). It is seen in unilateral as well as in bilateral cases. With the posterior capsular barrier breached, the elements of the developing crystalline lens are exposed to outside fluids. With the ingress of even the scanty previtreous fluid into the crystalline lens, a chain of events starts. There is local hydration, opacification, liquefaction and absorption, and posterior migration of the lens material toward Berger's space, as well as changes in the rest of the lens and, often, even changes in the anterior capsule. The suggested culpability of the posterior capsule break/partial absence as a trigger factor for the myriad lenticular changes is based on general principles of physiology and pathology. Besides, there are other posterior capsule abnormalities that present during the course of pediatric cataract surgery.[1]

Some of the observed changes, based on >6,500 pediatric cataract cases during the past 23 years, are as follows.

1. There may be *near-total absorption of the lens*, so that a semitransparent membrane is seen. The anterior capsule may show some opacification. The posterior capsule may be very thin and fragile, with or without telltale signs of a leakage to be described later.

2. The lens looks membranous, sometimes even transparent, while most of the lens matter lies outside the posterior capsule, on the anterior vitreous. There is an unquestionable opening in the posterior capsule.

3. The opaque fetal nucleus appears out of place. The nucleus gets displaced backward since the supporting posterior cortex and the capsule are deficient/absorbed. On moving the eyeball, one can make out a dense white round or oval ring on the posterior surface. The ring may be fairly large. It marks the edge of a same-sized opening in the posterior capsule. As soon as anterior capsulotomy is performed, the lens material starts flowing anteriorly and the vitreous follows.

4. A milk bag cataract with or without signs of hypermaturity on the anterior capsule can result from the dissolution of the lens and fluid collection by osmotic forces. The presence of any kind of scar on the posterior capsule is an indication that the process was likely initiated there (Fig. 34-2).

5. A cataractous posterior lenticonus, be it small or large, may show localized opacification and signs of leakage that call for very careful handling during surgery. There are some cases in which the cataract extends into the deep cortex and the nucleus. In such cases a posterior capsule defect, even a large one, is detected only when the lenticonus comes into view. The lenticonus area has a tendency to bulge anteriorly when the lens matter is removed. If there is a capsular dehiscence, the vitreous becomes prolapsed (Fig. 34-3).

6. The cortical material around the defective leaking posterior capsule attracts blood vessels and develops into a dense fibrovascular membrane (Fig. 34-4).

7. Very large ciliary processes may be found adherent to the posterior surface of the lens and may even reach the center. The opaque lens may be absorbed to a varying extent.

8. There may exist a large, thick, pearly white membrane behind a completely transparent lens. We do not know if this is a legacy of persistent fetal vasculature or an independent entity. The vitreous in these cases may be fluid, so that the eye tends to collapse the moment this membrane is breached (Fig. 34-5).

9. A posterior polar or subcapsular cataract may be attached to a persistent hyaloid artery. When cut, this artery has a tendency to bleed profusely.

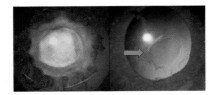

FIGURE 34-1. At age 7 months a congenital cataract shows only a small amount of lens matter and a dense white membrane in the central position, the removal of which reveals a posterior capsular opening with a thickened margin. The thickened margin suggests that the opening was preexisting, since it cannot be a result of surgical injury.

10. A peculiar, dumbell-shaped cataract may occur. The periphery is like a Sommering ring, while the central one third is thick and membranous. The major contributor to this membrane is the thickened anterior capsule; when it is carefully removed, absence of the posterior capsule may be noted, or it may look like a thin, crumpled or broken membrane atop the vitreous.

11. An onion ring–like posterior polar cataract may occur. A dense white opacity is an ominous sign that the underlying capsule is fragile or absent. If it shows concentric rings, it should be examined carefully. The posterior capsule in the direct proximity of the opacity undergoes certain changes.

a. It becomes thin and fragile.
b. The capsule becomes adherent to the overlying lenticular opacity.
c. Actual cracks develop near the edge of the opacity, which result in the formation of chalky white spots.

In scenario a, it is possible to preserve the posterior capsule with careful surgery. In situation b and c, it is usually not possible to avoid a posterior capsular hole. Onion ring cataract increases in size over years, increasing the fragility of the posterior capsule at the same time.

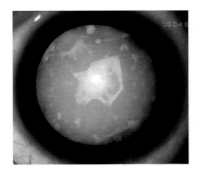

FIGURE 34-2. An 11-month-old child with a milk bag cataract. There are multiple patches of anterior capsular thickening, the one in the center being the largest.

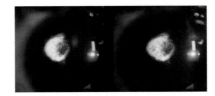

FIGURE 34-3. Three-dimensional picture of a posterior lenticonus showing dense opacification along the edges and base of the conus deformity.

12. A *posterior capsular plaque* is seen quite often. It varies in size, shape, thickness, and density. Often it seems to occupy Berger's space. Its origin is not understood. It might arise de novo or it may be related to PPCD. Sometimes blood vessels are seen, suggesting that it may be related to the tunica vasculosa lentis. In general, the more severe the changes in the lens as a result of posterior capsular crack or absence, the longer has been the process of interaction between the crystalline lens and the outside fluids. Severe changes in a newborn baby lead us to conclude that the process started in the early period of lens development.

The clinical presentation of PPCDs can be extremely varied due to the numerous possible combinations of primary and secondary changes in the lens and the posterior capsule. However, the surgeon's main concern is to remove the opacity without disturbing the vitreous and be able to implant an intraocular lens (IOL) at the same time or prepare a safe ground for later secondary IOL implantation. Besides the developmental posterior capsule defects, the posterior capsule also gets ruptured by blunt

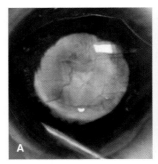 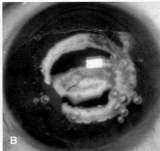

FIGURE 34-4. A 1-year-old patient with a unilateral opaque thick membrane showing a number of blood vessels that are derived from the numerous ciliary processes adherent to the edge of the opacity. A few of them are shown by retracting the pupil (**A**) with a cannula. The membrane was cut (**B**) with a Fugo Blade, and an iris-claw lens (Singh version) implanted. Manual iridectomy was not done, for fear of bleeding from the underlying ciliary processes. Instead Fugo Blade iridotomy was performed at the midperiphery of 5 o'clock. Adherent ciliary processes are also visible in the iridotomy area.

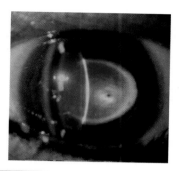

FIGURE 34-5. Thick, pearly white membrane on the posterior capsule.

and perforating injuries. Immediately after the injury, the capsular opening has a sharp clean edge. Soon, the tell-tale secondary reactive changes develop in and around the area of the posterior capsule opening. The consequences of the posterior capsular dehiscence/opening on the adjoining capsule and the nearby lens–cortex form the basis of the following *Singh signs.*

1. A deep anterior chamber is an important sign that results from the absorption of part of the crystalline lens.

2. White to chalky-white spots are produced, which are seen in front of and around the posterior capsular defect. The number of spots varies from a few to a great many. Their size is also variable. Most of them are like the spots of asteroid bodies in the vitreous. They have the same appearance that we often see around a traumatic perforation of the anterior capsule.

3. The capsule behind the opaque lens may show a partial or a complete white ring-shaped opacity. This opacity is contained within the posterior cortex, while the posterior capsule shows a hole with chalky-white spots on and around the defect.

4. Rarely, an opening in the posterior capsule shows pigment along the margins. Fine dustlike pigment along with fine dense white opacities may be seen in the Berger space. The presence of pigment suggests widespread movement of the fluid beyond the posterior capsular defect.

DIAGNOSIS

The diagnosis of a posterior capsule defect rests on the following clinical findings.

Preoperative

If the cortex anterior to the defective posterior capsule is partially or wholly clear, it is possible to visualize the hallmark of a posterior capsule break—dense white or chalky-

white spots. A lens that is thinner than normal, as evidenced by an abnormally deep anterior chamber, should further heighten suspicion. Dense white opacity behind an opaque fetal nucleus points to the defect. The best case to study is one of posterior lenticonus, if the opacity is limited to the ectatic area and the rest of the lens is clear. Posterior capsule rent can be suspected from the various abnormal manifestations that are seen in the lens and the capsule.

B-Scan ultrasound is necessary when a thorough slit-lamp examination cannot be done due to dense opacity. It might suggest a break in the posterior capsule if the posterior edge of the lens is not sharp and the adjacent vitreous space shows new shadows. In trauma cases the lens masses may reach a greater depth.

Intraoperative

If surgeons are not aware of the clinical entity of a preexisting posterior capsule/rent/rupture/absence/leakage/defect, they are surprised and shocked to see the vitreous prolapse, when everything seemed to be proceeding normally.

SURGICAL MANAGEMENT

Pars Plana Approach

We do not use the pars plana approach, for there are possibilities of damage to the vitreous cisterns and the creation of a lens–vitreous mix, which may give rise to vitreoretinal problems, glaucoma, and inflammation.

Anterior Approach

For any pediatric cataract in which the deeper layers of the opaque lens cannot be visualized or that shows the anatomical features of a possible PPCD, the surgery should proceed as follows.

1. The pupil should be dilated fully with preoperative local mydriatics. It may be reinforced by intracameral, 0.25% preservative-free phenylepherine. The lens should be examined under coaxial light as well as oblique light.

2. During surgery a pull on the anterior capsule in an eye with a defective posterior capsule can produce a tear in the capsule. Extreme caution should be used to avoid transmission of capsulotomy force to the vulnerable posterior capsule. A better way is to perform capsulotomy with Fugo Blade, which provides a truly traction-free incision.[2–5] Capsulotomy in the following specific circumstances can be quite demanding.

a. *Membranous cataract.* It is a good idea to inflate the capsular bag with a viscoelastic material. Any type of capsulotomy requires care, as the posterior capsule is very near. If a planned in-the-bag implantation is not possible, the posterior chamber lens is placed on the anterior capsule and the central part of the anterior as well as the posterior capsule is removed with a vitrector or, preferably, a Fugo Blade, followed by a small anterior vitrectomy. There is always some lens cortex that needs to be removed.

b. *Mostly empty capsular bag.* When the unabsorbed part of the cataract is outside the posterior capsule, a traction-free anterior capsulectomy is followed by aspiration of the prolapsed lens matter. Usually no vitreous gets disturbed. If the capsular bag is small, as is quite frequent, in-the-bag implantation is out of the question, unless special small posterior chamber IOLs can be obtained. An iris-fixated artisan lens is suitable for such a case. A small anterior vitrectomy needs to be done from under the optic of an implanted lens.

c. *Opaque posteriorly displaced fetal nucleus.* This happens either when the cortex is partly liquefied or when a PPCD allows the posterior cortex to migrate outside the capsule. The important thing is to proceed cautiously with the surgery, keeping an eye out for the possibility of a PPCD. After a large anterior capsulotomy, we lift the lens mass by injecting viscoelastic underneath it, from the sideport. The lift is started from the upper edge, by injecting viscoelastic material in the upper fornix. Every part of the fornix receives the same treatment to push out the cortex by positive pressure. Very little may be left for removal by aspiration or irrigation/aspiration. There is no danger of a large rupture of the posterior capsule, as it is well supported by healthy vitreous. The lens masses get lifted up and move in the direction of least resistance, i.e., anteriorly. The PPCD may remain preserved in its original form.

d. *Milk bag cataract.* The bag is intact at the time of surgery. One may or may not find a scar on the posterior capsule. PPCD as the cause of the milk bag cataract is a presumption in the latter case.

As soon as an anterior capsule is opened the capsular bag empties the milky fluid and capsulotomy becomes a problem. When a Fugo Blade is used the following steps are taken. A small puncture is made in the anterior capsule and the milky fluid is allowed to escape. The capsular bag is filled with high-viscosity viscoelastic. The Fugo Blade is used to do the desired capsulotomy, while simultaneously viscoelastic material is pushed from the sideport to prevent any undesired capsular movement. The capsulotomy is often completed in two or three stages. The final cutting is usually done with a scissors. No effort is made to speed up a capsulotomy in a collapsing bag or the anterior chamber; otherwise the posterior capsule may be nicked.

e. *Partial or complete opacification of the lens.* Capsulotomy is followed by dry aspiration using viscoelastic material that displaces and lifts the lens material anteriorly. Aspiration is done with a 23-gauge cannula connected to a 1-mL syringe. A 25-gauge cannula is safer from the point of view of vitreous safety. It aspirates only the lens matter. When vitreous blocks the port, it becomes nonfunctional. Gentle aspiration is recommended.

f. *Posterior lenticonus.* When it is transparent, or only the conus part is opacified, the surgery is simple. After continuous curvilinear capsulorhexis or Fugo Blade capsulotomy, the transparent lens is removed by dry aspiration after repeated injection of viscoelastic under the capsular fornices. At no time is the anterior chamber allowed to collapse, since the weakened posterior capsule in the conus can protrude and rupture, allowing the vitreous to escape.

If the posterior capsule shows typical signs of PPCDs and their significance is understood, management is the same as above, except that greater caution is required. The anterior vitreous face can be preserved.

If the central part of the lens is opaque and posterior lenticonus and PPCD are not suspected, one may encounter a situation in which the vitreous starts prolapsing as soon as the anterior capsulotomy is done. The vitreous dominates the scene, while the lens matter is still entrapped in the capsular fornices. Management is done from the sideport incisions. The vitreous is pushed back with viscoelastic. The lens matter in the fornices is displaced by injecting viscoelastic and is then aspirated with a 25-gauge cannula connected to a 1-mL syringe. The process is repeated until most or all the lens matter is removed. Vitrectomy is reserved until the end. It may be done before or after lens implantation. If a situation warrants the use of a vitrector to remove the lens matter and the vitreous, it is done as follows. The vitrector tip is directed toward the collection of lens matter. It is aspirated manually with a 1-mL syringe. As soon as the port gets blocked with vitreous, aspiration is stopped and the vitrector is turned on to chop the small amount that caused the blockage. This way, it is possible to remove most or all of the lens matter with minimum sacrifice of the vitreous.

g. *Thick fibrovascular membrane in the pupil in place of a cataract.* The membrane may or may not be adherent to the pupil margin. This condition is uncommon. Earlier we treated two cases by applying bipolar cautery to the potential bleeding sites, followed by manual dissection and cutting of the membrane. Yet bleeding did occur; it poured into the vitreous and took many weeks to become absorbed. We have also managed two cases using a Fugo Blade. In these cases the cutting, actually ablation, of the fibrovascular membrane was rather easy and bloodless.

h. *Large ciliary processes attached to the back of a normal-sized lens.* These, or similar processes attached to the edges of a shrunken cataract, need to be handled carefully for fear of bleeding and pull to the ciliary body. A Fugo Blade is ideal for this situation since there is no bleeding in the ablation path and the cutting is traction-free. Once the lens is free of the uveal tissues, it is managed according to the pathoanatomy of the case.

i. *Pearly white thick membrane presentation of the posterior capsule.* In these cases, the entire lens is transparent, and its removal is no problem. Once the membrane is reached, it is cut either manually or with a Fugo Blade. Beware of the possibility of a hyaloid vessel present on the back of the membrane. In each of the few cases we have operated on, the globe collapsed the moment the membrane was cut. This means that the vitreous gel was absent.

j. *Posterior subcapsular cataract with attached hyaloid vessel.* This diagnosis is most often known before surgery, from slit-lamp examination and from B scan. Bleeding can be confidently avoided by using bipolar cautery or, more confidently, by using a Fugo Blade.

k. *Dumbell cataract.* This is encountered frequently and is tackled in two stages. First, the large peripheral ring-like cataract is managed as follows. A circular capsulotomy is performed. Viscoelastic material is injected into the fornices of the peripheral bag (there is no bag in the center), which lifts what is practically a large Sommering's ring. It is delivered in two or more parts. The peripheral capsular bag is cleared by irrigation and aspiration. If Fugo Blade capsulotomy is done, an intact peripheral capsular bag is assured, wherein the loops of a posterior chamber lens can be engaged. The central part of the lens, which is densely membranous and has vitreous underneath, should be managed after an IOL has been implanted, which may be a posterior chamber IOL or an artisan lens. One way is to find and cut the edge of the opacity and deal with the rest with a vitrector or with forceps and scissors, depending on the case. The other is to use a Fugo Blade. There are two options available. One is to go around the edge of the opaque membrane and remove it completely. The other is to "erase" it with a small, flat Fugo Blade tip. The erasure is continued slowly until a translucent thin membrane is left, which can later be cut with a Nd:YAG laser. Or when the membrane has become thin, sodium hyaluranate is injected between the capsule and the vitreous.

Then the membrane is erased completely without causing injury to the vitreous face.

l. *Onion ring cataract.* This is sometimes seen as a familial case but, more often, as an isolated one. It seems to grow in diameter with age and the opacification also becomes denser. When white spots are seen along the edge of the onion ring, the strong possibility of a posterior capsular defect should be considered.

m. *Posterior capsular plaque.* This can be easily separated from the lens cortex. However, peeling it off the anterior vitreous is not always easy. Peeling it off may preserve the anterior vitreous face, but many times the anterior vitreous face gets ruptured. The plaque may be removed with a vitrector, along with the inevitable anterior vitrectomy. A plaque can be cleared without disturbing the vitreous, by repeatedly touching it with the flat tip of a Fugo Blade.

n. *Other abnormalities.* Microcornea and megalocornea are other abnormalities besides the lens that dictate the mode of cataract extraction and the choice of IOL.

CONCLUSION

To summarize, when a posterior capsular abnormality is diagnosed from slit-lamp examination and from B scan, the surgeon should prepare to deal with an expected problem. Whenever the posterior lens and the capsule cannot be reasonably visualized during pediatric cataract surgery, the surgeon should be prepared for the possibility of a PPCD and utilize the techniques discussed in this chapter.

REFERENCES

1. Singh D, Worst J, Singh R, Singh IR. Cataract and IOL. In: *Posterior Capsular Abnormalities.* New Delhi: JP Brothers, 1993:160–167.
2. Fugo RJ, DelCampo DM. The Fugo Blade™: the next step after capsulorhexis. *Ann Ophthalmol* 2001;33(1):12–20.
3. Fugo RJ, Singh D, Fine IH. Automated Fugo Blade capsulotomy: a new technique and a new instrument. *Eyeworld* 2002;7(9):49–54.
4. Singh D. Use of the Fugo Blade in complicated cases. *J Cataract Refract Surg* 2002;28(4):573–574.
5. Singh SK. Fugo Blade capsulotomy: a new high tech cutting technology. *Trop Ophthalmol* 2001;1(1):14–16.

Anterior Lenticonus in Alport Syndrome

Rupal H. Trivedi and M. Edward Wilson, Jr.

Anterior lenticonus is a rare bilateral condition wherein the anterior surface of the lens protrudes to assume a conical form. Usually the raised portion consists of clear cortex, while the lens nucleus remains intact and undistorted. Therefore, the deformity is thought to originate in late intrauterine or postnatal life.[1] It is less common than posterior lenticonus and most often found in association with Alport syndrome (AS).[2,3] However, isolated cases have been reported, as well as a rare association with Lowe syndrome and Waardenburg syndrome.[4-6]

AS, a hereditary nephritis accompanied by high-tone sensorineural deafness and distinctive ocular signs, was first reported in the early 1900s (quoted in Ref. 2). Guthrie described several cases of familial idiopathic hematuria and suggested maternal genetic transmittance.[2,7] In 1927, Cecil A. Alport described three generations of a family with a combination of progressive hereditary nephritis and deafness. He linked the hematuria with the auditory defects and noted that the severity of the disease corresponded to gender.[8] Many more families were subsequently described and the eponym AS was coined in 1961.[8,9] The anomalous basement membranes of the ocular, auditory, and renal systems cause the characteristic triad of abnormalities in patients with AS (i.e., ocular signs, sensorineural deafness, and hereditary nephritis).

The ocular signs were initially discussed by Sohar.[2,10] Anterior lenticonus is a distinctive feature in patients with AS, and its presence in any individual is highly suggestive of AS. Anterior lenticonus is an important indicator of a poor systemic prognosis because of renal disease in these patients. Anterior lenticonus is more common in male than female patients with AS.[11] The inheritance is predominantly X linked (85%), although it can be autosomal recessive (10%) or autosomal dominant (5%).[12]

CLINICAL FEATURES

Diagnosis of anterior lenticonus is made by slit-lamp examination. When using a parallelepiped or optic section during slit-lamp biomicroscopy, the lenticonus is seen as an axial protrusion, often conical or nipplelike, within the pupillary zone of the lens. Minor degrees of lenticonus are difficult to detect but are suggested by a distinctive *"oil drop"* appearance (effect produced by *oil globules in water*) of the red reflex on slit-lamp examination. This is due to the fact that none of the rays from the fundus reaches the observer's eye owing to prismatic reflection in the axial region.[1] Examination with a retinoscope can sometimes detect anterior lenticonus even when it is difficult to see with the slit lamp.

Associated Ocular Findings

These may include the following.

Refractive Error

Slowly progressing myopia and astigmatism may occur. A recent publication described the use of wavefront sensing to evaluate lenticular irregular astigmatism in eyes with lenticonus.[13] The authors noted that irregular astigmatism induced by lenticonus is a relatively symmetrical, spherical-like aberration, in contrast to irregular astigmatism in typical keratoconus, which is an asymmetrical, comma-like aberration.[13]

Corneal Abnormalities

Posterior polymorphous dystrophy (PPMD) and arcus juveniles are frequently encountered. Thickening of Descemet's layer with later endothelial cell changes can lead to PPMD. It should be noted that certain corneal abnormalities may be observed in all renal failure patients regardless of etiology. These include a white limbal girdle of Vogt and band keratopathy.[2] Care must be taken to ensure a complete differential diagnosis of the etiology of the patient's renal disease.

Glaucoma

Iridocorneal adhesions and transparent membranes owing to PPMD result in an increase risk for glaucoma in these patients.

Lens

Although cataracts are not a specific finding for AS, certain lens opacities are significant for these patients. First, *anterior subcapsular cataracts* can occur secondarily to lens capsule rupture. Second, *posterior subcapsular cataracts* may appear because of steroid use with post–renal transplant therapy. Third, internal lenticonus may be seen as a *posterior lamellar opacity* with a posterior projection along the visual axis.[11] Rarely lens coloboma has been reported associated with AS.[14]

Fundus

Yellow–white to silver flecks within the macular and midperipheral regions of the retina can be seen.

ANTERIOR CAPSULE AND LENTICONUS

AS is caused by a genetic defect within one of the α chains of Type IV collagen, which is a major constituent of basement membranes throughout the body.[15–17] In the eye, it mainly affects the anterior capsule of the lens. The primary defect for lenticonus lies within the lens capsule. Streeten et al.[18] identified specific histological structures that are affected in the crystalline lens capsule. They[18] inferred that the appearance of the lens capsule lesion was similar to the Bowman's capsule basement membrane defect in the renal system of AS patients. The anterior lens capsule was noted to be one third the normal thickness centrally and to be more fibrillar than usual, as well as to be associated with large numbers of partial capsular dehiscences containing fibrillar material and vacuoles. The pathological thinning in eyes with lenticonus as well as the abnormal epithelial cells and fibers may allow bulging of the anterior capsule. Kato et al.[17] also noted that the thickness of the anterior lens capsule was decreased, and there were many vertical capsular dehiscences localized in the inner part of the lens capsule. Besides the anatomical problems with the capsule, manipulation of the lens because of accommodation and normal growth causes added stress on the already weakened structure. A recent study showed abnormal composition of α (IV) chains in the anterior lens capsule of a patient with anterior lenticonus caused by a mutation in the COL4A5 gene.[19] Further studies are necessary to investigate the phenotype–genotype relationship to provide a better understanding of the molecular pathogenesis of anterior lenticonus.

The weakness in the anterior capsule can cause the capsule to rupture, with subsequent formation of an anterior subcapsular cataract. Traumatic and nontraumatic rupture of the lens capsule has been reported in the literature.[20] In contrast, some reports have noted that the anterior capsule is not so fragile (when performing capsulotomy) in these eyes.[21,22] These authors theorize that fragility and thinness may present in some AS patients only in the advanced stage of the disease.[21,22]

TREATMENT

Our current recommendation for treating an eye with anterior lenticonus is described in Figure 35-1.

Conservative Management

Even if there are no lens opacities, associated refractive errors may affect vision significantly. Glasses and/or contact lenses should be the first line of treatment in such cases. Patients with AS should be warned about the possible complication of spontaneous traumatic or nontraumatic rupture of the anterior capsule, leading to total cataract requiring surgery, and informed of the need for prompt evaluation if any sudden change in vision occurs.

Optionally, reduced vision secondary to lenticular changes is treated with topical mydriatics. Topical phenylephrine can be administered if the patient has axial opacities. If the patient has systemic hypertension, care must be taken when prescribing topical phenylephrine drops, and a diluted concentration can be a viable option.

Surgical Approach

Despite all efforts, often conservative management fails to improve vision satisfactorily. In such cases clear lens extraction with intraocular lens (IOL) implantation is the first reasonable option.[4,21] Occasional reports of traumatic and nontraumatic rupture of the anterior capsule have prompted some surgeons to treat this disease more aggressively. Rupture of the anterior capsule may require more urgent intervention and the torn anterior capsule adds to intraoperative difficulties.

Although clear lens extraction may be a viable alternative when treating such eyes, care must be taken to document the best corrected visual acuity (BCVA) and discuss the options with the patient or parents. In the rare case of a severe complication (e.g., endophthalmitis) it may be difficult to justify the indication for clear lens extraction. Documenting the decision-making process is very important in these cases.

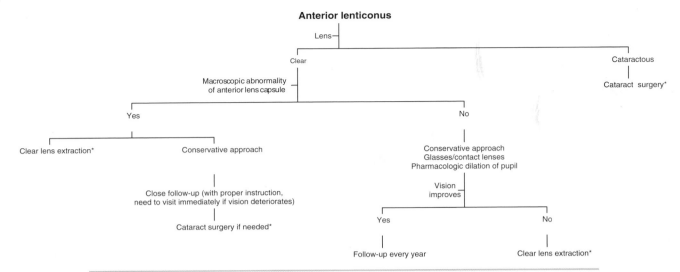

FIGURE 35-1. Flow diagram showing our current recommendation for treating an eye with lenticonus. *The other eye generally requires surgery within a few weeks.

Whether operating on a clear lens or a cataractous one, extra care is needed when performing anterior capsulotomy, as the anterior capsule is fragile. Some authors, however, have reported that they did not notice any extra difficulty when performing anterior capsulotomy in such cases.[5] Probably anterior capsule fragility is a concern in advanced cases of anterior lenticonus, but not when early intervention is attempted. In our experience, the anterior capsulorhexis is not distinguishable from that of other patients of a similar age. Undoubtedly the center of the capsule is fragile, but if care is taken to control the capsulorhexis peripheral to the fragile center (using ample viscosurgical agent), a strong capsulotomy edge can be created. For the remaining surgical steps, general surgical principles (as outlined elsewhere in this book) should be followed. Once one eye is operated on, the other eye will likely require surgery, to achieve better binocular vision and often to prevent the crisis of a ruptured anterior capsule in the fellow eye.

Supportive Treatment

Appropriate genetic counseling is essential for the management of AS. Due to the high risk for developmental delay and decreased social integration, management of AS patients requires a team effort from medical, behavioral, psychosocial, and educational specialists. Patients with AS should also consider the use of protective lenses during participation in contact sports.

CASE REPORT

We witnessed two cases of anterior lens capsule rupture in eyes with AS.

Case 1

A 13-year-old African-American boy presented to us in March 1992 with a diagnosis of AS. His medical

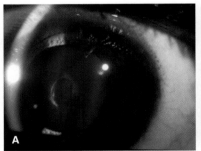
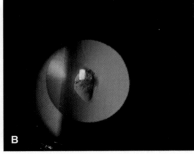
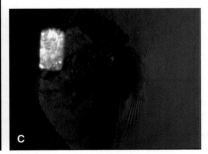

FIGURE 35-2. Right eye of a 12-year-old African-American boy with anterior lenticonus secondary to Alport syndrome. On slit-lamp examination, the paracentral anterior capsule was noted to have findings of early spontaneous rupture. **A.** Direct split illumination. **B.** Retroillumination. **C.** High magnification of spontaneous rupture.

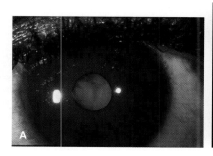
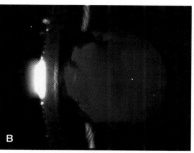

FIGURE 35-3. Same eye as described in Fig. 35-2. Note the total cataract following nontraumatic rupture of the anterior capsule.

history included hemorrhagic nephritis requiring a kidney transplant. We diagnosed anterior lenticonus in both eyes. His subjective refraction was difficult, but he preferred +1.25 D (diopters) in both eyes. The BCVA was 20/40 OD and 20/30 OS. Retinoscopy through the central lenticonus revealed an objective refraction of −11 OD and −7 OS. By July 1992, the patient's BCVA had dropped to 20/70 OD and 20/60 OS.

In December 1992 (age 14 years), he presented to a nephrologist with an acute decrease in vision in the left eye, which was diagnosed as leukocoria of the left eye, and sent to us for further management. He denied any trauma. On examination, vision was 20/60 OD and 20/640 OS. Slit-lamp examination revealed a ruptured anterior lens capsule, with cortex protruding through the pupil and into the anterior chamber. The lens had become hypermature, but the anterior chamber was quiet. The boy was taken to surgery; a ruptured anterior lens capsule was noted, with expulsed cortical material. Cortical material was removed by aspiration, and then capsulorhexis forceps were used to enlarge the opening in the anterior capsule. A posterior chamber IOL was implanted within the capsular bag. The boy's uncorrected visual acuity improved to 20/20. His other eye was operated on for clear lens extraction to avoid repetition of the crisis in the fellow eye as well as to provide better binocular vision. He now has 20/20 vision in both eyes.

Case 2

A 12-year-old African-American boy (nephew of case 1, described above) presented to us (July 2003) with anterior lenticonus secondary to AS. On slit-lamp examination, small "cracks" were seen in the anterior lens capsule of the right eye at the apex of the lenticonus (Figs. 35-2A–C). These were interpreted as early areas of spontaneous anterior lens capsule rupture. Vision was 20/125 OD and 20/80 OS. BCVA was 20/25 OD and 20/40 OS. We advised the family to watch for any sign/symptom related to cataract (leukocoria, sudden decrease in vision). In September 2003, the patient presented to us with total cataract (Figs. 35-3A and B). The patient was brought to surgery. After entering the anterior chamber, bimanual irrigation/aspiration was used to aspirate the lens substance. The torn anterior capsule had extended from equator to equator but no vitreous prolapse was seen. In-the-bag IOL implantation was achieved successfully. The fellow eye had a clear lens capsule (Fig. 35-4). It was operated on 1 month later. At surgery, this left eye was seen to have developed early "cracks" in the anterior lens capsule much like those seen originally in the right eye. Both eyes now have a BCVA of 20/20.

Lessons Learned

1. Close follow-up is necessary in patients with anterior lenticonus.

2. If signs of early lens capsule splitting, "cracking," or rupture are seen at examination, consider a clear lens extraction to avoid an uncontrolled lens rupture and hydration.

CONCLUSION

To summarize, AS offers many challenges to the ophthalmologist. Patients will present with the characteristic triad of hereditary nephritis, hearing loss, and ocular manifestations. A thorough investigation of the hereditary nature of this syndrome within a family is essential. A multidisciplinary approach in the management of these

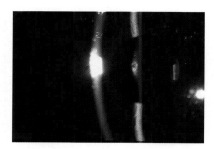

FIGURE 35-4. Left eye of the same child as in Fig. 35-2.

patients, including assistance with developmental and social deficiencies, is necessary to minimize detrimental effects on their quality of life and improve management outcomes. Close follow-up by an ophthalmologist is essential in patients with AS. If signs of early anterior lens capsule rupture are observed, clear lens extraction may be considered to avoid an uncontrolled rupture of the anterior lens capsule and subsequent cataract formation necessitating urgent intervention.

REFERENCES

1. Duke-Elder SS. Anterior lenticonus. In: Duke-Elder SS, ed. *Normal and Abnormal Development. Part 2. Congenital Deformities.* St. Louis: C. V. Mosby, 1964:696–700.
2. McCarthy PA, Maino DM. Alport syndrome: a review. *Clin Eye Vision Care* 2000;12:139–150.
3. Amaya L, Taylor D, Russell-Eggitt I, Nischal KK, Lengyel D. The morphology and natural history of childhood cataracts. *Surv Ophthalmol* 2003;48:125–144.
4. Basti S, Rathi V, Reddy MK, Gupta S. Clear lens extraction for anterior lenticonus. *J Cataract Refract Surg* 1995;21:363–364.
5. van Setten G. Anterior lenticonus: histological evaluation and approach for cataract surgery. *J Cataract Refract Surg* 2001;27:1071–1075.
6. Stevens PR. Anterior lenticonus and the Waardenburg syndrome. *Br J Ophthalmol* 1970;54:621–623.
7. Guthrie LG. Idiopathic or congenital, hereditary and family hematuria. *Lancet* 1902;1:1243–1246.
8. Alport AC. Hereditary familial congenital haemorrhagic nephritis. *Br Med J* 1927;1:504–506.
9. Saxena R. Alport syndrome. In: *Emedicine*, 2002. http://www.imedicine.com/displaytopic.asp?bookid=6&topic=110 (last update Nov 2004).
10. Sohar E. Renal disease, inner ear deafness, and ocular changes. *Arch Intern Med* 1956;97:627–630.
11. McCartney PJ, McGuinness R. Alport's syndrome and the eye. *Aust NZ J Ophthalmol* 1989;17:165–168.
12. Colville DJ, Savige J. Alport syndrome. A review of the ocular manifestations. *Ophthalm Genet* 1997;18:161–173.
13. Ninomiya S, Maeda N, Kuroda T, Saito T, Fujikado T, Tano Y, et al. Evaluation of lenticular irregular astigmatism using wavefront analysis in patients with lenticonus. *Arch Ophthalmol* 2002;120:1388–1393.
14. Amari F, Segawa K, Ando F. Lens coloboma and Alport-like glomerulonephritis. *Eur J Ophthalmol* 1994;4:181–183.
15. Junk AK, Stefani FH, Ludwig K. Bilateral anterior lenticonus: Scheimpflug imaging system documentation and ultrastructural confirmation of Alport syndrome in the lens capsule. *Arch Ophthalmol* 2000;118:895–897.
16. Takei K, Furuya A, Hommura S, Yamaguchi N. Ultrastructural fragility and type IV collagen abnormality of the anterior lens capsules in a patient with Alport syndrome. *Jpn J Ophthalmol* 2001;45:103–104.
17. Kato T, Watanabe Y, Nakayasu K, Kanai A, Yajima Y. The ultrastructure of the lens capsule abnormalities in Alport's syndrome. *Jpn J Ophthalmol* 1998;42:401–405.
18. Streeten BW, Robinson MR, Wallace R, Jones DB. Lens capsule abnormalities in Alport's syndrome. *Arch Ophthalmol* 1987;105:1693–1697.
19. Ohkubo S, Takeda H, Higashide T, Ito M, Sakurai M, Shirao Y, et al. Immunohistochemical and molecular genetic evidence for type IV collagen alpha5 chain abnormality in the anterior lenticonus associated with Alport syndrome. *Arch Ophthalmol* 2003;121:846–850.
20. Olitsky SE, Waz WR, Wilson ME. Rupture of the anterior lens capsule in Alport syndrome. *J AAPOS* 1999;3:381–382.
21. John ME, Noblitt RL, Coots SD, Boleyn KL, Ballew C. Clear lens extraction and intraocular lens implantation in a patient with bilateral anterior lenticonus secondary to Alport's syndrome. *J Cataract Refract Surg* 1994;20:652–655.
22. Mavrikakis I, Zeilmaker C, Wearne MJ. Surgical management of anterior lenticonus in Alport's syndrome. *Eye* 2002;16:798–800.

Aniridia and Cataracts

Rupal H. Trivedi and M. Edward Wilson, Jr.

Congenital aniridia (Greek; absence of iris) is a rare (1 in 64,000 to 1 in 96,000 live births) panocular syndrome in which the most dramatic manifestation is partial or nearly complete absence of the iris.[1] It was first described by Barrata in 1818 (quoted in reference 1). Aniridia is bilateral in 98% of cases.[1,2]

The term *aniridia* is actually a misnomer, for two reasons.

1. The condition rarely occurs in its pure form and usually presents with a rudimentary stump of iris. Since a small portion of iris tissue can almost always be found on gonioscopic examination or histologically, the term *iridemia* better describes the condition than does *"aniridia."*[1] The term aniridia came from earlier reports in which the iris appeared to be completely missing. However, complete gonioscopic examination was not performed.[1]

2. The term aniridia has also been misused to describe a group of conditions as if they were one.[1] Aniridia syndrome is not just partial or complete absence of the iris. Optic nerve hypoplasia, corneal vascularization, and cataract often accompany the iris abnormality. Glaucoma is a secondary problem adding to aniridia syndrome.

The exact defect in iris morphogenesis giving rise to aniridia is unknown. Although it is possible that a primary mesodermal defect is causative, it is also believed that a primary neuroectodermal defect is causative since the iris pigment epithelium is of neuroectodermal origin, as are the retina and optic nerve, which also have primary developmental defects in this disorder.[1]

GENETICS

1. An *autosomal dominant* inheritance pattern is the most common (85%).[1]

2. Congenital *sporadic* aniridia can be an isolated condition or a part of WAGR (Wilm's tumor–nephoroblastoma, aniridia, genitourinary anomalies, and retardation) (13%). A deletion of chromosome 11 at band p13 can involve the gene for sporadic aniridia as well as the Wilm's tumor suppressor gene located near the aniridia gene. Larger deletions at 11p13 are responsible for the full WAGR syndrome.

3. *Autosomal recessive* aniridia (2%) is associated with cerebellar ataxia and mental retardation (Gillespie's syndrome).

CATARACTS AND ANIRIDIA

Cataracts occur frequently and at a young age in aniridia.[1] Cataracts develop in 50 to 85% of patients with familial aniridia, usually during the first two decades of life.[1] Frequently small anterior and posterior lens opacities are noted at birth, but these do not usually cause significant visual difficulty. Cortical, subcapsular, and lamellar opacities often develop by the teenage years and may require lens extraction. In those families whose members maintain good vision throughout life, there appears to be a lower incidence of visually significant lens opacities.[1]

Partial dislocation of the lens, usually due to "weak" zonules (due to a molecular defect of the zonules), is more common in aniridic patients. Ectopia lentis has been reported in from 0 to 56% of patients with aniridia.[1,3] Superior lens dislocation in 12 members of a family in which 28 members had aniridia has been reported. The upward displacement of the lens is caused by loss of inferior zonules. The authors noted a disproportionately increased risk for glaucoma in the family members with dislocated lenses.

Yoshikawa et al.[4] reported a membranous cataract in association with aniridia in a 52-year-old female patient. The membranous cataract was associated with a high intraocular pressure (IOP). A seton procedure was carried out. During the follow-up period, the membranous cataract in the right eye spontaneously moved from its original position and floated in the vitreous, maintaining its shape.

Mehta and associates[2] noted an abnormal lens shape on computed tomography (CT) in a patient with aniridia and cataract. The lens shape appeared reversed; that is, the anterior lens surface was more, and the posterior lens surface less, convex.[2] A B-mode scan showed that the lens capsule shape was normal. In addition, it showed that the cataract was the same shape as the CT image. The CT had imaged the cataract of the patient as opposed to the lens capsule, hence giving the abnormal appearance. The authors cautioned clinicians about misinterpretation when assessing patients with aniridia and cataract by CT scan.[2]

Other clinical features include the following.

1. *Decreased vision.* Although iris hypoplasia is the most common ophthalmic manifestation of the aniridic eye, it is usually not the major determinator of visual function. Poor visual acuity (VA) appears to be correlated with absence of the macular reflex, optic nerve hypoplasia, and the development of cataracts, glaucoma, and corneal opacification. Vision is usually in the 20/100 to 20/200 range in patients with aniridia secondary to macular hypoplasia and optic nerve hypoplasia.

2. *Photophobia.* Photophobia may occur secondary to excessive light stimulation because of poor pupillary constriction. A characteristic facial expression in many children consists of narrowing of the palpabral fissures and furrowing of the brow.

3. *Glaucoma.* Glaucoma in infants with aniridia is rare, although it is relatively common later in childhood. Routine gonioscopic examination is important to detect anatomical changes in angle structure that may progress to angle closure. A small stump of iris can gradually produce angle closure by mechanically covering the trabecular meshwork. Patients with more residual iris (often up to where the collarette would be) seem to be at lower risk of glaucoma from this mechanism.

4. *Corneal vascularization and pannus.* Corneal epithelium changes eventually occur in all patients with aniridia. A superficial, slightly elevated, faint gray pannus with fine radially oriented blood vessels that stain positive with fluorescein is characteristic. Defects appear in the corneal periphery and progress to the center with age. Corneal erosions and frank ulceration occur in some cases. These lesions may progress to end-stage corneal scarring involving all layers.

Brandt et al.[5] reported a markedly increased central corneal thickness in eyes with aniridia. The authors noted an average central corneal thickness at least 100 μm greater than literature-derived normal values.[5] This may lead to incorrect estimates of IOP by applanation techniques and highlights the importance of monitoring patients with aniridia for the development of glaucoma by gonioscopy and optic nerve examination.

5. *Optic nerve hypoplasia, strabismus, and nystagmus.* Macular hypoplasia is usually accompanied by noticeable optic nerve hypoplasia. Nystagmus and strabismus are common as well.

6. *Hyphema.* Theobald and associates[6] have published a case report of a 2-month-old infant with known hemophilia A and aniridia who presented with spontaneous hyphema and severe IOP elevation. IOP remained uncontrolled with medical intervention. Anterior chamber wash was performed; at that time extensive pupillary plexus was noted over the anterior lens of both eyes, consistent with persistent iris structures associated with aniridia.

7. *Type 2 aniridia with preserved ocular function.* One of us (M.E.W.) has reported two cases of so-called "Type 2 aniridia with preserved ocular function."[7]

MANAGEMENT OF ANIRIDIA AND CATARACTS

Detailed preoperative assessment of ocular structures including careful evaluation of the zonular apparatus is essential. In the preoperative assessment of the aniridic patient with a cataract, it is important to attempt to ascertain whether the progressing visual loss arises from increasing lens opacification and not from other factors, such as worsening glaucoma or corneal opacification.[8] The guarded prognosis for visual outcome needs to be explained to the patients/parents/legal guardian.

The optical correction of aphakia in aniridic patients is difficult because concomitant corneal pannus may be a relative contraindication to contact lenses, and nystagmus may exacerbate the optical aberration of aphakic spectacles. Conventional intraocular lens (IOL) implantation in eyes with congenital aniridia has been reported in several studies.[8,9] Several reports have reported a successful anatomical outcome from IOL implantation in eyes with aniridia.[8]

The lack of a normal iris presents difficulties in placement of an IOL. Accurate positioning of an angle-fixated anterior chamber IOL would be problematic, and the lens might be at higher risk of dislocation. In the absence of an iris, an iris-fixated lens is out of the question. Ciliary sulcus fixation of an IOL is potentially unstable.[8] Segal and Li[10] reported a case with a successful outcome of transscleral ciliary fixation of a posterior chamber lens in an eye with congenital aniridia. All attempts should be made to achieve capsular fixation of the posterior chamber IOL. One aspect of an aniridic eye that can be an advantage when performing cataract surgery is that the absence of iris tissue gives better visualization while performing cataract and IOL surgery.

There are literature reports of thinning of the anterior capsule in association with congenital aniridia.[11] However, caution is required, as all aniridic eyes with a thin anterior capsule were in younger patients in this series compared with the control group. The younger the age, the thinner is the anterior capsule. It is not clear whether younger age or aniridia led to the thinner capsules in this series.

PROSTHETIC DEVICES

Many attempts have been made historically to compensate for lack of iris diaphragm, including eyelid surgery, use of colored contact lenses, and coloring of the cornea. Choyce[12] reported the implantation of colored diaphragm IOLs more than 40 years ago. Most studies have described the use of prosthetic devices in adult or adolescent populations. Thus, pertinent discussion of the subject will include adult literature as well. We recommend that interested readers visit manufacturers' Web sites to see the available designs and their dimensions (www.morcher.com and www.ophtec.com).

A modern artificial iris implant was introduced in Europe in 1994 by Sundmacher et al.[13,14] who reported using the black diaphragm IOL in aniridia. Morcher single-piece iris-diaphragm IOL styles 67F and 67G are the most commonly used designs, which have a full iris diaphragm 10.0 mm in diameter surrounding a central optic 5.0 mm in diameter. They differ only in overall diameter (67F, 13.5 mm; 67G, 12.5 mm) and are inserted through an incision at least 10.0 mm long. Ophtec aniridia lenses have colored haptics and additional optical correction, available from +10 to +30 D (diopters).

Encouraging short-term results for iris-diaphragm lens were reported in 1994.[13,14] Reinhard et al.[15] reported long-term follow-up of eyes with black iris diaphragm IOLs. As of 2000, these authors prefer to use the 67G model. Almost 75% (14/19) of patients with congenital aniridia and cataracts had increased VA after implantation of the black diaphragm aniridia IOL. Eleven of 14 patients (79%) reported reduced glare. However, these authors feel that this functional improvement in vision was achieved at the (presumed) risk of a variety of complications in some patients. The main postoperative problem noted was chronic IOP elevation, in 42% (8/19). In four of these eyes, chronic glaucoma had been diagnosed and well controlled preoperatively. In the other 4 eyes (29% of the 14 eyes without evident preoperative glaucoma), chronic glaucoma became evident after implantation of the black diaphragm aniridia IOL. In two, glaucoma could only be controlled by trabeculectomy, cyclodestruction, and explantation of the aniridia IOL. Although glaucoma is a common complication of congenital aniridia, the blood–aqueous barrier may be altered by the black diaphragm aniridia IOL, accelerating glaucoma progression. The authors hypothesized several reasons for chronic alteration of the blood–aqueous barrier. (1) The IOL is too large to be implanted in the capsular bag. Thus, the haptics and the diaphragm are in direct contact with uveal remnants in front of the capsular bag and may cause continuous irritation. (2) Proper placement of an IOL is difficult in an aniridic patient. Improper fixation of haptics may have accelerated the problem. (3) The black diaphragm IOL might have greater mobility than conventional IOLs after sulcus implantation behind the intact iris of "normal" eyes. (4) The blood–aqueous barrier in eyes with congenital aniridia may be much more vulnerable to all types of trauma than that in normal eyes. The authors recommended caution when using the aniridia IOL in eyes with existing glaucoma.

Osher and Burk[16] reported seven eyes of six patients with congenital aniridia, traumatic iris loss, or chronic mydriasis. All patients noted a marked reduction of glare symptoms and qualitative improvement in their vision after implantation of these prosthetic devices.

One drawback of placing the optic within an iris diaphragm is that a relatively large incision is required to obtain a full iris diaphragm. To avoid the drawbacks of large incisions, Heino Hermeking, MD, of Germany, proposed a system in which the optic portion and the iris diaphragm are inserted separately and then assembled in the eye. His Iris Prosthetic System (IPS) consists of different standard combinable elements and is used for artificial iris reconstruction. It provides occlusion of partial or total iris defects and creates a new iris diaphragm (Ophtec). Capsular tension rings with integrated tinted sector shields have been developed to compensate for aniridia (Morcher Type 50C).[17] Two rings are implanted. When adequately positioned, the interspaces of the first ring are covered by the sector shields of the second, forming a contiguous artificial iris. The Type 50C Morcher endocapsular ring with iris diaphragm, developed by Volker Rasch, MD, of Potsdam, Germany, provides a method for combining iris diaphragm implantation with modern small-incision surgery. The 50C aniridia ring can be inserted through the same small incision as the foldable IOL. This approach offers the advantages of a full iris diaphragm and separate optical system, both of which may be inserted through a small incision. The iris diaphragm produces a pupil size of approximately 6.0 mm, which is compatible with excellent fundus viewing. The disadvantage of the 50C is that the device is brittle and susceptible to fracture.[16]

Burk and associates[18] have reported their experience with prosthetic iris implantation. Glare disability was assessed by questioning patients directly and recording their subjective appraisal of the preoperative and postoperative impairment in bright-light and high-contrast settings. The subjective glare disability was reduced from a mean of 2.8 preoperatively to 1.3 postoperatively in eyes with congenital aniridia. The authors recommend the single-piece iris diaphragm IOL (type 67) when the capsular bag is absent or damaged. Of the two models, the 67G is more readily available and well suited for suture fixation. For implantation in the ciliary sulcus, the authors prefer the greater overall diameter of the 67F. The endocapsular devices were generally implanted at the time of cataract surgery. When a full iris diaphragm was needed, two multiple-fin rings (Type 50C) were inserted and rotated within the capsular bag until the fins interdigitated, creating a confluent diaphragm.

CATARACTS AND GLAUCOMA

Congenital glaucoma in patients with aniridia is rare; the risk for glaucoma increases with age. Angle closure as well as an open-angle mechanism can be causative in these eyes.

Khaw[19] has raised a question in the 2002 issue of *Journal of glaucoma*: *"If the patient presents at 29 years of age, not only with raised IOP (28 mm Hg), but also a dense cortical lens opacity, how should he be managed?"* Although the patient described there was 29 years of age, we thought it would be interesting for the reader of this text on pediatric surgery. David S. Walton replied, *"I should attempt medical therapy and, if necessary, surgery to control the glaucoma. A combined procedure at 29 years of age would seem reasonable, but I have no personal experience with such management."* Comments by Eugenio Maul suggested, *"This combination is best treated by a procedure combining an Ahmed valve with phacoemulsification and a foldable acrylic intraocular lens."* The authors further noted, *"Glare and edge effects may be reduced by the anterior capsule remaining peripheral to the capsulorhexis, which generally opacify soon after surgery."* Khaw noted, *"I carry out drainage tube surgery with MMC. I personally try not to carry out simultaneous surgery and usually do the tube implant first unless the lens is hypermature and swollen, when I will do the cataract alone if the glaucoma can be medically controlled."* The authors prefer Baerveldt with Mitomycin-C (MMC).

Arroyave and coworkers[20] have reported that glaucoma drainage device placement for glaucoma associated with aniridia achieves IOP control and vision preservation in most patients.

Most series have reported a significant improvement in VA after cataract surgery in aniridic patients, even though it is subnormal compared to that of patients with cataract without aniridia. Despite a successful outcome of cataract surgery, poor vision in an aniridic child is correlated with absence of the macular reflex, optic nerve hypoplasia, development of glaucoma, and corneal opacification.[1]

CONCLUSION

To summarize, operating on a congenitally aniridic eye presents special challenges, and implantation of an artifi-

cial iris device appears to be a reasonably effective method for reducing the subjective perception of glare resulting from the iris deficiency. While the currently available devices have limitations, these prosthetic iris devices provide a novel way to rehabilitate these symptomatic eyes for which there has been no alternative. As we move forward with the development of artificial irises, the design, availability, and flexibility, as well as insertion techniques, will likely continue to improve and provide better benefits to these eyes.

REFERENCES

1. Nelson LB, Spaeth GL, Nowinski TS, Margo CE, Jackson L. Aniridia. A review. *Surv Ophthalmol* 1984;28:621–642.
2. Mehta JS, Moseley IF, Restori M, Plant GT. Abnormal lens shape on CT in a patient with aniridia. *Eye* 2004;18:209.
3. David R, MacBeath L, Jenkins T. Aniridia associated with microcornea and subluxated lenses. *Br J Ophthalmol* 1978;62:118–121.
4. Yoshikawa K, Asakage H, Inoue Y. Membranous cataract in association with aniridia. *Jpn J Ophthalmol* 1993;37:325–329.
5. Brandt JD, Casuso LA, Budenz DL. Markedly increased central corneal thickness: an unrecognized finding in congenital aniridia. *Am J Ophthalmol* 2004;137:348–350.
6. Theobald T, Davitt BV, Shields SR. Hemorrhagic glaucoma in an infant with hemophilia, spontaneous hyphema, aniridia, and persistent iris vessels. *J AAPOS* 2001;5:129–130.
7. Traboulsi EI JM, Wilson ME, Parks MM. Hypoplasia of the iris: The aniridia spectrum—Two isolated cases and review of the literature. *Int Pediatr* 1990;5:275–278.
8. Johns KJ, O'Day DM. Posterior chamber intraocular lenses after extracapsular cataract extraction in patients with aniridia. *Ophthalmology* 1991;98:1698–1702.
9. Lewallen WM Jr. Aniridia and related iris defects; a report of twelve cases with bilateral cataract extraction and resulting good vision in one. *AMA Arch Ophthalmol* 1958;59:831–839.
10. Segal EI, Li HK. Transscleral ciliary sulcus fixation of a posterior chamber lens in an eye with congenital aniridia. *J Cataract Refract Surg* 1997;23:595–597.
11. Schneider S, Osher RH, Burk SE, Lutz TB, Montione R. Thinning of the anterior capsule associated with congenital aniridia. *J Cataract Refract Surg* 2003;29:523–525.
12. Choyce P. *Intra-ocular Lenses and Implants*. London: H. K. Lewis, 1964.
13. Sundmacher T, Reinhard T, Althaus C. Black diaphragm intraocular lens in congenital aniridia. *German J Ophthalmol* 1994;3:197–201.
14. Sundmacher R, Reinhard T, Althaus C. Black-diaphragm intraocular lens for correction of aniridia. *Ophthalm Surg* 1994;25:180–185.
15. Reinhard T, Engelhardt S, Sundmacher R. Black diaphragm aniridia intraocular lens for congenital aniridia: long-term follow-up. *J Cataract Refract Surg* 2000;26:375–381.
16. Osher RH, Burk SE. Cataract surgery combined with implantation of an artificial iris. *J Cataract Refract Surg* 1999;25:1540–1547.
17. Menapace R, Findl O, Georgopoulos M, Rainer G, Vass C, Schmetterer K. The capsular tension ring: designs, applications, and techniques. *J Cataract Refract Surg* 2000;26:898–912.
18. Burk SE, Da Mata AP, Snyder ME, Cionni RJ, Cohen JS, Osher RH. Prosthetic iris implantation for congenital, traumatic, or functional iris deficiencies. *J Cataract Refract Surg* 2001;27:1732–1740.
19. Khaw PT. Aniridia. *J Glaucoma* 2002;11:164–168.
20. Arroyave CP, Scott IU, Gedde SJ, Parrish RK, 2nd, Feuer WJ. Use of glaucoma drainage devices in the management of glaucoma associated with aniridia. *Am J Ophthalmol* 2003;135:155–159.

Lowe Syndrome

Stacey J. Kruger, M. Edward Wilson, Jr., and Rupal H. Trivedi

The oculocerebrorenal syndrome of Lowe is an X-linked recessive hereditary disorder. The syndrome was first described by Lowe in 1952 and is characterized by mental retardation, Fanconi syndrome of the proximal renal tubules, and congenital cataract.[1] Other findings include glaucoma, corneal opacity (keloid), enophthalmos, hypotonia, metabolic acidosis, proteinuria, and amino aciduria. Patients with Lowe syndrome often exhibit typical facial features that include frontal bossing, deep-set eyes, chubby cheeks, a fair complexion, and blonde hair (Figure 37-1).[2,3]

Lowe syndrome patients have bilateral cataracts that are usually deemed visually significant at or near birth. The appearance of the lens is marked by multiple gray–white opacities present in all the layers of the cortex, often in wedge-shaped segments.[4] Tripathi et al.[5] suggested that the characteristic lens opacities in Lowe syndrome result from a genetic defect in the lens cells. This defect manifests early in embryogenesis, and the progression of the lens opacities is related to both the inherent genetic abnormality and the prevailing extralenticular environment. The defective formation and subsequent degeneration of the primary posterior lens fibers account for their loss and for the flattened, discoid, or ring-shaped cataract. The other findings, such as anterior polar cataract, subcapsular fibrous plaque, capsular excrescences, bladder cells, and posterior lenticonus, are not necessarily specific for Lowe syndrome. The authors further noted that the pathogenesis of Lowe cataract can be explained by Lyon's hypothesis, which implies that, very early in embryogenesis (at the stage of the primitive streak), one of the two X chromosomes in females is deactivated. They considered the high incidence of lens opacities in female carriers to be due to this random deactivation. In male probands, since there is no normal X chromosome to nullify the effect of the Lowe gene, all lens cells are affected. Female carriers can be clinically identified solely on the basis of lens examination. The gene responsible for this syndrome has been localized to the Xq25 region using restriction fragment length polymorphism analysis.[6]

We have recently published a retrospective review of the outcome of cataract surgery in patients with Lowe syndrome.[3] Seven patients (14 eyes) with bilateral cataracts associated with Lowe syndrome were identified and reported. The mean age at cataract surgery was 1.2 months (range, 0.5 to 4 months; median, 1.1 months). All but one patient underwent cataract surgery in the first 2 months of life (see Table 37-1).

General principles of pediatric cataract surgery should be followed. Spierer and Desatnik have noted spontaneous intracameral bleeding at the end of cataract surgery in both eyes of two patients.[7] We noted that intraocular lens (IOL) placement was used less frequently in this population. Age at surgery, glaucoma propensity in these eyes, and poor pupil dilation were recorded as reasons the other patients did not get IOL implantation at the time of surgery. Glaucoma, common in these patients, can cause marked axial length changes, which would make primary IOL power selection very difficult.

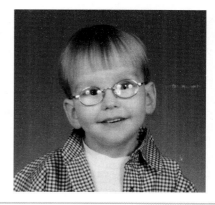

FIGURE 37-1. An 8-year-old patient who demonstrates the typical facial features of Lowe syndrome. (Reprinted with permission from Kruger SJ, Wilson ME Jr, Hutchinson AK, Peterseim MM, Bartholomew LR, Saunders RA. Cataracts and glaucoma in patients with oculocerebrorenal syndrome. *Arch Ophthalmol* 2003;121(9):1234–1237.)

▶ **TABLE 37-1** Overview of Cataracts and Glaucoma in Patients with Lowe Syndrome

Patient Code	Eye	Age at CE (mo)	IOL	Age at GD	IOP at GD (mm Hg)	Latest IOP (mm Hg)	No. Medications	Latest VA	GST	Other Surgery	Postop Follow-up (mo)
1	OD	1	No	Not yet	No	19	None	CUSM	None	None	190
	OS	4	No	5 yr 10 mo	25	25	None	CUSM	None	None	186
2	OD	1.25	No	10 mo	40	20	3	CUSM	None	None	38
	OS	1.50	No	10 mo	34	20	3	CUSM	None	None	38
3	OD	1.25	Yes	4.5 yr	23	23	1	CUSM	None	None	63
	OS	1.25	Yes	4.5 yr	24	24	1	CUSM	None	None	63
4	OD	1	No	2.5 yr	25	15.5	3	CUSM	None	None	96
	OS	1	No	3 yr	28.5	19	3	CUSM	None	None	96
5	OD	0.25	No	5 d	24	17	2	20/40	Cyclocryo	CTX aspir	118
	OS	0.5	No	5 d	25	9	2	LP	Cyclocryo	CTX aspir	118
6	OD	0.5	No	6 d	37	19	2	CSM	Trab 180°	Baerveldt	47
	OS	0.25	No	6 d	31	17	2	CSM	Trab 180°	Baerveldt	47
7	OD	1.25	No	Not yet	No	14	None	20/60	None	None	156
	OS	1.75	No	Not yet	No	17	None	20/70	None	None	156

Reprinted with permission from Kruger SJ, Wilson ME Jr, Hutchinson AK, Peterseim MM, Bartholomew LR, Saunders RA. Cataracts and glaucoma in patients with oculocerebrorenal syndrome. *Arch Ophthalmol* 2003;121(9):1234–1237.
CE—cataract extraction; IOL—intraocular lens; IOP—intraocular pressure; GD—glaucoma diagnosis; VA—visual acuity; GST—glaucoma surgical treatment; CUSM—central, unsteady, maintained; d—day; Cyclocryo—cyclocryotherapy; CTX aspir—lens cortex aspiration; LP—light perception; CSM—central, steady, maintained; Trab 180°—trabeculotomy, 180°.

It is very crucial to follow these eyes for glaucoma. Age at glaucoma diagnosis and treatment were variable in our series. Mean age (11 eyes) at glaucoma diagnosis was 24.1 months (range, 0.2 to 70 months). Many of the eyes were diagnosed with glaucoma at the time of cataract surgery when they underwent examination under anesthesia in the first week of life. As is generally true in pediatric glaucoma management, patients who were diagnosed within the first few weeks of life required surgery, while patients diagnosed later were better able to be managed medically.

It is difficult to assess the visual outcome in this group of patients, as many of them are severely developmentally delayed (Table 37-1). Literature has reported that the best visual outcome that can be expected is in the range of 20/100.[5] In our series, only three patients had a mental status that was amenable to Snellen letter visual acuity. Even with early surgery and early optical replacement of the crystalline lens, visual acuity is not likely to be normal in these patients and nystagmus usually develops. It is reported in the literature that children who underwent congenital cataract surgery developed poorer visual acuity if the cataract was part of a systemic disease compared with children without a systemic syndrome.[8]

To summarize, early identification and surgical removal of cataracts in patients with Lowe syndrome are recommended. Despite this, vision is not expected to be better than 20/70 and nystagmus is likely. IOL implantation at the time of cataract surgery can be performed, but the lack of eye growth predictability in these infants with glaucoma makes power selection very difficult. Patients with or without IOL placement should be monitored closely for changes in intraocular pressure, optic nerve cupping, and refractive error, so that glaucoma can be detected and treated promptly.

REFERENCES

1. Lowe CU, Terrey M, MacLachlan EA. Organic aciduria, decreased renal ammonia production, hydrophthalmos and mental retardation: A clinical entity. *Am J Dis Child* 1952;83:164–184.
2. Cibis GW, Waeltermann JM, Whitcraft CT, Tripathi RC, Harris DJ. Lenticular opacities in carriers of Lowe's syndrome. *Ophthalmology* 1986;93:1041–1045.
3. Kruger SJ, Wilson ME Jr, Hutchinson AK, Peterseim MM, Bartholomew LR, Saunders RA. Cataracts and glaucoma in patients with oculocerebrorenal syndrome. *Arch Ophthalmol* 2003; 121:1234–1237.
4. Silver DN, Lewis RA, Nussbaum RL. Mapping of the Lowe oculocerebrorenal syndrome to Xq24-q26 by use of restriction fragment length polymorphisms. *J Clin Invest* 1987;79:282–285.
5. Tripathi RC, Cibis GW, Tripathi BJ. Pathogenesis of cataracts in patients with Lowe's syndrome. *Ophthalmology* 1986;93(8):1046–1051.
6. Lavin CW, McKeown CA. The oculocerebrorenal syndrome of Lowe. *Int Ophthalmol Clin* 1993;33:179–191.
7. Spierer A, Desatnik H. Anterior chamber hemorrhage during cataract surgery in Lowe syndrome. *Metab Pediatr Syst Ophthalmol* 1998; 21:19–21.
8. Spierer A, Desatnik H, Rosner M, Blumenthal M. Congenital cataract surgery in children with cataract as an isolated defect and in children with a systemic syndrome: a comparative study. *J Pediatr Ophthalmol Strabismus* 1998;35:281–285.

Chapter 38

Dislocated Crystalline Lenses

Daljit Singh, Kiranjit Singh, Indu R. Singh, and Ravijit Singh

Ectopia lentis is a feature of a variety of systemic disorders including Marfan syndrome, homocysteinuria, and Weill Marchesani syndrome.[1–3] In the latter condition the lens is microspheric. Ectopia lentis is not uncommon. We operate on such cases quite frequently. Most often, it is a manifestation of Marfan syndrome. Rarely, it is part of other syndromes. Blunt ocular trauma also causes subluxation, besides causing many other problems.

A dislocated lens is one of the toughest surgical problems in pediatric ophthalmology. A number of questions arise when a diagnosis of this condition is made.

1. *Does it require surgery?* In most cases, the decision for surgery is made on the basis of physical examination of the eye. The benefit of surgery to the child is known later, on the basis of improved visual interaction with people and confidence in day-to-day activity. The visual acuity records become the guide when the child grows up.

2. *What is the right age for operation?* A familial case is spotted early and this question is posed at a very early age.

3. *What approach is correct for removing the dislocated lens?* The right approach is the one that the surgeon is most confident with. It may be the anterior route or the pars plana route. Does the inevitable damage to the vitreous body via the pars plana approach require extra thought?

4. *What will the visual gain be if the surgical goal is mere aphakia?* Is an intraocular lens (IOL) desirable? If yes, what design of artificial lens is suitable for a particular case?

5. *What should the follow-up strategy be?* How should postsurgical and visual problems be managed?

For the ophthalmologist, the main focus is the dislocated lens, which, in the presence of symptoms, needs to be removed.

BASIC PHILOSOPHY

Most often, we are dealing with an eye that has a healthy vitreous. The subluxated lens lies decentered on one side or the other, supported by a few to many zonular fibers, on the surface of the vitreous. The vitreous has a cisternal structure as we know from the descriptions by Jan Worst.[4] A lens will not fall in the vitreous, as long as the cisterns are unbroken and the vitreous has a gel form. The same is true of lens matter that may fail to be removed at the time of surgery. Every effort should be made to preserve the integrity of the vitreous face, which is a composite face of multiple cisterns. This is possible only if an anterior surgical approach is used. Myopia is a common development among Marfan cases. A thorough fundus examination before surgery is mandatory. A disturbed vitreous means a higher risk of retinal problems, whether cystoid macular edema (CME) or retinal detachment. For lens implantation, the ideal would be to have a lens sequestrated inside the capsular bag, whenever safely possible. A scleral-fixated posterior chamber intraocular lens (IOL) has the potential to cause vitreoretinal problems. An iris-fixated lens is a sensible option, if it is available and legal and the surgeon is conversant with its use. Manual capsulotomy is difficult to perform in cases of subluxated lenses. This often results in the rupture of whatever zonule is present, with the inevitable rupture and prolapse of vitreous, and the added risk of lens–vitreous mixing as the operation proceeds. Fugo Blade automated traction-free capsulotomy can improve the ease of lens extraction and the preservation of the zonule and vitreous (Figure 38-1).[5–7]

EXAMINATION OF THE PATIENT

Age

At our institution most patients are brought in after the age of 5 or 6 years. If pupil block glaucoma develops, the patient may be brought in earlier. In advanced countries,

205

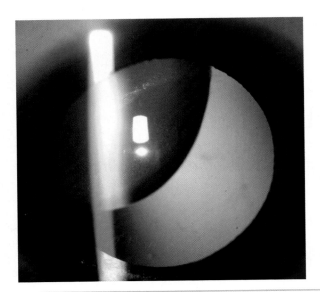

FIGURE 38-1. Dislocated lens in Marfan syndrome. There are no zonular fibers on the visible edge of the lens. The trio of lens extraction, vitreous preservation, and lens implantation requires a trauma-free surgical plan.

educated parents (especially if one of the parents is also affected) are more concerned about early diagnosis and treatment.

Ophthalmic Examination

a. *Cornea.* The cornea may be normal, or there may be a microcornea or megalocornea. A small cornea necessitates the use of a small iris-fixated lens, if a lens is desired. The capsular bag may be so small that it cannot accommodate any posterior chamber IOL. In cases of megalocornea, a suitably sized posterior chamber or angle-supported lens is not available. Besides, there is risk to the integrity of the overstretched zonules and the underlying vitreous, if it has been preserved during the surgery.

b. *Anterior chamber.* The depth of the anterior chamber is uneven owing to subluxation of the lens. It may be shallow in the case of microspherophakia.

c. *Pupil.* The pupil is often small and difficult to dilate even with a combination of mydriatics.

d. *Iris.* The iris is tremulous in most cases. This sign is helpful when the eye is examined without dilating the pupil. Lenses that are mobile under the iris rub against the pigment epithelium. There is shedding of some pigments, which may be found in the angle. Rarely the pupillary margin may lose its pigment. Iris bombe results when a microspheric lens blocks the pupil.

e. *Lens.* In pediatric patients, the crystalline lens is mostly clear. When the lens is not in its normal position, it is said to be dislocated. When it is decentered but remains in the pupillary area, it is subluxated. A luxated lens is completely displaced from the pupillary aperture. A totally dislocated lens floating in the vitreous or lying on the retina is very rare in our experience. We have seen only one case, a 14-year-old girl, who had an axial length of 30 mm and bilateral presence of the lens on the retina. One eye was blind owing to retinal detachment. A dislocated lens is frequently seen in cases of aniridia.

f. *Zonule.* Zonular fibers should be examined under full mydriasis. Our primary concern during surgery is the integrity of the zonular fibers. Therefore every available part of the zonule is studied under the microscope. Are the zonules merely stretched? Are there gaps? or Are they totally absent and the vitreous visible? The answers determine from which direction we should approach the dislocated lens for capsulotomy and lens extraction.

g. *Vitreous and retina.* This examination is done by a vitreoretinal surgeon, who looks for any evidence of vitreous liquefaction, the presence of lattices and holes in the retinal periphery, and the presence of a macular disease or retinal disease, especially detachment. Retinal treatment is a must before lens surgery is undertaken. Since myopia is frequent among cases of ectopia lentis, fundus examination by indirect ophthalmoscopy is most important. A disease like retinitis pigmentosa should be ruled out.

h. *Intraocular pressure.* Measurement of the intraocular pressure should be part of the full ophthalmic examination in these patients.

i. *Uncorrected and corrected visual acuity, with and without mydriasis.* This determination assures that an unnecessary surgery is not suggested to the patient. Potential visual acuity may be judged by blue-field entoptoscopy or by a potential acuity meter.

j. *IOL power calculation.* This is done by any of the standard formulas, from axial length, depth of the anterior chamber, and keratometry reading. It should be decided beforehand what kind of lens will be used, as well as what lens will be the stand-by if the first option proves unusable during surgery. Use of a capsule tension ring should also be decided on before hand. A capsule tension ring is useful in cases of aniridia cataracts with dislocation.

INITIAL MANAGEMENT

Refraction

The aim of management is for the eye to realize its full potential. The first step in this direction is checking the refraction and prescription of suitable glasses. Next, orthoptic and pleoptic exercises are given to improve amblyopia. Surgery for removal of the dislocated lens and lens implantation is advised only when it appears to be the best way to overcome the disability of dislocation and aphakia.

Preoperative Preparation

Atropine eye ointment, 1%, is applied twice on the day before the operation. Before surgery, a combination of tropicamide and 5% phenylepherine is instilled three times. General anesthesia is mandatory after a thorough assessment by a physician and an anesthesiologist.

Pars Plana Lensectomy and Vitrectomy

We neither use nor advise using a pars plana approach. It is difficult to avoid damage to the vitreous body. Further, a certain amount of lens–vitreous mixing as a result of surgery is a distinct possibility. Surgery-induced problems in the macula are not easy to gauge in children. The best course is to minimize the incidence and severity of vitreoretinal problems by adopting an anterior approach. An understanding of the highly organized system of vitreous cisterns, premacular bursa, and ciliomacular canal, as researched by Jan Worst, helps the surgeon to prevent or minimize damage to this vital "ecosystem" of the eye.

Anterior Approach

This is our favorite approach for lens extraction and iris-fixated lens implantation. The steps are as follows.

1. Incisions

Two sideport incisions (1 mm) and a main top incision (3.25 to 4.5 mm) to accommodate the passage of the IOL are made. They are all pocket incisions that are best made with diamond knives. The top incision is the last one made, after filling the anterior chamber with viscoelastic material. Sodium hyaluranate is a good material for this purpose, especially when zonular fibers are absent and the vitreous fills part of the anterior chamber. If the zonular fibers are intact, 2% methylcellulose is quite good.

2. Dilation of the Pupil

Every case needs additional dilation at the time of surgery. This is best obtained with intracameral 0.25% preservative-free phenylepherine. Full dilation does not occur in many cases. These cases may require the use of iris hooks in one or two places.

3. Anterior Capsulotomy and Lens Aspiration

a. *Manual capsulotomy.* When the lens is less well fixed by the zonule or is mobile to some degree, it is difficult to do a manual capsulotomy. Instead of making a puncture, the needle pushes the lens away. To succeed in puncturing the capsule, the method is to push a sharp, thin, disposable (28- or 30-gauge) needle with a sudden jab, which opens the capsule without moving the lens. It can then be extended with a fine long scissors, and some sort of anterior capsular hole is made. In these cases, removal of lens matter from the capsular bag is tedious, since the capsulotomy edge may at times get torn, and the zonule breached, so the vitreous starts bulging. If zonular fibers are missing at the start of the operation, a vitreous problem is unavoidable. When a vitreous problem is expected, perhaps surgery from the pars plana side is a better approach. However, using the anterior approach, vitreous disturbance can be minimized as follows. No irrigation is done at any time. The lens is alternatively aspirated and filled with viscoelastic material (dry aspiration). The quantity dealt with in the beginning is very small, and it increases as more space is created inside the capsular bag. The aspiration cannula is 23 or 24 gauge and is attached to a tuberculin syringe. Saline may be used in the very end when one is sure of the stability of the zonular fibers. The opening in the empty capsular bag is increased to the maximum using a long thin scissors and the posterior capsule is laid bare. In a fair number of cases, it is essential to manage the prolapsed vitreous. If an iris-fixated lens is to be used, this may be done after contracting the pupil with a miotic. Vitrectomy is done either before or after lens implantation. In the latter case the tip of the vitrector is passed under the optic of the lens. In some pediatric Marfan cases, a capsule tension ring may be utilized. This is extremely useful when dealing with a young aniridia patient with a dislocated cataract.

b. *Mechanical vitrector capsulotomy.* After making an opening in the anterior capsule, a vitrectomy tip is introduced under the capsule and a suitably sized anterior capsulotomy is done. The vitrector handpiece is sometimes also used for lens aspiration.

c. *Automated capsulotomy with a Fugo Blade.* The Fugo Blade performs well in dislocated lenses, because it cuts without any traction, and it cuts even when the lens is moving. There is no movement of the lens during the cutting (actually ablating) process. There is no disturbance of the vitreous during capsulotomy either. Any size capsulotomy can be done, but it is better to make the capsulotomy only about 3 mm in diameter. Usually there is no danger of the capsulotomy running out. Details on technical aspects of Fugo capsulotomy are described in Chapter 18.

4. Lens Implantation

a. Prior to lens implantation, the anterior chamber is observed again to look for any vitreous. A strand going toward the incision line is pushed back to the pupil, with a thin cannula passed through the sideport. The anterior chamber is then filled with air to observe any trace of vitreous. If need be, additional vitrectomy is done.

b. For the purpose of peripheral iridectomy, the iris is not pulled out of the pocket incision, as there is a risk of iris-root tear and bleeding. A Fugo Blade iridectomy is done inside the anterior chamber. No attempt is made to push fluid into the iridectomy opening for the purpose of verification, lest vitreous gets disturbed.

c. We prefer to implant an iris-claw lens. The surgical steps are described in Chapter 25. Other types of IOLs include the following. The best indication for a posterior chamber lens in-the-bag implantation is a case of aniridia with a dislocated cataract. A capsule tension ring and in-the-bag implantation are the only sensible solution. We perceive scleral fixation of a posterior chamber lens to be highly traumatic to the uvea and the vitreous; it also presents many question marks, especially biodegradation of the fixing nylon or Prolene suture. An angle-supported lens designed for pediatric use is not available.

SPECIAL SITUATIONS

Depending on the degree and direction of the dislocation, the degree of integrity of the zonules, the amount of vitreous presenting through the gap, and the mobility of the crystalline lens, a great variety of surgical situations can be created, each requiring a partly planned and partly innovative approach as dynamic conditions change during the course of the surgery. The sample situations below illustrate this point.

1. The lens is highly mobile, the zonules are barely existent, and the vitreous is beginning to prolapse. The pupil is moderately or well dilated. In this situation, it is preferable not to do a capsulotomy right away, but to try bring the lens into the anterior chamber. For this purpose two cannulas are used from the sideports, both carrying viscoelastic material. The cannulas are maneuvered under the lens in such a way that they sweep every part of the edge of the lens. At the same time the lens is gently lifted forward into the anterior chamber. If support is withdrawn, the lens is likely to fall back. To succeed, the assistant injects a miotic into the anterior chamber. When it is certain that the pupil is contracted enough, the cannulas are withdrawn. The lens, secured in the anterior chamber, is opened with the Fugo Blade and its contents are removed by aspiration or viscoinjection or by irrigation and aspiration. When the capsular bag becomes small, it is pulled out with the remaining contents.

It should be understood that most very mobile lenses still have many zonular fibers attached. If the pupil is not contracted well in time, the lens has a tendency to fall back, creating a difficult situation, because the pupil rapidly constricts over it.

In the case of a highly mobile lens that cannot be brought into the anterior chamber, the two-cannula technique described above should be abandoned if there is risk of damaging the vitreous face. The pupil is dilated maximally by intracameral 0.25% preservative-free phenylepherine. However, it still remains smaller than the lens diameter (that is why the lens does not deliver spontaneously in the first place). Thereafter, the top pocket incision is tapped to let the aqueous escape. The mobile crystalline lens also moves toward the direction of least resistance and gets stuck in the pupil, although it resists entering the anterior chamber. At this point the anterior chamber is deepened with viscoelastic and the Fugo Blade is used for an easy anterior capsulotomy, followed by dry aspiration to reduce the volume of the lens. The lens is delivered into the anterior chamber as soon as it becomes smaller than the pupil.

2. The patient has microspherophakia. A patient presenting with a crystalline lens in the anterior chamber, but no glaucoma, is treated as a special emergency. It is important not to let the lens go back into the posterior chamber. The patient is kept in the prone position and the pupil is contracted by instilling miotic as a jet from a cannula into the conjunctival sac. Once the pupil is well contracted, the case is operated on as a surgical emergency. Lens implantation is done at the same time.

If the patient is already suffering from pupil block glaucoma, or gives a history of other such attacks that resolved spontaneously, the crystalline lens is removed. Secondary lens implantation is done at a later date.

3. The lens is positioned up–out or up–in and the zonular fibers are stretched but intact. They are best seen by coaxial illumination at the highest magnification. Management is relatively simple. A Fugo Blade capsulotomy of about 3 to 4 mm is done a short distance from the insertion of the zonule. The viscoelastic is injected underneath the capsule. Most of the soft lens pops out of the capsulotomy opening into the anterior chamber. It does not rupture the posterior capsule, since the vitreous jelly provides support. The lens matter flows in the direction of least resistance—the anterior chamber and the incision line. The remaining lens matter is carefully dislodged with viscoelastic and dry-aspirated with a 23-gauge cannula. If the posterior capsule gets close to the cannula, aspiration is stopped. A careful irrigation/aspiration is possible without disturbing the vitreous, since the zonular fibers are intact. If some of the zonular fibers get broken, a careful dry aspiration is continued until the bag is clear. The deepest part of the fornix is the most difficult area to clean up. Therefore attention should be directed to it from the beginning. All work on the cannula is done from the sideports.

4. The lens is dislocated up–in, up–out, or in a directly upward position, and the lower zonular fibers are not visible. In this case the surgical steps are basically the same as described above (iii), but the surgery is done at a more leisurely pace, letting the vitreous remain settled by repeated deepening of the anterior chamber with viscoelastic. When the lens matter comes out of the bag and is lying in the anterior chamber, it should be aspirated with a 26-gauge cannula. This cannula aspirates the lens matter but becomes nonfunctional when vitreous blocks the port.

Sometimes when it is difficult to separate the vitreous from the lens matter by dry aspiration, the use of a vitrector becomes necessary. We proceed as follows.

a. The aspiration port is connected to a tuberculin syringe via silicone tubing. It is held by the assistant.

b. The surgeon holds the vitrector in one hand and an irrigating cannula in the other. The two operate through the main upper incision. The system works as follows. We make sure that aspiration and vitrectomy do not occur simultaneously. When the assistant aspirates, the vitrector is at a standstill. Some lens matter gets aspirated. The moment the aspiration port gets blocked with vitreous, aspiration is stopped and cutting is done to remove the tiny bit of vitreous in the port; as and when the need arises to fill the anterior chamber, the saline stream is directed toward the incision line from outside the incision line, just enough to keep the chamber formed. The primary aim is lensectomy, not vitrectomy. Patience is an important ingredient in this technique.

If the vitreous cisterns are not damaged during surgery and some lens matter is inadvertently left inside the capsular fornix or under the iris (because the pupil has contracted), there is no need to panic. It will not fall into the vitreous but will be seen as swollen lens matter in the pupillary area in a day or two. This material can be easily aspirated with a 30-gauge cannula from the sideport, or when there is only a small amount, it can be allowed to absorb spontaneously.

SECONDARY LENS IMPLANTATION IN MARFAN CASES

The surgical steps for artisan lens implantation are the same as those for primary implantation. But there is no struggle involved with removal of the dislocated lens. Vitreous in the anterior chamber, if present, is removed before or after lens implantation.

A thorough preoperative examination includes careful slit-lamp examination, refraction, endothelial cell counts, binocular indirect ophthalmoscopy, and intraocular pressure measurement.

An iris-claw lens is our choice for secondary implantation. There is minimal disturbance to the tissues duration implantation. However, lens implantation is not easy in eyes that have previously undergone pars plana lensectomy and vitrectomy. When incisions are made, the eyeball has a tendency to collapse, due to lack of vitreous support. Attempts to push the iris into the claw of the lens often fail, because the iris tends to fall back and is difficult to bring into the claw. In this situation, the solution is to use a disposable 28- or 30-gauge needle, suitably bent to pick up the iris. The sharp needle tip is pushed into the iris, practically puncturing it, to enable its lifting and passing into the claw. Clumsy attempts or the use of a blunt needle can tear the root of the iris and cause bleeding. Blood trickling into the vitreous delays the recovery of vision.

Scleral fixation of a posterior chamber lens is fraught with a number of problems, such as dealing with a small pupil, vitreous disturbance, surgical trauma to the vitreous or uvea, and vitreous hemorrhage. Postoperatively, one must deal with frequent cases of uveitis, glaucoma, and even retinal detachment. The possible late absorption of nylon or prolene sutures should be kept in mind.

It is very important that the anterior chamber should not go flat at any time during surgery. A flat anterior chamber encourages the appearance of fibrin from near the angle of the anterior chamber, whence it rapidly spreads toward the pupil. Sheets of fibrin form rapidly in complicated cases, for example, with a crystalline lens in the anterior chamber and an increased intraocular pressure. Once formed, fibrin is difficult to manage during surgery. It should be watched carefully in the postoperative period, for signs of pupil block, formation of anterior synechiae, and increases in intraocular pressure. The fibrin may disappear within a few days. Rarely, another intervention is necessary to restore the aqueous flow and clear the pupil. The best plan to minimize or prevent the formation of fibrin during surgery is to keep the anterior chamber formed at all times, not merely with saline but with viscoelastic, which is cleared at the end of the surgery.

POSTOPERATIVE MANAGEMENT

Watch for signs of inflammation and the presence of blood or fibrin and monitor the depth of the anterior chamber, the state of the pupil and the peripheral iridectomy, the presence of any lens matter, the intraocular pressure, vitreoretinal disturbance, and the fundus (if not visible, B scan should be performed). Postoperative medication is no different from that for routine cases of cataract surgery.

OUR RESULTS

In a series of 175 ectopia lentis patients between 2.5 and 16 years of age (average, 9.7 years), with a follow-up of 4 to 140 months (average, 18.4 months), the final refractive error was between +1.5 and −5.5 D (in 103 cases), the average being −1.61 D. The best corrected vision varied between 6/60 and 6/6, the average being 6/23 ($n = 103$). Four patients were treated for retinal detachment, and three for glaucoma.

CONCLUSION

In summary, management of a dislocated lens requires an understanding of the cisternal anatomy of the vitreous and the need for a traction-free clean capsulotomy, evacuation of the lens matter more by positive pressure of viscoelastic and less by irrigation or irrigation/aspiration, and the choice of a lens that requires no support from the capsule for fixation.

REFERENCES

1. Koenig SB, Mieler WF. Management of ectopia lentis in a family with Marfan syndrome. *Arch Ophthalmol* 1996;114:1058.
2. Maumenee IH. The eye in the Marfan syndrome. *Trans Am Ophthalmol Soc* 1981;79:684.
3. Nelson LB, Maumenee IH. Ectopia lentis. *Surv Ophthalmol* 1982; 27:143.
4. Worst JGF, Los LI. *Cisternal Anatomy of the Vitreous.* London: Kugler, 1995:1,9–29.
5. Fugo RJ, DelCampo DM. The Fugo Blade™: The next step after capsulorhexis. *Ann Ophthalmol* 2001;33(1):12–20.
6. Fugo RJ, Singh D, Fine IH. Automated Fugo Blade capsulotomy: A new technique and a new instrument. *Eyeworld* 2002;7(9): 49–54.
7. Singh SK. Fugo Blade capsulotomy: A new high–tech cutting technology. *Trop Ophthalmol* 2001;1(1):14–16.

Pediatric Cataract Surgery in Eyes with Uveitis

Suresh K. Pandey, Rupal H. Trivedi, and M. Edward Wilson, Jr.

Cataract surgery in children is usually associated with an increased risk of inflammation, as well as intraoperative and postoperative complications, in comparison to routine adult cataract surgery. Pediatric cataract surgery in eyes with uveitis may be associated with the highest rate of complications owing to the greater technical difficulty during surgery and, potentially, an even greater postoperative intraocular inflammatory response than is seen with other children. It is important to adopt strategies before, during, and after such surgery to minimize these complications.

Uveitis in children may occur for several reasons, the details of which are beyond the scope of this chapter. In brief, the main causes of uveitis in children are juvenile idiopathic arthritis (JIA), inflammatory bowel disease, ankylosing spondylitis, Reiter's disease, and sarcoidosis. Perhaps the most severe entity is JIA.

JIA is defined as an arthritis of unknown origin, of at least 6 weeks' duration, diagnosed before the age of 16 years.[1–5] The term JIA is now preferred over juvenile rheumatoid arthritis (JRA), the term most familiar to ophthalmologists in the United States.[1–5] The criteria of the European League of Associations of Rheumatology have been widely used in Europe, where the disease became known as juvenile chronic arthritis, whereas the American College of Rheumatology preferred the term JRA.[1–5] The term JRA implies a similarity to adult rheumatoid arthritis, whereas only a fairly small subset in fact has its counterpart in adult rheumatoid arthritis.[1] In 1994, the International League of Associations for Rheumatology proposed a new classification system, which was subsequently modified.[2–4] It avoids use of the terms *rheumatoid* and *chronic*, instead substituting the term *idiopathic*. Thus, arthritis of unknown cause occurring in a child is designated JIA. Table 39-1 compares the classification systems of arthritis in children (adapted from Ref. 2). In this chapter, we use the term JIA, although many of the publications referred to here use the older term, JRA.

Patients with JIA may present with a dense cataract at the time of initial ophthalmologic evaluation or they may develop a cataract slowly over the course of uveitis treatment. Cataracts associated with JIA are usually associated with other ocular complications, which make the cataract surgery more difficult and the results of such surgery more uncertain. In one study,[6] the prevalence of uveitis was 9.3% among 760 patients of JIA; other complications, such as band keratopathy, cataract, synechiae, or glaucoma, developed in 31% of patients with uveitis. In another study, of children with rheumatoid-related disease,[7] up to 10% had at least one episode of uveitis and other associated ocular complications observed were cataract, synechiae, band-shaped keratopathy, secondary glaucoma, and retinal diseases. It has also been observed that children with JIA-associated uveitis are younger, demonstrate an active intraocular inflammation for an extended period after surgery, and tend to develop secondary membranes postoperatively, necessitating a second surgical intervention.[8]

Cataracts develop in uveitic eyes for a number of reasons. Severe and recurrent anterior chamber inflammation can lead to posterior synechiae and/or anterior subcapsular lens opacities. Corticosteroid treatment of uveitis leads to formation of posterior subcapsular cataracts. Kanski and Shun-Shin[9] reported 46% secondary cataracts, which may be related to chronic inflammation, corticosteroid use, or both. Narayana et al.[10] studied the patterns of uveitis in children at a referral eye care center in South India and reported that approximately 25% (8/31) developed cataracts. In another study, cataract was noted in 35% (43/123) of children with uveitis.[11] In a study of 51 JIA patients by Wolf et al.,[12] cataract was noted in 46%. In a large series of children with anterior uveitis, Foster and Barrett found that, even with aggressive therapy to control

▶ **TABLE 39-1** **Comparison of Classification Systems of Arthritis in Children**

	Classification System		
	American College of Rheumatology	European League Against Rheumatism	International League of Associations for Rheumatology
Designation	Juvenile rheumatoid arthritis (JRA)	Juvenile chronic arthritis	Juvenile ankylosing spondylitis (JAS)
Types	Systemic	Systemic	Systemic
	Pauciarticular	Pauciarticular	Oligoarticular
	Polyarticular	RF-negative polyarticular	RF-negative polyarthritis
		RF-positive polyarticular (JRA)	
		Psoriatic	Psoriatic
		JAS	Enthesitis-related
			Undefined

Adapted from Fink CW. Proposal for the development of classification criteria for arthritides of childhood. *J Rheumatol* 1995;22:1566–1569.
RF, rheumatoid factor.

inflammation, 18% of patients with JIA-associated uveitis developed secondary cataracts.[13] In eyes with Behçet diseases one recent study has reported 46.9% incidence of cataract in involved eye.[14]

TIMING OF SURGERY

Cataract surgery in these cases should be performed only with valid indications, given the high complication rate. It is advisable to refer such complicated patients to an experienced pediatric cataract surgeon. Some authors have suggested that cataract surgery combined with pars plana vitrectomy should be performed on those eyes with cataracts sufficient to limit visual acuity to 20/200 or less, after maintenance of complete freedom from inflammation for at least 3 months.[13]

The most important caveat to follow in these eyes is the adequate control of inflammation before undertaking surgery, with intensive topical and, sometimes, systemic steroid therapy. The topical steroids should be started preferably 2 weeks before surgery.[15]

PREOPERATIVE CONSIDERATIONS

Elective cataract surgery should only be undertaken in uveitic eyes when intraocular inflammation has been minimized and intraocular pressure controlled. It may not be possible to completely inhibit all uveitis activity. However, every effort should be made to reduce inflammation prior to surgery. This will usually require systemic immunosuppressive therapy prescribed in conjunction with a pediatric rheumatologist. Systemic steroid prophylaxis should be considered if macular edema is a significant risk, such as in eyes with previous uveitis-related macular edema.

SURGICAL TECHNIQUE

It is debatable whether the older technique of lensectomy plus anterior vitrectomy, or extracapsular cataract surgery (ECCE) with intraocular lens (IOL) implantation, or ECCE plus anterior vitrectomy through posterior capsulotomy plus IOL implantation provides better results in children. The trend is now toward performing ECCE plus posterior capsulotomy plus anterior vitrectomy and IOL implantation.[16] However, this may be a demanding surgery in children with uveitis. A lensectomy with anterior vitrectomy and a peripheral iridectomy may be justified, followed by contact lenses for visual rehabilitation.[17] This technique has shown good results in many hands.[18]

USE OF INTRAOCULAR LENSES

There is no consensus on whether or not IOLs should be implanted in cases of cataract with uveitis.[19] Until recently, most considered IOL implantation to be contraindicated in children with JIA-associated uveitis because an IOL may act as a scaffolding agent and probably creates a higher risk for inflammatory membranes. However, increasing evidence is now available that the appropriate use of IOLs in carefully selected patients may be helpful for better visual rehabilitation[20] even when associated with JIA or when simultaneous trabeculectomy is done.[15] BenEzra and Cohen[8] evaluated the use of IOLs in children with both JIA-associated and non-JIA-associated uveitis. The authors concluded that IOL implantation seems preferable to correction with contact lenses in young children needing surgery in one eye, as their tolerance of contact lenses is poor and their use is generally discontinued, resulting in strabismus in some of the children on long-term follow-up.

In another study, Lam and associates[15] observed that with adequate long-term preoperative and postoperative control of intraocular inflammation with systemic immunosuppressive therapy in addition to intensive topical corticosteroid treatment, a final postoperative Snellen visual acuity of 20/40 or better could be achieved after cataract surgery with IOLs in JIA.

There is also controversy over the best type of lens in cases of uveitis. Foldable lenses have been evaluated in adult patients and found to be safe, but the authors concluded that the optimal biomaterial for these uveitic eyes has yet to be found.[21] The use of heparin-surface-modified (HSM) polymethylmethacrylate (PMMA) IOLs has also been advocated in these high-risk cases. A covalent surface linkage of heparin to synthetic polymeric materials is achieved by reductive amination, and this coating has been shown to be stable in the long term as well, based on some experimental studies.[22] It has been suggested that implantation of HSM IOLs in cataract patients with chronic uveitis may decrease the number and severity of deposits on the surface of the IOL. However, in a clinical study on adult patients with inactive uveitis or diabetes,[23] no statistically significant difference was found between HSM and uncoated PMMA IOLs in the number of cellular deposits found on the anterior IOL surface, the number of adhesions between the iris and the IOL, or the incidence of capsular opacification. Similar results were seen in another study of similar design comparing HSM and uncoated PMMA IOLs in eyes with uveitis.[24] However, these results may not be strictly applicable to children with uveitis where the inflammation is much more severe.

At the same time, it must be remembered that the use of IOLs in uveitis may lead to increased inflammation postoperatively in some cases, in which the IOL may even have to be explanted. In these cases, IOL explantation may salvage or stabilize the vision, provided that inflammation has not resulted in irreversible damage to the macula or optic nerve prior to explantation.[25]

INTRAOPERATIVE DIFFICULTIES

There are many potential complications in pediatric cataract surgery in children with uveitis. First, associated ocular complications such as synechiae may make the surgery difficult and the pupil may not dilate well (Figs. 39-1 and 39-2). Similarly, the associated band keratopathy may impair visualization. There is also a greater tendency toward bleeding during surgery.[20]

Maneuvers to increase the pupillary aperture include synechiolysis, iris stretching, use of self-retaining iris retractors (Fig. 39-2B–D), sphincterotomy, and iridotomy. The least iris manipulation consistent with adequate pupillary access should be the aim. A large capsulorhexis reduces the risk of synechia formation between the iris and the anterior capsular margin. A HSM IOL is less likely to be associated with deposits/giant cell formation on the lens surface, as mentioned earlier.

POSTOPERATIVE COMPLICATIONS

Various postoperative complications may occur, such as uveitis, which may even be of the severe fibrinous exudation type, macular edema, and hypotony, even leading to maculopathy. In a study by Kanski,[26] the results of lensectomy were reviewed retrospectively in 131 patients with JIA (187 eyes). The main operative complication was accidental loss of lens material into the vitreous cavity, and the postoperative complications were glaucoma (23 eyes; 15%), phthisis (14 eyes; 8%), secondary pupillary membranes (11 eyes; 6%), and retinal detachment (6 eyes; 3%). The main causes of a postoperative visual acuity of 20/200 or less were glaucoma, amblyopia, and phthisis. Later studies have reported a slightly lower incidence of complications, yet many children did not attain good vision after surgery owing to complications such as glaucoma and macular disease (chronic cystoid macular edema,

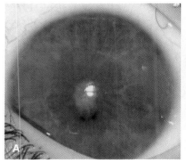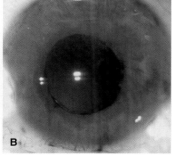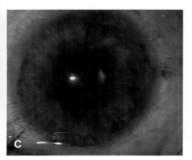

FIGURE 39-1. Cataract secondary to JIA-related uveitis in a 7-year-old child. Band-shaped keratopathy removed 2 months before cataract surgery. **A.** Preoperative photograph showing nondilated oval pupil secondary to irido-lenticular synechiae. **B.** In-the-bag fixation of a single-piece AcrySof IOL. **C.** Recurrence of band-shaped keratopathy; photograph taken 6 months after cataract surgery.

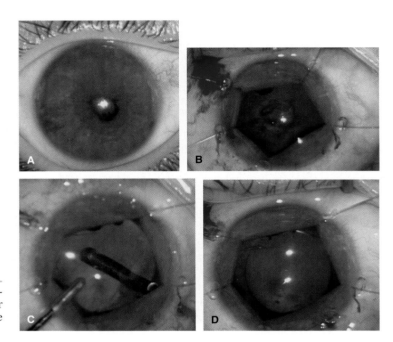

FIGURE 39-2. A. Cataract secondary to uveitis associated with a small pupil. The pupil failed to dilate after synechiolysis. **B–D.** Iris retractors were used to facilitate visualization during surgery.

macular hole, hypotony maculopathy, and recurrent macular pucker)[27] and other serious problems such as severe postoperative uveitis, hypotonia oculi, and phthisis bulbi.[18] In other studies, the reasons for lower visual acuity postoperatively were cystoid macular edema, band keratopathy, amblyopia, and floaters in the vitreous,[5] perilental membrane, chronic low-grade inflammation not responding to anti-inflammatory treatment, and cyclitic membrane resulting in hypotony and maculopathy.[25]

Fibrinous uveitis should initially be treated with intensive topical steroids, but if it persists, intracameral injection of recombinant tissue plasminogen activator (rtPA) should be considered. It has been suggested that intracameral rtPA may be used for fibrinolysis after cataract surgery in children when severe fibrin formation is seen despite intensive topical steroid therapy.[28] Ten micrograms of rtPA was applied 7.18 ± 2.04 days after intraocular surgery. Complete resolution of fibrin formation occurred in 90% of the patients, and in these cases no recurrent fibrinous reaction or adverse effects were noted. However, fibrin clot dissolution was incomplete in two eyes, in the same patient, with a history of JIA and chronic uveitis.

In a series of seven patients with JIA who underwent cataract extraction and IOL implantation, Probst and Holland[29] described less favorable results among children compared with adults. The major complications included membrane and synechia formation as well as elevated intraocular pressure. In a recent study, Lam et al.[15] did not observe any such complications. They believe that the lack of such complications may be attributed to the use of aggressive systemic methotrexate and corticosteroid immunosuppression. Four of five children in their study underwent systemic immunosuppression for a median length of 1.25 years before eye surgery.

Visually significant posterior capsule opacification or secondary membrane formation should be treated surgically or by YAG laser posterior capsulotomy. The rate of visual axis opacification requiring a secondary procedure has been reported as 100% by Probst and Holland,[29] 83% by Lam and associates,[15] 70.0% by Lundvall and Zetterstrom,[30] and 80% by BenEzra and Cohen.[8]

Posterior synechiae developed in 100 and 66%, respectively, of eyes with uveitis and IOL in the studies by BenEzra and Cohen[8] and Probst and Holland.[29] In contrast, Lam and associates[15] did not find any posterior synechiae. The incidence of glaucoma has been reported as 56%,[8] 60%,[30] 83%,[15] and 100%.[29] Severe band keratopathy can be associated in such eyes. In cases with band keratopathy chelating agents or excimer laser can be used to clear the cornea, however, the deposition of calcium tends to recur (see Fig. 39-1C).

CONCLUSION

In summary, pediatric cataract surgery in eyes with uveitis may be associated with increased ocular morbidity owing to the greater technical difficulty during surgery and increased intraocular inflammation in the postoperative period. Standard surgery with IOL implantation may be feasible if preoperative anti-inflammatory medications are used and the inflammatory condition is inactive. Lensectomy or anterior vitrectomy without IOL may be beneficial in some situations, such as a dense cataract associated with

JIA uveitis, which has been difficult to control. The surgical approach must always be individualized to consider the symptoms, visual acuity, or etiology of uveitis and to maintain the clarity of the visual axis. Postoperative control of inflammation, by long-term careful follow-up, is mandatory in these cases.

REFERENCES

1. Kotaniemi K, Savolainen A, Karma A, Aho K. Recent advances in uveitis of juvenile idiopathic arthritis. *Surv Ophthalmol* 2003;48:489–502.
2. Fink CW. Proposal for the development of classification criteria for idiopathic arthritides of childhood. *J Rheumatol* 1995;22:1566–1569.
3. Petty RE, Southwood TR, Baum J, Bhettay E, Glass DN, Manners P, Maldonado-Cocco J, Suarez-Almazor M, Orozco-Alcala J, Prieur AM. Revision of the proposed classification criteria for juvenile idiopathic arthritis: Durban, 1997. *J Rheumatol* 1998;25:1991–1994.
4. Cleary AG, Sills JA, Davidson JE. Revision of the proposed classification criteria for juvenile idiopathic arthritis: Durban, 1997. *J Rheumatol* 2000;27:1568.
5. Petty RE, Smith JR, Rosenbaum JT. Arthritis and uveitis in children. A pediatric rheumatology perspective. *Am J Ophthalmol* 2003;135:879–884.
6. Chalom EC, Goldsmith DP, Koehler MA, et al. Prevalence and outcome of uveitis in a regional cohort of patients with juvenile rheumatoid arthritis. *J Rheumatol* 1997;24:2031–2034.
7. Moller DE, Urban A, Kraft HE, Schontube M. Eye complications in 458 children with rheumatoid arthritis. *Klin Monatsbl Augenheilkd* 2001;217:15–22.
8. BenEzra D, Cohen E. Cataract surgery in children with chronic uveitis. *Ophthalmology* 2000;107:1255–1260.
9. Kanski JJ, Shun-Shin GA. Systemic uveitis syndromes in childhood: an analysis of 340 cases. *Ophthalmology* 1984;9:1247–1252.
10. Narayana KM, Bora A, Biswas J. Patterns of uveitis in children presenting at a tertiary eye care centre in south India. *Indian J Ophthalmol* 2003;51(2):129–132.
11. de Boer J, Wulffraat N, Rothova A. Visual loss in uveitis of childhood. *Br J Ophthalmol* 2003;87:879–884.
12. Wolf MD, Lichter PR, Ragsdale CG. Prognostic factors in the uveitis of juvenile rheumatoid arthritis. *Ophthalmology* 1987;94:1242–1248.
13. Foster CS, Barrett F. Cataract development and cataract surgery in patients with juvenile rheumatoid arthritis-associated iridocyclitis. *Ophthalmology* 1993;100:809–817.
14. Tugal-Tutkun I, Urgancioglu M. Childhood-onset uveitis in Behcet disease: a descriptive study of 36 cases. *Am J Ophthalmol* 2003;136:1114–1119.
15. Lam LA, Lowder CY, Baerveldt G, et al. Surgical management of cataracts in children with juvenile rheumatoid arthritis-associated uveitis. *Am J Ophthalmol* 2003;135:772–778.
16. Basti S, Ravishankar U, Gupta S. Results of a prospective evaluation of three methods of management of pediatric cataracts. *Ophthalmology* 1996;103:713–720.
17. Paikos P, Fotopoulou M, Papathanassiou M, et al. Cataract surgery in children with uveitis. *J Pediatr Ophthalmol Strabismus* 2001;38:16–20.
18. Verbraeken H. Pars plana lensectomy in cases of cataract with juvenile chronic uveitis. *Graefes Arch Clin Exp Ophthalmol* 1996;234:618–622.
19. Morgan KS. Cataract surgery and intraocular lens implantation in children. *Curr Opin Ophthalmol* 1993;4:54–60.
20. Samochowiec-Donocik E, Koraszewska-Matuszewska B, Stangrecka-Matelska K. Intraocular correction of aphakia after cataract extraction for uveitis in adolescents. *Klin Oczna* 2000;102:413–416.
21. Rauz S, Stavrou P, Murray PI. Evaluation of foldable intraocular lenses in patients with uveitis. *Ophthalmology* 2000;107:909–919.
22. Dick B, Greiner K, Magdowski G, Pfeiffer N. Long-term stability of heparin-coated PMMA intraocular lenses. Results of an in vitro study. *Ophthalmology* 1997;94:920–924.
23. Tabbara KF, Al-Kaff AS, Al-Rajhi AA, et al. Heparin surface-modified intraocular lenses in patients with inactive uveitis or diabetes. *Ophthalmology* 1998;105:843–845.
24. Lardenoye CW, van der Lelij A, Berendschot TT, Rothova A. A retrospective analysis of heparin-surface-modified intraocular lenses versus regular polymethylmethacrylate intraocular lenses in patients with uveitis. *Doc Ophthalmol* 1996;92:41–50.
25. Foster CS, Stavrou P, Zafirakis P, et al. Intraocular lens removal from patients with uveitis. *Am J Ophthalmol* 1999;128:31–37.
26. Kanski JJ. Lensectomy for complicated cataract in juvenile chronic iridocyclitis. *Br J Ophthalmol* 1992;76:72–75.
27. Fox GM, Flynn HW Jr, Davis JL, Culbertson W. Causes of reduced visual acuity on long-term follow-up after cataract extraction in patients with uveitis and juvenile rheumatoid arthritis. *Am J Ophthalmol* 1992;114:708–714.
28. Klais CM, Hattenbach LO, Steinkamp GW, et al. Intraocular recombinant tissue-plasminogen activator fibrinolysis of fibrin formation after cataract surgery in children. *J Cataract Refract Surg* 1999;25:357–362.
29. Probst LE, Holland EJ. Intraocular lens implantation in patients with juvenile rheumatoid arthritis. *Am J Ophthalmol* 1996;122:161–170.
30. Lundvall A, Zetterstrom C. Cataract extraction and intraocular lens implantation in children with uveitis. *Br J Ophthalmol* 2000;84:791–793.

Intraoperative Complications and Postoperative Sequelae

Intraoperative Complications of Pediatric Intraocular Lens Surgery and Their Management

Suresh K. Pandey and M. Edward Wilson, Jr.

The surgical management of cataracts in children is markedly different from that in adults. Not only are the eyes smaller because of age, but also many are microphthalmic. Decreased scleral rigidity and increased vitreous upthrust make surgical manipulations within these eyes more difficult. The anterior chamber is often unstable, the capsule management requires special considerations, and the propensity for postoperative inflammation is increased.[1–3] These special patients are uniquely challenging. The best surgical techniques for children will evolve most efficiently with optimal cooperation and collaboration between pediatric ophthalmologists and adult cataract surgeons.

OPERATIVE PROBLEMS, COMPLICATIONS, AND THEIR MANAGEMENT

Incision-Related Complications

Collapse of the anterior chamber and prolapse of iris tissue are also much more common when operating on pediatric eyes. Incisions should be constructed to provide a snug fit for the instruments that pass into the anterior chamber. Smaller wounds and tunnel configurations decrease the incidence of iris prolapse into the wound during surgery and assist the surgeon in preventing collapse of the anterior chamber, which occurs with greater frequency in the soft eyes of children. Since anterior chamber instability and wound leaks are such frequent problems in pediatric cataract surgery, the move to foldable lenses, which allow smaller incisions, has been a very welcome advance for the pediatric cataract surgeon. Also, bimanual surgery through two 20-gauge "tight-fit" tunneled "stab" incisions has been the norm in infantile cataract surgery for almost 20 years for the very reason of anterior chamber stability. Contrary to adult cataract surgery, scleral or corneal tunnel incisions and even paracentesis incisions do not self-seal in children.[2,3] Small paracentesis openings used to place iris retractors, 10.0 Prolene sutures for iris repair or scleral fixation of an intraocular lens (IOL), or ophthalmic viscosurgical devices (OVDs) usually do not need to be sutured. However, 20-gauge (or even 23-gauge) openings through which round irrigating or aspirating cannulas and vitrector handpieces have been placed usually leak if not sutured. Absorbable synthetic sutures (10.0 vicryl or Biosorb) are usually used since they do not need to be removed. However, more foreign body symptoms occur with them compared to nylon sutures because the synthetic absorbable sutures are usually braided and the knots do not bury easily. At the end of a pediatric cataract surgery, all wounds should be carefully tested to make sure no leakage is present. Since children rub their eyes after surgery, even when told not to, tightly sealed wounds are needed. Even if the closure is so tight that marked astigmatism is present on the first day after surgery, this is acceptable if it avoids a wound leak. The sutures will dissolve and the astigmatism will be temporary. A poorly sealed wound, however, will leak when the child rubs the eye. This leads to shallowing of the anterior chamber, which causes fibrin formation and may result in iris adhesion to the wound's internal lip. The parents should be instructed to have the child wear an eye shield until the wound is well healed.

Interested readers should refer to Chapter 11 for details on incision and suturing.

Formation of the Capsulorhexis

Because of the elasticity of the anterior capsule in young children, it is relatively difficult to achieve capsulorhexis without radial tear formation.[1] Use of high-density viscoelastic (e.g., Healon-GV and Healon-5; AMO Inc., Santa Ana, CA, USA) and newer techniques helps to achieve complete capsulorhexis. The most common anterior capsulotomy complication is the so-called "runaway rhexis," where the elasticity of the capsule causes the tear to extend suddenly out toward the lens equator (Figure 40-1). When this begins, the surgeon should stop tearing, place more OVD, regrab close to the tear edge, and pull toward the center of the pupil. If this does not recover the capsulotomy easily, conversion to a vitrectorhexis or to a Kloti diathermy capsulotomy has been successful for us. The Fugo Plasma Blade also works well for this recovery

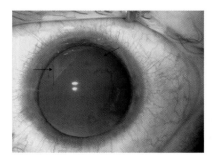

FIGURE 40-1. Photograph illustrating peripheral extension of the anterior capsule tear ("runaway rhexis" shown by arrows) during the vitrectorhexis procedure. This is not uncommon during pediatric cataract surgery owing to the elasticity of the lens capsule.

maneuver. To avoid this complication, the vitrectorhexis method is utilized worldwide most commonly in the first 2 years of life. After that age the manual tear capsulotomy is most commonly used, but with care to regrasp frequently, pull more toward the center of the pupil, reapply OVD often to keep the capsule surface flattened, and aim for a slightly smaller capsulorhexis since the elastic capsule stretches before it tears, often making the capsulotomy size bigger after release than it appeared during tearing.

Inappropriate size and shape are also complications of the anterior capsulotomy that are seen more often with children than with adults. Surgeons are urged to go slow and pay particular attention to size, shape, and centration each time the capsulotomy edge is released. If the capsulotomy opening is too small, it can be enlarged after the IOL is inserted, using any of the methods mentioned above. If it is too large or poorly shaped, take care to get the haptics of the IOL under the capsulorhexis edge and place the haptics where the capsulotomy edges can be most easily seen. Every attempt should be made to cover the edge of the IOL optic with the capsulorhexis edge when possible.

A round capsulotomy in children can still develop a radial tear during surgery. While the vitrectorhexis and the other alternatives to the standard manual-tear capsulorhexis have improved the surgeon's ability to control the size, shape, and centration of the capsulotomy in children, they are more easily torn during surgical manipulation. Most of the radial tears we have seen in children have occurred at previously identified "right-angle" edges in the capsulotomy. These small "squared-off" imperfections in an otherwise circular capsulotomy are not always obvious but can be detected if looked for carefully. With experience, the surgeon forms fewer of these weak areas inadvertently. Also, if identified, these areas can be rounded out by reapplying whatever instrument was used to cut around the "squared-off" edge. If, during this recovery maneuver, a prominent scalloped edge is created, no weakness results as long as the scalloped "point" is aiming at the center of the pupil. Right-angle edges, on the other hand, have a "point" aimed at the lens equator. This is the point at which tearing occurs.

The use of the single-piece AcrySof IOL and the Monarch II injector (Alcon Inc., Fort Worth, TX, USA) has decreased the incidence of intraoperative radial tears in the capsulotomy edge even when imperfections in the edge exist. The unfolding of the three-piece AcrySof IOL would sometimes occur more anteriorly than desired and strike the capsulotomy edge. Also, dialing of the IOL to place the trailing haptic into the capsular bag can be more traumatic when performed in the soft pediatric eye. This maneuver placed added stress on the capsulotomy edge but has been eliminated, for the most part, with use of the newer single-piece foldable lenses. Finally, the sudden flat anterior chamber that can occur after the OVD is removed from a pediatric eye before the wounds are sutured can cause the IOL to move anteriorly and place stress on the capsulotomy edge. Every effort should be made to sew the wounds prior to complete removal of the OVD if possible. Readers should also refer to Chapter 13 to learn about the various surgical techniques for anterior capsule management.

Positive Vitreous Pressure

A high intraoperative vitreous pressure is produced as a result of scleral collapse due to low scleral rigidity, which results in forward movements of the iris lens diaphragm.[2,3] An appropriate and safe hypotony can be achieved by inducing hyperventilation during anesthesia. A small incision helps to reduce the chances of a high intraoperative posterior vitreous pressure, as the surgery is performed practically in a closed chamber. Use of high-density viscoelastic (e.g., Healon-GV or Healon-5; AMO Inc.) helps to maintain a deep anterior chamber and keep the iris lens diaphragm backward. Pars plana approach removal of the OVD and vitreous can, at times, be needed as well.

Intraoperative Miosis

Among the operative challenges faced by the pediatric cataract surgeon, the miotic pupil is one of the most common obstacles that is associated with the greatest likelihood of intraoperative complications. Intraoperative miosis in young children is often due to a combination of congenital anterior segment maldevelopment and surgical manipulation/touch of the iris.

There are many regimens to provide adequate pharmacologic dilation in all patients. Most of these regimens are followed in adult cataract surgery and these may also be suitable for pediatric cataract surgery. One recommended guideline is 1% cyclopentolate (Cyclogel), 2.5% neosynephrine (Mydfrin), and 0.5% ketorolac tromethamine (Acular) given three times at 5-min intervals prior to surgery. Use of 0.5 mL of 1:1,000 adrenaline in 500 mL of irrigating fluid is essential to maintain pupillary dilation throughout the surgery.

If the pupil does not dilate to a size deemed adequate to allow safe cataract–IOL surgery, the surgeon can try other methods to dilate the pupil. Methods reported in the literature, mostly for adult cataract cases, include stretching with iris hooks, using the Beehler dilator (Moria, Doylestown, PA, USA), performing multiple sphincterotomies with microscissors, using iris retractors, and using the Graether pupil expander.[4,5] Surgeons have attempted to use some of these devices in pediatric cataract surgery, however, there are no published reports comparing the efficacy and pros and cons of various methods. Viscodilation is often helpful during capsulotomy and during IOL insertion. Highly viscous OVDs can often open the pupil wider than possible using pharmacological means.

Unique to pediatric cataract surgery is the infant with a dense nuclear congenital cataract and a pinpoint pupil that does not dilate at all. These infants usually have nearly cryptless irises with a poorly formed pupillary ruff and no collarette. Stretching these irises will sometimes provide enough visualization to perform the cataract surgery, but in our experience, severe miosis recurs after surgery despite the use of atropine. The vitrector is used, in these infants, to remove the central portion of the pupil. The new pupil is made round and midsized. Remarkably, little bleeding results and the cosmetic appearance is acceptable. These pupils have no ability to dilate in dim light or constrict in bright light. Therefore, these actions are not being sacrificed by the vitrector pupiloplasty.

A new device that does not share the disadvantages of the mechanical stretching, cutting, and iris retainer pupil dilating methods is the Perfect Pupil Injectable (Milvella Pty., Ltd., Sydney, Australia), which was developed by E. John Milverton, MD, for small pupil cataract surgery. The Perfect Pupil Injectable is a sterile, disposable, and flexible polyurethane ring with an integrated arm designed to allow easy insertion and removal through the smallest of incisions (<100 μm). Because of its unique, open ring design, the device captures the pupillary margin, protects the sphincter, and does not cause tears or stretching of the iris, bleeding, or pigment dispersion.[6] Capsulorrhexis, hydrodissection, phacoaspiration, and IOL insertion are performed with the device in place. The Perfect Pupil Injectable can be inserted through a small incision using an injector and then removed at the end of the surgery by reversing the steps used for insertion (Figure 40-2).

Intraoperative Complications of the Posterior Capsule

The surgeon can recognize a *torn posterior capsule* during lens aspiration by signs such as a sudden deepening of the anterior chamber. This occurs instantaneously as a rent appears in the capsule. As this occurs, the pupil will dilate in response to the deepening anterior chamber. Finally, during aspiration, lenticular particles/residual cortical matter falls away from, and will not come toward, the tip of the aspirator, as the flow dynamics in the anterior chamber have been altered by the tear in the posterior capsule. Sometimes the presence of vitreous in the anterior chamber may also indicate a torn posterior capsule. The posterior capsule can tear during hydrodissection, phacoaspiration, irrigation and aspiration, capsular polishing, lens insertion, and OVD removal.

In all cases, if the posterior capsular tear is entirely within view, a posterior capsulorhexis can be attempted. If the vitreous face is intact, this is done by placing viscoelastic above and below the tear, pushing the vitreous face back, and allowing room to grasp the torn capsule. If the vitreous face is already broken, viscoelastic is

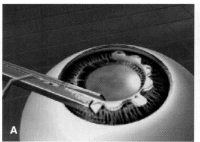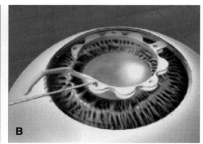

FIGURE 40-2. The Perfect Pupil device can be inserted via a small incision using an injector. Owing to its unique, open ring design it may be helpful for intraoperative pupillary dilation without causing tears or stretching of the iris. **A.** Schematic illustration showing insertion of the Perfect Pupil device. **B.** Schematic illustration showing removal of the Perfect Pupil device. (Courtesy of E. John Milverton, MD, FRANZCO, Sydney, Australia.)

necessary only to stabilize the anterior chamber and make room for the forceps. Using a capsulorhexis forceps, the capsule is then gently torn to create a 360° posterior capsulorhexis. As the posterior capsule is more fragile than the anterior capsule, frequent regrasping of the tearing capsular flap is necessary to provide adequate control of the direction of the tear. This procedure is made difficult due to difficulty with visualization of the tearing capsule and difficulty with forceps manipulation deep in the anterior chamber. Failed attempts may result in extension of the tear and, if not already present, vitreous loss.

Alternatively, the vitrector handpiece can be used to round out the posterior capsule tear, remove residual cortex, and remove prolapsed vitreous. Pediatric surgeons are more likely to use this approach since the use of the vitrector is often more familiar than the use of a capsulorhexis forceps on the posterior capsule. Care should be taken to begin with a low flow so that the anterior chamber dynamics are not changed drastically when the instruments are placed in the eye. This could lead to an extension of the posterior capsule tear. Once rounded out, the posterior vitrectorhexis can be quite stable and resistant to further tearing. The advantage of the vitrector handpiece is that it can safely remove cortex when it is mixed with vitreous. It can also cut the capsule and vitreous simultaneously without undue traction of the vitreous base or retina. A vitrector handpiece driven by a Venturi pump works best when used in this way.

When the surgeon chooses to perform a primary posterior capsulotomy and an anterior vitrectomy, the most common complication encountered intraoperatively is a vitreous strand to the anterior wound. When this occurs, the vitrector must be reinserted and the strand removed. A second instrument may be needed, through a paracentesis, to sweep the vitreous strand away from the wound so that the vitrector handpiece can remove it. A taut strand of vitreous will not easily enter the vitreous cutter until its connection to the wound it broken. A pars plana approach to the anterior vitrectomy avoids this possible complication and is recommended. The risk to the retina is very minimal as long as the proper placement is selected for the entry wound.

Two complications of pars plana posterior capsulotomy and anterior vitrectomy need to be mentioned here, how-

ever. The most common is laceration of the equator of the capsular bag with the micro vitreoretinal (MVR) blade. The entry with the MVR blade should be aimed toward the center of the vitreous cavity to avoid hitting the capsular bag. The capsule may still be distended with an OVD or irrigation fluid. Surgeons like to see the tip of the MVR blade in the pupillary space through the operating microscope before withdrawing it. The tendency is to advance the MVR blade too anteriorly. In very young infants, the entry is even closer to the limbus. In these cases, the MVR blade must be aimed at the optic nerve to avoid hitting the capsular bag. The second, less commonly encountered complication is bleeding into the vitreous cavity. The vitrector cutter must be turned off before the handpiece is withdrawn. If not, the cutter may engage the tip on a ciliary process during handpiece withdrawal, causing profuse bleeding. If this occurs, intraocular cautery will likely not be needed but a full-core vitrectomy will be needed to clear the blood. A retinal specialist will need to be consulted unless the surgeon is experienced in core vitrectomy techniques.

Interested readers should also refer to Chapters 16 and 19 to read about the surgical management of vitreous loss including technique for vitrectomy.

Zonular Dialysis: Recognition and Management

A complete discussion of preoperative zonular dialysis is beyond the scope of this chapter. It may be pertinent to refer to Chapter 38 for some details on zonular dehiscence. It should be noted that zonular dialysis greatly increases the risk of both vitreous loss and lenticular material sinking into the vitreous. Obviously IOL implantation may be more difficult. The surgeon needs to evaluate the number of clock hours involved with the zonular dialysis and the surgeon's ability to perform phacoaspiration in this setting. When inserted into the capsular sac, an endocapsular ring provides a circumferential expansile force to the capsular equator. However, the endocapsular ring does not always stabilize the lens position and often entraps the lens cortex between itself and the lens capsule. Removal of the trapped cortex can be difficult, and in fact, attempts to do so can cause further zonule dehiscence. Nonetheless, expansion of the capsule sac is often desirable either during

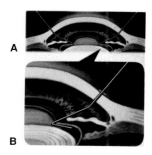

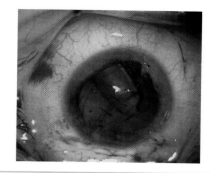

FIGURE 40-3. (A & B) Schematic illustration showing intraoperative placement of capsular retraction devices in the eye. (Courtesy of Richard J. Mackool, MD, New York, NY, USA.)

FIGURE 40-4. Photograph illustrating intraoperative decentration/misplacement of the IOL within the capsular bag in a case of traumatic cataract with repaired corneal laceration.

or after lens removal, and these devices enhance implant centration and reduce postoperative pseudophacodonesis. Intracapsular rings (e.g., Cionni's ring[7] and capsular tension ring segments[8]) are available and used frequently in adult cataract surgery. However, experience with them is still very limited in cataract surgery in children, and they are not approved by the Food and Drug Administration for pediatric cataract surgery.

The relatively short length of the iris retractor hook and the single-plane design may cause them to slip off the capsule easily during manipulation of the nucleus. In addition, short iris retractors do not extend into the capsular fornix and, therefore, do not offer support to this region. Because of some of these disadvantages, R. J. Mackool, MD, designed *capsule retraction devices* specifically shaped for the purpose of retracting the anterior capsule (Figure 40-3). According to experience during adult cataract surgery, as many as seven retractors can be placed at 45° intervals to provide reliable support to the capsule and the enclosed lens. The elongated return of the retractor extends into the capsular fornix and therefore functions to prevent attraction of the equatorial capsule to the phaco tip (Figure 40-3B). After lenticular material and cortex removal is complete, an endocapsular ring (standard or Cionni design) can be inserted prior to removal of the retractors and insertion of an IOL.[9]

Intraocular Lens Complications

The most common intraoperative complication related to the IOL is malplacement or malpositioning of the implant on entry into the eye (Figure 40-4). When polymethylmethacrylate (PMMA) IOLs were used most commonly in children, the leading haptic could easily be placed into the capsular bag, but the trailing haptic would commonly end up in the ciliary sulcus inadvertently, especially in infants. Placing an oversized rigid IOL into a small soft eye was a real challenge. After the leading haptic entered the capsular bag, the OVD often exited the eye through the large wound, the pupil became miotic, and the surgeon

was pleased just to get the trailing haptic somewhere posterior to the iris. Posterior vitreous upthrust made dialing the lens into the capsular bag more difficult. A second instrument was placed through the paracentesis site so that the optic of the lens could be pushed posteriorly during the dialing process. Nonetheless, the IOL was more likely to be dialed "out" of the capsular bag rather than into it. The use of foldable IOLs has made this complication less frequent but has not eliminated it. The trailing haptic of the single-piece AcrySof IOL can be manually placed under the capsulotomy edge using a push–pull instrument. A second hook can be used to pull the iris edge back for better visualization if needed. Care should be taken to place the haptics into the capsular bag before they have unfolded completely. Once the single-piece AcrySof haptics have unfolded outside the capsular bag, they are more difficult to place into proper position manually. If this happens, the IOL optic should be displaced eccentrically within the capsular bag as much as possible before an attempt is made to pull the haptic out of the ciliary sulcus. The single-piece AcrySof IOL does not dial easily.

Displacement of the IOL through a primary posterior capsulotomy is an intraoperative complication that almost never occurs in adult cataract surgery but is a real concern in pediatric cases. Many pediatric surgeons choose to perform a primary posterior capsulotomy and an anterior vitrectomy prior to implantation of an IOL. An OVD is then used to inflate the remaining capsular "tire." The IOL must be carefully aimed on entry so that it enters the capsular bag. Fearing the deep entry, some surgeons aim too anteriorly and the IOL enters the ciliary sulcus. Unlike the situation mentioned earlier, where IOLs dial up into the ciliary sulcus due to vitreous upthrust, IOLs often dial through the posterior capsulotomy when a vitrectomy has already been performed. Even gentle dialing and gentle posterior force on the optic will send a soft foldable IOL through an even modestly sized posterior capsulotomy. In this situation, the IOL is best removed and reinserted, rather than dialed. To avoid this complication and make IOL insertion easier, we recommend IOL insertion into an intact capsular bag prior to the posterior capsulotomy. The IOL haptics should be oriented 90° away from the wound. This allows the vitrector to be placed under the IOL optic more easily for OVD removal or for primary posterior capsulotomy and anterior vitrectomy. To avoid the possibility of dragging a strand of vitreous back to the wound, we recommend removing the OVD after the IOL is in place but performing the primary posterior capsulotomy and anterior vitrectomy through the pars plana, leaving the irrigation cannula in the anterior chamber.

Miscellaneous Intraoperative Complications

Intraoperative complications such as rupture of the posterior capsule may occur during the surgical step of hydrodissection. Chapter 14 addresses the details of hydrodissection and the techniques used to avoid them. Readers should refer to Chapter 12 regarding techniques to avoid retained viscoelastic material in the early postoperative period.

CONCLUSION

In *summary*, intraoperative complications during cataract surgery in children may occur as a result of the smaller size of the eye, sometimes poorly dilating pupil, highly elastic anterior capsule, low scleral rigidity, and dense vitreous, giving rise to increased intravitreal and intralenticular pressure. The complications may occur during various steps in cataract surgery in children. The surgeon should identify these complications and proceed accordingly.

REFERENCES

1. Wilson ME. Anterior capsule management for pediatric intraocular lens implantation. *J Pediatr Ophthalmol Strabismus* 1999;6:1–6.
2. Wilson ME, Pandey SK, Werner L, at al. Pediatric cataract surgery: Current techniques, complication and management. In: Agarwal A, Agarwal S, Apple DJ, Burato L, Agarwal A, eds. *Text Book of Ophthalmology*. New Delhi, Jaypee, 2000:370–378.
3. Wilson ME, Pandey SK, Werner L, et al. Pediatric Cataract Surgery: Current Techniques, Complications and Management. In: Agarwal S, Agarwal A, Apple DJ, Buratto L, Alio J, Pandey SK, Agarwal A, eds., *Textbook of Ophthalmology*, Jaypee Brothers, New Delhi, India 2002;1861–1879.
4. Nichamin LD. Enlarging the pupil for cataract extraction using flexible nylon iris retractors. *J Cataract Refract Surg* 1993:19:793–796.
5. Graether JM. Graether pupil expander for managing the small pupil during surgery. *J Cataract Refract Surg* 1996;22:530–535.
6. Kershner RM. Management of the small pupil for clear corneal cataract surgery. *J Cataract Refract Surg* 2002;28:1826–1831.
7. Cionni R, Osher R. Management of zonular dialysis with the endocapsular ring. *J Cataract Refract Surg* 1995;21:245–249.
8. Ahmed II, Crandall AS. Ab externo scleral fixation of the Cionni modified capsular tension ring. *J Cataract Refract Surg* 2001;27:977–981.
9. Mackool RJ. Capsule retraction device. Presented at ASCRS Symposium on Cataract, IOL, and Refractive Surgery, San Francisco, CA, May 2003.

Postoperative Complications of Pediatric Cataract–Intraocular Lens Surgery and Their Management

Suresh K. Pandey and M. Edward Wilson, Jr.

Cataract surgery with intraocular lens (IOL) implantation in children has undergone dramatic changes during the last three decades, largely as a result of advances in technological and microsurgical techniques.[1] However, postoperative complications associated with pediatric cataract–IOL surgery continue to be a major concern.[2] Addressing this concern, Ellis[3] aptly mentioned, *"Young children with an IOL in place are a unique clinical responsibility of an ophthalmologist. Long-term follow-up is especially important."* The risk of postoperative complications is higher due to the greater inflammatory response after pediatric intraocular surgery. While amblyopia from delayed treatment remains the most common cause of a poor visual outcome, these complications are the primary reason for poor vision in many cases. In some cases, the complications appear to be intrinsically related to associated ocular anomalies that coexist with the developmental cataract. Close follow-up and early detection and management of the complications are mandatory.

In this chapter we discuss common postoperative complications of pediatric cataract–IOL surgery and, also, address their management. Interested readers can also refer to other relevant chapters of the book that provide comprehensive details on selected postoperative complications, such as opacification of the visual axis, postoperative glaucoma, cystoid macular edema, and retinal detachment. We have arbitrarily classified the postoperative complications into two subgroups—early onset and delayed onset—for the sake of easy understanding.

EARLY-ONSET POSTOPERATIVE COMPLICATIONS

Postoperative Anterior Uveitis

Postoperative anterior uveitis (fibrinous or exudative) is a common complication owing to increased tissue reactivity in children. In comparative studies, the reported incidence of postoperative fibrinous anterior uveitis ranged from 81.8 to 19.0%.[4,5] Uveitis results in fibrinous membrane formation, pigment deposits on the IOL, and posterior synechia formation. Frequent topical steroids and even systemic steroids may be needed in selected cases to reduce uveitis-related complications. Brady et al.[6] recommend 5 units of intravenous heparin in 500 mL of irrigating solution. According to recent studies, implantation of heparin-surface-modified (HSM) polymethylmethacrylate (PMMA) IOLs in children reduces postoperative inflammation. Mullaney et al.[7] reported dissolution of pseudophakic fibrinous exudates with the use of intraocular streptokinase (500–1,000 IU) without any adverse effect. Similarly, Klais and coworkers[8] performed fibrinolysis in 11 eyes of 10 children who developed severe fibrin formation despite intensive topical steroid therapy. A complete resolution of fibrin formation was seen in 90% of the children after using 10 μg of recombinant tissue plasminogen activator (rtPA).[8] Besides incomplete resolution and recurrence of membranes, other complications of rtPA use include hyphema, dysfuction of corneal endothelial cells, and corneal band keratopathy. Other possibilities for treating fibrin formation after pediatric IOL surgery are Nd:YAG laser discission, simple mechanical discission, and an intraocular steroid (e.g., dexamethasone) delivery system (Surodex).[9] However, modern surgical techniques that limit iris manipulation and ensure capsular bag fixation of the IOL have resulted in less postoperative inflammation even in small children.

Corneal Edema

Transient corneal edema may occur in pediatric cataract surgery but bullous keratopathy is rare.[10] Cataract surgery does not cause significant endothelial cell loss in children. Reports on corneal endothelial cell counts in pediatric aphakia and IOL implantation have shown no significant loss of endothelial cells.[11,12] Corneal decompensation may occur if detergents (e.g., glutaraldehyde) are used for sterilization of cannulas or instruments and are not rinsed thoroughly before use in the anterior chamber. Indeed, cannulas or tubing should not be sterilized in glutaraldehyde solution, as, even after thorough rinsing, residual chemicals may remain.

Endophthalmitis

Endophthalmitis does occur after cataract extraction in children. It is a rare complication and appears to occur with the same frequency as in adult cataract patients. The prevalence of endophthalmitis after pediatric cataract surgery reported by Wheeler and associates[13] was 7 in 10,000 cases. Common organisms are *Staphylococcus aureus, Staphylococcus epidermidis,* and *Staphylococcus viridence.* Nasolacrimal duct obstruction, periorbital eczema, and upper respiratory tract infections have been cited as additional risk factors.[14]

Techniques to avoid the complication of endophthalmitis remain controversial in all cataract procedures. Some surgeons advise the use of topical antibiotic ophthalmic solutions applied to the cataractous eye for 24 hr preoperatively. However, it is unclear whether this decreases the incidence of infectious complications. Other authorities emphasize the need to use an undiluted povidone–iodine (Betadine) solution not only applied to the skin but also instilled in the eye at the time of the operation to reduce the bacterial flora in the operative field.

Identifying endophthalmitis in the young child is often much more difficult than in the adult aphakic patient. Careful slit-lamp examination may not be possible, even with a handheld device. It should be recalled that the most likely time for endophthalmitis to become clinically apparent in the postoperative period is between 48 and 96 hr postoperatively. Postoperative schedules for evaluating these patients should be drafted with this fact in mind in this era of ambulatory surgical therapy.

Noninfectious Inflammation

Jameson and colleagues[15] have described a benign syndrome of excessive noninfectious postoperative inflammatory response in young aphakic children. This syndrome presents with excessive photophobia, tearing, and even the inability to open the eyes postoperatively. It may persist for days or even weeks and may preclude early contact lens fitting in aphakic patients. It is not clear whether steroids applied topically or injected into the sub-Tenon's space are efficacious in shortening this benign inflammatory process.

LATE-ONSET POSTOPERATIVE COMPLICATIONS

Capsular Bag Opacification

Comprehensive details on opacification of the visual axis after pediatric cataract–IOL surgery and management options are provided in Chapter 43. In brief, opacification of the capsular bag universally occurs following pediatric cataract surgery. It includes opacification of the anterior, equatorial, and posterior capsules. Excessive anterior capsule fibrosis and shrinkage of the continuous curvilinear capsulorhexis opening can lead to difficulty in examining the retinal periphery and, occasionally, decentration of the IOL. Fig. 41-1 shows examples of capsular bag opacification after pediatric cataract-IOL surgery.

Posterior capsule opacification (PCO) is the most common complication after pediatric cataract surgery with or without IOL implantation.[16] A recent report has indicated an age-independent dramatic rise in the incidence of PCO beginning at 18 months after surgery and reaching nearly 100% over time.[17] PCO is amblyogenic if it occurs during the critical period of visual development in younger children. In cases of dense, thick PCO, surgical posterior capsulotomy combined with anterior vitrectomy may be required to clear the visual axis. Nd:YAG laser can also be used to perform posterior capsulotomy when PCO is not dense.[18] The use of newer surgical techniques such as primary posterior capsulotomy and anterior vitrectomy,

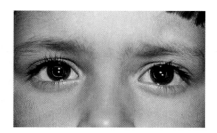

FIGURE 41-1. Anterior capsule opacification after phacoemulsification and implantation of an AcrySof IOL in a 7-year-old child. Both eyes had a best corrected visual acuity of 20/40. (Courtesy of Jagat Ram, MD, Chandigarh, India.)

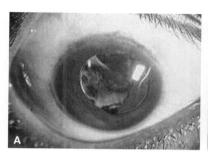
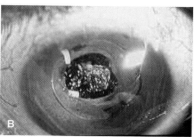

FIGURE 41-2. Pupillary capture and posterior capsule opacification (PCO) after pediatric cataract surgery and IOL implantation. **A.** Slit-lamp photograph of the anterior segment of a 12-year-old female child 13 months after ciliary sulcus fixation of a posterior chamber intraocular lens. Note the marked pupillary capture of the IOL optic, extending from 12 to 5 o'clock, associated with pupillocapsular synechia and marked PCO. Best corrected visual acuity was 20/80 in this eye due to PCO. It required Nd:YAG laser posterior capsulotomy. **B.** Clinical photograph of the eye of a 10-year-old girl, post PMMA posterior chamber intraocular lens implantation. There is a marked pupillary capture. This is associated with marked posterior capsule opacification. An attempt to perform Nd:YAG laser failed, resulting in multiple pits on the IOL optic. This type of dense PCO is an indication of surgical posterior capsulotomy with anterior vitrectomy. (Courtesy of Jagat Ram, MD, Chandigarh, India.)

posterior capsulorhexis with optic capture, and posterior capsulotomy performed with endodiathermy of the capsule has shown encouraging results in reducing PCO.[19,20]

Secondary Membrane Formation

Formation of secondary membranes is a common complication of pediatric cataract surgery, particularly after infantile cataract surgery.[21–23] We define secondary membrane here as a closure across a previously open space such as the pupillary membrane after anterior capsulotomy or a posterior membrane after posterior capsulotomy. Nd:YAG laser capsulotomy may be sufficient to open the secondary membrane in the early stage. More dense secondary membranes usually need surgical membranectomy.[24] Pupillary membranes can occur postoperatively in children whether or not an IOL has been implanted. Microphthalmic eyes with microcoria operated on in early infancy are at greatest risk, especially when mydriatic/cycloplegic agents have not been used postoperatively. When an IOL is in place, secondary membranes may form over the anterior and/or posterior surface of the implant. The incidence of secondary membranes after neonatal or infantile cataract surgery has been reduced dramatically by the "no-iris-touch" aspect of the closed chamber surgery, by application of topical corticosteroids and cycloplegic agents at frequent intervals postoperatively, and by performance of a posterior capsulectomy and an adequate anterior vitrectomy.

Pupillary Capture

Placing the IOL in the capsular bag with an anterior capsulotomy smaller than the IOL optic helps to prevent pupillary capture, a complication that is much more common in children than in adults. It often occurs in association with posterior synechia formation and PCO. The incidence of pupillary capture after pediatric cataract surgery varies from 8.5 to 41%. These data come from reports by several authors: Vasavada and Chouhan[25] report a rate of 33% (7 of 21 eyes); Basti et al.,[20] 8.5% (7 of 82 eyes); Brady et al.,[6] 14.2% (3 of 20 eyes); and Bustos et al.,[26] 10.5% (2 of 19 eyes). Pupillary capture occurs most often in children <2 years of age, when an optic size <6 mm is used and the lens is placed in the ciliary sulcus. In a series of 20 cases of traumatic cataracts with posterior chamber (PC-) IOL implantation in children, Pandey et al.[27] reported an incidence of pupillary capture as high as 40% in ciliary sulcus–fixated IOLs, while none of the eyes with in-the-bag fixation of the PCIOL had this complication (Fig. 41-2). Pupillary capture can be left untreated if it is not associated with decreased visual acuity, IOL malposition, or glaucoma. However, surgical repair recreates a more round pupil shape and IOL centration. Fixation of PCIOLs in the capsular bag (whenever possible) is recommended to decrease the incidence of this complication. Also, the anterior capsulotomy should be smaller than the IOL optic if possible. Prolapsing the optic of a secondary sulcus–fixated IOL through the anterior capsulorhexis opening can also prevent pupillary capture.

Deposits on the IOL Surface

Precipitates composed of pigments, inflammatory cells, fibrin, blood breakdown products, and other elements are often seen during the immediate postoperative period on the surface of an IOL optic implanted in a child (Fig. 41-3). The deposits can be pigmented or nonpigmented but are usually not visually significant. They occur much more commonly in children with a dark iris and when compliance with postoperative medications has been poor. HSM IOLs have been reported to decrease the

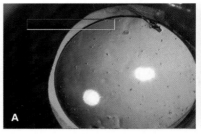 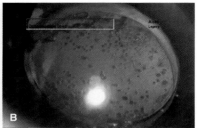

FIGURE 41-3. Slit-lamp photographs showing pigment deposition on the surfaces of two different IOLs. This complication is not uncommon after pediatric cataract surgery and usually does not cause a decrease in visual acuity. **A.** Foldable hydrophobic acrylic (Acarysof) IOL. **B.** Rigid PMMA IOL (Courtesy of A. R. Vasavada, MD, FRCS, Ahmedabad, India.)

incidence of these deposits. The site of IOL implantation can also influence the formation of deposits. Vasavada and Trivedi[28] found that the incidence of deposits was higher in eyes with the IOL optic captured through the posterior continuous curvilinear capsulorhexis in comparison with in-the-bag fixated IOLs. In a retrospective study, Wilson and associates[29] assessed the clinical biocompatibility of hydrophobic acrylic IOLs (AcrySof; Alcon Inc., Ft Worth, TX, USA) in a series of 230 children. Eyes implanted with PMMA implants were also reviewed and were used as a comparison group. The presence of synechiae, lens deposits, and PCO were evaluated from patient records. Results of this study suggested that IOL cell deposits were seen in 7 of 110 (6.4%) hydrophobic acrylic lenses, compared with 26 of 120 (21.75%) PMMA lenses. Posterior synechiae were seen in 5 of 110 (4.5%) hydrophobic acrylic lenses, compared with 23 of 120 (19.2%) PMMA implants. The authors concluded that hydrophobic acrylic implants appear clinically to be biocompatible when placed in the eyes of children despite the increased tissue reactivity known to occur in infants and young children.

IOL Decentration

Decentration of an IOL can occur because of traumatic zonular loss and/or inadequate capsular support. Capsular bag placement of the IOL is the most successful way to reduce this complication. Posterior capture of the IOL optic also resulted in better centration of the implanted IOL. The incidence of lens malposition in pediatric eyes following PCIOL implantation has been reported to be as high as 40%.[30] Asymmetric IOL fixation, with one haptic in the capsular bag and the other in the ciliary sulcus, can also lead to decentration and should therefore be avoided. Complete IOL dislocation can occur after trauma. Explantation or repositioning of the IOL may be necessary in some cases presenting with significant decentration/dislocation.

Delayed Postoperative Opacification of Foldable IOLs

Postoperative opacification of foldable hydrophilic acrylic lens designs is a major concern among surgeons and manufacturers. The majority of reports concern adult cases and are reported from Asia, Australia, Canada, Europe, Latin America, and South Africa. Three major hydrophilic acrylic lenses, explanted due to varying degrees of IOL opacification, secondary to different patterns of dystrophic calcification, include the Bausch and Lomb Hydroview, Medical Developmental Research SC60B-OUV, and Ophthalmic Innovations International Aqua-Sense. Recent reports indicate opacification of the Memory Lens (CibaVision, Duluth, GA, USA),[31] the BioComFold 92S (Morcher GmbH, Stuttgart, Germany), and the IOLTECH lens (IOLTECH Laboratories, Rochelle, France). Opacification of a plate-haptic silicone IOL caused by calcification in a diabetic patient with asteroid hyalosis was also recently reported.[32]

A recent report indicates opacification of hydrophilic acrylic IOLs in children, suggesting that there may be a special pattern of dystrophic calcification in this population. Kleinmann and associates[51] reported the clinicopathological and ultrastructural features of three hydrophilic acrylic IOLs, manufactured from two different biomaterials, explanted from children who had visual disturbances caused by progressive postoperative opacification of the lenses' optic component (Fig. 41-4). These lenses were explanted at 20, 22, and 25 months postoperatively, from children aged 10, 36, and 20 months, respectively, at lens implantation. Clinical data were obtained to correlate the findings with possible associated risk factors. The IOLs were examined by gross and light microscopy. They were further analyzed with a special stain for calcium (1% alizarin red). Additional analysis included scanning electron microscopy (SEM) and energy-dispersive x-ray spectroscopy (EDS). The primary reasons for cataract surgery were persistent hyperplastic primary vitreous, familiar bilateral congenital cataract, and congenital rubella cataract. Although they were of different designs, all lenses presented with deposits on the optic surfaces, especially on the anterior surface. The deposits had a unique pattern, with central foci surrounded by radial lines. They were of variable sizes and stained positive with alizarin red. Analysis of cut sections of the lenses' optics did not show any evidence of deposits within the lenses. EDS confirmed the presence of calcium and phosphate within the deposits.[51]

Ophthalmic surgeons, manufacturers, and scientists are working to explore the etiopathogenesis of the

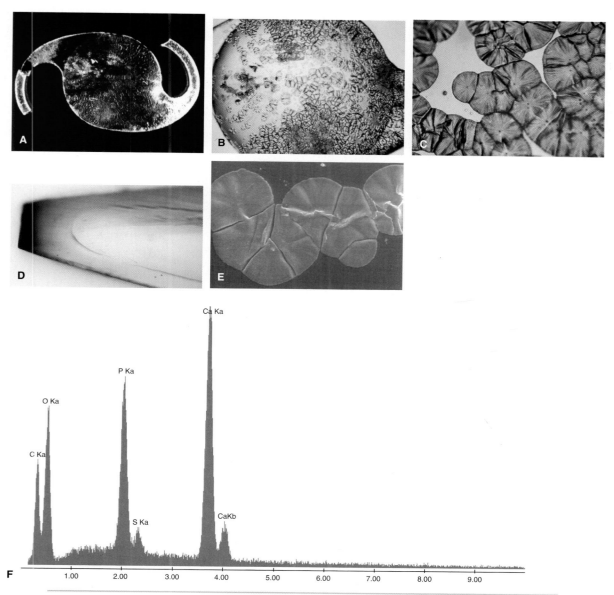

FIGURE 41-4. Clinicopathological and ultrastructural evaluation of an explanted hydrophilic IOL from a 10-month-old child. **A.** Gross photograph of the explanted lens presenting deposits on its surfaces (anterior surface). **B.** Photomicrograph of the anterior surface of the lens, showing the deposits original magnification, ×40. **C.** Photomicrograph of the deposits on the anterior surface of the lens, which stained positive with 1% alizarin red (original magnification, ×100). **D.** Photomicrograph of the sagittal view of the lens optic, with no evidence of deposits within the lens (alizarin red; original magnification, ×40). **E.** Scanning electron microscope image of the deposits on the anterior surface of the lens. **F.** Energy-dispersive x-ray analysis of the deposits demonstrating high peaks of calcium and phosphate. The peaks are related to an alizarin red area positive area. (Courtesy of Liliana Werner, MD, PhD, and Guy Kleinmann, MD.)

miniepidemic of IOL opacification. Contrary to the adult population, in which associated systemic diseases (e.g., diabetes mellitus) have been reported as a potential cause for the calcification, no metabolic systemic diseases have been reported in children. To prevent the occurrence of lens opacification, Bausch and Lomb, Medical Developmental Research, and Ophthalmic Innovations International modified the IOL packaging and/or changed the source of IOL polymers. They now believe that the problem is resolved. However, final verification will require further clinical study. IOL explantation/exchange is currently the only available treatment. Future clinical studies will determine the efficacy of modifications performed on polymers and packaging. Hydrophilic acrylic IOLs have a good uveal biocompatibility and appear to be appropriate in pediatric cases. However, surgeons should remain vigilant in careful follow-up of pediatric patients implanted with these lens designs.

Postoperative Glaucoma

Pediatric aphakic/pseudophakic glaucoma remains a challenge. Its etiopathogenesis, incidence, onset, diagnosis, and successful treatment are addressed in Chapter 44. The incidence of glaucoma varies from 3 to 32%.[33-41] Although microphthalmic eyes appear to be at the highest risk, cataract surgery before 1 year of age, congenital rubella, and poorly dilated pupils are other important risk factors and should alert the treating ophthalmologist.

Retinal Detachment

This complication is discussed thoroughly in Chapter 47. In brief, the incidence of retinal detachment following pediatric cataract surgery has been reported to be approximately 1 to 1.5%. The incidence appears to be decreasing as surgical techniques advance and evolve. The interval from infantile cataract surgery to retinal detachment can be as long as 23 to 34 years according to some authors.[42-44]

Cystoid Macular Edema

Clinical details of, and management options for, cystoid macular edema after pediatric cataract–IOL surgery are discussed in Chapter 46. In brief, this is a rare complication following pediatric cataract surgery, probably because of the healthy retinal vasculature and formed vitreous in children.[45,46] Because of the difficulty of performing fluorescein angiography in young patients, surgeons seldom evaluate children for this complication.

Hemorrhagic Retinopathy

This complication may occur following infantile cataract surgery in up to one third of eyes as reported by Mets and Del Monte.[49] It presents with flame-shaped retinal hemorrhages and may be associated with concurrent vitreous hemorrhage.[50] The hemorrhages develop during the first 24 hr following surgery, are nonprogressive, and resolve within a few weeks.

CONCLUSION

In summary, the main postoperative complications following pediatric cataract surgery–IOL implantation are PCO, secondary membrane formation, postoperative glaucoma, fibrinous anterior uveitis, pupillary capture, IOL precipitates, and decentration/dislocation of the implant. These complications may develop in the early postoperative period or after many years. Therefore, it is crucial to follow children closely on a long-term basis after pediatric cataract surgery.

REFERENCES

1. Wilson ME. Intraocular lens implantation: Has it become the standard of care for children? (Editorial). *Ophthalmology* 1996;103:1719–1720.
2. Pandey SK, Wilson ME, Trivedi RH, et al. Pediatric cataract surgery and intraocular lens implantation: current techniques, complications and management. *Int Ophthalmol Clin* 2001;41:175–196.
3. Ellis FD. Intraocular lenses in children. *J Pediatr Ophthalmol Strabismus* 1992;29:71–72.
4. Gupta AK, Grover AK, Gurha N. Traumatic cataract surgery with intraocular lens implantation in children. *J Pediatr Ophthalmol Strabismus* 1992;29:73–78.
5. Eckstein M, Vijayalakshmi P, Killedar M, et al. Use of intraocular lens in children with traumatic cataract in south India. *Br J Ophthalmol,* 1998;82:911–915.
6. Brady KM, Atkinson CS, Kilty LA, et al. Cataract surgery and intraocular lens implantation in children. *Am J Ophthalmol* 1995;120:1–9.
7. Mullaney PB, Wheeler DT, al-Nahdi T. Dissolution of pseudophakic fibrinous exudate with intraocular streptokinase. *Eye* 1996;10:362–366.
8. Klais CM, Hattenbach LO, Steinkamp GW, et al. Intraocular recombinant tissue-plasminogen activator fibrinolysis of fibrin formation after cataract surgery in children. *J Cataract Refract Surg* 1999;25:357–362.
9. Leung TSA, Lam DSC, Rao SK. Fibrinolysis of postcataract fibrin membranes in children. *J Cataract Refract Surg* 2000;26:4–5.
10. Rozenman Y, Folberg R, Nelson LB, Cohen EJ. Painful bullous keratopathy following pediatric cataract surgery with intraocular lens implantation. *Ophthalmic Surg* 1985;16:372–374.
11. Basti S, Aasuri MK, Reddy S, Reddy S, Rao GN. Prospective evaluation of corneal endothelial cell loss after pediatric cataract surgery. *J Cataract Refract Surg* 1998;24:1469–1473.
12. Hiles DA, Biglan AW, Fetherolf EC. Central corneal endothelial cell counts in children. *J Am Intra-Ocular Implant Soc* 1979;5:292–300.
13. Wheeler DT, Stagger DR, Weakley DR, Jr. Endophthalmitis following pediatric intraocular surgery for congenital cataracts and congenital glaucoma. *J Pediatr Ophthalmol Strabismus* 1992;29:139–141.
14. Good WV, Hing S, Irvine AR, et al. Postoperative endophthalmitis in children following cataract surgery. *J Pediatr Ophthalmol Strabismus* 1990;27:283–285.
15. Jameson NA, Good WV, Hoyt CS. Inflammation after cataract surgery in children. *Ophthalmic Surg* 1992;23:99–102.
16. Apple DJ, Solomon KD, Tetz MR, et al. Posterior capsule opacification. *Surv Ophthalmol* 1992;37:73–116.
17. Plager DA, Lipsky SN, Snyder SK, et al. Capsular management and refractive error in pediatric intraocular lenses. *Ophthalmology* 1997;104:600–607.
18. Atkinson CS, Hiles DA. Treatment of secondary posterior capsular membrane Nd:YAG laser in a pediatric population. *Am J Ophthalmol* 1994;118:496–501.
19. BenEzra D, Cohen E. Posterior capsulectomy in pediatric cataract surgery: the necessity of a choice. *Ophthalmology* 1997;104:2168–1674.
20. Basti S, Ravishankar V, Gupta S. Results of a prospective evaluation of three methods of management of pediatric cataracts. *Ophthalmology* 1996;103:713–720.
21. Parks MM, Johnson DA, Reed GW. Long term visual results and complications in children with aphakia: a function of cataract type. *Ophthalmology,* 1993;100:826–841.
22. Kugelberg U. Visual acuity following treatment of bilateral congenital cataracts. *Doc Ophthalmol* 1992;82:211–215.

23. Zetterström C, Kugelberg. After cataract formation in the newborn rabbits implanted with intraocular lenses. *J Cataract Refract Surg* 1996;22:85–88.

24. Menezo JL, Taboada JF, Ferrer E. Managing dense retropseudosphakos membranes with a pars plana vitrectomy. *J Am Intra-Ocular Implant Soc* 1985;11:24–27.

25. Vasavada A, Chauhan H. Intraocular lens implantation in infants with congenital cataracts. *J Cataract Refract Surg* 1994;20:592–597.

26. Bustos FR, Zepeda LC, Cota DM. Intraocular lens implantation in children with traumatic cataract. *Ann Ophthalmol* 1996;28:153–157.

27. Pandey SK, Ram J, Werner L, et al. Visual results and postoperative complications of capsular bag versus ciliary sulcus fixation of posterior chamber intraocular lenses for traumatic cataract in children. *J Cataract Refract Surg* 1999;25:1576–1584.

28. Vasavada AR, Trivedi RH. Role of optic capture in congenital cataract and intraocular lens surgery in children. *J Cataracts Refract Surg* 2000;26:824–829.

29. Wilson ME, Elliott L, Johnson B, et al. AcrySof acrylic intraocular lens implantation in children: clinical indications of biocompatibility. *J AAPOS* 2001;5:377–380.

30. Hiles DA. Intraocular lens implantation in children with monocular cataracts. 1974–1983. *Ophthalmology* 1984;91:1231–1237.

31. Tehrani M, Mamalis N, Wallin T, et al. Late postoperative opacification of MemoryLens hydrophilic acrylic intraocular lenses: case series and review. *J Cataract Refract Surg* 2004;30:115–122.

32. Wackernagel W, Ettinger K, Weitgasser U, et al. Opacification of a silicone intraocular lens caused by calcium deposits on the optic. *J Cataract Refract Surg* 2004;30:517–520.

33. Asrani SG, Wilensky JT. Glaucoma after congenital cataract surgery. *Ophthalmology* 1995;102:863–867.

34. Brady KM, Atkinson CS, Kilty LA, Hiles DA. Glaucoma after cataract extraction and posterior chamber lens implantation in children. *J Cataract Refract Surg* 1997;23(Suppl):669–674.

35. Chrousos GA, Parks MM, O'Neill JF. Incidence of chronic glaucoma, retinal detachment and secondary membrane surgery in pediatric aphakic patients. *Ophthalmology* 1984;91:1238–1241.

36. Egbert JE, Kushner BJ. Excessive loss of hyperopia: presenting sign of juvenile aphakic glaucoma. *Arch Ophthalmol* 1990;108:1257–1259.

37. Simon JW, Metge P, Simmons ST, et al. Glaucoma after pediatric lensectomy/vitrectomy. *Ophthalmology* 1991;98:670–674.

38. Walton DS. Pediatric aphakic glaucoma: a study of 65 patients. *Trans Am Ophthalmol Soc* 1995;93:403–420.

39. Vajapyee RB, Angra SK, Titiyal JS, et al. Pseudophakic pupillary block glaucoma in children. *Am J Ophthalmol* 1991;11:715–718.

40. Phelps CD, Arafat NI. Open-angle glaucoma following surgery for congenital cataracts. *Arch Ophthalmol* 1977;95:1985–1987.

41. Wallace DK, Plager DA. Corneal diameter in childhood aphakic glaucoma. *J Pediatr Ophthalmol Strabismus* 1996;33:230–234.

42. Jagger JD, Cooling RJ, Fison LG, et al. Management of retinal detachment following congenital cataract surgery. *Trans Ophthalmol Soc UK* 1983;103:103–107.

43. Kanski JJ, Elkington AR, Daniel R. Retinal detachment after congenital cataract surgery. *Br J Ophthalmol* 1974;58:92–95.

44. Toyofuku H, Hirose T, Schepens CL. Retinal detachment following congenital cataract surgery. *Arch Ophthalmol* 1980;98:669–675.

45. Morgan KS, Franklin RM. Oral fluorescein angioscopy in aphakic children. *J Pediatr Ophthalmol Strabismus* 1984;21:33–36.

46. Pinchoff BS, Ellis FD, Helveston EM, Sato SE. Cystoid macular edema in pediatric aphakia. *J Pediatr Ophthalmol Strabismus* 1988;25:240–243.

47. Hoyt CS, Nickel B. Aphakic cystoid macular edema: occurrence in infants and children after transpupillary lensectomy and anterior vitrectomy. *Arch Ophthalmol* 1982;100:746–749.

48. Gilbard SM, Peyman GA, Goldberg MF. Evaluation for cystoid maculopathy after pars plicata lensectomy-vitrectomy for congenital cataracts. *Ophthalmology* 1983;90:1201–1206.

49. Mets MB, Del Monte M. Hemorrhagic retinopathy following uncomplicated pediatric cataract extraction. *Arch Ophthalmol* 1986;104:975–979.

50. Christiansen SP, Munoz M, Capo H. Retinal hemorrhage following lensectomy and anterior vitrectomy in children. *J Pediatr Ophthalmol Strabismus* 1993;30:24–27.

51. Kleinmann G, Werner L, Pandey SK, et al. Opacification of surface of hydrophilic acrylic intraocular lenses in children. Presented at ASCRS Symposium on Cataract, IOL, and Refractive Surgery, San Diego, CA, May 2004.

Growth of Aphakic and Pseudophakic Eyes

Rupal H. Trivedi and M. Edward Wilson, Jr.

Pediatric eyes have a rapidly developing visual system.[1–4] The growth of different components of the eye is regulated by a process known as *emmetropization.*[5] Emmetropization occurs through both passive and active phenomena.[6] *Passive emmetropization* occurs with normal eye growth. As the eye size increases, the power of the optical component decreases proportionally. Thus despite axial elongation, we do not see large refractive changes. The term *active emmetropization* describes the role of visual feedback in controlling the growth of the eye.

The process of emmetropization after cataract surgery in children is complex and poorly understood. Both active and passive components of emmetropization process are different in these eyes compared with phakic eyes. The normal phakic lens retains accommodation and helps to reach the goal of emmetropia by *passive emmetropization.* Thus, although the axial length (AL) shows a huge increase, the refractive status does not change very much in phakic children. This is because the natural lens power declines from 34.4 to 18.8 D (diopters).[2] However, after cataract surgery, in the absence of the crystalline lens, these eyes are not able to compensate through this passive emmetropization process.[7–10] In aphakic eyes, the shift averages 10 D from infancy to adulthood, compared with 0.9 D in normal phakic eyes.[7,9] *Active emmetropization* (visual feedback) is also affected by several factors: age at cataract development, age at cataract surgery, aphakia/pseudophakia, laterality etc.

A tendency toward *axial elongation and a myopic refraction* change after pediatric cataract surgery has been reported.[7,8,10–36] Much of the myopic shift can be attributed to normal eye growth; however other factors—including age at surgery, visual input, presence or absence of an intraocular lens (IOL), and laterality—also play a role in this process. Studies on animals and humans have focused on various factors influencing axial and refractive growth of the eye after cataract surgery. Table 42-1 lists

factors that may affect the growth of the eye. Some of them are identified to affect growth after cataract surgery in children, while others have been reported in the literature to affect the growth of phakic eyes. In this chapter we discuss the available literature on ocular growth in aphakia and pseudophakia.

A cautionary note is needed at this point. Studies describing the growth of an eye can be problematic to interpret. Results from different studies are difficult to compare because of common inconsistencies in inclusion and exclusion criteria, surgical technique, and length of follow-up. Some studies report growth as axial growth[26]; others, as refractive change.[16,26–30] Some studies have reported growth as an absolute value (AL in millimeters or refraction in diopters), while others have reported rate of growth [Depending on refractive OR axial rate of growth—(Final refraction OR AL minus intial refraction OR AL) divided by log of ratio of age at which initial and final refraction OR AL are observed]. A word of caution is also needed here, as many of the factors described below may not occur individually. Aphakic eyes may have a poor visual outcome compared to pseudophakic eyes. Thus, two main factors are in effect simultaneously in this situation: aphakia versus pseudophakia and visual deprivation. In addition to, and perhaps more important than, the optical effect of an IOL, better visual input may have been responsible for retardation of growth in pseudophakic eyes.

GENERAL FACTORS

Age of the Child at the Time of Cataract Diagnosis and Cataract Surgery

It is well documented in the literature that the normal phakic human eye undergoes extensive growth in the postnatal period.[1,2,4] Larsen[1] reported a *rapid postnatal growth phase*, with an increase in AL of 3.7 to 3.8 mm in the first

▶ **TABLE 42-1 Factors That May Effect Growth of Aphakic and Pseudophakic Eyes**

I. General
  Age of the child at the time of cataract diagnosis and cataract surgery
  Gender
  Ethnicity
  Heredity
II. Ocular and related factors
  A. Preoperative
    Laterality
    Type of cataract
    Axial length, keratometry, interocular axial length difference
  B. Intraoperative
    Vitrectomy
    Aphakia versus pseudophakia
    ■ If aphakia—optical correction with glasses, contact lenses, or secondary IOLs?
    ■ If pseudophakia—primary versus secondary IOL, size of IOL, and IOL power
  C. Postoperative
    Duration of follow-up
    Glaucoma
    Visual axis opacification
III. Functional issues
  Visual deprivation; density of amblyopia and compliance with amblyopia therapy; compliance with residual refractive error
  Excessive near-work and optical correction of refractive error

year and a half, followed by a *slower infantile growth phase* from the second to the fifth year of life, with an increase in AL of 1.1 to 1.2 mm, and, finally, by a *slow juvenile growth phase* lasting until the age of 13 years, with an increase of 1.3 to 1.4 mm. Longitudinal growth terminates at the age of 13 years or is minimal after this age.[1] Gordon and Donzis[2] noted that the AL increases from an average of 16.8 mm at birth to 23.6 mm in adult life. Although most studies have observed rapid axial growth in infantile eyes, there is no sharp cutoff point when axial growth stabilizes.

It is reasonable to believe that eyes with cataracts follow a similar triphasic curve—before surgery as well as after surgery. However, we have noted that the mean AL of our patients' cataractous eyes is different (20.6 ± 2.9 mm) from that of the noncataractous eyes in Gordon's data (21.9 ± 1.6 mm). Not only did the mean values differ, but more importantly, the standard deviation was two to three times that of the normal population. Also, the younger the age at the time of measurement, the more variability existed (Trivedi RH, Wilson ME, et al. Axial length and keratometry in eyes with pediatric cataract. Poster presented at ASCRS, 2002).

The age at onset and duration of cataract (deprivation) also influence axial growth.

■ Lambert[19] reported that age at the time of lensectomy appears to be a critical factor in determining subsequent axial growth in monkeys.
■ Moore[16] noted that the refractive error of the aphakic eye of patients treated for unilateral congenital cataracts decreases most rapidly during infancy and less rapidly during the next few years of childhood.
■ McClatchey and Parks[7] reported that the average refraction tended to follow a logarithmic decline with age. The average rate of myopic shift was −5.5 D. The authors performed a stepwise regression and concluded that age at surgery had a small but significant effect on rate of the growth.[7] Much of the observed myopic shift in aphakic eyes is due to normal growth of the eye.
■ McClatchey and Parks[8] used aphakic refraction at last follow-up to calculate the final pseudophakic refraction, and these values were compared with the prediction of a logarithmic model of myopic shift. They reported a median calculated pseudophakic refraction at last follow-up of −6.6 D, with a range of −36.3 to +2.9 D. Children who underwent surgery in the first 2 years of life had a substantially greater myopic shift (11.9 D) than older children (4.7 D) and a larger variance in this myopic shift. The logarithmic model accurately predicated the final refraction within 3 D in 24% of eyes undergoing surgery before 2 years of age and in 77% of eyes undergoing surgery after this age.
■ Kampik et al. (cited in Ref. 8) also noted the large variance in children who underwent surgery before 1 year of age.
■ Dahan and Drusedau[14] reported an average elongation of 19% for age <18 months and 3.4% for age >18 months.
■ Enyedi et al.[31] reported that children operated on at years 0 to 2, 2 to 6, 6 to 8, and >8 years of age had refractive shifts of −3.0, −1.5, −1.8, and −0.38 D respectively. The authors noted a statistically significant difference in the average total change in refraction between the youngest age group (0 to 2 years) and the oldest age group (>8 years).
■ Flitcroft et al.[15] reported a mean increase in AL of 3.41 mm in congenital cataract (<1 year), versus 0.36 mm in developmental cataracts (>1 year).
■ Plager and associates[29] reported that children operated on at ages 2 to 3, 6 to 7, 8 to 9, and 10 to 15 years had mean myopic shifts of −4.60, −2.68, −1.25, and −0.61 D, respectively.
■ Crouch et al.[11] reported that children operated on at years 1 to 3, 3 to 4, 5 to 6, 7 to 8, 9 to 10, 11 to 14, and 15 to 18 years had mean myopic shifts of −5.96, −3.66, −3.40, −2.03, −1.88, −0.97, and −0.38 D, respectively, with an average follow-up of 5.45 years.
■ Postoperative refractive changes are highly variable and relatively unpredictable in infants <6 months of age undergoing primary IOL implantation. The greatest

refractive change is in the first years after surgery (4.2 D). On average, however, this is less than would be predicted by logarithmic scales or extrapolation of previously published refractive change curves (Plager D. Presentation at AAPOS, 2004).

Gender

Sex-linked differences in AL have been reported in the literature on normal phakic eyes. Larsen[1] reported that values in girls were, on average, 0.3 to 0.4 mm shorter than in boys. Gwiazda et al.[37] also noted a sex-linked difference in terms of AL.

In eyes with cataracts, we have noted that overall girls have a significantly shorter AL than boys (23.92 versus 24.36 mm). However, in the first year of life, males have a shorter AL than females (Trivedi RH, Wilson ME, et al. Axial length and keratometry in eyes with pediatric cataract. Poster presented at ASCRS, 2002). McClatchey and Parks[7] noted that gender had no effect on the rate of myopic shift in pediatric aphakic eyes.

Ethnicity

Several studies in normal phakic eyes have reported racial differences in relation to axial and refractive status. The prevalence of myopia is 37% among Chinese school-children,[38,39] versus only 7.5% among American school-children. Gwazda et al.[37] noted that they did not find a difference in axial dimensions in different ethnic groups. In our cataractous population we noted significantly longer eyes in African-American patients than in Caucasian patients (21.8 versus 20.1 mm) (Trivedi RH, Wilson ME, et al. Axial length and keratometry in eyes with pediatric cataract. Poster presented at ASCRS, 2002). We are not aware of any study showing the pattern of growth and its relation to ethnicity.

Heredity

Parental refractive error has also been shown to be an important predictor for the refractive errors of their children. For example, if both parents are myopic, 30 to 40% of their children become myopic, whereas if only one parent is myopic, 20 to 25% of their children will become myopic. If neither parent is myopic, fewer than 10% of their children will become myopic (cited in Ref. 5).

Moore[16] noted that 2 of 42 patients were highly myopic in their phakic eyes and were less hyperopic in their aphakic eyes than the group means. Both of these patients had a father with high bilateral myopia and can be presumed to have a hereditary form of myopia superimposed on their unilateral congenital cataract.

Plager and associates[29] noted an unexpected larger myopic shift in a genetically predisposed patient (moderate myopia in both parents).

OCULAR AND RELATED FACTORS

Preoperative

Laterality

Eyes with a unilateral cataract are known to have a longer AL than eyes with bilateral cataracts (21.0 versus 20.4 mm), even before cataract surgery secondary to deprivation amblyopia (Trivedi RH, Wilson ME, et al. Axial length and keratometry in eyes with a pediatric cataract. Poster presented at ASCRS, 2002). In eyes with a unilateral cataract, axial elongation and myopic shift relative to the unaffected eye have been well described in aphakic and pseudophakic eyes.

- Rasooly and BenEzra[20] reported that in cases of unilateral aphakia, the aphakic eye was consistently longer than the normal fellow eye.
- In their prospective study of children with congenital cataract, Lorenz and associates[21] reported that the mean decrease in refraction was 15 D in unilateral cataracts and 10 D in bilateral cataracts.
- In older children, Kora and coauthors[34] reported a longer AL in operated eyes than in normal fellow eyes.
- Eyes with unilateral cataracts tend to have a higher rate of myopic shift than eyes with bilateral cataracts; this effect was statistically significant among eyes with cataract removal after the age of 6 months.[7]
- Results of Hutchinson et al.[33] in a series of children <2 years old with IOL implantation showed that in eyes with a unilateral cataract, the operated eye grew an average of 0.35 mm more than the fellow noncataractous eye. (Calculation was done from data in reference 33, only nine eyes with a unilateral cataract were included here for analysis.) Operated eyes grew 1.49 (SD, 0.74) mm on average, while unoperated eyes grew 1.14 (SD, 0.88) mm.
- Griener and coauthors[18] concluded, in their retrospective study, that there was a reduction in axial growth in unilateral pseudophakic eyes compared to fellow normal eyes. The authors[18] noted that in seven patients receiving unilateral IOL implantation at between 2 and 4 months of age, the mean AL was 0.46 mm less in the pseudophakic eye than in the fellow eye (range, 0.15 to 0.70 mm).
- Crouch et al.[11] noted that there was a minimal myopic shift difference in patients with binocular implants, suggesting that both eyes grew similarly. In the unilateral case, they noted that the pseudophakic eye

showed a larger myopic shift than the unoperated fellow eye.

- Weakley et al.[32] noted that the difference in refractive rate of growth between good- and poor-seeing eyes was less in eyes with bilateral cataracts than in eyes with unilateral cataracts.

Type of Cataract

The type of cataract does not seem to influence the growth of aphakic eyes.[7]

Axial Length, Keratometry, and Interocular Axial Length Difference (IALD)

There is insufficient proof whether preoperative AL and keratometry affect subsequent growth in aphakic and pseudophakic eyes. However, regarding IALD, we have recently reported (Trivedi RH, Wilson ME, Facciani J. Interocular axial length difference. Presentation at ASCRS, 2004) that compensatory changes lead shorter eyes to grow more and longer eyes to grow less. Studies aimed at solving the mysteries of growth of an eye after pediatric cataract surgery may need to consider IALD as a covariate. Animal studies have shown that making the eyes of chicks functionally myopic with positive spectacle lenses or functionally hyperopic with negative spectacle lenses results in a compensatory change in the growth of the eye.[40] Troilo et al.[41] noted that growth stopped in eyes compensating for myopia and continued in eyes recovering from hyperopia.

Intraoperative

Vitrectomy

Theoretically, vitrectomy may affect the growth of the eye. Sorkin and Lambert[26] noted that while, in theory, vitrectomy may affect axial elongation, they did not find a correlation between axial elongation and vitreous management at the time of cataract surgery.

Aphakia Versus Pseudophakia

Several studies have reported that aphakic eyes grow more than pseudophakic eyes.[5,22] Why? We think several factors contribute to this retardation of growth in pseudophakic eyes and elongation of aphakic eyes. (1) Aphakic eyes may have a poorer visual outcome compared to pseudophakic eyes, which in turn leads to axial elongation. (2) Optical factors may have an impact on emmetropization and thus axial growth. (3) Aphakic eyes may be shorter to start with, so to "catch up" they grow more. (4) Most published series have a longer follow-up in aphakic eyes compared to pseudophakic eyes.

- Sinskey and associates[22] reported the case of an 18-year-old patient who had developmental cataracts treated at 7 years of age with bilateral cataract extraction and implantation of an IOL in one eye only. The AL increased in the eye with a contact lens compared with the eye with the IOL.

- Both aphakic and pseudophakic eyes have a slower rate of refractive growth after cataract surgery at from 3 to 6 months of age. Overall, pseudophakic eyes showed a lower rate of refractive growth than aphakic eyes (−4.6 versus −5.7 D; $P = 0.03$).[10]

- Superstein and associates[35] concluded that pseudophakic eyes show less postoperative myopic shift than aphakic eyes.

- Pan and Tang[36] analyzed 65 eyes of 65 patients from 5 to 12 years of age who underwent IOL implantation. Sixty-five healthy eyes were in the control group. The mean preoperative AL of the surgical group was (22.48 ± 0.44) mm, and that of the control group was 22.43 ± 0.41 mm. There was no statistically significant difference in AL after 10 years in either group: 23.45 ± 0.53 mm in the surgical group and 23.41 ± 0.50 mm in the control group. All the eyes showed a myopic drift, of 3.29 D in the surgical group and 1.75 D in the control group.

If Aphakia—Optical Correction with Glasses or Contact Lenses?

To the best of our knowledge, no studies have analyzed this issue.

If Pseudophakia, Primary Versus Secondary IOL, Size of IOL, and IOL Power

To the best of our knowledge the effect of primary versus secondary IOL implantation has not been reported in the literature.

Animal studies have shown that inappropriate size of an IOL can adversely influence ocular growth.[42] Implanting a regular-size IOL in a newborn rabbit eye retards eye growth.[42]

The mathematical analysis by McClatchey and Parks[8] showed that choosing an IOL to initially give moderate hyperopia results in less myopic shift as the eye grows than choosing an IOL to initially give emmetropia, for optical reasons alone. High-power IOLs result in a greater myopic shift for the same increase in AL.

Postoperative

Duration of Follow-up

Studies reporting a longer follow-up will show more myopic shift than studies reporting a shorter follow-up. Crouch et al. observed a myopic shift that ranged from plano to −2.25 D. With a longer follow-up of 5.45 years the same authors observed a more significant myopic shift.[11] Including eyes with insufficient follow-up time in such studies may lead to erroneous conclusions.

Glaucoma

Excessive eye elongation may be a presenting sign of aphakic glaucoma.[43,44] However, controlled glaucoma has been shown to have no effect on the rate of growth.[7]

Visual Axis Opacification

It is reasonable to assume that, in the amblyogenic age group, if visual axis opacification exists for a sufficient period of time, the eye may become elongated. It is difficult to document the exact onset of visual axis opacification. When it is noticed, the tendency is to clear it as soon as possible. Thus, it is not surprising that many studies did not find this to be a significant factor.

FUNCTIONAL ISSUES

Visual Deprivation, Density of Amblyopia and Compliance with Amblyopia Therapy, and Compliance with Residual Refractive Error

Emmetropization of the eye may be affected by visual experience. Excessive eye elongation may be induced in experimental animals by lid suturing, corneal opacification, or opaque contact lenses. These treatments resulted in axial elongation, whereas lesser degrees of visual deprivation were shown to retard axial growth.[45–48] Poor vision seems to influence the evolution of ocular growth away from emmetropization.[49] In humans, however, this is not always predictable.[50,51] In the case of cataracts in children, two main factors predict the pre–cataract surgery AL. Developmental anomalies may lead to microphthalmos and a shorter AL, while deprivation amblyopia may lead to axial elongation. In a case report of identical twins, Johnson et al. reported that the AL of the visually deprived eye was 2 mm longer.[52] The authors noted a statistically significant increase in AL in the fixating eye of patients with hypermetropia compared with the amblyopic eye. In patients with myopia, less of an increase in AL was found in the fixating eye compared with the amblyopic eye.[49]

Several investigators have examined the association between visual acuity outcome and myopic shift or axial elongation in both aphakic and pseudophakic eyes. McClatchey and Parks[7] noted that best corrected visual acuity had no significant effect on rate of myopic shift. Weakley et al.[32] noted that the rate of growth was significantly lower in eyes with better acuity.

Excessive Near-Work and Optical Correction of Refractive Error During Childhood

Near-work may increase the risk of myopia. Optical correction of refractive error during childhood may disturb the process of emmetropization. A higher percentage of children with moderate or high hyperopia remain hyperopic if their hyperopia is corrected with spectacles during infancy.[53] Emmetropization occurs more rapidly in the presence of high refractive errors.[54] Thus if we leave behind high residual refractive error, these eyes may grow more.

CONCLUSION

In summary, predicting ocular growth and postoperative refractive changes to appropriately calculate pseudophakic power has become one of the major challenges in pediatric cataract management. The surgeon who performs pediatric cataract surgery in young children must be prepared for a wide variation in long-term myopic shift. Both the magnitude of and the variance in this myopic shift are likely to be greater among children who undergo cataract surgery in the first few years of life. A significant body of evidence suggests that emmetropization is influenced by many factors. Some children with pseudophakia are likely to have a large amount of myopic shift; this myopic shift is due to growth of the eye. Cataract surgery with lens implantation after the age of 6 months appears to have little effect on the refractive growth of the eye. Eyes with unilateral cataracts tend to have a larger myopic shift than eyes with bilateral cataracts. Aphakic eyes tend to have a larger myopic shift than pseudophakic eyes.

REFERENCES

1. Larsen JS. The sagittal growth of the eye. IV. Ultrasonic measurement of the axial length of the eye from birth to puberty. *Acta Ophthalmol* 1971;49:873–886.
2. Gordon RA, Donzis PB. Refractive development of the human eye. *Arch Ophthalmol* 1985;103:785–789.
3. Inagaki Y. The rapid change of corneal curvature in the neonatal period and infancy. *Arch Ophthalmol* 1986;104:1026–1027.
4. Bluestein EC, Wilson ME, Wang XH, Rust PF, Apple DJ. Dimensions of the pediatric crystalline lens: implications for intraocular lenses in children. *J Pediatr Ophthalmol Strabismus* 1996;33:18–20.
5. Lambert SR. Ocular growth in early childhood: Implications for pediatric cataract surgery. *Op Techn Cataract Refract Surg* 1998;1:159–164.
6. Saunders KJ. Early refractive development in humans. *Surv Ophthalmol* 1995;40:207–216.
7. McClatchey SK, Parks MM. Myopic shift after cataract removal in childhood. *J Pediatr Ophthalmol Strabismus* 1997;34:88–95.
8. McClatchey SK, Parks MM. Theoretic refractive changes after lens implantation in childhood. *Ophthalmology* 1997;104:1744–1751.
9. McClatchey SK. Intraocular lens calculator for childhood cataract. *J Cataract Refract Surg* 1998;24:1125–1129.

10. McClatchey SK, Dahan E, Maselli E, Gimbel HV, Wilson ME, Lambert SR, et al. A comparison of the rate of refractive growth in pediatric aphakic and pseudophakic eyes. *Ophthalmology* 2000;107: 118–122.
11. Crouch ER, Crouch ER Jr, Pressman SH. Prospective analysis of pediatric pseudophakia: myopic shift and postoperative outcomes. *J AAPOS* 2002;6:277–282.
12. Vanathi M, Tandon R, Titiyal JS, Vajpayee RB. Case series of 12 children with progressive axial myopia following unilateral cataract extraction. *J AAPOS* 2002;6:228–232.
13. Inatomi M, Kora Y, Kinohira Y, Yaguchi S. Long-term follow-up of eye growth in pediatric patients after unilateral cataract surgery with intraocular lens implantation. *J AAPOS* 2004;8:50–55.
14. Dahan E, Drusedau MU. Choice of lens and dioptric power in pediatric pseudophakia. *J Cataract Refract Surg* 1997;23(Suppl 1):618–623.
15. Flitcroft DI, Knight-Nanan D, Bowell R, Lanigan B, O'Keefe M. Intraocular lenses in children: changes in axial length, corneal curvature, and refraction. *Br J Ophthalmol* 1999;83:265–269.
16. Moore BD. Changes in the aphakic refraction of children with unilateral congenital cataracts. *J Pediatr Ophthalmol Strabismus* 1989;26:290–295.
17. Huber C. Increasing myopia in children with intraocular lenses (IOL): an experiment in form deprivation myopia? *Eur J Implant Refract Surg* 1993;5:154–158.
18. Griener ED, Dahan E, Lambert SR. Effect of age at time of cataract surgery on subsequent axial length growth in infant eyes. *J Cataract Refract Surg* 1999;25:1209–1213.
19. Lambert SR. The effect of age on the retardation of axial elongation following a lensectomy in infant monkeys. *Arch Ophthalmol* 1998;116:781–784.
20. Rasooly R, BenEzra D. Congenital and traumatic cataract. The effect on ocular axial length. *Arch Ophthalmol* 1988;106:1066–1068.
21. Lorenz B, Worle J, Friedl N, Hasenfratz G. Ocular growth in infant aphakia. Bilateral versus unilateral congenital cataracts. *Ophthalmic Paediatr Genet* 1993;14:177–188.
22. Sinskey RM, Stoppel JO, Amin PA. Ocular axial length changes in a pediatric patient with aphakia and pseudophakia. *J Cataract Refract Surg* 1993;19:787–788.
23. Kugelberg U, Zetterstrom C, Lundgren B, Syren-Nordqvist S. Eye growth in the aphakic newborn rabbit. *J Cataract Refract Surg* 1996;22:337–341.
24. Tigges M, Tigges J, Fernandes A, Eggers HM, Gammon JA. Postnatal axial eye elongation in normal and visually deprived rhesus monkeys. *Invest Ophthalmol Vis Sci* 1990;31:1035–1046.
25. Wilson JR, Fernandes A, Chandler CV, Tigges M, Boothe RG, Gammon JA. Abnormal development of the axial length of aphakic monkey eyes. *Invest Ophthalmol Vis Sci* 1987;28:2096–2099.
26. Sorkin JA, Lambert SR. Longitudinal changes in axial length in pseudophakic children. *J Cataract Refract Surg* 1997;23(Suppl 1):624–628.
27. Spierer A, Desatnik H, Blumenthal M. Refractive status in children after long-term follow up of cataract surgery with intraocular lens implantation. *J Pediatr Ophthalmol Strabismus* 1999;36:25–29.
28. Plager DA, Lipsky SN, Snyder SK, Sprunger DT, Ellis FD, Sondhi N. Capsular management and refractive error in pediatric intraocular lenses. *Ophthalmology* 1997;104:600–607.
29. Plager DA, Kipfer H, Sprunger DT, Sondhi N, Neely DE. Refractive change in pediatric pseudophakia: 6-year follow-up. *J Cataract Refract Surg* 2002;28:810–815.
30. Hutchinson AK, Drews-Botsch C, Lambert SR. Myopic shift after intraocular lens implantation during childhood. *Ophthalmology* 1997;104:1752–1757.
31. Enyedi LB, Peterseim MW, Freedman SF, Buckley EG. Refractive changes after pediatric intraocular lens implantation. *Am J Ophthalmol* 1998;126:772–781.
32. Weakley DR, Birch E, McClatchey SK, Felius J, Parks MM, Stager D. The association between myopic shift and visual acuity outcome in pediatric aphakia. *J AAPOS* 2003;7:86–90.
33. Hutchinson AK, Wilson ME, Saunders RA. Outcomes and ocular growth rates after intraocular lens implantation in the first 2 years of life. *J Cataract Refract Surg* 1998;24:846–852.
34. Kora Y, Shimizu K, Inatomi M, Fukado Y, Ozawa T. Eye growth after cataract extraction and intraocular lens implantation in children. *Ophthalmic Surg* 1993;24:467–475.
35. Superstein R, Archer SM, Del Monte MA. Minimal myopic shift in pseudophakic versus aphakic pediatric cataract patients. *J AAPOS* 2002;6:271–276.
36. Pan Y, Tang P. Refraction shift after intraocular lens implantation in children. *Chin J Ophthalmol* 2001;37:328–331.
37. Gwiazda J, Marsh-Tootle WL, Hyman L, Hussein M, Norton TT. Baseline refractive and ocular component measures of children enrolled in the correction of myopia evaluation trial (COMET). *Invest Ophthalmol Vis Sci* 2002;43:314–321.
38. Chung KM, Mohidin N, Yeow PT, Tan LL, O'Leary D. Prevalence of visual disorders in Chinese schoolchildren. *Optometry Vis Sci* 1996;73:695–700.
39. Zadnik K, Satariano WA, Mutti DO, Sholtz RI, Adams AJ. The effect of parental history of myopia on children's eye size. *JAMA* 1994;271:1323–1327.
40. Schaeffel F, Glasser A, Howland HC. Accommodation, refractive error and eye growth in chickens. *Vis Res* 1988;28:639–657.
41. Troilo D, Wallman J. The regulation of eye growth and refractive state: an experimental study of emmetropization. *Vis Res* 1991;31:1237–1250.
42. Kugelberg U, Zetterstrom C, Syren-Nordqvist S. Ocular axial length in children with unilateral congenital cataract. *Acta Ophthalmol Scand* 1996;74:220–223.
43. Dietlein TS, Jacobi PC, Krieglstein GK. Assessment of diagnostic criteria in management of infantile glaucoma. An analysis of tonometry, optic disc cup, corneal diameter and axial length. *Int Ophthalmol* 1996;20:21–27.
44. Egbert JE, Kushner BJ. Excessive loss of hyperopia. A presenting sign of juvenile aphakic glaucoma. *Arch Ophthalmol* 1990;108:1257–1259.
45. Wiesel TN, Raviola E. Myopia and eye enlargement after neonatal lid fusion in monkeys. *Nature* 1977;266:66–68.
46. Wiesel TN, Raviola E. Increase in axial length of the macaque monkey eye after corneal opacification. *Invest Ophthalmol Vis Sci* 1979;18:1232–1236.
47. Yinon U. Myopia induction in animals following alteration of the visual input during development: a review. *Curr Eye Res* 1984;3:677–690.
48. Tejedor J, de la Villa P. Refractive changes induced by form deprivation in the mouse eye. *Invest Ophthalmol Vis Sci* 2003;44:32–36.
49. Burtolo C, Ciurlo C, Polizzi A, Lantier PB, Calabria G. Echobiometric study of ocular growth in patients with amblyopia. *J Pediatr Ophthalmol Strabismus* 2002;39:209–214.
50. Gee SS, Tabbara KF. Increase in ocular axial length in patients with corneal opacification. *Ophthalmology* 1988;95:1276–1278.
51. von Noorden GK, Lewis RA. Ocular axial length in unilateral congenital cataracts and blepharoptosis. *Invest Ophthalmol Vis Sci* 1987;28:750–752.
52. Johnson CA, Post RB, Chalupa LM, Lee TJ. Monocular deprivation in humans: a study of identical twins. *Invest Ophthalmol Vis Sci* 1982;23:135–138.
53. Ingram RM, Arnold PE, Dally S, Lucas J. Results of a randomised trial of treating abnormal hypermetropia from the age of 6 months. *Br J Ophthalmol* 1990;74:158–159.
54. Saunders KJ, Woodhouse JM, Westall CA. Emmetropisation in human infancy: rate of change is related to initial refractive error. *Vis Res* 1995;35:1325–1328.

Chapter 43

Opacification of the Ocular Media

Mohammad Ali Javadi and Hamid Ahmadieh

Visually significant cataracts in children call for prompt surgical intervention to clear the ocular media and provide optical correction; the *younger the child, the more urgent the operation.* Delayed intervention may lead to visual deprivation owing to lack of clear retinal image formation; this is of greater concern in unilateral cases and in dense bilateral cataracts not removed by 6 weeks of age.[1] Cataract surgery is the first stepping stone on the long road to visual rehabilitation; the main goal of surgery is relief of media opacity, its maintenance, and proper correction of refractive errors. Despite the numerous, differing views regarding the optimal treatment of pediatric cataracts,[2] no cataract surgeon can manage postoperative care without the cooperation of anesthesiologists, pediatricians, nurses, social workers, and parents.[3]

Pediatric cataract surgery is a complex issue best left to expert hands familiar with the long-term complications and the lengthy follow-up. There are a number of options in the treatment of pediatric cataracts; the choice depends to some extent on socioeconomic status. For instance, a family with suboptimal resources and a low income who have a long distance to travel may not be compliant with appropriate follow-up visits; in such a case it is best to remove the posterior capsule and perform anterior vitrectomy rather than risk posterior capsule opacification and amblyopia. The surgeon should choose the most suitable method with the lowest risks from which the patient will benefit most and should get involved in the teamwork required in postoperative management.

Media opacification after cataract surgery is more common in children than adults. This interferes with the main goals of the operation and is a potential cause of amblyopia, which should be prevented or treated at all costs. Media opacification may develop rapidly or insidiously. Examples of sudden-onset media opacification include corneal edema, inflammatory pupillary membranes, and vitreous hemorrhage; these events are usually identified promptly, sometimes by the parents or caretaker, and usually resolve with appropriate treatment and with time. In contrast, some types of media opacity are delayed and tend to be progressive, including posterior capsule or hyaloid face opacification and cellular, fibrinous, or pigmentary deposits on the intraocular lens (IOL). Since children may be unable to report decreased vision, these may go unnoticed and lead to irreversible visual damage. This chapter focuses on posterior capsule opacification (PCO) and its incidence, predisposing factors, prevention, and treatment and also reviews other, less common causes of media opacification.

POSTERIOR CAPSULE OPACIFICATION

Until the late 1960s the preferred method of pediatric cataract surgery was lens aspiration, leaving the posterior capsule intact as popularized by Scheie.[4] With this method, remaining lens epithelial cells proliferated and migrated on the intact posterior capsule, leading to opacification of the once-clear capsule. In some cases, the ensuing opacity caused more visual deterioration than the original cataract itself.[2] With the advent of vitrectomy in 1976, the majority of pediatric cataract surgeons performed lensectomy with anterior vitrectomy through a large opening in the posterior capsule, leaving only a 1- to 2-mm rim behind. This new trend resulted in superior media clarity, better correction of refractive errors, and a lower incidence of amblyopia.[5] Further refinements of surgical technique, improved IOL quality, and favorable results of IOL implantation in adults started a trend toward IOL implantation in children in the early 1990s. However, opacification of the retained lens capsule still led to poor vision and amblyopia.[5,6] The secondary opacification and fibrosis may be severe enough to cause IOL decentration and even break the optic–haptic junction.[7] Even in the era of modern cataract surgery, PCO still poses a challenge for ophthalmologists.[8–10]

PCO has been reported in 39 to 100% of cases in which the capsule is left intact.[2,3,8,9,11–34] Taylor[35] reported

32 reoperations for capsular opacity in 28 eyes with an intact posterior capsule following lens aspiration for pediatric cataracts. This opacity is caused by proliferation, metaplasia, and migration of equatorial lens epithelial cells on the posterior capsule.[36] The incidence of PCO depends on the age at surgery, the type of cataract (congenital, developmental, or traumatic), aphakia versus pseudophakia, ciliary sulcus versus capsular bag fixation, associated ocular abnormalities (e.g., persistent fetal vasculature, microcornea), and preexisting systemic conditions such as juvenile rheumatoid arthritis. Additionally, the duration of follow-up affects the incidence of PCO; the longer the follow-up, the more PCO is manifested.

The burden of PCO is reflected in numerous reports. Basti et al.[31] reported the mean time for PCO appearance to be 3 months after surgery. Jensen et al.[25] observed significant PCO 1–26 months after cataract surgery in children with a mean age of 7.3 years. The peak incidence of PCO was 18 months after surgery; thereafter the curve flattened considerably. In their study PCO was more common in younger children: 64% of children 1 to 6 years old, versus 19% of those 6 to 13 years old, developed PCO. Gimbel et al.[30] reported a cumulative rate for Nd:YAG laser capsulotomy of 17, 42, 52, and 59% at 1, 2, 3, and 4 years after surgery, respectively. Plager et al.[9] observed a mean duration of 2 years for PCO development. According to Crouch et al.,[16] PCO developed in 72% of 35 eyes of children 5 to 18 years of age undergoing cataract surgery and IOL implantation with retention of the posterior capsule. Plager et al.[9] reported PCO in 90% of 71 eyes with a retained posterior capsule by 3.5 years in children 10 months to 17 years of age. Mullner-Eidenbock et al.[37] observed PCO in 9 out of 15 eyes (60%) of children 6 to 16 years of age with an intact posterior capsule and acrylic IOL implant. In a retrospective study, Hosal and Biglan[24] observed secondary capsular membranes in 78.6% of operated eyes 3 weeks to 53 months after surgery; they reported a 10-fold risk of media opacity with posterior capsule retention. In the same study, eyes with an IOL implant had 3.6 times the risk for PCO that aphakic eyes did; age <1 year at surgery created a 4.7-fold risk.

Recent modifications in IOL design (i.e., square-edge profile) and improved biocompatibility (e.g., hydrophobic acrylic) have significantly reduced the incidence of PCO in adults, however, there are insufficient data and experience to support their use in children.[37,38] Therefore, current options for prevention of PCO include postoperative Nd:YAG laser disruption of the posterior capsule before or after opacification[39] and primary posterior capsulotomy. Disadvantages of the former method include the lack of sufficient cooperation by children and possible need for a second anesthesia, need for a special Nd:YAG laser capable of functioning with the patient in the supine position, risk of IOL damage, and, above all, risk of recurrent media opacity on the anterior vitreous or hyaloid face. The anterior hyaloid face not only serves as a scaffold for migration and metaplasia of lens epithelial cells, but also acts as a surface for deposition of inflammatory cells, debris, and pigment.[40] Atkinson and Hiles[20] reported on 32 eyes of 28 children undergoing cataract surgery with or without IOL implantation who received postoperative Nd:YAG laser capsulotomy with the Microruptor III, which is capable of rotating 90°. In 16 eyes in which laser capsulotomy was performed earlier than 4 weeks, the mean energy required was 114 mJ; however, in the remaining eyes the procedure was performed later than 4 weeks and the mean energy required was 324 mJ. Overall, the rate of membrane reformation was 25% in this series. Hutcheson et al.[26] compared the incidence of media opacity between pediatric cataract extractions with primary posterior capsulotomy (33 eyes) and those with postoperative laser disruption (23 eyes); 3 versus 57% of the eyes, respectively, developed media opacity needing treatment. Furthermore, in the second group, 17% required repeat laser treatment after the second laser session.

Primary posterior capsulotomy with or without anterior vitrectomy decreases the chance for PCO and it is believed to be safe and to lack many of the complications associated with laser capsulotomy. Dahan and Salmenson[41] suggested removal of the posterior capsule with a vitrector. Buckley et al.[42] observed no media opacity by 13 months in 20 eyes undergoing primary posterior capsulotomy and anterior vitrectomy through a pars plana approach. However, opponents of this approach believe that retention of the posterior capsule without concomitant vitrectomy may decrease the risk of cystoid macular edema, retinal detachment, and vitreous incarceration into the surgical wound, facilitate in-the-bag IOL implantation, and provide long-term IOL stability.[39]

Opinions differ regarding the effect of primary posterior capsulotomy on cystoid macular edema (CME). Hoyt and Nickel[43] operated on 27 children with bilateral cataracts: one eye of each patient underwent lensectomy and vitrectomy; the fellow eye was treated with lens aspiration and discision of the posterior capsule. In the first group, 10 eyes developed CME, while no instances were noted in the fellow eyes. On the other hand, other investigators have reported different results. Gilbard et al.[44] reported only one case of suspected CME on angiographic and angioscopic examination of 25 eyes of 17 patients undergoing lensectomy and anterior vitrectomy. Green et al.[45] observed no cases of CME in 52 eyes undergoing pars plicata lensectomy and vitrectomy. In a series of 24 children undergoing bilateral cataract surgery and IOL implantation, Gimbel et al.[34] reported only one case of bilateral CME in a patient with retinitis pigmentosa. Pinchoff et al.[46] reported on lensectomy and vitrectomy (12 eyes), extracapsular cataract extraction and discision (5 eyes), extracapsular cataract extraction (3 eyes), and secondary discision (3 eyes); in none of the eyes was CME detectable by angiography. Ahmadieh et al.[47] also reported no case of CME on the angioscopic examination of 38 eyes undergoing limbal or pars plana lensectomy, anterior vitrectomy, and posterior chamber IOL implantation.

Overall, current evidence supports the idea that primary posterior capsulotomy is a safe procedure in children and is effective in the prevention of media opacity. Primary posterior capsulotomy may be performed with a vitrectomy probe via the limbus, pars plicata, or pars plana; another method is to perform a posterior continuous curvilinear capsulorhexis with forceps. Following posterior capsulotomy the posterior chamber IOL may be implanted into the capsular bag or ciliary sulcus. In either case and to provide better lens centration or to decrease the risk of media opacity, posterior capture of the optic into the capsular opening may be performed.

Despite removal of the posterior capsule, numerous studies have shown that secondary membranes and media opacity can still develop.[2,10,12,14,15,17,19,28,29,38,48–50] An intact hyaloid face can serve as a scaffold for migration of lens epithelial cells and their subsequent proliferation and transformation.[1,17,38,49] This phenomenon is further enhanced in children by the more intense inflammatory response following surgery.[51] O'Keefe et al.[12] reported media opacity in 33.3% of cases following primary posterior capsulotomy when anterior vitrectomy was not performed. Metge et al.[52] also showed that primary posterior capsulotomy alone cannot prevent formation of secondary membranes. Cassidy et al.[15] reported on three patients in whom posterior capsulorhexis had been performed; in all patients PCO and anterior hyaloid opacification occurred, and two of them eventually required surgical membranectomy due to ineffective Nd:YAG laser treatment. Raina et al.[53] reported a 44.4% incidence of significant media opacity in 18 eyes of children 1.5 to 12 years of age in whom posterior capsulorhexis without anterior vitrectomy and in-the-bag implantation of a polymethylmethacrylate (PMMA) lens had been performed.

It seems that removal of the posterior capsule by itself is not sufficient to prevent secondary opacification of the visual axis. One alternative proposed for this problem is posterior capsulorhexis with optic capture without anterior vitrectomy. It has been hypothesized that obliteration of the capsular bag and the posterior location of the IOL optic prevent lens epithelial cell migration along the vitreous face. Gimbel[54] performed this technique in 16 eyes of patients 2.5 to 12 years of age and observed no cases of media opacity by 35.5 months. In this study heparin-surface-modified PMMA lenses were used. The same author reported use of this technique in a 2.5-year-old patient, which resulted in a clear media up to 5 months after surgery.[55] Raina et al.[53] also reported no media opacity in 16 eyes of children 1.5 to 12 years of age for up to 17.5 months with the same technique. Mullner-Eidenbock et al.[37] performed the same technique but using hydrophobic IOLs in seven patients older than 6 years and observed no media opacity by 20.7 months. Argento et al.[38] also implanted hydrophobic acrylic IOLs using the same technique and observed no secondary opacity in eight eyes of children 2 to 8 years old by 18 to 34 months.

Despite the favorable results described above, a number of investigators have reported conflicting results. In a study by Vasavada and Desai,[17] posterior capsulorhexis and optic capture were performed in children <5 years old, and subsequently 62.5% underwent pars plana membranectomy. In the same study, the incidence of secondary opacification in eyes that underwent concomitant anterior vitrectomy was only 10%, and none required additional surgery. Vasavada and Trivedi[48] compared posterior capsulotomy and optic capture with and without vitrectomy in 41 eyes of 25 patients aged 5 to 12 years. After a mean follow-up of 21 months, visual acuity was similar in the two groups; however, low-contrast sensitivity was significantly better in the vitrectomized group. The visual axis remained clear in this group, while in the nonvitrectomized group, 70% showed media opacity of a reticular pattern on the vitreous. Koch and Kohnen[22] reported visual axis opacity by 6 months in four of five eyes after posterior capsulorhexis and optic capture without vitrectomy.

Based on the above studies, posterior capsulorhexis and optic capture without vitrectomy cannot eliminate secondary opacification completely, especially in patients <5 years old. Further studies with acrylic IOLs may improve the results with this technique.

Another alternative to overcome the problem of secondary opacification following removal of the posterior capsule is anterior vitrectomy, which may be performed via the limbus after posterior capsulotomy or trans pars plana following IOL implantation.[5,17,31,47,55] Buckley et al.[42] reported no case of secondary opacification in 20 cases of lensectomy, posterior capsulotomy, and anterior vitrectomy. Awner et al.[13] also reported no opacification in 21 patients <4 years of age who underwent the same procedure together with posterior chamber IOL implantation. Vasavada and Trivedi[48] observed no media opacification after performing optic capture in addition to the above-mentioned procedure in 21 eyes of children 5 to 12 years old. Vasavada and Desai reported no media opacification in 10 eyes undergoing anterior vitrectomy in addition to primary posterior capsulotomy.[17] Green et al.[50] performed pars plana lensectomy and vitrectomy in 52 eyes of patients 2 weeks to 4.5 years of age and observed secondary membranes in 6 eyes, all of which had an axial length of <17.4 mm and a corneal diameter of <9.5 mm. Koch and Kohnen[22] performed lensectomy and anterior vitrectomy with or without optic capture in six eyes of children 1.5 to 2 years with no secondary opacification. Chrousos et al.[56] reported no opacification after lensectomy, posterior capsulotomy, and vitrectomy in 54 eyes of children 3 months to 17 years of age. Vasavada and Trivedi[57] performed lensectomy, posterior capsulotomy, and anterior vitrectomy in 40 eyes of patients 4 to 55 months of age; optic capture was performed in 14 cases. After a mean follow-up of 16.5 months, only one case of secondary membrane formation was noted anterior to the IOL optic. In a report by Zubcov et al.[28] on 12 eyes in patients 3 to 12 years of age, the incidence of clinically significant opacity was 25% by 17 months. Ahmadieh et al.[47] reported four cases of opacification in 38 eyes of pediatric patients (mean age, 6.3 years) who had undergone limbal or pars plana operation with IOL implantation, however, only one was significant. Basti et al.[31] compared cataract extraction and posterior chamber IOL implantation with (82 eyes) and without (87 eyes) anterior vitrectomy in children 2 to 8 years of age; secondary opacification occurred in 3.6 and 43.7% of the eyes, respectively, by 11 months.

Considering these results, primary surgical removal of the posterior capsule should now be considered the gold standard in pediatric cataract surgery, especially under age 7, when the risk of PCO is higher and the potential for amblyopia still exists. Our routine for pediatric cataract surgery is primary posterior capsulotomy together with anterior vitrectomy up to the age of 9 years.[47] Furthermore, we perform and recommend the same procedure under certain circumstances in older patients; factors such as type of cataract, overall ocular condition, and socioeconomic status may influence such a decision. For instance, in a 14-year-old patient with traumatic cataract and an open anterior capsule with no possibility for in-the-bag IOL implantation, the risk for PCO is high enough to warrant posterior capsulotomy and anterior vitrectomy.

PREDISPOSING FACTORS FOR RECURRENT OPACIFICATION

Despite posterior capsulotomy and anterior vitrectomy, secondary opacification may occur in the visual axis. Predisposing factors for recurrent opacification include the following: small-sized capsulotomy (<4 mm), young age, type of cataract, ciliary sulcus versus capsular bag fixation, reaction to IOL material, and associated ocular or systemic inflammatory conditions.

Capsulotomy Size

Chrousos et al.[56] reported opacification in 12% of cases in which the posterior capsule was minimally opened, however, when the capsulotomy size was adequate, no instance of opacification was reported. All cases had undergone vitrectomy, however, the authors failed to define what size capsulotomy was considered adequate. Ahmadieh et al.[47] reported four cases of opacity, all in which the capsulotomy

size was <3 mm, however, only one eye required surgical intervention.

Age at Surgery

The younger the age at surgery, the more intense the postoperative inflammation and risk for subsequent opacification. Morgan and Karcioglu[10] reported significant opacification in three of four eyes in infants 2 weeks to 2 months of age despite a capsulotomy size of at least 5 mm and anterior vitrectomy. Alexandrakis et al.[6] reported 7 cases of opacification among 66 eyes of 61 children (median age, 21 months); 6 of these cases occurred in children <6 months old. Peterseim and Wilson[27] also observed media opacification to occur much more frequently in children <2 months old compared to older children (4 of 8 cases versus 1 of 24). Lambert et al.[58] observed a significant correlation between age at surgery and rate of complications. In a study by Hosal et al.[24] relative risk for development of opacification was 4.7 times higher in children <1 year of age compared to older children.

Sulcus Versus Bag Fixation

In 1985 Apple et al.[59] described the advantages of capsular bag fixation in adults, including less risk of pupillary capture, reduced decentration, less trauma to pigmented uveal tissue, decreased disruption of the blood–aqueous barrier, and less inflammation. Pandey et al.[18] operated on 20 eyes with traumatic cataracts. Lens aspiration was performed, followed by IOL implantation either in the capsular bag or in the ciliary sulcus. Complications including postoperative uveitis, PCO, pupillary capture, and lens decentration occurred more frequently in the sulcus fixation group. However, Jensen et al.[25] found no significant difference in the rate of PCO in relation to IOL position.

Type of Cataract

Some investigators have reported the results for congenital, developmental, and traumatic cataracts to be different. Gimbel et al.[30] calculated the cumulative incidence of need for capulotomy to be 41% for congenital cataracts and 66% for traumatic cataracts over 2 years. Gupta et al.[60] operated on 22 eyes with traumatic cataracts in children 3 to 11 years old. A posterior chamber IOL was implanted in 18 eyes, however, whether sulcus or bag fixation was used was not stated. After 6 to 15 months, the most common postoperative complications included fibrinous uveitis, in 81.8%, and synechiae, in 54.4%. Kora et al.[32] compared the results of cataract surgery and IOL implantation among congenital, developmental, and traumatic cataracts. PCO was noted to occur more commonly and earlier in congenital cases than in the other two categories. However, patients were not age-matched, which may explain the higher incidence of PCO in congenital cases. Ahmadieh et al.[47] also reported no difference between traumatic and developmental cataracts. The apparently increased incidence of PCO in traumatic cataracts may be due to the lower possibility of in-the-bag IOL implantation and more severe inflammation following trauma.

Associated Ocular and Systemic Conditions

Anomalies such as PFV (persistent fetal vasculature) or microcornea; ocular conditions such as rubella syndrome, toxocariasis, toxoplasmosis, and pars planitis; and systemic diseases such as juvenile rheumatoid arthritis are associated with a higher incidence of complications and capsular opacity.[2,3,33,49,50,58] Green et al.[50] performed pars plana lensectomy and anterior vitrectomy in 52 cases and observed secondary opacification in 6 eyes, all of which had an axial length of <17.4 mm and a corneal diameter of <9.5 mm. According to Lambert et al.,[58] of eight complications, four were related to eyes with PFV. Ben Ezra and Cohen[33] observed retrolental membranes in 80% of eyes with juvenile rheumatoid arthritis despite posterior capsulotomy and vitrectomy, all of which required a second surgical intervention. Lundvall et al.[61] reported on cataract surgery with IOL implantation in 10 eyes with juvenile rheumatoid arthritis; in five eyes anterior vitrectomy was also performed. After a mean follow-up of 28 months, media opacification occurred in seven eyes (70%).

INFLAMMATORY MEMBRANES

Another cause of media opacification after cataract surgery is formation of inflammatory membranes in the pupil, anterior and/or posterior to the IOL surface, together with synechiae formation and pigment deposition. Iris manipulation, blood–aqueous barrier disruption, reaction to IOL material, younger age at surgery, and associated ocular or systemic inflammation predispose to greater postoperative inflammation. Fibrinous uveitis following pediatric cataract surgery has been reported in from 57.5%[3] to 81.8%[18] of cases.

These membranes may be transient, with varying degrees of resorption in several days or a few weeks. Some cases may persist, necessitating a second surgical intervention. Due to the more intense inflammatory reaction in children and the potential for amblyopia, this issue is of greater concern in children. Attempts may be directed toward prevention or immediate medical or surgical treatment once the membrane has developed.

The risk of inflammatory membranes may be decreased by the frequent use of topical and systemic steroids before and following cataract surgery. In cases of uveitic cataracts, preexisting intraocular inflammation must be controlled with topical and systemic steroids prior to surgery.[61] Postoperatively high-dose topical and systemic steroids must be continued and slowly tapered off. Intraoperative use of low molecular weight heparin in irrigation fluids may decrease the severity of postoperative inflammation.[62,63] Heparin-surface-modified (HSM) PMMA IOLs may also be useful in reducing inflammatory membranes.[54,55,64] However, recent studies have shown no significant difference between PMMA and HSM-PMMA IOLs in quiescent uveitis.[65,66] Hydrophobic acrylic IOLs may reduce lens epithelial cell migration,[67] PCO, and giant cell deposits.[68] In a study by Gatinel et al.[65] no significant difference was observed between HSM-PMMA and hydrophobic acrylic IOLs in diabetic patients. It is noteworthy that the above-mentioned studies were performed in adults, and generalization of the results to pediatric cases is uncertain.

Once inflammatory membranes have developed, timely initiation of topical and systemic steroids is necessary. Tissue plasminogen activator (TPA), first used in 1988,[69] has recently been used for dissolution of fibrin clots after pediatric cataract surgery. TPA is normally produced by vascular endothelial cells, corneal epithelium and endothelium, and the trabecular meshwork.[70] Significant reduction of TPA activity has been noted after cataract surgery, which, in combination with blood–aqueous barrier disruption, leads to fibrin deposition.[71] Recombinant TPA is a fibrinolytic serine protease produced genetically by cloning and expression of recombinant DNA.[72] Plasminogen activator causes fibrin lysis by localized transformation of plasminogen to plasmin in the presence of fibrin. The half-life of the intravenous TPA is 7 min.[73] No systemic effects have been noted with injection into the anterior chamber.[74] Recombinant TPA has no deleterious effect on corneal endothelium[74] and has been used for dissolution of fibrin clots after penetrating keratoplasty,[73] vitrectomy, and glaucoma surgery.[75] Mean time for effect is 3.3 hr. Complications of intraocular TPA are hyphema and increased intraocular pressure, therefore its use is not recommended earlier than 3 days after surgery.[76] The optimal dosing for TPA remains unsettled. Klais et al.[77] used 10 μg/100 μL TPA in the anterior chamber of 11 eyes of children aged 3 to 13 years who developed a severe fibrinous reaction unresponsive to conventional treatment. Dissolution of the fibrin and resolution of synechiae were observed in nine eyes by 6 days; no complications or recurrence of fibrin deposition was observed. Mehta and Adams[78] reported a 25-μg dose without any complications. TPA seems to be effective only up to 3 weeks after cataract surgery.[79]

Dense fibrin membranes may require surgical intervention. In the pupillary space, the membrane may be retracted with a sharp needle[80] or by Nd:YAG laser application in cooperative cases, however, dense membranes anterior or posterior to the IOL require membranectomy.

OTHER CAUSES OF MEDIA OPACITY

Vitreous condensation and opacification may follow excessive iris manipulation, inadequate vitrectomy, vitreous incarceration into the surgical wound, and admixture of lens material with vitreous. To prevent the latter complication the surgeon should try to avoid opening the posterior capsule prior to complete removal of lens material. In cases of uveitic cataracts such as juvenile rheumatoid arthritis, pars planitis, and rubella syndrome, complete anterior vitrectomy is mandatory to clear organized vitreous and to remove any remaining strands capable of causing secondary opacities. In some instances, hemorrhage may occur when performing peripheral iridectomy. It is best to avoid excessive stretch on the iris root to prevent hemorrhage and its seepage into the vitreous cavity. Vitreous hemorrhage after cataract surgery may also occur in cases with PFV; use of intraocular cautery may be useful in preventing this complication.[2]

Corneal edema is another cause of media opacification, which may be caused by irrigation fluids, toxic substances, excessive intraocular manipulations, IOL touch during implantation, or late corneal touch. In cases with microcornea there is a higher risk of corneal edema with limbal approaches. Hiles et al.[11] reported the overall incidence of corneal edema to be 4% in congenital and traumatic cataracts with posterior chamber, anterior chamber, and iris-fixated IOLs.

Perhaps the most serious condition that can lead to media opacity is glaucoma. This is a well-known complication of pediatric cataract surgery that has been reported by many investigators.[21,56,61,81,82] There seem to be multiple mechanisms involved including surgical trauma, inflammation, obliteration of angle structures by synechiae, and predisposing conditions. Media opacification caused by glaucoma is an end-stage condition indicating a poor visual prognosis.

CONCLUSION

The main goal of cataract surgery in children is relief of media opacity and proper correction of refractive errors with concomitant amblyopia therapy. All these depend on maintenance of clear ocular media. Opacification involving ocular media may be early or late onset. The latter may go unrecognized and lead to amblyopia. Another serious complication is secondary glaucoma, therefore attention to red reflex and IOP measurements are mandatory at all follow-up visits.

REFERENCES

1. Nelson LB. *Harley's Pediatric Ophthalmology.* Philadelphia: W. B. Saunders, 1998:269–273.

2. Lambert SR, Drack AV. Infantile cataract. *Surv Ophthalmol* 1996;40:427–428.
3. Pandey SK, Wilson ME, Trivedi RH, Izak AM, Macky TA, Werner L, et al. Pediatric cataract surgery and intraocular lens implantation: current techniques, complications, and management. In: Werner L, Apple DJ, eds. *International Ophthalmology Clinics: Complications of Aphakic and Refractive Intraocular Lenses. Vol 4.* Philadelphia: Lippincott, Williams and Wilkins, 2001:175–196.
4. Scheie HG. Aspiration of congenital or soft cataracts: a new technique. *Am J Ophthalmol* 1960;50:1048–1056.
5. Parks MM. Posterior lens capsulotomy during primary cataract surgery in children. *Ophthalmology* 1983;90:344–345.
6. Alexandrakis G, Peterseim MM, Wilson ME. Clinical outcomes of pars plana capsulotomy with anterior vitrectomy in pediatric cataract surgery. *J AAPOS* 2002;6:163–167.
7. Lambert SR, Fernandes A, Grossniklaus H, Drews-Botsch C, Eggers H, Boothe RG. Neonatal lensectomy and intraocular lens implantation: effects in rhesus monkeys. *Invest Ophthalmol Vis Sci* 1995;36:300–310.
8. Greenwald MJ, Glaser SR. Visual outcomes after surgery for unilateral cataract in children more than two years old: posterior chamber intraocular lens implantation versus contact lens correction of aphakia. *J AAPOS* 1998;2:168–176.
9. Plager DA, Lipsky SN, Snyder SK, Sprunger DT, Ellis FD, Sondhi N. Capsular management and refractive error in pediatric intraocular lenses. *Ophthalmology* 1997;104:600–607.
10. Morgan KS, Karcioglu ZA. Secodary cataracts in infants after lensectomies. *J Pediatr Ophthalmol Strabismus* 1987;24:45–48.
11. Hiles DA. Intraocular lens implantation in children with monocular cataracts. *Ophthalmology* 1984;91:1231–1237.
12. O'Keefe M, Mulvihill A, Yeoh PL. Visual outcome and complications of bilateral intraocular lens implantation in children. *J Cataract Refract Surg* 2000;26:1758–1764.
13. Awner S, Buckley EG, Varo JM, Seaber JH. Unilateral pseudophakia in children under 4 years. *J Pediatr Ophthalmol Strabismus* 1996;33:230–236.
14. Azar DT. *Intraocular Lenses in Cataract and Refractive Surgery.* Philadelphia: W. B. Saunders, 2001:99–111.
15. Cassidy L, Rahi J, Nischal K, Russell-Eggitt I, Taylor D. Outcome of lens aspiration and intraocular lens implantation in children aged 5 years and under. *Br J Ophthalmol* 2001;85:540–542.
16. Crouch ER, Crouch ER Jr, Pressman SH. Prospective analysis of pediatric pseudophakia: myopic shift and postoperative outcomes. *J AAPOS* 2002;6:277–282.
17. Vasavada A, Desai J. Primary posterior capsulorhexis with and without anterior vitrectomy in congenital cataracts. *J Cataract Refract Surg* 1997;23:645–651.
18. Pandey SK, Ram J, Werner L, Brar GS, Jain AK, Gupta A. Visual results and postoperative complications of capsular bag and ciliary sulcus fixation of posterior chamber intraocular lenses in children with traumatic cataracts. *J Cataract Refract Surg* 1999;25:1576–1584.
19. Zween J, Mullaney PB, Awad A, Al-Mesfer S. Wheeler DT. Pediatric intraocular lens implantation: surgical results and complications in more than 300 patients. *Ophthalmology* 1998;105:112–119.
20. Atkinson CS, Hiles DA. Treatment of secondary posterior capsular membranes with the Nd:YAG laser in a pediatric population. *Am J Ophthalmol* 1994;118:496–501.
21. Keech RV, Tongue AC, Scott WE. Complications after surgery for congenital and infantile cataracts. *Am J Ophthalmol* 1989;108:136–141.
22. Koch DD, Kohnen T. Retrospective comparison of techniques to prevent secondary cataract formation after posterior chamber intraocular lens implantation in infants and children. *J Cataract Refract Surg* 1997;23:657–663.
23. Ghosh B, Gupta AK, Taneja S, Gupta A, Mazumdar S. Epilenticular lens implantation versus extracapsular cataract extraction and lens implantation in children. *J Cataract Refract Surg* 1997;23:612–617.
24. Hosal BM, Biglan AB. Risk factors for secondary membrane formation after removal. *J Cataract Refract Surg* 2002;28:302–309.
25. Jensen AA, Basti S, Greenwald MJ, Mets MB. When may the posterior capsule be preserved in pediatric intraocular. *Ophthalmology* 2002;109:324–328.

26. Hutcheson KA, Drack AV, Ellish NJ, Lambert SR. Anterior hyaloid face opacification after pediatric Nd: YAG laser capsulotomy. *J AAPOS* 1999;3:303–307.

27. Peterseim MW, Wilson MW. Bilateral intraocular lens implantation in the pediatric population. *Ophthalmology* 2000;107:1261–1266.

28. Zubcov AV, Stahl E, Rossillion B, Nutzenberger A, Kohnen T, Ohrloff C, et al. Streopsis after primary in the bag posterior chamber implantation in children. *J AAPOS* 1999;3:227–233.

29. Simons BD, Siatkowski RM, Schiffman JC, Flynn JT, Capo H, Munoz M. Surgical technique, visual outcome and complications of pediatric intraocular lens implantation. *J Pediatr Ophthalmol Strabismus* 1999;36:118–124.

30. Gimbel HV, Frensowicz M, Raanan M, DeLuca M. Implantation in Children. *J Pediatr Ophthalmol Strabismus* 1993;30:69–79.

31. Basti S, Ravishankar U, Gupta S. Result of a prospective evaluation of three methods of management of pediatric cataracts. *Ophthalmology* 1996;103:713–720.

32. Kora Y, Inatomi M, Fukado Y, Marumori M, Yaguchi S. Long-term study of children with planted intraocular lenses. *J Cataract Refract Surg* 1992;18:485–487.

33. BenEzra B, Cohen E. Cataract surgery in children with chronic uveitis. *Ophthalmology* 2000;107:1255–1260.

34. Gimbel HV, Basti S, Ferensowicz M, DeBroff BM. Results of bilateral cataract extraction with posterior chamber intraocular lens implantation in children. *Ophthalmology* 1997;104:1737–1743.

35. Taylor D. Choice of surgical technique in the management of congenital cataract. *Trans Ophthalmol Soc UK* 1981;101:114–117.

36. Peng Q, Apple DJ, Visessook N, Werner L, Pandey SK, Escobar-Gomez M, et al. Surgical prevention of posterior capsule opacification. Part 2: Enhancement of cortical cleanup by focusing on hydrodissection. *J Cataract Refract Surg* 2000;26:188–197.

37. Mullner-Eidenbock A, Amon M, Moser E, Kruger A, Abela C, Schlemmer Y, et al. Morphological and functional results of acrysof intraocular lens implantation in children prospective randomized study of age- related surgical management. *J Cataract Refract Surg* 2003;29:285–293.

38. Argento C, Badoza D, Ugrin C. Optic capture of the Acrysof intraocular lens in pediatric cataract surgery. *J Cataract Refract Surg* 2001;27:1638–1642.

39. Wang XH, Wilson E, Bluestein EC, Auffarth G, Apple DJ. Pediatric cataract surgery and intraocular lens implantation techniques: a laboratory study. *J Cataract Refract Surg* 1994;20:607–609.

40. Oliver M, Milstein A, Pollak A. Posterior chamber lens implantation in infants and juveniles. *Eur J Implant Ref Surg* 1990;2:309–314.

41. Dahan E, Salmenson BD. Pseudophakia in children: Precautions, technique, and feasibility. *J Cataract Refract Surg* 1990;16:75–82.

42. Buckley EG, Klombers LA, Seaber JH, Scalise-Gordy A, Minzter R. Management of the posterior capsule during pediatric intraocular lens implantation. *Am J Ophthalmol* 1993;115:722–728.

43. Hoyt CS, Nickel D. Aphakic cystoid macular edema. occurrence in infants and children after transpupillary lensectomy and anterior vitrectomy. *Arch Ophthalmol* 1982;100:746–749.

44. Gilbard SM, Peyman GA, Goldberg MF. Evaluation for cystoid maculopathy after pars plicata lensectomy for congenital cataracts. *Ophthalmology* 1983;90:1201–1206.

45. Green BF, Morin JD, Brent HP. Pars plicata lensectomy vitrectomy for developmental cataract extraction: surgical results. *J Pediatr Ophthalmol Strabismus* 1990;27:229–232.

46. Pinchoff BS, Ellis FD, Helveston EM, Sato SE. Cystoid macular edema in pediatric aphakia. *J Pediatr Ophthalmol Strabismus* 1988;25:240–243.

47. Ahmadieh H, Javadi MA, Ahmady M, Karimian F, Einollahi B, Zare M, et al. Primary capsulectomy, anterior vitrectomy, lensectomy, and posterior chamber lens implantation in children: Limbal versus pars plana. *J Cataract Refract Surg* 1999;25:768–775.

48. Vasavada AR, Trivedi RH, Singh R. Necessity of vitrectomy when optic capture is performed in children older than 5 years. *J Cataract Refract Surg* 2001;27:1185–1193.

49. Hiles DA. Visual rehabilitation of aphakic children. *Surv Ophthalmol* 1990;34:371–379.

50. Green BF, Morin JD, Brent HP. Pars plicata lensectomy/vitrectomy for developmental cataract extraction: surgical results. *J Pediatr Ophthalmol Strabismus* 1990;27:229–232.

51. Sinskey RM, Amin PA, Lingua R. Cataract extraction and intraocular lens implantation in an infant with a monocular congenital cataract. *J Cataract Refract Surg* 1994;20:647–651.

52. Metge P, Cohen H, Chemila JF. Intercapsular implantation in children. *Eur J Cataract Refract Surg* 1990;2:319–323.

53. Raina UK, Gupta V, Arora R, Mebta DK. Posterior continuous curvilinear capsulorhexis with and without optic capture of the posterior chamber intraocular lens in the absence of vitrectomy. *J Pediatr Ophthalmol Strabismus* 2002;39:278–287.

54. Gimbel HV. Posterior continuous curvilinear capsulorhexis and optic capture of the intraocular lens to prevent secondary opacification in pediatric cataract surgery. *J Cataract Refract Surg* 1997;23:652–656.

55. Gimbel HV, DeBroff BM. Posterior capsulorhexis with optic capture: Maintaining a clear visual axis after pediatric cataract surgery. *J Cataract Refract Surg* 1994;20:658–664.

56. Chrousos GA, Parks MM, O'Neill JF. Incidence of chronic glaucoma, retinal detachment, and secondary membrane surgery in pediatric aphakic patiets. *Ophthalmology* 1984;91:1238–1241.

57. Vasavada AR, Trivedi RH. Role of optic capture in congenital cataract and intraocular lens surgery in children. *J Cataract Refract Surg* 2000;26:824–831.

58. Lambert SR, Buckley EG, Plager DA, Medow NB, Wilson ME. Unilateral intraocular lens implantation during the first six months of life. *J AAPOS* 1999;3:344–349.

59. Apple DJ, Reidy JJ, Googe JM, Mamalis N, Novak LC, Loftfield K, et al. A comparison of ciliary sulcus and bag fixation of posterior chamber intraocular lenses. *J Am Intraocular Implant Soc* 1985;11: 44–63.

60. Gupta AK, Grover AK, Gurha N. Traumatic cataract surgery with intraocular lens implantation in children. *J Pediatr Ophthalmol Strabismus* 1992;29:73–78.

61. Lundvall A, Zetterstrom C. Cataract extraction and intraocular lens implantation in children with uveitis. *Br J Ophthalmol* 2000;84:791–793.

62. Lambert SR, Fernandes A, Grossniklaus H, Drews-Botsch C, Eggers H, Boothe RG. Neonatal lensectomy and intraocular lens implantation: effects on rhesus monkey. *Invest Ophthalmol Vis Sci* 1995;36:300–310.

63. Kohnen T, Dick B, Hessemer V, Koch DD, Jacobi KW. Effect of heparin in irrigating solution on inflammation following small incision cataract surgery. *J Cataract Refract Surg* 1998;24:237–243.

64. Zetterstrom C, Kugelberg U, Lundgren B, SyrenNordqvist S. After cataract formation in newborn rabbits implanted with intraocular lenses. *J Cataract Refract Surg* 1996;22:85–88.

65. Gatinel D, Lebrun T, Le Toumelin P, Chaine G. Aqueous flare induced by heparin-surface-modified poly (mrthyl methacrylate) and acrylic lenses implanted through the same- size incision in patients with diabetes. *J Cataract Refract Surg* 2001;27:855–860.

66. Tabbara KF, Al-Kaff AS, Al-Rajhi AA, Al-Mansouri SM, Badr IA, Chavis PS, et al. Heparin surface-modified intraocular lenses in patients with inactive uveitis or diabetes. *Ophthalmology* 1998;105:843–845.

67. Hollick EJ, Spalton DJ, Ursell PG, Pande MV, Barman SA, Boyce JF, et al. The effect of polymethylmethacrylate, silicone, and polyacrylic intraocular lenses on posterior capsular opacification 3 years after cataract surgery. *Ophthalmology* 1999;106:46–54, discussion by RC Drews 54–55.

68. Hayashi H, Hayashi K, Nakao F, Hayashi F. Area reduction in the anterior capsule opening in eye of diabetes mellitus patients. *J Cataract Refract Surg* 1998;24:1105–1110.

69. Williams GA, Lambrou FH, Jaffe GA, Snyder RW, Green GD, Devenyi RG, et al. Treatment of postvitrectomy fibrin formation with intraocular tissue plasminogen activator. *Arch Ophthalmol* 1988;106:1055–1058.

70. Tripathi RC, Park JK, Tripathi BJ, Millard CB. Tissue plasminogen activator in human aqueous and is possible therapeutic significance. *Am J Ophthalmol* 1988;106:719–722.

71. Yoshitomi F, Utsumi E, Hayashi M, Futenma M, Yamada R, Yamada S. Postoperative fluctuation of tissue plasminogen activator (t-PA) in aqueous humor of pseudophakes. *J Cataract Refract Surg* 1991;18:252–264.

72. Collen D, Stassen JM, Marafino BJ Jr, Builder S, De Cock F, Ogez J, et al. Biological properties of human tissue-type plasminogen

activator obtained by expression of recombinant DNA in mammalian cells. *J Pharmacol Exp Ther* 1984;231:146–152.

73. Snyder RW, Lambrou FH, Williams GA. Intraocular fibrinolysis with recombinant human tissue plasminogen activator: experimental treatment in a rabbit model. *Arch Ophthalmol* 1987;105:1277–1280.

74. Gerding PA Jr, Hamor RE, Ramsey DT, Vasaune S, Schaeffer DJ. Evaluation of topically administered tissue plasminogen activator for intraocular fibrinolysis in dogs. *Am J Vei Res* 1994;55:1368–1370.

75. Jaffe GJ, Lewis H, Han DP, Williams GA, Abrams GW. Treatment of postvitrectomy fibrin pupillary block with tissue plasminogen activator. *Am J Ophthalmol* 1989;108:170–175.

76. Wedrich A, Menapace R, Muhlbauer-Reis E. The use of recombinant tissue plasminogen activator for intracameral fibrinolysis following cataract surgery. *Int Ophthalmol* 1995;18:277–280.

77. Klais CM, Hattenbach LO, Steinkamp GWK, Zubcov AA, Kohnen T. Intraocular recombinant tissue-plasminogen activator fibrinolysis of fibrin formation after cataract surgery in children. *J Cataract Refract Surg* 1999;25:357–362.

78. Mehta JS, Adams GGW. Recombinant tissue plasminogen activator following paediatric cataract surgery. *Br J Ophthalmol* 2000;84:983–986.

79. Moon J, Chung S, Myong Y, Chung S, Park C, Baek N, et al. Treatment of post-cataract fibrinous membranes with tissue plasminogen activator. *Ophthalmology* 1992;99:1256–1259.

80. Leung ATS, Lam DSC. Fibrinolysis of postcataract fibrin membranes in children. *J Cataract Refract Surg* 2000;26:4–5.

81. Lundvall A, Kugelberg U. Outcome after treatment of congenital bilateral cataract. *Acta Ophthalmol Scand* 2002;80:593–597.

82. Simon JW, Mehta N, Simmons ST, Catalano RA, Lininger LL. Glaucoma after pediatric lensectomy/vitrectomy. *Ophthalmology* 1991;98:670–674.

Postoperative Glaucoma

John Facciani, Rupal H. Trivedi, and M. Edward Wilson, Jr.

Aphakic glaucoma is the bane of cataract surgery. Laboratory scientists cannot submit an etiology that is accepted by all clinicians, clinicians cannot offer a treatment that is effective for all patients, and the onset of glaucoma can range from the immediate period to many years later. To make matters worse, children do not always cooperate for intraocular pressure (IOP) measurements, optic disc evaluation, or visual field documentations. Thus, defining when glaucoma is present and when a treatment is effective at halting the progression of damage is unusually challenging. The common factor for all of these patients is the fact that cataract surgery has been performed. Even with severe microphthalmia, glaucoma does not seem to occur in the absence of the cataract procedure. In the predisposed eye, surgery to remove the cataract must trigger a cascade of events that can lead to elevated IOP and/or glaucoma early on or even 5 to 15 years later.

In years past, all pediatric patients were left aphakic after cataract extraction. Today, intraocular lens (IOL) implantation is a reasonable alternative and arguably a better choice in many cases, and a trend toward implanting IOLs in patients <2 years old is becoming more common.[1] There have been many reports of pediatric patients with aphakic glaucoma, but few reports of pseudophakic glaucoma. Perhaps this represents a selection bias since the more severely maldeveloped and microphthalmic eyes are the ones least likely to be implanted with an IOL.

Ophthalmologists must be vigilant about assessing for postoperative glaucoma in children left aphakic or pseudophakic after uncomplicated cataract removal by the most sophisticated, modern techniques. This approach is mandated both by the disagreement regarding risk factors and by the lack of knowledge of the pathophysiology of postoperative pediatric glaucoma.

Scheie (2) introduced an aspiration technique for removing congenital cataracts that may have reduced the incidence of complications compared to the linear extraction method in 1960. The older method resulted in lens swelling and, at times, a prolonged flat anterior chamber.

Acute angle closure glaucoma and excessive inflammation often ensued.

Acute angle closure following pediatric cataract surgery with modern techniques is relatively uncommon, and peripheral iridectomies are performed less commonly today than in years past.[3–6] While some surgeons perform this procedure on every case, we do not perform peripheral iridectomies in routine cases. Good wound closure with 10-0 vicryl sutures for both keratome incisions and paracentesis sites militates against wound leak. A prolonged flat chamber will necessitate a return to the operating room to create a peripheral iridectomy and ensure that wounds are well closed.

Late-onset open-angle glaucoma is thought to occur much more commonly today than angle closure after pediatric cataract surgery.[3–6] Open-angle glaucoma can occur without the presence of any symptoms or gross changes in the appearance of the eye and has been described both in normal-appearing open angles and in angles that have undergone change.

How often does late postoperative glaucoma occur? Why does it occur? Which patients are more likely to develop glaucoma after surgery? What therapy is appropriate once this is recognized? These questions are discussed in this chapter.

ESTIMATE OF FREQUENCY OF POSTCATARACT GLAUCOMA IN CHILDREN

Knowledge of the incidence of a postoperative complication allows a clinician to establish the need for a reasonable program of surveillance for that condition. It is even more crucial if the condition presents insidiously and if this unrecognized process can cause significant morbidity or mortality. The incidence of glaucoma following pediatric cataract removal has been reported to be as low as 5% and as high as 41%.[3–8] In a review of 13 studies from the international literature on congenital cataract surgery in an earlier era, Francois[7] reported that delayed glaucoma following cataract surgery in children occurred in between 0 and 14% of cases. The majority of these data are available in reports from the 1940s or 1950s, when the linear aspiration technique was used.

While this report is interesting from a historical perspective, it cannot elucidate the likelihood that glaucoma may develop using more modern techniques. In 1984, Chrousos et al.[8] reported their 15-year experience with pediatric cataract surgery; the surgeons utilized Scheie's manual aspiration technique as well as automated styles of cataract removal. The standard needle-and-syringe technique was performed in 304 eyes, rotoextraction with a small opening in the posterior capsule was performed in 34 eyes, and Ocutome vitrector aspiration with wide posterior capsular excision was performed in 54 eyes. All patients had at least 3 months of follow-up. Overall, chronic glaucoma was found in 6.1% of the eyes; no patients with Ocutome aspiration developed glaucoma. Of the 11 eyes with glaucoma for which gonioscopic data were available, all had open angles.

Interestingly, the 6.1% overall rate of glaucoma reported by Chrousos et al.[8] using "modern" techniques was similar to the 5% rate achieved by Francois[7] before aspiration techniques were used. The authors of the 1984 study admitted that a limitation of the study is length of follow-up of some patients, which could have resulted in underreporting glaucoma. While the aspiration-only group was followed for a mean of 6.3 years, the Ocutome group was followed for only 2 years on average. Was there something remarkable about the vitrector that prevented glaucoma from forming or had not enough time elapsed since surgery to develop it? If glaucoma does occur in patients who have cataracts removed by vitrectomy, would the total incidence in the Chrousos study be significantly higher than the rates obtained by surgeons in the 1950s?

Making such a comparison is rather unreasonable for many reasons, including the variety of definitions of glaucoma that authors have used through the ages and the variety of instruments used to measure IOP. However, perhaps the most important factor in studies aiming to report the frequency of glaucoma in a postoperative population is the length of follow-up, as a study by John Simon and associates addresses below.

Simon et al.[5] invited their patients who had undergone pediatric cataract surgery back to their office to check for asymptomatic glaucoma, which was defined as an IOP ≥26. Twenty-six patients were examined of the 42 who were contacted. While almost a quarter of the patients examined had glaucoma, the interesting data involved length of follow-up. While only 1 of 14 eyes (7%) with ≤60 months of follow-up since lensectomy developed glaucoma, 7 of 17 eyes (41%) followed for >5 years had glaucoma. The message is clear that reports with <5 years of follow-up may significantly underestimate the frequency

with which glaucoma develops after pediatric cataract surgery.

Chrousos et al.[8] and Simon et al.[5] both pointed out an important finding in asymptomatic postoperative glaucoma—that although the onset is typically delayed until years after the surgery, the diagnosis may be made within the first year of surgery in some cases and surveillance of IOP must be initiated early.

Simon et al.[5] did not choose objective signs of glaucoma such as visual field loss or optic nerve head damage in their definition of glaucoma. Therefore, it is likely that some of his patients actually had ocular hypertension, and "true" glaucoma probably occurred less frequently than was reported. In adults, the Ocular Hypertension Treatment Study (OHTS)[9] recognized that only a small percentage of patients with an IOP >21 mm Hg will progress to develop glaucoma after several years. The lack of an equivalent randomized, prospective trial with adequate follow-up in children combined with the difficulty of obtaining objective evidence of glaucoma in children probably leads to a judicious overtreatment of elevated IOP in the pediatric population.

A prospective, nonrandomized study provides some valuable data on the rates of pediatric glaucoma and ocular hypertension after automated lensectomy and vitrectomy. Egbert et al.[10] reviewed records of patients with 5 years of follow-up after lensectomy. Of 159 patients, 52 were excluded because of trauma, microphthalmos, uveitis, or a similar complicating factor. Sixty-two of 107 patients (58%) participated, and participating and nonparticipating patients had no differences in average corneal diameter or age at the time of surgery. Glaucoma was defined as an IOP >21 with a cup/disk ratio >0.5 or a cup/disk asymmetry ≥0.2. Ocular hypertension (OHTN) was defined as an IOP >21 without the aforementioned optic nerve parameters. Six of 40 (15%) patients had glaucoma in their aphakic eye. OHTN was even more common. Thirteen of 40 (32.5%) patients had OHTN in their unilaterally aphakic eye, while 10 of 22 (45%) patients who previously had bilateral cataracts had OHTN in one (4 patients) or both (6 patients) eyes. Overall, 23 of 62 (37%) patients had aphakic ocular hypertension when examined ≥5 years after surgery. This report demonstrates that OHTN is a common long-term finding in patients with pediatric aphakia and glaucoma is an uncommon but not rare event. With time, more patients with a normal IOP or with OHTN may develop glaucoma. The true incidence of glaucoma is likely to be significantly above zero and justifies the authors' lifelong follow-up of these patients.

We believe that it is vital to examine patients on at least a yearly basis after uneventful pediatric cataract surgery with or without IOL implantation. Egbert and colleagues[10] concluded that good data can be obtained from patients >5 years of age in the clinic; we schedule examinations under anesthesia only when clinic examinations with IOP measurements or refractions are technically impossible.

PROPOSED MECHANISMS FOR THE DEVELOPMENT OF GLAUCOMA AFTER PEDIATRIC CATARACT SURGERY

The causes of pediatric aphakic open-angle glaucoma are as elusive today as they were years ago. Today, however, it is widely known that glaucoma *does* occur in a significant minority of patients. In 1977, Charles Phelps and Nour Arafat brought this to the attention of ophthalmologists as a "warning."[11] They were surprised to diagnose an insidious, asymptomatic type of glaucoma in 18 patients who had undergone congenital cataract removal years (6 to 56 years) before the patients manifested an elevated IOP. They expressed concern that although those patients had cataracts removed by simple needling, linear extraction, or intracapsular extraction, more modern techniques (such as needling and aspiration, phacoemulsification, and rotoextraction) may also produce glaucoma.

The authors discussed several of the mechanisms that could be at fault. Could an undescribed ocular syndrome involving both cataract and glaucoma be causal? Does early surgery promote such significant inflammation or expose the fledgling trabeculum to so much lens protein that it is irrevocably damaged? Is a vitreous component toxic to the trabeculum? Even today we do not know the answer to these questions or how much these factors contribute to the development of glaucoma, if at all.

What do we know about aphakic glaucoma? Is it an open-angle or closed-angle mechanism? In 1986, David Walton discussed pupillary block and chronic angle closure from peripheral anterior synechiae as the typical mechanism following cataract removal by the "aspiration" mechanism.[12]

A decade later, Walton's American Ophthalmological Society thesis[3] concluded that the asymptomatic, postoperative glaucoma in aphakic patients was actually an open-angle mechanism and that those who underwent surgery in the first year of life were at highest risk for this complication, but the etiology of the glaucoma was still speculative. Walton[3] studied the angle structure of 65 aphakic children with postoperative glaucoma from modern methods of pediatric cataract removal. Vitrectomy techniques were utilized in the majority (80%) of cases. Preoperatively, the majority of patients with available gonioscopy (19/29 eyes) had no angle abnormalities, while 10 patients did have "anomalous attachments from the iris root to Schwalbe's line and the trabecular meshwork." Postoperatively, the angles were open in 79 of 80 eyes, but in 76 of 79 (96%) eyes "circumferential repositioning of the iris insertion anteriorly at the level of the posterior or mid-trabecular meshwork with resultant loss to view

of the ciliary body band and scleral spur" occurred. Windows of visible scleral spur or ciliary body were visible in these eyes, confirming open angles. Phelps and Arafat[11] had described similar changes in the anterior chamber angles in their patients. Walton[3] observed scattered pigment deposits in the exposed anterior trabecular meshwork and, less frequently, white crystalline deposits suggestive of lens protein.

The mechanism does not appear to be related to clinically identifiable *late* postoperative inflammation. Walton[3] reported on slit-lamp examinations of 19 children performed after lensectomy and before glaucoma was diagnosed. In none of those patients was an anterior chamber cell or band keratopathy present; these patients had a different appearance than those with chronic inflammation. In addition, none of the patients examined after the diagnosis of glaucoma had evidence of active intraocular inflammation.

The absence of active intraocular inflammation years after surgery does not negate the possibility of acute postoperative inflammation causing significant, immediate damage to the trabecular meshwork that develops into a chronic, secondary open-angle glaucoma. Several authors have reported cases of bilateral cataracts that had subtle, bilateral angle abnormalities but developed glaucoma only in the operated eye.[3,13] We are curious whether the presence of "anomalous attachments from the iris root to Schwalbe's line and the trabecular meshwork" documented in 10 of Walton's[3] patients (but absent in 19 patients) before surgery implies that an abnormal process was already occurring subclinically in all patients. Perhaps cataract surgery simply amplified the process such that "circumferential repositioning of the iris insertion anteriorly" was observed at a later time. Phelps and Arafat,[11] observing similar gonioscopic findings in patients after surgery, implied that the uniformity of the angle findings "throughout its circumference" instead suggested that these findings were congenital and not related to the cataract surgery. There is no way to prove, however, that those angle findings were not indicative of subclinical dysfunction.

Walton himself, in the discussion following his study, lamented that despite his careful attention to gonioscopic detail in his patients, the cause of the glaucoma could not be inferred.[3] Whether or not the angle is described as open or closed is probably irrelevant if we cannot correlate microscopic, ultrastructural changes (by light microscopy or electron microscopy) in the trabecular meshwork with changes in aqueous outflow and increases in IOP in eyes of children with and without glaucoma who had cataract surgery in one or both eyes. Such a study may lead to the elucidation of the mechanism of the glaucoma and, ultimately, its true cause.

It is possible that cataract extraction may indeed damage a growing, vulnerable anterior chamber angle in an eye with a subclinically imperfect trabecular outflow in a way that creates high IOP years later.[4] This may be why patients with a preexisting ocular abnormality (such as trauma, dislocated lens, chronic uveitis, or anterior segment dysgenesis) may be at higher risk for postoperative glaucoma.[6]

If such a theory were correct, and if surgery were to be performed satisfactorily with modern techniques, the most important step in preventing glaucoma for these patients would be to minimize acute postoperative inflammation by applying various forms of anti-inflammatory preoperative and postoperative medications. The results of a randomized, prospective trial addressing this issue would be most helpful. Until then, we operate on eyes with significant cataracts and hope we are doing more good than harm. Then we treat glaucoma as we detect it.

RISK FACTORS HISTORICALLY ASSOCIATED WITH POSTCATARACT, PEDIATRIC GLAUCOMA

When the pathophysiologic mechanism of a disease is unclear, clinicians can care for their patients better by identifying those who appear to be at risk for developing the disorder.

A number of reports have discussed the following risk factors associated with postoperative glaucoma in children with cataracts: microcornea, poorly dilating pupils, surgery at <1 year of age, the presence of other ocular disease (e.g., congenital rubella syndrome), nuclear cataract, persistent fetal vasculature (PFV), and performance of a posterior capsulorhexis. Much disagreement accompanies these risk factors, and some authors found no association among glaucoma, age at surgery, microphthalmos, and surgical complications.[5]

Walton argues that the angle abnormalities previously discussed[3] are the result of cataract surgery—especially early surgery. The majority of his patients (77%) were operated on at <1 year of age. The author suggests that performing surgery on "small eyes ... with small corneas and often poorly dilating pupils ... must be considered ... a risk factor for the development of glaucoma." The author implies that cataract surgery is difficult to perform adequately on these eyes and cites residual lens tissue behind the iris in 78% of patients and a prominent need for secondary lens surgery (in 47% of patients) as evidence of technical inadequacy of the surgery in these patients.

Reproliferation of lens tissue is not unique to eyes with small corneas and poorly dilated pupils. Pediatric cataract surgeons recognize that residual lens cortex will appear in the capsular bag after extracapsular extraction performed as completely as possible even in the most widely dilated pupils. Potentially, the recognition of a significant amount

of "retained" [*sic*][a] lens material (41%) and the necessity of second membrane surgery (71%) in Chrousos and coworkers' glaucomatous patients discussed previously[8] may be more related to the type of eyes capable of producing such a vigorous reproliferative response rather than signifying causal factors of the glaucoma.

Mills and Robb[4] reported several risk factors for childhood glaucoma: cataract surgery at an age of <1 year (relative risk [RR] = 9.9; $P \leq 0.001$), microcornea (RR = 4.4; $P \leq 0.001$), poor pupillary dilation (RR = 5.2; $P \leq 0.001$), and congenital rubella syndrome (RR = 5.8; $P \leq 0.001$). Over a 25-year period, cataracts were removed for 125 eyes of 82 children <10 years of age using a variety of techniques, including simple aspiration, aspiration and discission, and lensectomy/capsulectomy/vitrectomy. After a minimum of 5 years of follow-up, chronic angle-closure and chronic open-angle glaucoma were diagnosed in 4 eyes (3%) and 14 eyes (11%), respectively. Acute angle closure occurred in one case after secondary membrane removal and resolved after peripheral iridectomy. The RR was notably high for patients undergoing surgery before the age of 6 months (RR = 5.4; $P \leq 0.001$) and 1 year (9.9; $P \leq 0.001$). No patient who had surgery after 1.25 years of age developed chronic open- or closed-angle glaucoma. The authors state,

> The time at surgery may not be independent of other pathologic factors ... [as] a disproportionate share of those patients who had early cataract surgery had other ocular abnormalities (congenital rubella syndrome (10.1% of 79 eyes operated on before 1 year of age), poorly dilating pupils (22.0%), microcornea (10.1%), or persistent fetal vasculature (6.3%)) ... or more complete lens opacity.

Congenital rubella syndrome, poor pupillary dilation, and microcornea were also determined to be independent risk factors in this report.

Wallace and Plager[14] evaluated corneal diameter as a potential risk factor in childhood aphakic glaucoma, which had been suggested by earlier reports.[4,15] In a retrospective analysis of all patients treated for aphakic glaucoma within a 5-year period, 48 eyes of 29 patients were identified. The authors defined glaucoma as an IOP of >21 with

---

[a] It is unlikely that this material was left behind at surgery. It most likely represents new cortex made by residual equatorial lens cells. The age at which surgery was performed may not be responsible for lens reproliferation—these eyes may possess characteristics that promote robust lens reproliferation after surgery. Whether or not glaucoma is caused by this response may or may not be related. Alternatively, these "small eyes" may be prone to develop cataracts at such an early age that they require surgery. Perhaps a gene that causes these eyes to be small also lends these eyes an increased propensity to develop glaucoma from a structural or biochemical abnormality. These are the main issues involved in the debate on causality of this postoperative glaucoma, which is pursued further below.

an increased cup-to-disk ratio or unexpected increases in axial length or decreases in hyperopia. Prior to this report, the authors had measured the corneal diameter of 200 patients of many ages to establish an age-related curve. Microcornea was defined as a corneal diameter smaller for that eye than the diameter established by the authors' age-related curve. Almost all of their patients (45/48 eyes = 94%) with childhood aphakic glaucoma had microcornea. The frequency of microcornea in their surgical population in general was unavailable.

The cataract types for the 18 eyes with such data were either nuclear (15/18 eyes) or PFV (3/18 eyes). Gonioscopy in 18 eyes revealed eight patients with completely open angles, four with partially open angles, and six with closed angles. In addition, 46 of 48 (96%) eyes were operated on within the first year of life; 45 of 48 (94%) eyes and 31 of 48 (65%) eyes were operated on within the first 9 and 3 months of life, respectively. Did the authors attribute the glaucoma to the early surgery or to other factors?

Wallace and Plager[14] argued that certain cataract types (nuclear and PFV) cause early visual axis opacification and necessitate early surgery, and these cataract types are in turn associated with glaucoma; microcornea is the unifying sign that anterior segment dysgenesis is present (including angle anomalies), which may lead to glaucoma. Wallace and Plager's work corroborates the conclusions of earlier work by Parks and coauthors[15] discussed below.

Ultimately, the victory for the cataractous child is not the absence of glaucoma but the presence of good vision years after surgery. Parks and colleagues[15] reported cataract type as the most important predictor of the long-term visual acuity (VA) of children. Records of 174 eyes of 118 children who underwent lensectomy and anterior vitrectomy for cataracts and were followed for a minimum of 6 months (but a mean of 5.54 years) were retrospectively reviewed. Of the cataract types with an adequate number of patients, the visual outcomes were the worst in two cataract types: nuclear (postoperative Snellen VA, 20/200; 53 eyes of 30 patients) and PFV (20/400; 18 eyes of 16 patients).

Which cataract types were associated with the highest rates of glaucoma? Excluding the anterior polar cataract type, in which three eyes of two patients developed glaucoma, the highest rates of glaucoma occurred in the nuclear (30.2%) and PFV (27.8%) types. Open-angle aphakic glaucoma occurred in 26 eyes of 18 patients.

Age at surgery and microcornea are two interesting data points to evaluate. Patients with nuclear and PFV cataract types underwent surgery at an average age significantly ($P = 0.0001$) younger (mean, 0.48 year for nuclear and 0.87 years for PFV) than patients with all other cataract types (mean, between 3.06 and 6.05 years). Microcornea existed in a very high percentage of eyes with nuclear (96.2%) and PVF (66.7%) cataract types.

Several explanations of glaucomatous risk are plausible. The immature trabecular meshwork of patients undergoing cataract surgery at a very young age were exposed to inflammation or direct surgical trauma and led to glaucoma. Another theory is that "high-risk" cataract types such as nuclear and PFV imply abnormal anterior segment development, and these defective angles lead to glaucoma. A combination of these two factors may be present.

Did *microcornea* appear to be a risk factor for glaucoma in Parks and coworkers' study.[15] Aphakic glaucoma occurred much more frequently in patients with microcornea (23/72 eyes = 31.9%) than in patients with normal corneal diameters (3/102 eyes = 2.9%). Parks et al. state,

> Of the patients who developed aphakic glaucoma, all those with PFV cataracts (5/5 eyes) and all but one with nuclear cataracts (15/16 eyes) had microcornea. However, all the remaining nuclear cataract patients (35/51 eyes = 69%) [and PFV patients (13/18 eyes = 72%)] had microcornea but did not develop glaucoma. Development of aphakic glaucoma is related to the two cataract types that are related to small cornea size.

Age at surgery in the Parks et al.[15] report was not significantly correlated with final VA. For the subgroup of patients with nuclear and PFV cataracts who had complications, no significant difference was recognized in age of surgery. For nuclear cataract types, a nonsignificant trend ($P < 0.09$) toward better vision with earlier surgery was recognized. Without increasing the number of patients to increase the power of the study, one cannot say whether a statistically significantly *better degree of vision* would have been achieved with earlier surgery as much as one cannot speculate whether more patients would have allowed detection of *more complications* with earlier surgery. The authors believe the data suggest that cataract type is an "important determinant" of both "long-term outcome and complications in aphakic children."[15]

Dr. Ron Keech, in an editorial immediately following the Parks et al. study,[15] discusses the limitations of retrospective analyses.[16] He also indicates that it may be difficult to identify independent influences on outcome if two factors are closely linked. For example, since microcornea occurred in 51 of 53 eyes with nuclear cataracts, it may be difficult to ferret out which factor had what particular effect on VA. He cautions the reader to recognize that other variables, while not found to be *independently* significant in this study, may also be important factors in achieving good *VA*. Among these factors are patient age at the onset of the opacity, patient age at the time of surgery, and postoperative treatment. Likewise, it follows that factors not identified by Parks et al.[15] may also be important risk determinants of *glaucoma*.

Magnusson et al.[17] prospectively followed a cohort of 137 patients in Sweden for an average of 9 years and concluded that cataract extraction in children <10 days old is associated with double the frequency of glaucoma. Twenty-nine percent (4/14) of patients operated on before the age of 10 days developed glaucoma; operations performed after 10 days of life had half the frequency of glaucoma. Small sample size and lack of randomization are limitations of this study.

Recently, an article by Peter Rabiah has made it more difficult to retain the belief that age at surgery is unrelated to the development of glaucoma.[18] He concluded, in a retrospective study of childhood aphakes, that *age at time of surgery* is an important determinant of chronic glaucoma.

Five hundred seventy eyes of 322 patients who underwent limbal approach surgery without IOL implantation in Saudia Arabia were analyzed. Patients were excluded if follow-up was for <5 years or if ocular trauma, PFV, prior eye surgery, or rubella or Lowe syndrome was present. Microcornea was not an exclusion criterion. Glaucoma was defined as an IOP ≥26 mm Hg on two occasions. Potential predictors of risk were entered into a univariate and multivariate model.

Glaucoma was diagnosed in 118 of 570 eyes (21%) at a mean age of 5.4 years after surgery (range, 2 weeks to 15.6 years); average total follow-up for eyes with and without glaucoma was 8.5 and 10.9 years, respectively. The vast majority (86%) of the glaucoma was diagnosed in patients who underwent surgery at or before 9 months of age. Of patients with cataracts in one or both eyes, *no unoperated fellow eye* developed glaucoma. The significant predictors of glaucoma in the multivariable analysis included microcornea, primary posterior capsulotomy/anterior vitrectomy, secondary membrane surgery, and surgery at ≤9 months of age. The risk appeared substantially lower in children operated on after 3 years of age.

The study did not address the influence of cataract type on the risk of developing glaucoma. The majority of patients with nuclear or PFV cataracts that develop glaucoma also have microcornea.[3,14]

An interesting comparison in the study by Rabiah is the rate of glaucoma in patients with microcornea operated on before or after 9 months of age.[18] Forty-one of 75 (55%) patients with microcornea developed glaucoma after early surgery, versus 1 of 12 (8%) patients with microcornea requiring late surgery. The significantly lower rate of glaucoma with late surgery in these patients lends credence to early age at cataract surgery (without IOL implantation) as an additional, independent risk factor for postsurgical glaucoma.

Finally, the fact that, in several studies, few or no patients with bilateral cataracts that went unoperated developed glaucoma in the unoperated eye suggests that surgery somehow promoted the development of glaucoma, perhaps in eyes already at high risk to develop this complication because of structural or humoral predisposition.

How should a clinician use these data? It may be reasonable to require more frequent anesthetized exams for children operated on at 3 months of age than for those operated on at 3 years. In our opinion, the data are not of sufficient strength to postpone surgery of a 7-month-old with a visually significant cataract to lower the presumed risk of future glaucoma. The ethics of performing a randomized, prospective trial involving delay of surgery beyond 9 months for visually significant cataracts seems questionable.

Is surgery performed in the first 9 months of life beneficial or harmful for children with cataracts? A balance of the best final VA and lowest incidence of complications has not been established by randomized prospective trials. It may be that a high complication rate (presence of glaucoma) may be justified by a good VA achieved by cataract surgery performed at a particular age.

A few authors[19,20] have discussed the critical period for binocular development beginning at about the fifth or sixth week of life. At our current level of knowledge, we feel it is reasonable to postpone surgeries in babies <10 days old (as well as neonates younger than 3 to 4 weeks) with unilateral or bilateral cataracts until about the fifth week of life in theory to reduce rates of glaucoma and other complications. It also allows the surgeon to operate on a firmer, more developed eye, which is technically easier to perform.

Whether or not the addition of an IOL increases the risk of glaucoma is unresolved. Assuming that the addition of a lens has no impact on the physiology of the eye is probably incorrect, but concluding that the absence of a lens radically lowers the risk of glaucoma in all eyes is likely to be inaccurate as well. It may be that the eyes at highest risk for developing aphakic glaucoma maintain the same level of risk after a synthetic lens is inserted. The fear of placing an IOL in young patients may originate from Francois's[7] study discussed previously, in which he reported the highest rates of glaucoma in patients operated on before 2 years of age. It cannot be ruled out that placement of a lens does not increase the risk of glaucoma, but in general materials used today such as acrylic and PMMA (polymethylmethacrylate) are well tolerated within the eye. Several reports document a surprisingly low rate of glaucoma after IOL implantation.[21,22] At present, we do not know if the relative absence of mention in the world literature of pseudophakic glaucoma in pediatric cataract surgery is related to a protective effect of the synthetic lens from a vitreous component, or alteration of the lens–iris–drainage angle relationship by the synthetic lens, or whether patients most at risk for developing glaucoma simply may be selected not to receive IOLs. The incidence of aphakic glaucoma has been reported to be higher when children are followed for a longer period after cataract surgery. We might expect the same trend with pseudophakic eyes, and the incidence may be higher as we have longer-term follow-up. A randomized, prospective trial of pseudophakia versus aphakia for cataractous children <1 year of age is eagerly awaited to answer these interesting questions. Meanwhile, as surgeons we must operate according to our convictions developed from the body of literature partially addressed above and seek to treat any glaucoma detected in the most efficacious manner.

TREATMENT

The treatment for a disease is aimed at altering the known pathophysiology of the disease by medical therapy or surgical manipulation of tissue. At present, it is unknown what causes the delayed-onset postsurgical glaucoma in children with or without IOL implantation.

Although pupillary block was once the leading cause of postoperative aphakic glaucoma,[23] acute angle closure rarely occurs in aphakic patients after modern surgery[4]; open-angle glaucoma occurs more frequently.[3–5] A surgical or laser peripheral iridectomy is standard treatment once pupillary block is recognized.

Pupillary block glaucoma may occur more commonly in pseudophakic rather than aphakic patients, especially in patients with significant amounts of inflammation or those with prior trauma or poor lens placement.[24,25] Posterior synechiae may attach to the lens capsule and promote acute angle closure. Although some surgeons perform peripheral iridectomy in every case,[4] we reserve this step for some patients with preexisting synechiae or with prior trauma in whom we are implanting an IOL.

The typical approach for treating open-angle glaucoma differs for adult and pediatric patients. Treatment of glaucoma in adults is typically first managed medically, and only when maximal medical management is exhausted is a surgical remedy attempted. Management of congenital glaucoma in children often demands a primary surgical treatment, as in goniotomy or trabeculotomy, followed by the addition of topical medications for refractory cases.

The management of children with postoperative aphakic or pseudophakic glaucoma differs from that of congenital glaucoma. There is a paucity of literature available on PUBMED on children with aphakic glaucoma treated with angle surgery in the face of myriad publications of congenital glaucoma treated with angle surgery. Although the number of patients treated was small, Walton's success rates for postoperative glaucoma were significantly lower after goniotomy (2/13 = 15%) than for trabeculectomy (9/14 = 64%) or for seton placement (3/6 = 50%).[3] It has not been demonstrated whether, for cataractous children thought to be at high risk of glaucoma, performing prophylactic angle surgery (or, more interestingly, endocyclophotocoagulation) at the time of cataract surgery would forestall aphakic glaucoma without introducing other complications.

Medical management is often initiated after aphakic glaucoma is diagnosed. One retrospective study of 64 eyes of 38 patients with glaucoma reported that medications alone controlled IOP in 63.6% (21/33 eyes) of patients, almost all of whom had open-angle glaucoma.[6]

When medical management fails, realistic surgical options include seton implantation, trabeculectomy, and cyclodestructive procedures. Aphakia has been previously reported as a significant risk factor for failure of trabeculectomy with mitomycin C (TMMC) not only in adult patients[26,27] but also in patients <1 year of age[28,29]; the latter studies are discussed below.

Freedman et al.[28] retrospectively evaluated results for 17 consecutive children (21 eyes) <17 years of age (median age, 2.6 years) who had failed maximum medical therapy, prior angle or filtration surgery (goniotomy, trabeculotomy, trabeculectomy), or both. TMMC with or without postoperative 5-fluorouracil (5-FU) or laser suture lysis or both was performed. Aphakic patients performed worse than phakic patients whether TMMC was performed before or after 1 year of age. Success was poor in all patients <1 year old, whether phakic (3/8 eyes; 38%) or aphakic (0/2 eyes). Success rates were higher in patients ≥1 year of age, for both the phakic (6/6 eyes) and the aphakic (2/5 eyes; 40%) groups. The authors contend that laser-suture lysis or 5-FU augmentation of TMMC did not improve success in younger, aphakic children and may have increased the complication rate. The study is limited by the small number of patients in each subgroup and limited (median, 23-month) follow-up of successful cases. Mandal et al.[30] also reported high success rates in older, phakic patients without identifying success in the subgroup of patients who were younger or aphakic.

Beck and colleagues[29] provide another report of failure of TMMC in aphakic patients <1 year of age. Records of 49 patients (60 eyes) ≤17 years of age (mean age, 7.6 years) who had undergone TMMC for various etiologies were retrospectively reviewed. Success (IOP ≤22 without glaucoma progression or visually devastating complications) rates were 67% at 1 year and 59% at 2 years. Young age (≤1 year) and aphakic status were statistically significant risk factors in multivariate analysis. Failure occurred in 60% of 20 aphakic eyes and in 24% of 29 phakic eyes. Failure occurred in 7 of 8 eyes of children <1 year old and in 29% of 41 eyes of patients 1 to 17 years of age. Late-onset, bleb-related endophthalmitis occurred in 5 of 60 (8%) eyes. Although TMMC demonstrated considerable efficacy in phakic patients >1 year old in this and other reports,[30] the authors express concern about the "substantial" risk of infection with TMMC in aphakic infants.

Age <1 year and aphakia are risk factors for failure of TMMC in the two aforementioned retrospective studies. How do aqueous shunt devices compare?

For children 2 years and younger, Beck et al.[31] recently reported greater efficacy of aqueous shunt devices over TMMC. Only the minority of these patients studied were aphakic or pseudophakic. In this retrospective, age-matched comparison of aqueous shunt devices and TMMC, Beck et al.[31] determined the likelihood of maintaining an IOP of <23 mm Hg in 46 eyes of 32 patients <2 years of age. According to the authors, pressure below this level provides clinical stability in very young patients with glaucoma. For the 46 eyes receiving aqueous shunts, 16 eyes (34.8%) were aphakic or pseudophakic, compared to 3 of 24 eyes (12.5%) in the TMMC group.

Beck and colleagues[31] employed Baerveldt implants for 32 eyes and Ahmed valves for 14 eyes. After the aforementioned procedures, success achieved at 1 and 3 years was 87 and 53% in the aqueous shunt device group, respectively, compared to 36 and 19% in the TMMC group at the same intervals. Interestingly, although the seton implantation group was comprised of more high-risk patients (16 of 46 [34.8%] eyes aphakic or pseudophakic) than the TMMC group (3 of 24 [12.5%] eyes), the seton group overall (no separate success rates were reported for aphakic and pseudophakic patients) fared better (72 versus 21% success in the TMMC group) and had no infections (versus 8.3% in the TMMC group). Infection is an even larger concern for contact lens–wearing aphakic patients.[32]

The poor success rates and potential for infection with TMMC for young, aphakic patients in the retrospective studies discussed previously corroborate the results of Beck and associates' work discussed above. For the first surgical procedure for aphakic or pseudophakic patients on maximal medical therapy, seton implantation appears more likely to succeed in controlling IOP than TMMC, especially in infants.

Seton implantation size and type are additional surgical considerations. Higher success rates have been reported for Ahmed glaucoma valve implants, Baerveldt implants, and double-plate Molteno implants than single-plate Molteno implants.[33–40]

An attractive feature of Ahmed valve implants is the immediate pressure lowering effect delivered to the glaucomatous eye without a high risk of hypotomy; the non-valved Baerveldt implants will not lower the pressure until the temporary tube occluder is removed at least 1 month after the original surgery. Without this temporary tube occlusion the Baerveldt implant would produce marked early hypotony. Rapid IOP reduction may be less crucial in aphakic glaucoma than in patients with congenital glaucoma who fail angle surgery—the latter patients depend on rapid clearing of the visual axis from lower pressure. Patients with aphakic glaucoma typically have clear corneas. It is easier to implant an Ahmed glaucoma valve than a Baerveldt in an infant due to eye and orbit size, but aphakic glaucoma is most commonly diagnosed 4 to 5 years after the cataract surgery is performed. The valve in the Ahmed implant may fail,[41] and there is a greater probability of having a hypertensive phase in an Ahmed valve than in a Baerveldt in pediatric patients. The hypertensive

phase tends to peak at 1 month and resolve by 6 months after Ahmed implantation in adults.[42]

In children, success has been reported with Molteno implants,[36,43–45] Ahmed valve glaucoma implants,[35,38,39] and Baerveldt implants.[34,46,47] Since all types of glaucoma implants will demonstrate a decline in success rates over time,[33,47,48] the ideal seton implant for the aphakic or pseudophakic child with glaucoma is not currently agreed on.

Cycloablative techniques have generally been reserved for refractory cases of glaucoma in children.[49–52] Reported success rates have been low when these techniques are used as the initial surgical option.[53] Cyclocryotherapy and laser cyclophotocoagulation in children may result in severe complications in some patients. Reported complications include retinal detachment, sympathetic ophthalmia, and phthisis.[54–56] Surgical revision or addition of a second tube implant can also be associated with high rates of complications such as new corneal edema.[57] Supplemental transcleral laser photocoagulation is a viable alternative for children suffering tube failure.[58] Several laser treatments may be required to achieve long-term control.

Endocyclophotocoagulation is a relatively recently applied technique that has demonstrated some promise in treating refractory glaucoma in children and adults. Would this be applicable to children with aphakic glaucoma?

Neely and Plager[52] reported on 51 endoscopic diode laser cyclophotocoagulation procedures performed on 36 eyes of 29 pediatric patients. The cumulative success rate after all procedures at a mean of 19 months of follow-up was 43%, which is similar to the 50% success rates achieved by Phelan et al.[56] and Bock et al.[55] with forms of transcleral Nd:YAG or diode laser. Severe visual complication rates were lowest with endocyclophotocoagulation (11% with the endoscope versus 50 or 19% of patients with transcleral Nd:YAG or diode, respectively). In fact, the authors point out that when combining their study with other studies of this procedure,[59–62] only 1 of 123 diode endolaser–treated eyes progressed to phthisis. In contrast, cyclocyrotherapy is historically associated with more morbidity, as 12 to 34% of patients treated with cyclocryotherapy progressed to phthisis in past reports.[63–69] Nonetheless, for aphakic patients especially, Neely and Plager[52] report that endocyclophotocoagulation is not undertaken without risk, as retinal detachment, hypotony, and decreased vision all have occurred. Long-term results are not available, so this procedure should still be used with caution in children with refractory aphakic glaucoma.

The methods we use to evaluate IOP and other relevant data points in children may be inadequate. The TonoPen, which is the easiest to use and the most portable of the devices commonly used, may be less valid than the pneumotonometer.[70] An ideal instrument for a child's eye would instantly, easily, and accurately measure IOP (and anterior chamber angle and optic nerve health, for that matter) and obviate diagnostic visits to the operating room. Ideally, we would want an instrument to determine whether removing a child's cataract will result in good vision and whether or not glaucoma will occur. Until the days of such magic wands arrive, surgeons must remove cataracts from the eyes of children according to available data and the principles of the Hippocratic Oath, search relentlessly for glaucoma based on clinical suspicion and knowledge of risk factors, and treat whatever glaucoma is found quickly and effectively.

REFERENCES

1. Wilson ME Jr, Bartholomew LR, Trivedi RH. Pediatric cataract surgery and intraocular lens implantation: practice styles and preferences of the 2001 ASCRS and AAPOS memberships. *J Cataract Refract Surg* 2003;29:1811–1820.
2. Scheie HG. Aspiration of congenital or soft cataracts: a new technique. *Am J Ophthalmol* 1960;50:1048–1056.
3. Walton DS. Pediatric aphakic glaucoma: A study of 65 patients. *Trans Am Ophthalmol Soc* 1995;93:403–413.
4. Mills MD, Robb RM. glaucoma following childhood cataract surgery. *J Pediatr Ophthalmol Strabismus* 1994;31:355–360.
5. Simon JW, Mehta N, Simmons ST. Glaucoma after pediatric lensectomy/vitrectomy. *Ophthalmology* 1991;98:670–674.
6. Asrani SG, Wilenski, JT. Glaucoma after congenital cataract surgery. *Ophthalmology* 1995;102:863–867.
7. Francois, J. Late results of congenital cataract surgery. *Ophthalmology* 1979;86;1586–1598.
8. Chrousos GA, Parks MM, O'Neill JF. Incidence of chronic glaucoma, retinal detachment, and secondary membrane surgery in pediatric aphakic patients. *Ophthalmology* 1984;91;1238–1241.
9. Gordon MO, Beiser JA, Brandt JD, Heuer DK, Higginbotham EJ, Johnson CA, Keltner JL, Miller JP, Parrish RK 2nd, Wilson MR, Kass MA. The Ocular Hypertension Treatment Study: baseline factors that predict the onset of primary open-angle glaucoma. *Arch Ophthalmol* 2002;120:714–720.
10. Egbert JE, Wright MM, Dahlhauser KF, Keithahn MA, Letson RD, Summers CG. A prospective study of ocular hypertension and glaucoma after pediatric cataract surgery. *Ophthalmology* 1995;102:1098–1101.
11. Phelps CD, Arafat NI. Open-angle glaucoma following surgery for congenital cataracts. *Arch Ophthalmol* 1977;95:1985–1987.
12. Walton DS. Glaucoma secondary to operation for childhood cataract. In: Epstein DC, ed. *Chandler and Grant's Glaucoma.* Philadelphia: Lea & Feiberger, 1986:521–525.
13. Keech RV, Tongue AC, Scott WE. Complications after surgery for congenital and infantile cataracts. *Am J Ophthalmol* 1989;108:136–141.
14. Wallace DK, Plager DA. Corneal diameter in childhood aphakic glaucoma. *J Pediatr Ophthalmol Strabismus* 1996;33:230–234.
15. Parks MM, Johnson DA, Reed GW. Long-term visual acuity results and complications in children with aphakia. A function of cataract type. *Ophthalmology* 1993;100:826–840.
16. Keech R. Discussion. Long term results and complications in children with aphakia. A function of cataract type. *Ophthalmology* 1993;100:840–841.
17. Magnusson G, Abrahamsson M, Sjostrand J. Glaucoma following congenital cataract surgery: an 18-year longitudinal follow-up. *Acta Ophthalmol Scand* 2000;78:65–70.
18. Rabiah PK. Frequency and predictors of glaucoma after pediatric cataract surgery. *Am J Ophthalmol* 2004;137:30–37.
19. Birch EE, Swanson WH, Stager DR, Woody M, Everrtt M. Outcome after early treatment of dense congenital unilateral cataract. *Invest Ophthalmol Vis Sci* 1993;34:3687–3699.
20. Birch EE, Stager DR. The critical period for surgical treatment of dense congenital unilateral cataract. *Invest Ophthalmol Vis Sci* 1996;37:1532–1538.
21. Asrani s, Freedman S, Hasselblad V, et al. Does primary intraocular lens implantation prevent "aphakic" glaucoma in children? *J AAPOS* 2000;4:33–39.
22. Zwann J, Mullaney PB, Awad A, et al. Pediatric intraocular lens implantation. Surgical results and complications in more than 300 patients. *Ophthalmology* 1998;105:112–119.
23. Chandler PA. Surgery of congenital cataract. *Am J Ophthalmol* 1968;65:663–673.
24. Vajpayee RB, Angra SK, Titiyal JS, Sharma YR, Chabbra VK. Pseudophakic pupillary-block in children. *Am J Ophthalmol* 1991;111:715–718.
25. Vajpayee RB, Talwar D. Pseudophakic malignant glaucoma in a child. *Ophthalmic Surg* 1991;22:266–267.
26. Greenfield DS, Suner IJ, Miller MP, et al. Endophthalmitis after filtering surgery with mitomycin. *Arch Ophthalmol* 1996;114:943–949.
27. Higginbotham EJ, Stevens RK, Musch DC, et al. Bleb-related endophthalmitis after trabeculectomy with mitomycin C. *Ophthalmology* 1996;103:650–656.
28. Freedman SF, McCormick K, Cox TA. Mitomycin C-augmented trabeculectomy with post-operative wound modulation in pediatric glaucoma. *J AAPOS* 1999;3:117–124.
29. Beck AD, Wilson WR, Lynch MG, et al. Trabeculectomy with adjunctive mitomycin C in pediatric glaucoma. *Am J Ophthalmol* 1998;126:648–657.
30. Mandal AK, Walton DS, John T, et al. Mitomycin C-augmented trabeculectomy in refractory congenital glaucoma. *Ophthalmology* 1997;104:996–1003.
31. Beck AD, Freedman S, Kammer J, Jin J. Aqueous shunt devices compared with trabeculectomy with mitomycin-C for children in the first two years of life. *Am J Ophthalmol* 2003;136:994–1000.
32. Bellows AR, McCulley JP. Endophthalmitis in aphakic patients with unplanned filtering blebs wearing contact lenses. *Ophthalmology* 1981;88:839–843.
33. Eid TE, Katz LJ, Spaeth GL, Augsburger JJ. Long-term effects of tube-shunt procedures on management of refractory childhood glaucoma. *Ophthalmology* 1997;104:1011–1016.
34. Fellenbaum PS, Sidoti PA, Heuer DK, Baerveldt G, Lee PP. Experience with the Baerveldt implant in young patients with complicated glaucomas. *J Glaucoma* 1995;4:91–97.
35. Englert JA, Freedman SF, Cox TA. The ahmed valve in refractory pediatric glaucoma. *Am J Ophthalmol* 1999;127:34–42.
36. Hill RA, Heuer DK, Baerveldt G, Minckler DS, Martone JF. Molteno implantation for glaucoma in young patients. *Ophthalmology* 1991;98:1042–1046.
37. Netland PA, Walton DS. Glaucoma drainage implants in pediatric patients. *Ophthalmic Surg* 1993;24:723–729.
38. Coleman AL, Smyth RJ, Wilson MR, Tam M. Initial clinical experience with the Ahmed glaucoma valve implants in pediatric patients. *Arch Ophthalmol* 1997;115:186–191.
39. Djodeyere MR, Calvo JP, Gomez JA. Clinical evaluation and risk factors of time to failure of Ahmed glaucoma valve implant in pediatric patients. *Ophthalmology* 2001;108:614–620.
40. Heuer DK, Lloyd MA, Abrams DA, et al. Which is better? One or two? A randomized clinical trial of single-plate versus double-plate Molteno implantation for glaucomas in aphakia and pseudophakia. *Ophthalmology* 1992;99:1512–1519.
41. Hill RA, Pirouzian A, Liaw L. Pathophysiology of and prophylaxis against late Ahmed glaucoma valve occlusion. *Am J Ophthalmol* 2000;129:608–612.
42. Ayyala RS, Zurakowski D, Smith JA. A clinical study of the Ahmed valve implant in advanced glaucoma. *Ophthalmology* 1998;105:1968–1976.
43. Molteno ACB. Children with advanced glaucoma treated by draining implants. *S Afr Arch Ophthalmol* 1973;1:55–61.
44. Lloyd MA, Sedlak T, Heuer DK, et al. Clinical experience with the single-plate Molteno implant in complicated glaucomas: update of a pilot study. *Ophthalmology* 1992;99:679–687.
45. Billson F, Thomas R, Aylward W. The use of two-stage Molteno implants in developmental glaucoma. *J Pediatr Ophthalmol Strabismus* 1989;26:3–8.
46. Donahue SP, Keech RV, Munden P, et al. Baerveldt implant surgery

in the treatment of advanced childhood glaucoma. *J AAPOS* 1997;1: 41–45.

47. Krishna R, Godfrey DG, Budenz DL, et al. Intermediate-term outcomes of 350 mm² Baerveldt glaucoma implants. *Ophthalmology* 2001;108:621–626.
48. Topouzis F, Coleman AL, Choplin N, et al. Follow-up of the original cohort with the Ahmed glaucoma valve implant. *Am J Ophthalmol* 1999;128:198–204.
49. Al Faran MF, Tomey KF, Al Mutlaq FA. Cyclocryotherapy in selected cases of congenital glaucoma. *Ophthalmic Surg* 1990;21:794–798.
50. Wagle NS, Freedman SF, Buckley EG, et al. Long-term outcome of cyclocryotherapy for refractory pediatric glaucoma. *Ophthalmology* 2002;109:316–323.
51. Kirwan JF, Shah P, Khaw P. Diode laser cyclohotocoagulation: role in the management of refractory pediatric glaucomas. *Ophthalmology* 2002;109:316–323.
52. Neely DE, Plager DA. Endocyclophotocoagulation for management of difficult pediatric glaucomas. *J AAPOS* 2001;5:221–229.
53. Aminlari A. A cyclocryotherapy in congenital glaucoma. *Glaucoma* 1981;3:331–332.
54. Wagle NS, Freedman SF, Buckley EG. Long-term outcome of cyclocryotherapy for refractory pediatric glaucoma. *Ophthalmology* 1998;105:1921–1926.
55. Bock CJ, Freedman SF, Buckley EG, Shields MB. Transscleral diode laser cyclophotocoagulation for refractory pediatric glaucomas. *J Pediatr Ophthalmol Strabismus* 1997;34:235–239.
56. Phelan MJ, Higginbotham EJ. Contact transscleral Nd:YAG laser cyclophotocoagulation for the treatment of refractory pediatric glaucomas. *Ophthalmic Surg Lasers* 1995;26:401–403.
57. Shah AA, WuDunn D, Cantor LB. Shunt revision versus additional tube placement after failed tube shunt surgery in refractory glaucoma. *Am J Ophthalmol* 2000;129:455–460.
58. Semchyshyn TM, Tsai JC, Joos KM. Supplemental transscleral diode laser cyclophotocoagulation after aqueous shunt placement in refractory glaucoma. *Ophthalmology* 2002;109:1078–1084.
59. Uram, M. Ophthalmic laser microendoscope ciliary process ablation in the management of neovascular glaucoma. *Ophthalmology* 1992;99:1823–1828.
60. Chen J, Cohn RA, Lin SC, Cortes AE, Alvarado JA. Endoscopic photocoagulation of the ciliary body for treatment of refractory glaucomas. *Am J Ophthalmol* 1997;124:787–796.
61. Mora JS, Iwach AG, Gaffney MM, Wong PC, Nguyen N, MA AS, et al. Endoscopic diode laser endoyclophotocoagulation with a limbal approach. *Ophthalmic Surg Lasers* 1997;28:118–123.
62. Gayton JL. Traumatic aniridia during endoscopic laser cycloablation. *J Cataract Refract Surg* 1998;24:134–135.
63. Shields, MB. Cyclodestructive surgery for glaucoma: past, present, and future. *Trans Am Ophthalmol Soc* 1985;83:285–303.
64. Bellows AR, Grant WM. Cyclocryotherapy in advanced inadequately controlled glaucoma. *Am J Ophthalmol* 1973;75:679–684.
65. De Roeth A. Cryosurgery for the treatment of advanced chronic simple glaucoma. *Am J Ophthalmol* 1968;66:1034–1041.
66. Chee CK, Snead MP, Scott JD. Cyclocryotherapy for chronic glaucoma after vitreoretinal surgery. *Eye* 1994;8:414–418.
67. Benson MT, Nelson ME, Cyclocryotherapy: a review of cases over a 10-year period. *Br J Ophthalmol* 1990;74:103–105.
68. Brindley G, Shields MB. Value and limitations of cyclocryotherapy. *Graefes Arch Clin Exp Ophthalmol* 1986;224:545–548.
69. Krupin T, Mitchel DB, Becker B. Cyclocryotherapy in neovascular glaucoma. *Am J Ophthalmol* 1978;86:24–26.
70. Eisenberg DL, Sherman BG, McKeown CA, Schuman JS. Tonometry in adults and children. A manometric evaluation of pneumatonometry, applanation, and TonoPen in vitro and in vivo. *Ophthalmology* 1998;105:1173–1181.

Strabismus in Pediatric Aphakia and Pseudophakia

M. Edward Wilson, Jr. and Rupal H. Trivedi

Children with cataracts in one or both eyes may experience enough disruption in binocular sensory and motor fusion mechanisms to lose proper ocular alignment. The frequent association of strabismus and cataracts in children has been well known for many years.[1-3] It appears to present in all age groups and at a greater incidence than in the general population. Strabismus is common when deprivation amblyopia is present but may occur even in the absence of amblyopia, as in dense bilateral lens opacities. Furthermore, strabismus can also have its onset after the cataracts have been removed, especially if the proper optical correction is not worn or if occlusion therapy leaves little time for binocular viewing. Overall, approximately 50% of all children with cataracts will develop strabismus.[2] Earlier-onset unilateral cataracts have the highest risk for strabismus and late-onset bilateral cataracts have the least risk. Also, as a general rule, patients with partial cataracts and relatively good preoperative visual acuity have less strabismus. Long delays in detection and treatment of visually significant cataracts increase the risk of strabismus, even when the cataracts are incomplete. Strabismus at presentation is often an indication that the cataract is long-standing and that significant amblyopia is likely to be present.

In a retrospective study, France and Frank[4] found that strabismus was present in 40% of their patients with cataracts or dislocated lenses at the time of initial diagnosis. After surgery and amblyopia therapy, 86% of the congenital cataract patients and 61% of the acquired cataract patients had strabismus at their latest post-therapy visit. Unilateral congenital cataract patients had esotropia or exotropia at about equal proportions. However, bilateral congenital cataract patients, when strabismic, were all esotropic. The acquired cataract patients had mostly exotropia.

Hiles and Sheridan[2] also reported a retrospective analysis of strabismus in children operated on for cataracts.

Records of 350 consecutive children having cataract surgery over a 10-year period were reviewed. Follow-up ranged from 1 to 9 years. Unilateral cataracts were present in 212 (61%) patients. Bilateral cataracts were present in the remaining 138 (39%) children. Strabismus was present in 161 (46%) patients prior to or following cataract surgery. The overall incidence of strabismus in patients with unilateral cataracts was 59%. In bilateral cataract patients the incidence was 41%. Unexpectedly, Hiles and Sheridan[2] found that the children with cataracts who remained orthophoric were very similar to the patients who developed strabismus. They had the same constellation of ocular and/or systemic physical findings, the same cataract types, and similar ages at surgery. Aphakic correction and amblyopia therapy were also similar in the strabismic and nonstrabismic children. Sixty-two percent of the nonstrabismic patients had unilateral cataracts and 38% had bilateral cataracts. These values are almost identical to the percentages quoted above for the strabismic group. The authors concluded that early cataract surgery and vigorous optical rehabilitation did not seem to ensure against strabismus or guarantee orthophoria.

Parks and Hiles,[3] in contrast, found a strong correlation between cataract type and risk for strabismus. In their study, strabismus was found in 100% of persistent fetal vasculature cataracts and 65.5% of nuclear cataract patients, but in only 48.4% with posterior lentiglobus and 21.8% in the lamellar group ($P = 0.0001$). Ocular misalignment was found in 66.7% of patients with unilateral cataracts but only 37.9% of patients with bilateral cataracts ($P = 0.0018$).

We have reported strabismus in 50% of our patients preoperatively, while it occurred in 45% of patients after cataract surgery in eyes with monocular cataract.[5] In our review of the literature since 1980 we found that strabismus was present in 33.3% of patients preoperatively and in 78.1% of patients postoperatively.[5] The higher incidence of strabismus after treatment than before may reflect the intensity of the occlusion prescribed, the ongoing susceptibility of the infantile eye to amblyopia owing to an uncorrected refractive error, or the easier detection of strabismus in older children. Preoperative strabismus was especially common among older patients at the time of surgery. In reviewing the literature we must remember that it is difficult to compare individual studies because of the variations among the inclusion criteria, exclusion criteria, prescription of occlusion, and compliance to occlusion, however, certain general conclusions can be drawn.

In monocular aphakia corrected with contact lenses, the incidence of strabismus with congenital cataract ranges from 34 to 100% (average, 74%). With traumatic and nontraumatic acquired monocular aphakia the incidence of strabismus ranges from 13 to 100% (average, 60%). In all the series that documented preoperative strabismus in acquired pediatric cataracts, the incidence of strabismus either stayed the same or increased after treatment.[6]

The popular use of intraocular lens (IOL) implantation and the trend toward earlier surgery for partial or complete cataracts in children had brought with it the hope for a decrease in the incidence of strabismus. BenEzra and Cohen noted that only 9% of children with unilateral pseudophakia developed strabismus, compared to 71% of children with unilateral aphakia treated with contact lenses.[7] The reduced incidence of strabismus in children with unilateral pseudophakia compared to unilateral aphakia is probably because of the constancy of the optical correction and the improved visual outcome in pseudophakic children.

Reports of primary and secondary IOLs in children with monocular congenital, traumatic, and nontraumatic acquired cataracts list the incidence of strabismus as from 0 to 88% (average, 31%). While most of the series that documented pre-IOL strabismus reported either an increase or no change in the incidence of strabismus, three authors reported a spontaneous improvement of strabismus after treatment.[6]

Greenwald and Glaser[8] reported better binocularity and stereopsis in patients implanted with an IOL compared to age-matched controls who were left aphakic and wore contact lenses.

Lambert and coworkers,[9] however, found a high rate of strabismus in patients operated on for unilateral congenital cataracts whether or not an IOL was implanted. Nine of the 12 patients in the IOL group had strabismus (4 esotropia, 4 exotropia, 1 hypertropia), compared with 12 of 13 in the contact lens group (5 esotropia, 5 exotropia, 2 hypertropia; $P = 0.24$).

Weisberg and associates presented results on strabismus associated with pediatric pseudophakia (poster presented at 30th AAPOS meeting, Washington, DC, 2004). The authors identified 94 patients, and 37 (39%) had strabismus. Exotropia was found in 46% of eyes, and esotropia in 41% of eyes.

Strabismus surgery is often delayed until after the initial amblyopia treatment has improved the visual acuity somewhat. Occasionally, an intermittent strabismus will resolve as the visual acuity improves. However, this is the exception rather than the rule. Strabismus associated with cataracts in children usually requires surgery. At times, strabismus surgery is performed prior to cataract surgery. Hiles and Sheridan[2] found that strabismus surgery was equally successful when performed either before or after cataract surgery, provided that the best possible visual acuity was attained and maintained. However, it has been our experience that stability of ocular alignment is not often achieved when strabismus surgery precedes cataract surgery. The preferred route is to rehabilitate the optical system of the eye or eyes and strive for the best possible vision prior to strabismus correction. That said, strabismus correction can still be done during, rather than at the completion of, amblyopia treatment. Normally, the strabismus is measured several times during the postoperative follow-up after cataract surgery. If the strabismus angle and pattern are stable, correction is planned at an elective time such as during a scheduled examination under anesthesia where intraocular pressure, retinal examination, and serial axial length measurements are planned.

Stability of alignment after strabismus surgery in aphakic or pseudophakic children is difficult to predict. Generally, children with better visual outcomes and better binocularity have better stability of ocular alignment. Dense deprivation amblyopia lessens the chance of long-term correction of strabismus, but despite this, a cosmetically acceptable alignment is often maintained for many years. Overall, the success of strabismus surgery is higher for strabismus that develops after cataract surgery compared to strabismus that is present preoperatively, at initial presentation. Although occlusion therapy for amblyopia must usually be continued after surgical realignment of the eyes, full-time occlusion is not recommended since it carries a high risk for recurrence of strabismus.

REFERENCES

1. Deweese MW. A survey of the surgical treatment of congenital cataracts. *Am J Ophthalmol* 1962;53:853–858.
2. Hiles DA, Sheridan SJ. Strabismus associated with infantile cataracts. *Int Ophthalmol Clin* 1977;17:193–202.
3. Parks MM, Hiles DA. Management of infantile cataracts. *Am J Ophthalmol* 1967;63:10–19.
4. France TD, Frank JW. The association of strabismus and aphakia in children. *J Pediatr Ophthalmol Strabismus* 1984;21:223–226.
5. Wilson ME Jr, Trivedi RH, Hoxie JP, Bartholomew LR. Treatment

outcomes of congenital monocular cataracts: the effects of surgical timing and patching compliance. *J Pediatr Ophthalmol Strabismus* 2003;40:323–329, quiz 353–354.

6. http://www.sph.emory.edu/IATS. Accessed May 25, 2004.

7. BenEzra D, Cohen E. Posterior capsulectomy in pediatric cataract surgery: the necessity of a choice. *Ophthalmology* 1997;104:2168–2174.

8. Greenwald MJ, Glaser SR. Visual outcomes after surgery for unilateral cataract in children more than two years old: posterior chamber intraocular lens implantation versus contact lens correction of aphakia. *J AAPOS* 1998;2:168–176.

9. Lambert SR, Lynn M, Drews-Botsch C, Loupe D, Plager DA, Medow NB, et al. A comparison of grating visual acuity, strabismus, and reoperation outcomes among children with aphakia and pseudophakia after unilateral cataract surgery during the first six months of life. *J AAPOS* 2001;5:70–75.

Cystoid Macular Edema

Srinivas K. Rao

The presence of fluid in the macula was first described in diabetic retinopathy by Appolinaire Bouchardat from Paris in 1875.[1] Subsequently, a similar appearance of the retina was noted in a number of other conditions, and in 1950, Hruby drew attention to the occurrence of macular edema after cataract extraction.[1] This was followed 3 years later by Irvine's classical paper on cystoid macular edema (CME), occurring after intra- and extracapsular cataract extraction complicated by incarceration of vitreous in the anterior segment.[1] These changes in the macula were further described by Gass and Norton, a decade later, using fluorescein angiography.[1] In this condition, fluid accumulation in the internal retinal layers around the fovea causes a thickening of the retina in a characteristic cystic pattern[2] (Fig. 46-1). Clinically, this appears as cystoid changes radiating in a petal pattern from the fovea. Histopathologically, fluid is present in the outer plexiform and inner nuclear layers of the retina, centered on the fovea. It is accepted that this is a result of a breakdown in the blood–retinal barrier (BRB), with subsequent leakage from the small paramacular capillaries.[2] Electron microscopy has also revealed accumulation of fluid within expanded Muller cell processes, which can result in cell degeneration.[3] In a recent study, Lardenoye et al.[4] used scanning laser ophthalmoscopy to assess the macular status in eyes with macular edema secondary to diabetes mellitus or inflammatory causes. They reported decreased directional sensitivity and visual pigment density at the macula in these eyes, reflecting retinal damage due to the edema.[4]

Defining this entity has proved difficult over the years, since the changes at the macula are only discernible in some patients using techniques such as fluorescein angiography and angioscopy. Such changes have little impact on visual function and have been termed *angiographically determined CME*. In these subtle forms of the condition, clinical examination using indirect ophthalmoscopy may be normal except for an alteration of the foveal reflex. Slit-lamp microscopy is more helpful and may demonstrate mild retinal thickening. The characteristic cystoid space formation at the macula is seen in more advanced stages of the disease, in which loss of visual acuity occurs—this is termed *clinical CME*.[2] Vitreous fluorophotometry, a measure of blood–retinal permeability has also been used to evaluate CME,[5] while focal macular electroretinograms can characterize and classify this condition.[6] Recently, more sophisticated methods such as optical coherence tomography have been used to describe the retinal changes in this condition.[7]

Several criteria have been suggested for the grading of CME—clinical severity is based on the ophthalmoscopic findings of retinal edema and extent of visual acuity loss. Using fluorescein angiography, the following classification has been suggested: 0 = no edema; 1 = capillary leakage; 2 = partial petalloid ring; 3 = complete petalloid ring[2] (Fig. 46-2A and B). Another classification scheme has been proposed using focal macular electroretinograms. Eyes with a type I response have reduced amplitudes of the oscillatory potentials with normal a- and b-wave responses. In type II, the eyes have reduced amplitudes of the oscillatory potentials and b-waves, while in type III reduced amplitudes of the oscillatory potentials, a-waves, and b-waves are observed. The least reduction in visual acuity is seen in type I, while the most severe reduction is present in type III.[6]

Typically CME is noted 4 to 16 weeks after cataract surgery. There have been isolated reports of late-onset CME, 7 to 16 years after cataract surgery, although its occurrence more than 2 years after the surgical procedure is considered unusual.[8] If angiography is performed, the incidence of this entity can be as high as 70%. However, there are no clinical consequences in many of these eyes. If the definition of clinical CME is used, the reported incidence varies from 0.1 to 12.0%.[9–12] The wide variation in the reported rates is due to several factors, including the definition of the disease used, different surgical techniques and procedures followed, rates of surgical complications, methods used for diagnostic assessment, types of patients,

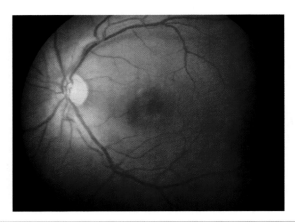

FIGURE 46-1. Fundus photograph of posterior pole showing cystic spaces in the macular region.

and follow-up criteria used after surgery. Recent studies in patients undergoing cataract surgery with modern techniques report an incidence of CME of between 0.2 and 0.4%.[13,14] It is, however, generally accepted that vitreous loss during cataract surgery is an important risk factor in the causation of this disease, and in such eyes the prevalence of CME increases to 10 to 20%.[9–12] It also appears that the type of surgical technique may affect the occurrence of this outcome. In a retrospective study of vitreous loss cases, clinical CME was found in 18.7% of patients undergoing phacoemulsification and in 30.8% of patients undergoing conventional extracapsular cataract extraction.[15] It has been suggested that the closed nature of phacoemulsification surgery confers the advantage of keeping the vitreous body contained following posterior capsule rupture. This may minimize the traction on the vitreoretinal interface, thereby decreasing the occurrence of CME.[16] Posterior capsulotomy has traditionally been considered a risk factor for the postoperative occurrence of CME. In a recent study, Zaczak et al.[17] compared the

incidence of CME in eyes undergoing phacoemulsification and in-the-bag implantation of a foldable silicone intraocular lens (IOL). In one group of patients the procedure was followed by posterior continuous curvilinear capsulorrhexis (CCC). No significant difference was found in the occurrence of CME in the two groups. This suggests that the occurrence of CME following disruption of the posterior capsule may be related to the accompanying vitreous disturbance that often accompanies capsule rupture during cataract surgery.

These factors assume importance in the context of cataract surgery and IOL implantation in children. In very young children, there is a 100% incidence of posterior capsular opacification if the posterior capsule is retained during the primary surgical procedure.[18,19] Performing a posterior CCC does not prevent this complication, since the condensed anterior hyaloid provides an adequate scaffold for the migration of Elschnig pearls across the visual axis. Hence it is considered important to perform an anterior vitrectomy to destroy the anterior hyaloid face and maintain a clear visual axis in children younger than 6 years of age.[20] However, violating the vitreous in a growing eye may have untoward effects on the normal development of the eye, and Gimbel proposed the technique of posterior *optic capture* of the IOL, which allows preservation of the anterior hyaloid face.[21] There have, however, been conflicting reports of its efficacy in maintaining a clear visual axis. Dada et al.[22] and Argento et al.[23] have reported good outcomes with this procedure with a mean follow-up of up to 28.9 to 38.0 months. However, the purpose of Dada and coworkers' study was to study the efficacy of primary posterior capsulorhexis with optic capture and intracameral heparin. The series compared two techniques: (1) posterior capsulorhexis and optic capture and (2) no posterior capsulorhexis. The better outcome in Group 1 may relate to the posterior capsulorhexis. Similarly, Argento and coworkers' series described outcomes using

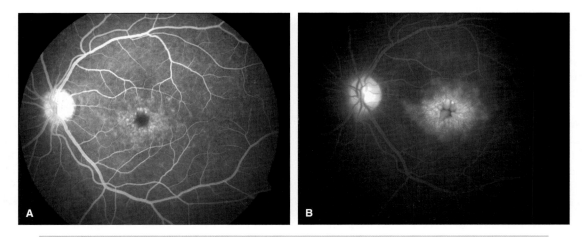

FIGURE 46-2. A. Fluorescein angiogram showing early leakage of the dye. **B.** Late-stage fluorescein showing the classical *"petalloid pattern"* of pooling of the dye consistent with cystoid macular edema.

optic capture with AcrySof IOL, but it is not clear whether the advantage was provided by optic capture or by the AcrySof material. The study did not have a control group (AcrySof implantation with no optic capture). Vasavada et al.[24] reported in a randomized study that anterior capsule fibrosis occurred in 70% of 20 eyes of children aged 5 to 12 years when optic capture was performed without anterior vitrectomy. In contrast, all 21 eyes in which optic capture was accompanied by anterior vitrectomy maintained a clear visual axis, with a mean follow-up of 21.04 months. In another study of children younger than 5 years of age, all eyes underwent posterior capsulectomy and anterior vitrectomy, while optic capture was assigned randomly. The authors reported that one eye in the optic capture group developed a membrane in front of the IOL that required a secondary procedure. Posterior synechia formation was significantly greater in the optic capture group, as were deposits on the IOL optic. Although all eyes in both groups (optic capture/no capture) maintained a clinically centered IOL, geometric decentration was more common in the no-capture group. They concluded that although optic capture allowed the maintenance of a clear visual axis in young children, it predisposed these eyes to an increased uveal inflammatory response.[25] Optic capture of the IOL is also a technically challenging procedure and is not performed by many pediatric cataract surgeons today. The current procedure of choice to maintain a clear visual axis after cataract extraction and IOL implantation in children is a posterior CCC and anterior vitrectomy. As mentioned above, one of the important concerns when performing this procedure is the possibility of CME.

The natural history of CME is variable. Pseudophakic CME in adults often resolves spontaneously, and a visual acuity of 20/40 is attained in 90% of cases. However, in some patients, repeated remissions and exacerbations can result in a prolonged course of the disease, with subsequent permanent loss of visual function owing to foveal receptor damage and macular degeneration. It is, therefore, important to understand the epidemiology of this condition in children undergoing cataract surgery, since an improved understanding of its pathophysiology and potentiating factors would allow better strategies for prevention and treatment of this potentially serious complication.

Current evidence indicates that the main etiologic factors for CME include direct vitreous traction on the macula, ocular inflammation, increasing age, and other contributory factors such as hypotony.[2] In patients undergoing cataract surgery, adherence of vitreous to the wound,[10] presence of iris adhesions to the surgical section,[26] inflammation,[27] prostaglandin release,[28] retained cortical material, previous uveitis,[29] use of adrenaline and ocular hypotensive lipids in the pre- and postoperative periods,[30,31] use of intracameral vancomycin (10 μg/mL) as infection prophylaxis,[32] and presence of systemic vascular diseases such as hypertension, ischemic heart disease,[33] and diabetes mellitus[34] have been postulated as risk factors. Many of the factors postulated above appear to cause CME secondary to intraocular inflammation, and prostaglandins and leukotrienes have been identified as possible mediators. Prostaglandins have vasoactive effects causing vasodilation, increased capillary permeability, and breakdown of the BRB. This results in a weakening of tight endothelial junctions in retinal capillaries and decreased pumping of fluid from the retinal pigment epithelium. The role of leukotrienes in this process is less clear. This chapter focuses on the occurrence of CME in children undergoing cataract surgery with IOL implantation and reviews evidence that can help minimize CME in these eyes.

CME is considered to be uncommon in children. Although the reasons for this are not clear, it may be due to a healthier vasculature, a general lack of systemic vascular disease, possible differences in prostaglandin physiologic structure, and differences in operative techniques in children.[35] Early reports of cataract surgery in children indicated that the incidence of CME may be lower in these eyes.[29,36–38] Hoyt and Nickel,[39] however, reported a CME incidence of 37% in children undergoing lensectomy and vitrectomy. All of these early studies were in aphakic eyes, while the use of an IOL is considered standard-of-care in pediatric cataract surgery today. Current studies appear to indicate that with present techniques of cataract surgery and IOL implantation, the occurrence of this complication in children is quite rare.[40,41] Assessment of CME in children can be complicated by poor cooperation of young children for slit-lamp biomicroscopy. Inaccuracies in visual acuity estimation in the early postoperative period in these young children, many of whom also have amblyopia, would reduce the effectiveness of clinical CME assessment. Angiographic CME has thus been used as a measure of the occurrence of this complication. Standard fluorescein angiography using 5 mL of 10% fluorescein may require the use of general anesthesia to obtain good-quality fundus pictures. To avoid injecting fluorescein, which can lead to occasional serious complications,[42] oral fluorescein can be used. For children weighing <25 kg, 0.5 g of the dye (one vial of the 10% solution) is mixed with 50 mL of iced fruit juice, while for children weighing 26 to 50 kg, 1 g of the dye is mixed with 100 mL of iced fruit juice. Serum levels of orally administered fluorescein approximate late intravenous levels by 30 min, and the concentration persists for 2 hr.[43] The maximal intensity of dye leakage at the macula in CME occurs 45 to 60 min after ingestion of the dye, when it can be visualized with indirect ophthalmoscopy using a cobalt blue filter. The safety and efficacy of this procedure have been validated in previous studies.[27,44,45] Ahmadieh et al. evaluated 45 eyes of 31 children undergoing cataract surgery and IOL implantation, using intravenous fluorescein and fundus fluorescein angiography, and did not detect CME in any eye at 6 weeks after surgery.[40] Rao et al.[41] performed a similar evaluation 4 to 6 weeks after surgery, using oral fluorescein and angioscopy, in 25 eyes of children and did not detect CME in any of them. However, other studies in high-risk populations, such as children with uveitis, indicate that the rate of postoperative CME can be higher.[46,47]

In a child with developmental cataract, attention to pre-, intra-, and postoperative issues may help to decrease the incidence of postoperative CME. The use of topical nonsteroidal eye drops prior to cataract surgery has been shown to decrease the occurrence of intraoperative miosis and also reduce the incidence of postoperative CME.[48] There is as yet no evidence of the effectiveness of this approach in pediatric cataract surgery. Other precautions regarding the preoperative preparation of children undergoing cataract surgery include the cessation of antiglaucoma medications such as pilocarpine for 2 weeks prior to surgery and of the newer ocular hypotensive lipids such as latanoprost for 8 weeks prior to surgery.[30] In patients with uveitis, surgery is best performed after clinical resolution of ocular inflammation. It is also recommended that such eyes be treated with a subtenon injection of 20 mg triamcinolone 3 days prior to surgery and topical steroids and cycloplegics for 3 days prior to surgery.

Intraoperatively the use of incisions that are multiplanar, with a corneal rather than a limbal entry into the eye, help prevent repeated iris prolapse during surgery. This minimizes uveal trauma, reduces the chance of intraoperative miosis and poor visualization, and also helps decrease the incidence of iris adhesion to the wound postoperatively. The use of small incisions that fit snugly around the instrumentation used and high-flow phaco instrumentation reduces the occurrence of intraoperative hypotony. This also minimizes the chance of pupillary miosis, which increases surgical trauma to the iris. The larger bore of the phaco instrumentation and the higher vacuum used allow rapid, efficient removal of the cataractous lens material, compared to devices using manual suction. Vitrectomy, if required, is performed within the opening provided by a controlled curvilinear opening in the posterior capsule. This limits the amount of vitreous that needs to be removed. The rest of the posterior capsule prevents the uncontrolled egress of the vitreous gel into the anterior chamber and out of the surgical wound. This is aided by the use of a closed bimanual approach, which allows greater flexibility in removal of the vitreous gel and prevents vitreous prolapse out of the eye. A limited vitrectomy performed in this manner decreases the vitreous-induced traction on the posterior ocular structures, which results in a reduced incidence of retinal complications and CME. The use of the anterior capsulorhexis has revolutionized cataract surgery in adults and many of the benefits are evident in pediatric cataract surgery as well. Most importantly, it allows secure placement of the IOL within the confines of the capsular bag and limits its contact with the reactive uveal tissue in a child's

eye. Secure wound closure is also critical to the success of cataract surgery in children and can be achieved either by sutures or by the creation of a sutureless tunnel incision.

A better understanding of the mechanisms of post–cataract surgery intraocular inflammation and the availability of newer pharmacological agents like the nonsteroidal anti-inflammatory drugs have improved the postoperative care of the pediatric eye. Studies have shown the efficacy of 0.1% diclofenac eye drops in the prevention of postoperative CME.[49,50] Indomethacin (1.0%) eye drops and ketorolac (0.5%) eye drops have also been shown to be effective in the treatment of CME, although prolonged use is required.[51,52] These studies report outcomes in adults, but the use of these medications is efficacious in pediatric cataract surgery as well (*personal observation*). In addition to nonsteroidal anti-inflammatory eye drops, topical steroids form the mainstay in postoperative treatment. If the IOL is securely placed within the capsular bag, the use of a strong cycloplegic like atropine can be considered in the initial postoperative period to reduce the uveal response. With current techniques, the use of postoperative systemic steroids is not required in the majority of surgical procedures.

In the event of persistent CME following surgery, traditional methods of treatment include the use of topical, oral, and transseptal steroids,[53] topical and oral nonsteroidal agents,[53] and carbonic anhydrase inhibitors.[54] Other options that have been suggested include high-dose intravenous methylprednisolone,[55] intravitreal injection of triamcinolone,[56] and pars plana vitrectomy.[57]

In conclusion, it is now clear that retention of the posterior capsule during cataract surgery has a protective effect on the occurrence of postoperative CME. However, it is also becoming clear that with current approaches to IOL implantation in eyes of children after cataract extraction, it is imperative to create a central opening in the posterior capsule, through which a limited anterior vitrectomy must be performed to maintain a clear visual pathway. Performing an optic capture through the posterior CCC may help avoid the need for an anterior vitrectomy, but current evidence indicates that this procedure may need to evolve further before finding universal acceptance. Despite the need to violate the vitreous in young children, it appears, based on available evidence, that such a procedure, using modern technology and techniques, does not predispose the child to an increased risk of CME. The reasons for this are not clear, since similar procedures in adults tend to show a higher occurrence of CME. It may be that the pediatric eye is structurally more resistant to the effects of anterior segment manipulations. Improved understanding of the pathophysiology of intraocular inflammation and its role in the causation of CME has resulted in better treatment approaches in the postoperative period. This has led to improved outcomes of cataract surgery in children. Despite these advances, there are still many unanswered questions. These include the possibility of late-onset changes in the macula of these eyes, sequelae of posterior vitreous detachments as these children grow older, and the relevance of some of the newly described methods to treat CME, such as intravitreal triamcinolone injections and pars plana vitrectomy, in children.

REFERENCES

1. Wolfensberger TJ. The historical discovery of macular edema. *Doc Ophthalmol* 1997;97:207–216.
2. Cunha-vaz JG, Travassos A. Breakdown of the blood-retinal barriers and cystoid macular edema. *Surv Ophthalmol* 1984;28:485–492.
3. Alexandrakis G. Macular edema—Irvine-Gass. www.emedicine.com
4. Lardenoye CW, Probst K, DeLint PJ, Rathova A. Photoreceptor function in eyes with macular edema. *Invest Ophthalmol Vis Sci* 2000;41:4048–4053.
5. Zeimer RC, Cunha-Vaz JG, Johnson ME. Studies on the technique of vitreous fluorophotometry. *Invest Ophthalmol Vis Sci* 1982;22:668–674.
6. Miyake Y, Miyake K, Shiroyama N. Classification of aphakic cystoid macular edema with focal macular electroretinograms. *Am J Ophthalmol* 1993;116:576–583.
7. Antcliff RF, Stanford MR, Chauhan DS, Graham EM, Spalton DJ, Schilling JS, Ffytche TJ, Marshall J. Comparison between optical coherence tomography and fundus fluorescein angiography for the detection of cystoid macular edema in patients with uveitis. *Ophthalmology* 2000;107:593–599.
8. Mao LK, Holland PM. 'Very late onset' cystoid macular edema. *Ophthalmic Surg* 1998;19:633–635.
9. Flach AJ. The incidence, pathogenesis and treatment of cystoid macular edema following cataract surgery. *Trans Am Ophthalmol Soc* 1998;96:557–634.
10. Irvine SR. A newly defined vitreous syndrome following cataract surgery. *Am J Ophthalmol* 1953;36:599–619.
11. Holekamp NM. The treatment of pseudophakic CME. *Ocul Immunol Inflamm* 1998;6:121–123.
12. Milch FA, Yanuzzi LA. Medical and surgical treatment of aphakic cystoid macular edema. *Int Ophthalmol Clin* 1987;27:205–217.
13. Norregaard JC, Bernth-Petersen P, Bellan L, Alonso J, Black C, Dunn E, Andersen TF, Espallargues M, Anderson GF. Intraoperative clinical practice and risk of early complications after cataract extraction in the United States, Canada, Denmark, and Spain. *Ophthalmology* 1999;106:42–48.
14. Wegener M, Alsbirk PH, Hojgaard-Olsen K. Outcome of 1000 consecutive clinic- and hospital-based cataract surgeries in a Danish county. *J Cataract Refract Surg* 1998;24:1152–1160.
15. Ah-Fat FG, Sharma MK, Majid MA, Yang YC. Vitreous loss during conversion from conventional extracapsular cataract extraction to phacoemulsification. *J Cataract Refract Surg* 1998;24:801–805.
16. Koch PS. Anterior vitrectomy. In: Nordan LT, Maxwell WA, Davidson JA, eds. *The Surgical Rehabilitation of Vision: An Integrated Approach to Anterior Segment Surgery.* London: Gower; 1992:chap 17.
17. Zaczak A, Petrelius A, Zetterstrom C. Posterior continuous curvilinear capsulorhexis and posterior inflammation. *J Cataract Refract Surg* 1998;24:1339–1342.
18. Vasavada A, Desai J. Primary posterior capsulorhexis with and without anterior vitrectomy in congenital cataracts. *J Cataract Refract Surg* 1997;23:645–651.
19. Koch DD, Kohnen T. Retrospective comparison of techniques to prevent secondary cataract formation after posterior chamber intraocular lens implantation in infants and children. *J Cataract Refract Surg* 1997;23:657–663.
20. Jensen AA, Basti S, Greenwald MJ, Mets MB. When may the posterior capsule be preserved in pediatric intraocular lens surgery? *Ophthalmology* 2002;109:324–327.
21. Gimbel HV. Posterior capsulorhexis with optic capture in pediatric cataract and intraocular lens surgery. *Ophthalmology* 1996;103:1871–1875.
22. Dada T, Dada VK, Sharma N, Vajpayee RB. Primary posterior capsulorhexis with optic capture and intracameral heparin in pediatric cataract surgery. *Clin Exp Ophthalmol* 2000;28:361–363.
23. Argento C, Badoza B, Ugrin C. Optic capture of the Acrysof intraocular lens in pediatric cataract surgery. *J Cataract Refract Surg* 2001;27:1638–1642.
24. Vasavada AR, Trivedi RH, Singh R. Necessity of vitrectomy when optic capture is performed in children older than 5 years. *J Cataract Refract Surg* 2001;27:1185–1193.
25. Vasavada AR, Trivedi RH. Role of optic capture in congenital cataract and intraocular lens surgery in children. *J Cataract Refract Surg* 2000;26:824–831.
26. Spaide RF, Yanuzzi LA, Sisco LJ. Chronic cystoid macular edema and predictors of visual acuity. *Ophthalmic Surg* 1993;24:262–267.
27. Irvine AR, Bresky R, Crowder BM, Forster RK, Hunter DM, Kulvin SM. Macular edema after cataract extraction. *Ann Ophthalmol* 1971;3:1234–1240.
28. Waitzman MB. Topical indomethacin in treatment and prevention of intraocular inflammation—with special reference to lens extraction and cystoid macular edema. *Ann Ophthalmol* 1979;11:489–491.
29. Gilbard SM, Peyman GA, Goldberg MF. Evaluation for cystoid maculopathy after pars plicata lensectomy-vitrectomy for congenital cataracts. *Ophthalmology* 1983;90:1201–1206.
30. Yeh PC, Ramanathan S. Latanoprost and clinically significant cystoid macular edema after uneventful phacoemulsification with intraocular lens implantation. *J Cataract Refract Surg* 2002;28:1814–1818.
31. Wand M, Gaudio AR. Cystoid macular edema associated with ocular hypotensive lipids. *Am J Ophthalmol* 2002;133:403–405.
32. Axer-Siegel R, Stiebel-Kalish H, Rosenblatt I, Strassmann E, Yassur Y, Weinberger G. Cystoid macular edema after cataract surgery with intraocular vancomycin. *Ophthalmology* 1999;106:1660–1664.
33. Jain R, Stevens JD, Bunce CV, Garrett C, Hykin PG. Ischemic heart disease may predispose to pseudophakic cystoid macular edema. *Eye* 2001;15:34–38.
34. Oliver M. Posterior pole changes after cataract extraction in elderly subjects. *Am J Ophthalmol* 1966;62:1145–1148.
35. Poer DV, Helveston EM, Ellis FD. Aphakic cystoid macular edema in children. *Arch Ophthalmol* 1981;99:249–252.
36. Schulman J, Peyman GA, Raichand M, Jebnock N. Aphakic cystoid macular edema in children after vitrectomy for anterior segment injuries. *Ophthalmic Surg* 1983;14:848–851.
37. Morgan KS, Franklin RM. Oral fluorescein angioscopy in aphakic children. *J Pediatr Ophthalmol Strabismus* 1984;21:33–36.
38. Pinchoff BS, Ellis FD, Helveston EM, Sato SE. Cystoid macular edema in pediatric aphakia. *J Pediatr Ophthalmol Strabismus* 1998;25:240–243.
39. Hoyt CS, Nickel B. Aphakic cystoid macular edema; occurrence in infants and children after transpupillary lensectomy and anterior vitrectomy. *Arch Ophthalmol* 1982;100:746–749.
40. Ahmadieh H, Javadi MA, Ahmady M, Karimian F, Einollahi B, Zare M, Dehghan MH, Mashyekhi A, Valaei N, Soheilian M, Sajjadi H. Primary capsulectomy, anterior vitrectomy, lensectomy, and posterior chamber lens implantation in children: limbal versus pars plana. *J Cataract Refract Surg* 1999;25:768–775.
41. Rao SK, Ravishankar K, Sitalakshmi G, Ng JSK, Yu C, Lam DSC. Cystoid macular edema after pediatric intraocular lens implantation: fluorescein angioscopy results and literature review. *J Cataract Refract Surg* 2001;27:432–436.
42. Ascaso FJ, Tiestos MT, Navales J, Iturbe F, Palomar A, Ayala JI. Fatal acute myocardial infarction after intravenous fluorescein angiography. *Retina* 1993;13:238–239.
43. Kelley JS, Kincaid M. Retinal fluorograms using oral fluorescein. *Ophthalmology* 1980;87:805–811.
44. Hara T, Inami M, Hara T. Efficacy and safety of fluorescein angiography with orally administered sodium fluorescein. *Am J Ophthalmol* 1998;126:560–564.
45. Kelley JS, Kincaid M. Retinal fluorography using oral fluorescein. *Arch Ophthalmol* 1979;97:2331–2332.

46. Turno-Krecicka A, Nizankowska MH, Oficjalska-Mlynczak J, Koziorowska M. Cataract surgery in adults and children with chronic uveitis. *Klin Oczna* 2000;102:427–430.

47. Paikos P, Fotopoulou M, Papathanassiou M, Choreftaki P, Spryopoulos G. Cataract surgery in children with uveitis. *J Pediatr Ophthalmol Strabismus* 2001;38:16–20.

48. Flach AJ. Topical nonsteroidal anti-inflammatory drugs in ophthalmology. *Int Ophthalmol Clin* 2002;42:1–11.

49. Miyake K, Masuda K, Shirato S, Oshika T, Eguchi K, Hoshi H, Majima Y, Kimura W, Hayashi F. Comparison of diclofenac and fluorometholone in preventing cystoid macular edema after small incision cataract surgery: a multicentered prospective trial. *Jpn J Ophthalmol* 2000;44:58–67.

50. Rossetti L, Butjar E, Castoldi D, Torrazza C, Orzalesi N. Effectiveness of diclofenac eyedrops in reducing inflammation and the incidence of cystoid macular edema after cataract surgery. *J Cataract Refract Surg* 1996;22:794–799.

51. Peterson M, Yoshizumi MO, Hepler R, Mondino B, Kreiger A. Topical indomethacin in the treatment of chronic cystoid macular edema. *Graefes Arch Clin Exp Ophthalmol* 1992;230:401–405.

52. Weisz JM, Bressler NM, Bressler SB, Schachat AP. Ketorolac treatment of pseudophakic cystoid macular edema identified more than 24 months after cataract extraction. *Ophthalmology* 1999;106:1656–1659.

53. Rojas B, Zafirakis P, Christen W, Markomichelakis NN, Foster CS. Medical treatment of macular edema in patients with uveitis. *Doc Ophthalmol* 1999;97:399–407.

54. Wolfensberger TJ. The role of carbonic anhydrase inhibitors in the management of macular edema. *Doc Ophthalmol* 1999;97:387–397.

55. Conway MD, Canakis C, Livir-Rallatos C, Peyman GA. Intravitreal triamcinolone acetonide for refractory chronic pseudophakic cystoid macular edema. *J Cataract Refract Surg* 2003;29:27–33.

56. Abe T, Hayasaka S, Nagaki Y, Kadoi C, Matsumoto M, Hayasaka Y. Pseudophakic cystoid macular edema treated with high-dose intravenous methyl prednisolone. *J Cataract Refract Surg* 1999;25:1286–1288.

57. Fung WE. Vitrectomy for chronic aphakic cystoid macular edema. Results of a national, collaborative, prospective, randomized investigation. *Ophthalmology* 1985;92:1102–1111.

Chapter 47

Retinal Detachment

Suresh K. Pandey

Retinal detachment (RD) occurs when subretinal fluid accumulates in the potential space between the neurosensory retina and the underlying retinal pigment epithelium. Depending on the mechanism of subretinal fluid accumulation, RDs traditionally have been classified into rhegmatogenous, tractional, and exudative. Retinal detachment can result in a poor visual outcome after cataract surgery in children as well as in adults. The RD may be preexistent or may occur anytime in the postoperative period, sometimes many years later.[1] RD complicating previous congenital cataract surgery poses problems in management, especially related to difficulties in localization of retinal breaks.[2] However, the introduction of closed microsurgical techniques has significantly improved the prognosis in such cases.

Observations on the incidence and management of RD after pediatric cataract surgery are limited by the lack of studies with a long-term follow-up after the cataract surgery. Previous studies reporting this complication relate to the older techniques of cataract surgery and may not be strictly applicable to the currently performed modern cataract techniques.

In this chapter, we attempt to provide an overview of the incidence, predisposing factors, management, and prognosis of RD following pediatric cataract surgery. Wherever appropriate, we also compare this rare complication of pediatric cataract surgery to the occurrence of RD following adult cataract surgery.

INCIDENCE OF RETINAL DETACHMENT: ADULT CATARACT SURGERY VERSUS PEDIATRIC CATARACT SURGERY

A review of the literature suggests that most RDs after cataract surgery occur in persons aged 40 to 70 years. In a retrospective population-based incidence study, the estimated cumulative probability of RD 10 years after phacoemulsification or extracapsular cataract extraction was 5.5 times as high as would have been expected in a similar population not undergoing cataract surgery.[3] In another study,[4] the incidence of RD was 0.79% with intracapsular cataract extraction and 0.44% after extracapsular cataract extraction with a follow-up of 2.5 to 4.5 years. The incidence did not vary between those <60 years old and those >60 years old at the time of surgery. Other authors[5] have noted RD rates in extracapsular cataract extraction of 2.98% with anterior chamber intraocular lens (IOL) implantation and 0.56% with posterior chamber IOL implantation. The authors identified high myopia, peripheral retinal degenerations, and vitreous loss as risk factors for the development of RD.

Keech and associates[6] evaluated the complications after surgery for congenital and infantile cataracts (operated before 30 months of age) and found a 1% rate of RD. A study that evaluated three older techniques of congenital cataract surgery found a 1.5% incidence of RD with a mean follow-up of 5.5 years.[7] However, all these studies are limited by the lack of really long-term follow-up, as RD after pediatric cataract surgery is known to occur even decades after the surgery.[8–10] In one study, the time interval between congenital cataract surgery and onset of RD ranged from 1 month to 46 years and was 10 to >30 years in 60% of patients. Up to 30% of eyes with fresh detachment have a history of prior cataract surgery.[11]

CHARACTERISTICS OF RETINAL DETACHMENT

The RD that develops after cataract surgery varies in many respects from the commonly seen idiopathic RD. A 1980 study evaluated 114 eyes with RD occurring after congenital cataract surgery and found a higher incidence of RD in males, myopes (determined by a lower than expected aphakic refractive error), those in the second and fourth decades of life, and those with a longer interval after cataract surgery.[1] They also frequently observed undetected retinal breaks (most commonly small oval or round holes in the upper nasal quadrant near the ora serrata), RD in more than one quadrant, and extensive vitreous and preretinal traction. A study done to evaluate the characteristics and results of phakic and pseudophakic RDs found that proliferative vitroretinopathy (PVR) was present in 30% of the patients.[12] Another study done exclusively on RD after pediatric cataract surgery also found a 36% rate of PVR grades B to D3.[13] It has also been observed that the factors that predispose patients to PVR in aphakia include a history of inadvertent vitreous loss during cataract surgery, RD developing within 3 months after cataract extraction, a duration of RD longer than 3 months, a break larger than three disc diameters, and choroidal detachment.[14] These observations were duplicated in another study[15] on the same topic, which identified the risk factors for developing PVR as choroidal detachment, a duration of RD longer than 1 month, the occurrence of RD within 1 year following cataract surgery, and a history of vitreous loss during cataract surgery (in order of significance).

An important problem in RD occurring after cataract surgery relates to the inability to find a retinal break,[1] which makes management difficult. In a study evaluating RD without detectable breaks, the most common cause of failure to find retinal breaks was aphakia/pseudophakia, seen in 22 of 45 eyes.[16] Another additional problem seen after pediatric cataract surgery arises due to the almost-universal opacification of the posterior capsule seen after this type of surgery, which hampers the visualization of the posterior segment.[13] The preoperative examination is at times also hampered by a small, bound-down pupil, nystagmus, extreme photophobia, or an inability to move the eye in desired directions.[1]

ROLE OF SURGICAL/NEODYMIUM:YAG LASER POSTERIOR CAPSULOTOMY

Recent studies suggest that in young children, a primary opening in the posterior capsule is a required step in pediatric cataract–IOL surgery to prevent opacification of the visual axis. It is also necessary in these children to perform an anterior vitrectomy to maintain a clear visual axis. However, possible long-term complications such as RD or vitreous or macular changes that may not occur for several decades after pediatric cataract–IOL surgery have not been studied extensively.

Opacification of the posterior capsule occurs frequently in children when the posterior capsule is left intact. In these cases, YAG laser capsulotomy may be needed. In adults, retinal complications including rhegmatogenous RD and acute symptomatic retinal tear have been shown to develop in 2.5% of eyes followed up for 1 year after a YAG laser capsulotomy and 3.6% of eyes followed up for 2 years. These complications were significantly correlated with

axial myopia, preexisting vitreoretinal disease, male gender, younger age, vitreous prolapse into the anterior chamber, and spontaneous extension of the capsulotomy.[17] Lin and associates[18] found a 1.36% incidence of rhegmatogenous RD with a mean follow-up of 10.5 months after the laser capsulotomy. The highest risk for development of RD after laser capsulotomy is seen in patients with an axial eye length of 26.1 to 28.0 mm.[19] In the case of children with a longer life expectancy after the surgery, the incidence of RD after YAG laser is unknown but a long follow-up is needed.

SURGICAL MANAGEMENT OF RETINAL DETACHMENT

The goal is to identify and close all retinal breaks. Several techniques, as they pertain to repair of RD, can be used, based on the type and location of the hole/tear. Surgical management often involves a scleral buckle with or without vitrectomy.

Scleral Buckle

An encircling band is often used in aphakic or pseudophakic detachments. The band helps to close retinal holes near the vitreous base and can relieve vitreous traction that might lead to new break formation.

Vitrectomy

This may be an ideal procedure for these cases, as vitreoretinal traction may be relieved in an efficient manner without regard to potential damage to the lens by scleral depression. The major complication of vitrectomy with intraocular tamponade is formation of a lenticular opacity, which is a nonissue in these aphakic/pseudophakic eyes. Fluid–air exchanges in pseudophakic eyes with an open capsule may pose a problem. Fluid condensation on the surface of the IOL may impair the visibility of the retina, making completion of the fluid–air exchange challenging.

Vitrectomy and Scleral Buckling

Pars plana vitrectomy, an encircling band, internal drainage, and intraocular tamponade are effective and efficient methods of repairing primary pseudophakic RDs.

PROGNOSIS OF RETINAL DETACHMENT

The overall anatomically successful reattachment rate for RD after pediatric cataract surgery has been reported to be as high as 88% by Bonne and Delage[13] in a series of 25 eyes with at least a 6-month follow-up. Negative prognostic indicators for reattachment include poor preoperative visual acuity, extension of the RD to the macula, and grade B, C, or D PVR. Additional factors predictive of poor visual outcome include eyes with inadvertent vitreous loss, aphakia, and a greater extent of RD.[13]

CONCLUSION

In summary, the incidence of RD following pediatric cataract surgery appears to be decreasing as surgical techniques advance and evolve. Most reported cases have a history of multiple reoperations performed in the years prior to the introduction of automated lensectomy and vitrectomy. A long-term follow-up is critical in children, as the RD can occur many years after cataract surgery. A detailed retinal examination is recommended after cataract surgery at least yearly. This is especially important for those eyes at higher risk for RD by virtue of a long axial length for age, persistent fetal vasculature, or multiple surgeries. The use of a modern high-speed vitreous cutter reduces the traction on the retina. The increased use of a pars plana approach to the anterior vitreous (with anterior irrigation) has also decreased vitreous prolapse or incarceration into an anterior chamber, thus further decreasing the rate of late RD.

REFERENCES

1. Toyofuku H, Hirose T, Schepens CL. Retinal detachment following congenital cataract surgery. I. Preoperative findings in 114 eyes. *Arch Ophthalmol* 1980;98:669–675.
2. Jagger JD, Cooling RJ, Fison LG, Leaver PK, McLeod D. Management of retinal detachment following congenital cataract surgery. *Trans Ophthalmol Soc UK* 1983;103:103–107.
3. Rowe JA, Erie JC, Baratz KH, Hodge DO, Gray DT, Butterfield L, Robertson DM. Retinal detachment in Olmsted County, Minnesota, 1976 through 1995. *Ophthalmology* 1999;106:154–159.
4. Urbak SF, Naeser K. Retinal detachment following intracapsular and extracapsular cataract extraction. A comparative, retrospective follow-up study. *Acta Ophthalmol (Copenh)* 1993;71:1782–1786.
5. Nicula C, Nicula D. Etiopathogenic consideration in the development of retinal detachment in aphakic and pseudoaphakic eye. *Oftalmologia* 2000;50:28–31.
6. Keech RV, Tongue AC, Scott WE. Complications after surgery for congenital and infantile cataracts. *Am J Ophthalmol* 1989;108: 136–141.
7. Chrousos GA, Parks MM, O'Neill JF. Incidence of chronic glaucoma, retinal detachment and secondary membrane surgery in pediatric aphakic patients. *Ophthalmology* 1984;91:1238–1241.
8. Pavlovic S. Cataract surgery in children. *Med Pregl* 2000;53:257–261.
9. McLeod D. Congenital cataract surgery: a retinal surgeon's viewpoint. *Aust NZ J Ophthalmol* 1986;14:79–84.
10. Kanski JJ, Elkington AR, Daniel R. Retinal detachment after congenital cataract surgery. *Br J Ophthalmol* 1974;58:92–95.
11. Algvere PV, Jahnberg P, Textorius O. The Swedish Retinal Detachment Register. I. A database for epidemiological and clinical studies. *Graefes Arch Clin Exp Ophthalmol* 1999;237:137–144.
12. Berrod JP, Sautiere B, Rozot P, Raspiller A. Retinal detachment after cataract surgery. *Int Ophthalmol* 1996–97;20:301–308.
13. Bonnet M, Delage S. Retinal detachment after surgery of congenital cataract. *J Fr Ophtalmol* 1994;17:580–584.
14. Nagasaki H, Ideta H, Uemura A, Morita H, Ito K, Yonemoto J. Comparative study of clinical factors that predispose patients to proliferative vitreoretinopathy in aphakia. *Retina* 1991;11:204–207.
15. Nagasaki H, Ideta H, Mochizuki M, Shibata A. A case-control study of risk factors for proliferative vitreoretinopathy in aphakia. *Jpn J Ophthalmol* 1993;37:187–191.
16. Kocaoglan H, Unlu N, Acar MA, Sargin M, Aslan BS, Duman S. Management of rhegmatogenous retinal detachment without detectable breaks. *Clin Exp Ophthalmol* 2002;30:415–418.
17. Koch DD, Liu JF, Gill EP, Parke DW 2nd. Axial myopia increases the risk of retinal complications after neodymium:YAG laser posterior capsulotomy. *Arch Ophthalmol* 1989;107:986–990.
18. Lin ZD, Yang WH, Liu YZ. Complications following Nd:YAG laser posterior capsulotomy. *Zhonghua Yan Ke Za Zhi* 1994;30:325–327.
19. Dardenne MU, Gerten GJ, Kokkas K, Kermani O. Retrospective study of retinal detachment following neodymium:YAG laser posterior capsulotomy. *J Cataract Refract Surg* 1989;15:676–680.

Functional Issues

Chapter 48

Management of Residual Refractive Error After Intraocular Lens Implantation

*M. Edward Wilson, Jr. and
Suresh K. Pandey*

Management of residual refractive error is a very important part of pediatric cataract management. Uncorrected refractive error after pediatric cataract surgery can cause or worsen amblyopia. When a child is left aphakic, every effort should be made to minimize time intervals when the prescribed aphakic glasses or aphakic contact lenses are not worn. Even short intervals of uncorrected aphakia are potentially very damaging to the prognosis.[1-5] When an intraocular lens (IOL) is implanted, a smaller amount of residual hyperopia may be present. However, correction of this residual hyperopia and any significant astigmatic error is necessary to optimize visual development and recovery from amblyopia. Some surgeons prefer to correct children to emmetropia with an IOL even at young ages to minimize the amblyogenic effects of residual hyperopia. Since young children's eyes continue to grow axially after cataract surgery and IOL implantation, significant late myopia will be more and more common as the years pass, especially if emmetropia is achieved early in life with an IOL.[6-8] Glasses or contact lenses will be used for correction of secondary myopia in most cases. However, the development of new corneal and intraocular refractive procedures will provide new options for correcting significant late myopia.

In this chapter, we present a brief overview of our practice pattern and philosophy when treating residual refractive error *after an IOL has been implanted. Interested readers should also consult Chapters 27 and 51 to become familiar with some of the surgical methods used to minimize or treat residual refractive error.*

MANAGEMENT OF RESIDUAL REFRACTIVE ERROR

After Surgery in Infancy

Nearly all infants will have residual refractive error after cataract and IOL surgery. On the first postoperative day, however, these small soft eyes will not yield a reliable refraction by which this residual refractive error can be determined. Even with small-incision surgery and careful control of the placement and tying of synthetic absorbable suture, marked temporary astigmatism (often 3 to 5 D [diopters]) will be seen initially. This resolves quickly over the first 2 to 4 weeks after surgery. After that, the goal for prescribing glasses to correct the residual hyperopia should be 1 to 2 D of overcorrection (myopia) in single-vision (not bifocal) glasses. This end point amounts to a neutralized retinoscopic reflection without any working lens held before the eyes.

When a single IOL is implanted in infancy, marked axial growth must be expected over the first 1 to 2 years after surgery. On average, axial growth in a normal eye is 4.5 mm over the first 2 years of life. With an IOL in place, this growth is likely to change the refraction by ≥ 10 D. Therefore, IOLs implanted in infancy are usually selected to produce a $\geq 20\%$ undercorrection. The closer to birth, the more marked this undercorrection will need to be. We have, in general, selected the target refractive error of $+12.00$ D in the first month of life, $+8.00$ D to $+10.00$ in the second to third months of life, $+6.00$ D in the fourth to sixth months, and $+5.00$ D in the remainder of the first year of life. With this said, however, the range of microphthalmia and the variability of growth we have documented in the first year of life are marked. Therefore, residual refractive errors over a wide range will need to be managed in these patients.

When the eyes are microphthalmic at surgery, the targeted refractive error may not be achievable with the maximum single IOL available. Therefore, more residual hyperopia will be present. Until recently, 30 D was the maximum power available in the AcrySof IOL series. Lenses up to 40 D can now be ordered in many IOL designs (including AcrySof) if desired to achieve the refractive goal in very small eyes. However, the surgeon must realize that the higher the power of the implant, the greater the refractive error change will be per millimeter of eye growth.

Variability in growth and refractive change after IOL implantation is much more marked in infants than in older children. In a report of a series of 47 eyes of 33 patients implanted in the first year of life, we found an average first postoperative refraction of +7.98 D when a single IOL was implanted. The range, however, was from −0.50 to +18.25 D.[9] In one patient implanted bilaterally with 30-D IOLs, a marked residual refractive error of +16.00 D in the right eye and +18.25 D in the left eye was recorded 1 week after surgery. Remarkably, the refraction recorded 28 months after surgery was − 4.00 D in the right eye and +2.50 D in the left eye. There was no evidence of glaucoma and the visual acuity appeared to be normal in each eye. For this patient, contact lenses were used initially to correct the high residual hyperopia but a switch to glasses was made when the refraction fell (with further eye growth) to the single digits.

At the other extreme, two infants in that same series had postoperative refractions of −0.50 D after implantation of a single IOL. In these patients (both with unilateral surgery), dense amblyopia was already present, and a posterior staphyloma was seen in one. Emmetropia was aimed for in hopes of simplifying a difficult battle for improved vision, although high myopia would probably develop later. Surprisingly, over the next 1.5 years, neither eye underwent substantial growth. One patient has remained at −0.5 D and the other increased only to −1.00 D.

Most patients, however, demonstrated eye growth that more closely matched the predicted normal growth curve, especially if they were operated on near the end of infancy. Even for these patients, a sizable residual refractive error was present and needed to be corrected. The correction was changed frequently during the first 2 years after surgery, after which the changes slowed considerably. Contact lenses should be considered if the residual hyperopia is very large initially. We fit these infants with a Silsoft silicone contact lens if possible, with an aim for mild myopia of −1.00 to −2.00 D. Silsoft contact lenses are only available down to a +12.00-D power, however. For power needs less than +12.00 D, a daily-wear contact lens is chosen. Since these daily-wear lenses are more difficult to fit, we most often transition the babies into glasses as soon as the power needs are less than the minimum available in the Silsoft line. For bilateral surgeries, this transition is less troublesome. However, for unilateral pseudophakia, high residual refractive error requires a marked anisometropic glasses prescription. When good visual and binocular potential exists, contact lenses (or piggyback IOLs) are more aggressively pursued to reduce the anisokonia that can result from anisometropic glasses. When dense amblyopia is present, however, the chance of achieving high-grade stereopsis is poor. In these patients, marked anisometropic glasses are tolerated very well and may help achieve good visual acuity when contact lenses are unsuitable.

If compliance with glasses or contacts for the residual refractive error is poor, amblyopia may worsen or improve more slowly even when appropriate patching is being done. However, it is reasonable to conclude that *undercorrected* aphakia is less amblyogenic than *uncorrected* aphakia. In our experience, the former interferes less with amblyopia progress than the later. In fact, we have been amazed by how well some children can see (when old enough to read or match letters), for both distance and near vision, when moderate amounts of residual hyperopia are not corrected. This degree of "pseudoaccommodation" with monofocal IOLs is not seen in aphakic children corrected with contact lenses and it is not seen in adults with similar amounts of residual refractive error.

Some surgeons advocate aiming for emmetropia after surgery regardless of age. In infancy, however, this cannot usually be achieved without placing piggyback IOLs in the eye. Myopic change after infantile surgery is marked. Glasses for residual refractive error are often changed three or four times in the first year after surgery.

After Surgery in Toddlers and Pre-School–Aged Children

On average, the eye grows 4.5 mm in the first 2 years of life and then growth slows considerably. However, growth from age 2 to age 6 years is still substantial, averaging 0.4 mm per year. In a survey we published in 2003, nearly 90% of the surgeons responding from the American Association for Pediatric Ophthalmology and Strabismus (AAPOS) recommended leaving residual hyperopia at age 2 years.[10] This recommendation dropped to 45% when the surgery was done at age 5 years.[10] Plager and coworkers[11] recommended leaving 5 D of hyperopia at age 3 years, 4 D at age 4, 3 D at age 5, 2.25 D at age 6, 1.5 D at age 7, 0.5 D at age 10, and plano at age 13. For each individual case, however, we customize the residual postoperative refractive aim based on many characteristics including the laterality (one eye or both), amblyopia status (dense or mild), likely compliance with glasses, and family history of myopia. More hyperopia is left when the surgery will be done bilaterally since noncompliance with glasses is less amblyogenic in these children. Dense amblyopia may prompt a decision to leave less hyperopia (or even emmetropia) in an effort to help recover vision by emphasizing the occlusion therapy but minimizing the glasses need. In this instance, late myopia is acceptable if it helps to recover vision during the amblyopia treatment years.

Toddlers and preschool children are usually given glasses about 2 weeks after surgery. Initially, temporary astigmatism is usually present from the synthetic absorbable suture used to close the wounds. Young children have much more early postoperative astigmatism than adults. It tends to fade away over the first 2 to 4 weeks after surgery. Unlike infants, these children are prescribed their full cycloplegic refraction for distance and a +3.00-D bifocal for near viewing. In the past, many surgeons waited until school age to prescribe bifocals for aphakic or pseudophakic children. However, toddlers are often much more active with near tasks and school activities these days. We feel that bifocals should be added to the glasses as soon as the child is 2 years old.

After Surgery in School-Aged and Older Children

More than 85% of the surgeons from AAPOS who responded recommended a plano refractive aim when surgery was done at age 10 years. On average, axial eye growth form age 10 to age 20 years will be <1 mm or approximately 1 to 2 D of myopic shift. We have seen that some children in this age group do not show any eye growth, and others (especially those with a family history of myopia) grow twice the expected amount.

Since growth can be difficult to predict for an individual school-aged child, many surgeons choose to aim for emmetropia for all patients from age 6 or 7 through the end of childhood. If eye growth continues, mild myopia develops initially and this may not need to be corrected with spectacles. Moderate degrees of myopia are usually corrected with spectacles. When the pseudophakia is bilateral, bifocals (usually lineless progressive bifocals) are prescribed. However, with unilateral pseudophakia, the bifocal can be placed unilaterally, bilaterally, or not at all. This is left up to the preference of the surgeon and the patient.

Multifocal IOLs are being implanted more commonly in children who are not likely to demonstrate significant eye growth after surgery. These IOLs work better when implanted bilaterally, but in older children they are also sometimes placed unilaterally. It is expected that the use of multifocal IOLs in children will increase with the availability of mutifocality within an acrylic (rather than a silicone) IOL.

When Young Adulthood Is Near

Residual refractive error in the late teenage years is usually myopia or astigmatism or both. Glasses or contact lenses can be used when needed. Laser refractive surgery will likely be very popular with this group of patients to minimize the use of glasses. IOL exchanges are also becoming more commonplace when the myopia is moderate to severe.

REFERENCES

1. Birch EE, Stager DR. Prevalence of good visual acuity following surgery for congenital unilateral cataract. *Arch Ophthalmol* 1988;106:40–42.
2. Birch EE, Stager DR. The critical period for surgical treatment of dense, congenital, unilateral cataracts. *Invest Ophthalmol Vis Sci* 1996;37:1532–1538.
3. Birch EE, Swanson WH, Stager DR, et al. Outcome after very early treatment of dense congenital unilateral cataract. *Invest Ophthalmol Vis Sci* 1993;34:3687–3699.
4. Bradford GM, Keech RV, Scott WE. Factors affecting visual outcome after surgery for bilateral congenital cataracts. *Am J Ophthalmol* 1994;117:58–64.
5. Catalano RA, Simon JW, Jenkins PL, Kandel GL. Preferential looking as a guide for amblyopia therapy in monocular infantile cataracts. *J Pediatr Ophthalmol Strabismus* 1987;24:56–63.
6. Enyedi LB, Peterseim MW, Freedman SF, Buckley EG. Refractive changes after pediatric intraocular lens implantation. *Am J Ophthalmol* 1998;126:772–781.
7. Huber C. Increasing myopia in children with intraocular lenses: An experiment in form deprivation myopia? *Eur J Implant Ref Surg* 1993;5:154–158.
8. Hutchinson AK, Drews-Botsch C, Lambert SR. Myopic shift after intraocular lens implantation during childhood. *Ophthalmology* 1997;104:1752–1757.
9. Wilson ME, Peterseim MW, Englert JA, Lall-Trail JK. Pseudophakia and polypseudophakia in the first year of life. *J AAPOS* 2001;5:238–245.
10. Wilson ME, Bartholomew LR, Trivedi RH. Pediatric cataract surgery and intraocular lens implantation: practice styles and preferences of the 2001 ASCRS and AAPOS memberships. *J Cataract Refract Surg* 2003;29:1811–1820.
11. Plager DA, Kipfer H, Sprunger DT, et al. Refractive change in pediatric pseudophakia: 6-year follow-up. *J Cataract Refract Surg* 2002;28:810–815.

Aphakia

Rupal H. Trivedi and M. Edward Wilson, Jr.

Despite the continuing threat of amblyopia, the prognosis for a good visual outcome after cataract surgery in children has improved dramatically over the last decade. Not only have we improved our understanding of the sensitive period for the development and reversal of amblyopia, but also we have refined both the surgical techniques used during cataract removal and the option for optical correction of the resulting aphakia.[1] The use of primary intraocular lens (IOL) implantation has become increasingly common in recent years and is now the standard of care for older children undergoing cataract surgery. Although more and more surgeons implant IOLs in older children, the use of an IOL still remains controversial in infants and young children.[1-4] As a result, many very young children presenting with congenital cataracts (especially when bilateral or complicated by other ocular or systemic conditions) are left aphakic initially, with the hope that an IOL can be implanted a later time.

Situations where an IOL implant may not be the primary surgical procedure (relative contraindication to IOL implantation), necessitating aphakic correction, are listed in Table 49-1. Because the resulting residual refractive error is amblyogenic, it is crucial to correct this aphakia. Various modalities have been suggested in the literature to correct pediatric aphakia.[5-8] Table 49-2 describes the arguments *for and against* these approaches. For complete description, this table includes details for IOL implantation as well.

Although many of the problems of aphakic spectacles can be overcome by the use of contact lenses, preference for one modality over the other depends on several considerations, listed in Table 49-3.[5-8]

APHAKIC GLASSES

Aphakic glasses are still often used for the correction of bilateral aphakia in children (Fig. 49-1). Pros and cons of aphakic correction are listed in Table 49-2.

Since IOL implants are commonly used for aphakic correction in adults, the availability of and advancement in technology for high-power plus-lenses (generally over 10 D [diopters]) have declined. Thus options are very limited for the child requiring prescription eyewear following cataract surgery. Details of aphakic eyeglass design and optics can be found in basic textbooks on optic and refraction, and are beyond the scope of this book.[9,10] Instead, we furnish information designed to provide guidelines for parents and practicing clinicians published on the MORIN formation section of PGCFA Web site.[11]

In general, three primary types of high-power plus-lenses are in use. Ultraviolet protection should be added to any lenses used.

- *Lenticular lenses.* These lenses have the prescribed power at the center of the lens surrounded by a "ring" of little or no power. Although these lenses are inferior to other types, they are necessary for power over +20 D.
- *Aspheric lenticular lenses.* These have a nonspherical (aspheric) central area surrounded by a ring with little or no power. Power ranges for the aspheric lenticular lens is in the range of +10 to +20 D. The optical properties of this lens type are superior to the lenticular lens.
- *Multidrop lenses.* These lenses have a spherical central zone that flattens into an aspheric zone and then is blended into an area of lesser power. The lens resembles the aspheric lenticular lens without the noticeable "ring." It is far superior to other lens designs. However, it is only available in the range +10 to +16 D.

Frame Selection

It is important that the line of vision rests ideally at the vertical center of the frame. Since the central portion of the lens has the greatest thickness and curvature, the depth of the frame should be sufficient to prevent exposure of the lens thickness along the top of the frame. Frame selection

▶ **TABLE 49-1 Relative Contraindications to Intraocular Lens Implantation**

1. *Institutional factor*: Nonavailability of an IOL
2. *Surgical factor*: Surgeon prefers not to implant a lens in the patient.
3. *Patient factors*: Minimum age at surgery for an IOL implantation varies from surgeon to surgeon and varies between unilateral and bilateral cataracts.
4. *Ocular factors*: Vary from surgeon to surgeon: associated uveitis, severe microphthalmia such that IOL size is not feasible to implant, persistent fetal vasculature, inadequate anterior and/or posterior capsular support, etc.
5. *Parental factor*: Permission/consent denied

▶ **TABLE 49-3 Factors to Consider When Deciding Between Aphakic Eyeglasses and Contact Lenses**

1. *Unilateral aphakia versus bilateral aphakia factors:* Aphakic spectacles are not appropriate for monocular aphakia because of relative magnification differences; if possible, contact lenses should be tried in such a situation. Eyeglasses can be used for bilateral aphakia with reasonable success.
2. *Institutional and compliance factors:* When good contact lens care is not available, eyeglasses can be offered.
3. *Cost factors:* Available silicone contact lenses are expensive. The need for repeated lens purchase because of changing refractive error or lost lenses makes the cost even higher.

is therefore very important. When it can be used, multidrop lenses positioned correctly in a small frame will offer the child the best optics and the best appearance. Some additional considerations for frame selection are listed in Table 49-4. Whenever possible, it is important to involve the child in the decision-making process.

CONTACT LENSES

Pediatric aphakia can be successfully treated with contact lenses (Fig. 49-2). A major advantage is that their power can be easily adjusted as the child's eye grows (Table 49-3). Such lens wear can be both safe and effective with appropriate lens fit, good lens care, and compliance with proper hygiene. Otherwise, it may become hazardous.[12–17] *Compliance* and *complications* are major factors that may limit

the routine use of contact lenses for pediatric aphakia in some settings.

The development of binocular vision and stereopsis has been reported after early removal of infantile cataracts in patients who show excellent compliance with contact lens use and occlusion regimens.[18] When contact lenses fail, they tend to do so at between 2 and 4 years. Lambert et al.[19] reported preliminary results comparing IOL implantation to primary aphakia with contact lens correction. The authors found that fewer reoperations were needed in the contact lens group, but the IOL group had slightly better visual acuity on average. We recently reported that although the incidence of secondary surgery for visual axis opacification (VAO) in the aphakic group was lower compared to that in the pseudophakic group, if all reoperations are considered (VAO, glaucoma,

▶ **TABLE 49-2 Arguments For and Against Different Modalities to Correct Aphakia**

	Arguments For	*Arguments Against*
Aphakic glasses	Safe Power can be easily adjusted Inexpensive	Restriction of visual field to approximately 30° Because of marked retinal size disparity (approximately 30% magnification), not suitable for long-term monocular aphakia Distortion of image and prismatic effect Heavy weight of the glasses may be cumbersome Debilitating visually, cosmetically, and psychologically
Contact lenses	Power can be easily adjusted Relatively safe Suitable for unilateral aphakia Image size differences lessened compared to glasses Field of vision better than with glasses	Noncompliance of both parents and patients Difficulty of insertion Psychologically traumatic 5 to 9% magnification Frequency of lens loss Corneal complication
Epikeratophakia	Reversible Extraocular No damage to recipient's cornea	Tissues not readily available Graft failure Difficult to achieve target refractive power Delays amblyopia therapy
Intraocular lens	Immediate and constant visual input Maximum compliance with amblyopia therapy Minimum anisometropia, which is especially important in unilateral cataract	Frequent changes of residual refractive error Correct sizing still a problem in severe microphthalmic eyes Concern for long-term safety of IOL High incidence of visual axis opacification in infantile eyes

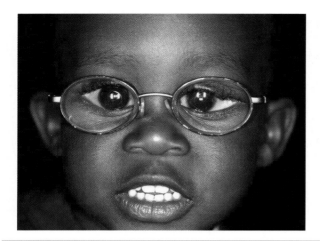

FIGURE 49-1. This 3-year-old boy is bilaterally aphakic and has aphakic glaucoma controlled with topical medications. He is shown wearing aphakic spectacles.

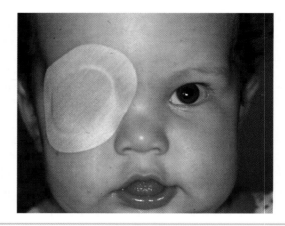

FIGURE 49-2. A 6-month-old child with a unilateral cataract operated on at 2 weeks of age. Patching (OD) and a Silsoft contact lens (OS) are tolerated well.

secondary IOL, strabismus surgery), the incidence of total reoperations was similar in the two groups.[20]

Lambert et al.[21] recently published the results of their study ascertaining whether American Association for Pediatric Ophthalmology and Strabismus (AAPOS) members have equipoise regarding contact lens and IOL implantation for unilateral congenital cataract. During 1997 survey of AAPOS members, only 4% had implanted an IOL in an infant <7 months old with a unilateral congenital cataract. Silsoft (Bausch & Lomb, Rochester, NY, USA) contact lens correction was the preferred treatment choice for 84% of the respondents. In 2001, 21% of the respondents had implanted an IOL in an infant. On a scale of from 1 to 10, with 1 strongly favoring an IOL implant and 10 strongly favoring a contact lens, the median score was 7.5. The main concerns about IOL implantation were poor predictability of power changes, postoperative complications, inflammation, and technical difficulty of surgery. The main

concerns about contact lens correction were poor compliance, high lens loss rate, high cost, and keratitis. The authors concluded that although most AAPOS members still favor contact lens correction after cataract surgery for a unilateral congenital cataract in infants, five times as many had implanted an IOL in an infant in 2001 compared with the number in 1997. Parents were almost equally divided in their preference for IOL implant versus contact lens correction.

How Pediatric Contact Lens Practice Differs from That in the Adult

Pediatric contact lens practice is quite challenging, as well as different from adult lens practice. The dissimilarities arise mainly from the anatomical differences between the pediatric and the adult eye. The conjunctival fornix is shallower, the globe is smaller, and the sclera has a stepper curvature than in the adult eye. The infant cornea is smaller and steeper and the vault is less than in the adult cornea. The continuously changing refraction in pediatric eyes is primarily related to the increasing axial length, and progressive corneal flattening provides an additional challenge. Repeated insertion and removal of a contact lens can be psychologically traumatic to a child as well as to the parents.

Although there are differences between pediatric and adult contact lens practice, there are also some similarities between the two. The similarities include the basic fitting principles used to obtain well-fitted lenses and the physiological requirements of the cornea and anterior segment. The optical lens characteristics and materials are essentially the same regardless of the age of the person wearing the lens. Lens care techniques are identical for children and adults, although the method of handling the lens is modified for the pediatric patient.

▶ **TABLE 49-4** **Factors to Consider When Selecting a Frame for Pediatric Eyes**

- The *smallest* frame is the best choice for children.
- A frame with *strong color* will help direct attention to the frames and away from the lens.
- The *bridge of the frame* should carefully conform in shape to that of the child. If the bridge of the frame is too high, the child's nose will appear longer. A lower bridge will make the child's nose appear shorter.
- *Cable temples* (earpieces) that wrap around the back of the ear are recommended. This will help to keep heavier lenses positioned correctly in front of the child's eyes. Temples should not extend past the ear lobe.
- *Spring hinges* will absorb a lot of abuse and are considered a must-have for children.

▶ **TABLE 49-5** Arguments For and Against Various Contact Lens Material

	Arguments For	*Arguments Against*
PMMA	Available in a wide range of prescriptions Can be customized to power and base curve Comparatively inexpensive Good optical performance (in most cases neutralizing astigmatic and spherical components of refractive error) More durable and easy to handle.	Must be removed daily Some initial discomfort Occasional lens breakage and loss
Soft material	Comfort	Frequent and rapid lens loss Poor correction of residual refractive astigmatism Difficulty in lens insertion
Silicone	Superior corneal oxygenation Easy to handle, durable Relatively low loss rate Can be fitted using either ocular measurements or trial techniques.	High cost Inability to obtain full optical correction because available in limited powers

PMMA, polymethylmethacrylate.

Contact Lens Choices

There are three types of contact lens: the hard lens (including polymethylmethacrylate [PMMA] lens and rigid gas-permeable lens), the hydrogel extended-wear or daily-wear lens, and the silicone lens.[22–24] Advantages and disadvantages of various contact lens materials are listed in Table 49-5.[25] Some commercially available, flexible contact lenses above +20 D are compared in Table 49-6.

The silicone contact lens (Fig. 49-3) combines the best features of hard and soft lenses. They are reported to mask up to +2 D of astigmatism. Lens movement with blinking is the most critical and important factor for evaluating fitting characteristics. If too much movement is seen, a steeper lens can be tried. If little or no movement is seen, a flatter lens is indicated. Silsoft Super-Plus Kids, manufactured by Bausch and Lomb (Silsoft), are available in base curve 7.5 mm (45.0 D) to 8.3 mm (40.62 D) in 0.2-mm steps. The Silsoft lens can be fitted on OR near the flat keratometry reading. Most children <1 year old can be fitted with a lens of 7.5-mm (45 D) base curve in the 11.3 mm diameter. Older children are most often fit with a base curve

of 7.7 mm. A fluorescein pattern may be used during the fitting sequence as needed. Lens power varies from 12 to 20 D (in 1-D increments) and 23 to 32 D (in 3-D increments). Aasuri et al.,[24] from India, reported that these lenses are safe, provide satisfactory optical correction, and are easy to handle. The limited availability of contact lenses and the financial cost (ca. US $150/unit) associated with frequent lens replacement are limitations to contact lens use in developing countries. A disadvantage of silicone contact lenses in older children and adults is that they may be uncomfortable initially. Other disadvantages are their hydrophobicity and adhesion effects. Since infants have more watery tear layers and produce less mucus, the drying and discomfort of the silicone elastomer lens, as noted with adult wearers, are not as common with children. Silicone lenses also have a tendency to acquire deposits when drying, which can alter the lens surface characteristics.

If a silsoft contact lens cannot be worn by a child, a rigid gas permeable lens can be tried. Base curve should be selected 1 to 1.5 mm steeper than flattest keratometry reading (infantile aphakia treatment study protocol). Lens power should be determined by retinoscopy over the

▶ **TABLE 49-6** Manufacturers of Flexible Contact Lenses with Power >20 D

Manufacturer	*Lens Name*	*Material*	*Available Powers (D)*
Bausch & Lomb	Silsoft	Silicone elastomer	+12 to +32
Flexlens	Flexlens	45% Hydrogel, water	−50 to +50
Optech	Fre-flex	55% Hydrogel, water	−40 to +40
Strieter	Accugel	47% Hydrogel, water	+21 to +36
Vision Tech	VT-79 pediatric aphakic	79% Hydrogel, water	+20 to +35
	VT-45 pediatric aphakic	45% Hydrogel, water	+20 to +35

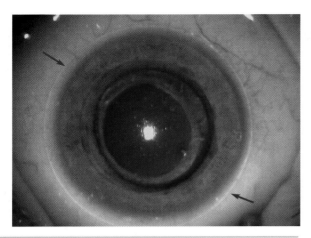

FIGURE 49-3. A silicone contact lens in pediatric aphakia.

diagnostic lens. The diagnostic set of lenses used is based on a formula of base curve radius plus 1.3 mm equals the lens diameter.

Daily-Wear Versus Extended-Wear Lenses

Most clinicians and parents agree that extended-wear contact lens would be ideal for children with aphakia. However, owing to the increased incidence of severe complications (e.g., acute red eye reaction, giant papillary conjunctivitis, neovascularization, abrasion, infective keratitis) associated with the use of some designs and materials for extended-wear lenses, daily wear is instead recommended for all lens types, for pediatric patients >6 years old. However, the majority of pediatric ophthalmologists in the United States use SilSoft extended-wear lenses for children <6 years old, with a high degree of safety and rewarding results.

Contact Lens Fitting Techniques

Most children are initially examined under anesthesia. If the practitioner decides to fit the contact lenses in the office, the child can be seated on the caregiver's lap for the examination. An examination includes an external examination, corneal measurements, examination of the media and retina, careful accurate keratometry (especially if hard lenses are going to be fitted), and refraction by retinoscopy. Although keratometry can be revealing in many cases, it usually is not essential for fitting silicone soft contact lenses. Final contact power for the infant and young child is most easily determined by retinoscopy through trial contact lenses. If the child is to undergo cataract surgery, initial diameter and power of the contact lens are selected by knowledge of age norms or from a keratometry reading and, perhaps, axial length measurements made dur-

ing surgery. Infants who are aphakic should be fitted with contact lenses preferably immediately after the cataract surgery. Otherwise, they should be fitted as early in the postoperative course as possible. Strict hygiene is important for any contact lens use, but it is especially important with recent surgery.

For hard lens fitting, a set of trial lenses (all 10 mm in diameter) with base curves varying from 7.2 to 8.2 mm at 0.1-mm increments is often used. For hard lenses, a study of the fluorescein pattern is made and the lenses changed if indicated. Fluorescein evaluation with these template lenses in situ allows an experienced observer to determine the lens that best aligns with the underlying cornea. A "steep" lens produces distinct central pooling of fluorescent tears, perhaps with bubbles; a "flat" lens produces an absence of fluorescence centrally; and a lens in alignment with the corneal curvature produces a uniform distribution of the dye. The major problem with fitting young children is stability. To overcome displacement due to the small size of the eye and high tonicity of the lids, it is necessary to fit a lens that is both tight and relatively large in comparison with the fitting criteria for an adult eye. In one report, it was found necessary to fit as steep as 0.1 mm flatter than the flattest corneal reading, with an overall diameter 2–3 mm greater than the horizontal diameter.[26]

Contact Lens Insertion and Removal

The success of the contact lens fitting, and ultimately of the child's vision correction, often depends on the training and understanding of the parents or caregivers who will be responsible for the child's eyes and lenses. The parent who is going to take the most responsibility for the lens-wearing schedule during insertion (Fig. 49-4), removal (Fig. 49-5), storage, and disinfections should be encouraged to attend the clinics as much as possible to learn these techniques and to develop a relationship with the practitioner, thus aiding communication should any problems arise in the future. From the outset, parents should always be present and included in such procedures as insertion and removal of a contact lens. In this way, they will learn about the handling of the contact lens and their responsibilities toward the success of their child's contact lens treatment. Each step should be practiced in the office, under supervision. It is the physician's responsibility not only to make sure the parents learn to apply, remove, and care for the lenses, but also to help them make these activities a simple daily or weekly routine. Furthermore, it is the parents who must scrutinize the child daily and report any change at the earliest possible moment. Written instructions regarding the fundamentals of hygiene, handling, insertion, and removal of the lenses should be given to reinforce oral instructions. The clinician should tell the parents what to observe in terms of a steep (nonmoving) lens, which may induce injection or a sectorial or complete compression "ring"

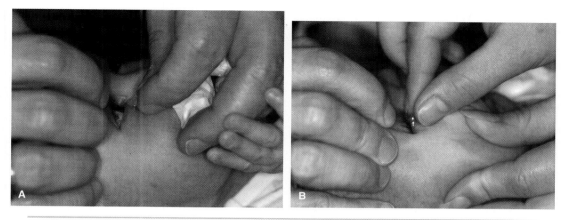

FIGURE 49-4. Insertion of contact lens. **A.** Teaching mom to insert a silicone contact lens. **B.** Parent successfully inserts a silicone contact lens in the office.

indentation in the sclera (e.g., when using the hydrogel lens); or a loose lens, which can produce some edge-lift, increased lens excursions, and poor centering. The parents should also be told that the child's eye should "quiet" quickly after contact lens insertion; but if the child continues to cry for more than about 5 min, the lens may be torn, chipped, cracked, or inside-out, or there may be a foreign body underneath it. If the child continues to be uncomfortable, the lens should be removed and inspected.

When the clinician is convinced that the parents can adequately care for the lenses, they can be given a lens-wearing schedule for the child and a return appointment. Wearing time for daily wear lenses is rapidly increased to all waking hours if no particular problems are encountered. Parents should be certain that the lenses are always adequately cleaned and disinfected before reinsertion. For silicone lenses, weekly removal for cleaning is usually recommended.

Topical anesthetics are never used to facilitate either the evaluation of the fitting of contact lenses or the teaching of *insertion and removal techniques.* The greatest obstacle to the insertion of a lens is the child's fear. Topical anesthetics have little effect on this critical issue, and they also give a false impression as to what the child will experience when the lenses are inserted at home. Some suggestions follow.

- *When the patient is <2 years of age.* Insertion in this age group is easily managed, as there is a minimum of struggle. The practitioner should pull up the baby's upper lid and insert the lens under it, then pull the lower lid over the lower edge of the lens. The lens should then be checked to ensure that it has not folded during insertion.

   To remove silicone or soft contact lenses in a child, the lids are pulled apart as much as possible and gentle pressure is put on the superior and inferior lens edges; this produces an interruption of the suction and allows the lens to be lifted out by the lids. If there is struggling, the lids may be squeezed tightly shut and this may

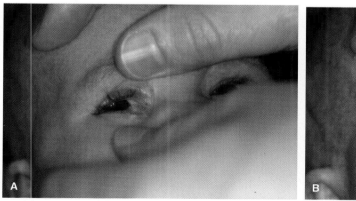
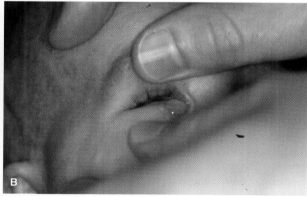

FIGURE 49-5. Removing a silicone contact lens. **A.** The eyelids are gently pulled apart. **B.** Pressure is applied to the superior and inferior lens edge as the thumbs are brought together. The lens lifts out onto the skin.

actually help ejection of the lens as the practitioner pulls the lids apart. Once the child is old enough, the lens can be pinched off in the conventional way.

- *When the patient is between 2 and 5 years of age.* Insertion may be easier if the child is laid on a bed. With time, no holding is required, and eventually the lenses can be inserted while the child is sitting in the chair. To remove the lenses, the same method as described for younger children can be used, although sometimes holding the head may be necessary.
- *When the patient is >5 years old.* It may be possible to encourage the children to begin to manage insertion and removal themselves. Insertion is not always easily achieved at this age, so initially help is required from parents to hold the lids or guide the child's finger. Once children have gained confidence and appreciate the advantages of being independent, their insertion technique improves, enabling them to handle the lenses without any assistance. To remove the lenses, children may pinch off soft contact lenses.

Contact Lens Follow-up

Care of the patient after the contact lenses are fitted is a shared responsibility between the parent or caregiver and the practitioner. Questions should be directed at the care regimen: Have there been any difficulties handling the lens since the last visit? Lens loss? Any irritation of the eyes? Was any visual progress observed. Excessive blinking, photophobia, tearing, conjunctival injection, or discharge may indicate the possible presence of conjunctival or corneal pathology. Careful slit-lamp examination after contact lens removal, with and without fluorescein staining, is essential. Parents should be queried regarding any untoward reaction. Lens-wearing time is gradually increased, starting with a few hours at first. Follow-up keratometry should be practiced by anyone fitting contact lenses. The corneal radius and diameter change very rapidly over the first few years. The possibility therefore exists that if an extended-wear lens is deliberately fitted tight and is left in situ for too long, the cornea will grow beneath it and the fit will become tighter still, which can lead to complications. Such a tight lens will cause corneal edema and conjuctival chemosis and, in turn, cause embarrassment of the limbal capillaries. If a regular follow-up pattern is maintained, little difficulty will arise.

As the eye grows, the aphakic power requirements will decrease. Also, the cornea changes rapidly in children, increasing in overall diameter and decreasing in radius of curvature. Thus the importance of frequent early visits cannot be overemphasized. When corneal changes are found, wearing of the lens should be stopped and keratometric measurements taken weekly, until the values stabilize. Measurements that stabilize at a curvature other than the original will require refitting of the lens. Sometimes,

minor corrections are possible when using hard contact lenses but not when using soft lenses.

Considerations and Complications of Contact Lenses

- *Lens Loss.* Morris[15] reported an average loss of 9.0 lenses in the first year and 2.4 lenses each year thereafter. The major loss was by ages 1 to 2 years. Babies only a few months of age can easily rub the lenses out during sleep. Jacobs[26] reported that one mother even attempted to recover a lens from an infant who was seen to remove it and then swallow it; fortunately or unfortunately, her efforts were unrewarded. For continued optical correction to prevent amblyopia, a spare set of lenses should always be available through the clinic, and with the parents. An up-to-date pair of spectacles must be available in case of contact lens loss or any other contact lens problems. Once on a daily-wear schedule, the problem of loss decreases, and eventually lens deterioration becomes the major cause of lens replacement, occurring approximately every 6 months.
- *Noncompliance.* Noncompliance of both the parents and the child is the major obstacle in contact lens practice. Loss of contact lenses, conjunctival erythema, and poor lens fit are reasons for noncompliance in pediatric patients. Assaf et al.[27] reported that only 44% of children in Saudi Arabia with unilateral aphakia were wearing their contact lens when they returned for follow-up (quoted in Ref. 21). Poor compliance in children with unilateral aphakia is multifactorial, but contributing factors include the high cost of contact lenses, the inability of children to discern a visual benefit from contact lens use if the fellow eye has normal vision, and the difficulty of caregivers inserting and removing contact lenses in a small child.[21]
- *Infection.* Minor infections can occur from time to time, especially if the child is using soft lens extended-wear contacts. The parents must always be carefully alerted to the removal of a lens if they see the slightest redness of the bulbar conjunctiva. If at this stage they are unable to handle the lens, then they must get ophthalmic help. If the infant is bilaterally aphakic, removal of both lenses is advisable, as amblyopia can quickly develop in the eye without the lens. Aphakic spectacles should then be worn until refitting of the contact lenses.
- *Corneal vascularization.* Due to various degrees of anoxia in soft contact lens wearers, corneal vascularization can occasionally be observed with contact lens use. In such a situation, a child using extended-wear lenses must be refitted with daily-wear lenses, or a child using daily-wear soft lenses, with hard gas-permeable lenses. Otherwise, spectacles are often the preferred choice. This is also true for contact lens–induced giant

papillary conjunctivitis. Problems with contact lens use that are more commonly encountered in patients from a developing country (i.e., patients who often come from rural communities with poor socioeconomic and educational backgrounds) include infectious keratitis, corneal vascularization, hypoxic corneal ulceration, and red eye without ulcerations.

- *Power changes.* Frequent follow-up is needed, as the power changes occur very rapidly. The younger the child, the more frequent the follow-up.
- *Parental stress.* Psychological stress (to parents, caregivers, or patient) is one of the most important obstacles when prescribing contact lens to children. However, Ma et al.[28] recently reported that contact lenses seemed to be well tolerated by most patients, as assessed by caregivers. Although initial resistance to contact lens use is high, this decreases with time. Relative to other events in the treatment of pediatric cataracts, contact lens use is not a major stressor for most caregivers and patients.

EPIKERATOPHAKIA

Epikeratophakia is a potentially reversible corneal surgical procedure that can correct residual aphakia. With *epi [on top of] kerato [cornea] phakia [lens]*, a donor cornea is lathed, shaped, and sterilized and then sewn on top of the cornea.[8,29–31] Graft failure and other problems currently make it a less than optimal approach for pediatric aphakia correction. The only theoretical indication for this procedure is probably a patient with unilateral aphakia who cannot have an IOL implant (because of serious intraocular inflammation, uveitis) and is intolerant of contact lenses.

SUMMARY

In cases in which it is not feasible to implant an IOL, contact lenses can be the first line of treatment, at least in unilateral cases. However, in bilateral cases, aphakic glasses are still a reasonable option. When patients are not compliant with either aphakic eyeglasses or contact lenses, it may be necessary to implant a secondary IOL (see Chapter 29).

REFERENCES

1. Wilson ME. Management of aphakia in childhood. *Focal Points Am Acad Ophthalmol* 1999:1–18.
2. Wilson ME, Bluestein EC, Wang XH. Current trends in the use of intraocular lenses in children. *J Cataract Refract Surg* 1994;20:579–583.
3. Wilson ME. Intraocular lens implantation: Has it become the standard of care for children? *Ophthalmology* 1996;103:1719–1720.
4. Wilson Jr ME, Bartholomew LR, Trivedi RH. Pediatric cataract surgery and intraocular lens implantation: Practice preferences of the 2001 ASCRS and AAPOS memberships. *J Cataract Refract Surg* 2003;29:1811–1820.
5. Dutton JJ. Visual rehabilitation of aphakic children. *Surv Ophthalmol* 1990;34:365.
6. Baker JD. Visual rehabilitation of aphakic children. II. Contact lenses. *Surv Ophthalmol* 1990;34:366–371.
7. Hiles DA. Visual rehabilitation of aphakic children. III. Intraocular lenses. *Surv Ophthalmol* 1990;34:371–379.
8. Morgan KS. Visual rehabilitation of aphakic children. IV. Epikeratophakia. *Surv Ophthalmol* 1990;34:379–384.
9. Piippo LJ, Coats DK. Pediatric spectacle prescription. *Comp Ophthalmol Update* 2002;3:113–122.
10. Cho MH, Wild BW. Spectacles for children. In: Rosenbloom AA, Morgan MW, eds. *Principles and Practice of Pediatric Optometry.* Philadelphia: Lippincott, 1990:192–206.
11. Schramm KD. Pediatric cataracts: post-surgical eyewear options. In: MORIN formation, Winter ed., 2002. www.pgcfa.org/files/MORIN_02_FEB.pdf (page 3–4)
12. Stenson SM. Pediatric contact lenses. *Ophthalmol Clin North Am* 1996;9:129–136.
13. Halberg GP. Contact lenses for infants and children. In: Harley RD, ed. *Pediatric Ophthalmology.* 2nd ed. Philadelphia: W. B. Saunders, 1975:1280–1288.
14. Epstein RJ. Contact lenses for the correction of pediatric aphakia. In: *International Ophthalmology Clinics.* Boston, MA: Little, Brown, 1991:53–60.
15. Morris J. Pediatric contact lens practice. In: Barnard S, Edgar D, eds. *Pediatric Eye Care.* Cambridge, MA: Blackwell Science, 1995:312–323.
16. Weissman BA. Contact lenses for children. In: Rosenbloom AA, Morgan MW, eds. *Principles and Practice of Pediatric Optometry.* Philadelphia: Lippincott, 1990:207–218.
17. Neumann D, Weissman BA. Use of contact lenses in infants. In: Isenberg SJ, ed. *The Eye in Infancy.* 2nd ed. St. Louis, MO: Mosby, XXXX:374–379.
18. Brown SM, Archer S, Del Monte MA. Stereopsis and binocular vision after surgery for unilateral infantile cataract. *J AAPOS* 1999;3:109–113.
19. Lambert SR, Lynn M, Drews-Botsch C, et al. A comparison of grating visual acuity, strabismus, and reoperation outcomes among children with aphakia and pseudophakia after unilateral cataract surgery during the first six months of life. *J AAPOS* 2001;5:70–75.
20. Trivedi RH, Wilson ME, Bartholomew LR, et al. Opacification of the visual axis after cataract surgery and single acrylic intraocular lens implantation in the first year-of-life. *J AAPOS* 2004;8:156–164.
21. Lambert SR, Lynn M, Drews-Botsch C, et al. Intraocular lens implantation during infancy: perceptions of parents and the American Association for Pediatric Ophthalmology and Strabismus members. *J AAPOS* 2003;7:400–405.
22. Pe'er J, Rose L, Cohen E, BenEzra D. Hard and soft contact lens fitting in infants. *CLAO J* 1987;13:46–49.
23. McQuaid K, Young TL. Rigid gas permeable contact lens changes in the aphakic infant. *CLAO J* 1998;24:36–40.
24. Aasuri MK, Venkata N, Preetam P, Rao NT. Management of pediatric aphakia with silsoft contact lenses. *CLAO J* 1999;25:209–212.
25. Jacobs DS. The best contact lens for baby. In: Jakobiec FA, ed. *International Ophthalmology Clinics.* Boston, MA: Little, Brown, 1991:173–179.
26. Ellis P. The use of permanent wear contact lenses on young aphakic children. *Contact Lens J* 1977;5:23.
27. Assaf AA, Wiggins R, Engel K, Senft S. Compliance with prescribed optical correction in cases of monocular aphakia in children. *Saudi J Ophthalmol* 1994;8:15–22.
28. Ma JJ, Morad Y, Mau E, et al. Contact lenses for the treatment of pediatric cataracts. *Ophthalmology* 2003;110:299–305.
29. Morgan KS, McDonald MB, Hiles DA, et al. The nationwide study of epikeratophakia for aphakia in children. *Am J Ophthalmol* 1987;103:366–374.
30. Morgan KS, McDonald MB, Hiles DA, et al. The nationwide study of epikeratophakia for aphakia in older children. *Ophthalmology* 1988;95:526–532.
31. Uusitalo RJ, Uusitalo HM. Long-term follow-up of pediatric epikeratophakia. *J Refract Surg* 1997;13:45–54.

Assessment of Visual Functions (Acuity, Contrast Sensitivity) and Amblyopia Management

Catherine M. Suttle and Suresh K. Pandey

The accurate and reliable assessment of visual function in infants and young children is important for ensuring evaluation and optimal visual rehabilitation after pediatric cataract surgery. Visual acuity is the aspect of visual function most commonly assessed clinically and can be measured in infants and children using appropriate techniques. Acuity measurements obtained using different techniques may show considerable disagreement and may mislead when monitoring acuity development. With any technique, performance of a visual assessment in an infant or young child requires flexibility in approach.

A communication barrier exists between the ophthalmologist and very young patients. With different methods and levels of communication, the ophthalmologist and infant patient are not easily able to understand each other. It is particularly important to assess visual function in young patients because, during infancy and childhood, the visual system is undergoing developmental changes that depend on the quality of visual input. Amblyopia may be treated within the first few years of life, when the visual system is sufficiently plastic to respond to modifications in visual input, such as partial or total occlusion therapy. Beyond this period, treatment becomes increasingly difficult.[1] Thus, it is essential to assess visual function effectively for all patients, and particularly those with altered visual input following cataract implant surgery and subsequent vision therapy.

In this chapter, we present an overview of some of the techniques used in pediatric visual assessment. We also briefly discuss contrast sensitivity and amblyopia management.

VISUAL FUNCTION ASSESSMENT

Visual Acuity

As mentioned previously, visual acuity is the measure of visual function most commonly used by eye care practitioners in practice. In children and infants, acuity should be measured monocularly if possible, since interocular differences, such as those arising in anisometropic or strabismic amblyopia, may be masked by binocular visual function assessment. Two types of visual acuity, resolution and recognition acuity, are widely measured in clinic. Resolution acuity provides an indication of the patient's ability to resolve the spatial separation of contrasting visual stimuli (such as lines on a grating acuity test) while recognition acuity indicates ability not only to resolve the spatial elements of the stimulus, but also to perceive the elements as a whole, and in many cases to recognize the shape formed by the elements (such as a letter).[2] A recognition acuity task is relatively complex, since it requires knowledge of the stimulus shape and/or ability to match the shape, in addition to the ability to communicate in some way that the shape is recognized. Communication may be verbal (e.g., reading out letters on a Snellen chart as they are read) or by pointing (to a matching shape, such as Sheridan-Gardner letters).

Symbol and Letter Recognition

One of the most important aspects of the pediatric eye examination is the assessment of visual acuity in each eye. Letter acuity measurement is normally possible in children from about 5 years of age. In younger children (from about 3 years), recognition acuity may be assessed using symbols.[3] Depending on age and level of understanding, the child may be asked to name the symbol or to point to an identical symbol on a card he or she is holding.

LEA symbols and the New York Lighthouse Acuity Test,[4] for example, offer this means of acuity assessment. The practitioner presents simple symbols (such as a circle or an apple) from a viewing distance of 3 m and the child is asked to name the symbol or to point at the corresponding symbol on the card he or she is holding. Another recognition acuity test for children, Glasgow acuity cards, involves the presentation of letters rather than symbols but is designed for use with children.[5] In a way similar to the Bailey–Lovie test chart,[6] Glasgow cards minimize limitations of the Snellen test chart format by ensuring progression of letter size in equal steps, equivalent letter spacing on each line, and an equal number of letters per line. In addition, Glasgow cards and LEA symbols have a number of features specifically aimed at testing acuity in children. For example, letters on Glasgow cards are horizontally symmetrical, to minimize confusion in younger children. In addition, LEA symbols and Glasgow cards are designed for use at a viewing distance of 3 m, aimed at increasing cooperation in poorly motivated children.

When high-contrast symbols or letters (optotypes) are presented in isolation, recognition acuity is higher than when presented in a crowded format, flanked by other optotypes.[7–9] This acuity difference is known as the crowding phenomenon and is thought to be due to a number of factors, including contour interaction and fixation instability. Crowding reduces recognition acuity significantly, when stimuli are at high contrast (as is the case for most letter and symbol charts) but at low contrast the effect of crowding is negligible.[9] Crowding also depends on the separation of adjacent optotypes, having little or no effect when separation is greater than 1 optotype diameter and reaching a maximum at about 0.4-diameter separation.[7–9] There is some disagreement on the question of whether crowding is a reliable tool in the diagnosis and assessment of amblyopia.[10]

The Preferential Looking Technique

The preferential looking (PL) technique is commonly used in the form of acuity cards, such as Keeler and Teller cards. A black-and-white grating pattern is presented on one half (left or right) of a gray card and the other half is a uniform gray, of the same space-average luminance as the pattern. This means that, if the infant is unable to discriminate the black-and-white elements of the pattern, the patterned region will appear identical to the uniform region, with the same luminance level. If the infant observer is able to distinguish the pattern, he or she will tend to look toward it, in preference to the plain region.[11] One disadvantage of printed acuity cards is that the pattern may not be well

blended into the uniform surround. As a result, the pattern stops abruptly at its edge. In this case, it is possible that the visual system may be able to detect the edge but not the pattern.[12] In an attempt to resolve this problem, printed acuity cards now have an identical band around the patterned region and the corresponding region of the uniform half, so that the abrupt transition at the edge will be seen on both halves of the card. In this case, the observer is not able to distinguish the patterned half on the basis of the edge and discrimination must be based on the pattern itself.

The PL stimulus may also be computer generated and presented on a cathode ray tube (CRT) monitor. In this case, the stimulus appearance is very similar to that of the cards described above, with a pattern on one half of the screen and a luminance-matched uniform field on the other half. One advantage of computer presentation is that a wide range of stimulus parameters (spatial frequency, contrast, etc.) may be specified precisely and the edges of the patterned stimulus may be blended with the uniform surround. Computer presentation is widely used in research on infant visual function, because it allows excellent control of stimulus specifications. However, a computerized system of PL stimulus presentation may not be feasible for use clinically, perhaps due to cost and the difficulties involved in accurate calibration of such a system. Thus, while a set of printed PL cards can be an expensive item for a nonspecialist practice, cards are more commonly used than computerized presentation in clinical practice.

Whether stimulus presentation is by card or CRT monitor, the PL technique requires an adult observer to note the infant's behavioral responses to the stimulus presentation. The adult is usually positioned out of the infant's sight during presentation, behind the acuity card or a screen, and views the infant through a peephole positioned midway between the pattern and the uniform field. The adult is unaware of the position of the pattern, so that judgment is not biased. The adult may use any aspect of the infant's behavior to determine whether the pattern was perceived.

For example, infants may turn their head and/or eyes toward the pattern. Alternatively, they may spend more time looking at the pattern than at the uniform field. Each infant will respond in a different way, and the adult observer initially uses a few trial presentations of stimuli that the infant is expected to be able to discriminate, to determine which aspect of the infant's behavior most closely relates to his or her perception of the pattern. For this purpose, feedback may be provided to inform the adult whether the judged behavior corresponds with the position of the pattern. For example, the adult may have judged that the infant is looking to the left and subsequently learns that the pattern appeared on that side. If the infant was attentive and the pattern was within the infant's expected visual range, this result would help to confirm that the adult had used appropriate behavioral cues to judge the infant's preference.

The PL technique may be used in a forced-choice paradigm, in which case the procedure is known as forced-choice PL.[13] The forced-choice element reflects the fact that when the infant shows no preference, the adult must guess where the stimulus was presented on the display. As a result, if only two options are presented (for example, left and right) the recorded response will be correct on approximately 50% of presentations when the infant is unable to discriminate the pattern and, thus, shows no preference. If an infant appears to prefer the patterned stimulus on most of the presentations, this behavior may be accepted as an indication that the pattern is discriminated by the infant, implying function of the visual pathway from retina to visual cortex and beyond to regions of the brain responsible for a motor response (eye or head turn, for example).

If the infant shows no preference for the pattern, there are at least three possibilities. First, the infant may be unmotivated or bored with the procedure so that when the pattern is presented, even if the infant is able to distinguish it, he or she may not choose to look toward it. Perhaps the infant is preoccupied with thoughts of feeding, sleeping, or simply wanting a change of activity. Second, a lack of preference for the pattern may indicate a genuine inability to distinguish the pattern. In this case, the left and right halves of the presentation will appear identical to the infant because the pattern is designed with the same average luminance and color as the uniform region. Third, it is feasible that the visual pathway is functioning perfectly well, allowing the infant to discriminate the pattern, but that motor regions of the brain or connections with those regions are immature, preventing the infant from making an appropriate behavioral response.

As explained above, the PL technique requires attention from the young observer. As infants develop, they become increasingly interested in and curious about their environment. The simple grating stimulus may be sufficient to maintain the attention of most infants during the first year of life but beyond this age a more interesting stimulus and task may be required. The Cardiff Acuity test was introduced with the intention of providing a more engaging stimulus for older infants and young children.[14] Instead of a grating pattern, the stimuli consist of simple, recognizable shapes. The stimuli are known as "vanishing optotypes," because the shapes disappear at the observer's resolution limit. The shape is drawn as a white outline with a black boundary. The average luminance of this black–white outline is identical to that of the uniform (gray) surround, so that the shape is not distinguishable from the surround beyond the observer's resolution limit. This test is used in a forced-choice PL paradigm and children may be encouraged to point toward the pattern or to name the shape if they can. The adult observer's judgment must be based on the child's behavioral response (for example, eye movement or head turn) to maintain a consistent procedure within and between patients.

Visual Electrophysiology

Function of the visual system may be assessed using electrophysiological techniques, such as the electroretinogram (ERG) to assess retinal function and the visual evoked potential (VEP) to assess function of the retino-cortical visual pathway. The VEP is affected by optical abnormalities, such as cataract, and by abnormal visual pathway function such as amblyopia. The VEP is a useful means of visual assessment in infants and children, because it is an objective technique, and thus overcomes much of the communication barrier discussed earlier. The VEP is recorded at the scalp surface and reflects activity of a large number of cortical neurons in the vicinity of the recording site. The VEP will also depend, to some extent, on the intervening tissues. Skull and skin tissues are interposed between the cortical source of the electrical activity and the electrode. In infants, a fontanelle exists at the skull region underlying the typical VEP recording site. This means that there is probably a lower signal impedance in early infancy than in later infancy (as the fontanelle closes) or in adults. It is possible that a signal may be apparent in early infancy but diminish or even disappear at a later stage in development.[15] While this type of change may reflect a higher signal impedance due to increased thickness of intervening (skull) tissue, it could also have one of at least two other causes. First, it could reflect a number of cortical developmental changes, such as a change in orientation of the striate cortex, with respect to the electrode position. Alternatively, it could mean that the signal no longer arises, implying that the visual pathway is less responsive to the stimulus in question than it was at an earlier age.

It should be noted that the VEP provides an indication of retino-cortical function, but for at least two reasons it may not accurately reflect the patient's visual perceptual ability. Firstly, the VEP does not involve neurons at high levels, such as those involved in recognition, so in the patient with a normal VEP it is possible that stimuli may be resolved but not recognized. Secondly, VEP electrodes are positioned according to skull landmarks, in an attempt to record from locations over specific regions of the occipital cortex. However, measured locations may not correspond well with the anticipated cortical regions, due to interindividual variation in cortical topography. Thus, the VEP is a very useful technique for fast, objective assessment of infant visual function but, as with other techniques, its limitations must be taken into account when analyzing VEP findings.

Optokinetic Nystagmus

Optokinetic nystagmus (OKN) is a series of repetitive eye movements, consisting of a slow pursuit phase, during which a moving target is smoothly tracked, followed by a fast saccadic phase, allowing refixation when the eye meets its limit of movement in the direction of pursuit. OKN is elicited by pattern movement. When used in clinical or research assessment of infant vision, the stimulus for OKN is usually a vertical grating pattern, moving laterally. For research purposes, the moving pattern may be presented on a CRT monitor. In the clinic, a simpler alternative is the Catford drum.

The Catford drum is a cylinder (drum) with a handle, which the practitioner can use to spin the drum. The drum is covered with a vertical grating pattern, so that when it spins, the gratings move to the right or left. The drum may be presented at a range of viewing distances so that a range of spatial frequencies may be presented, using gratings of constant width. One criticism of the Catford drum is that as the drum is presented at greater viewing distances, the region of visual field covered by the pattern is reduced and the likelihood of eliciting an OKN response may vary. Computerized presentation is preferable because the grating width (spatial frequency) may be altered without changing viewing distance. In addition, this method allows precise specification of a wide range of stimulus parameters, such as spatial frequency and contrast. In binocular viewing, infants demonstrate OKN eye movements from birth.

Acuity Measures Using Different Techniques

PL, OKN, and VEP estimates of visual acuity show considerable disagreement during the first few years of life, with VEP acuity up to four times higher than PL acuity in early infancy[16] and PL acuity two to three times higher than OKN acuity during the first 3 years.[17] The VEP–PL difference diminishes during development until, by the end of the first year, the two methods show reasonable agreement.[18] Agreement is also found in adulthood, when the VEP provides acuity estimates comparable to those provided by psychophysical techniques.[19]

CONTRAST SENSITIVITY

Visual acuity is a useful means of assessing one aspect of visual function, but it provides a very limited indication of the patient's visual perception. Most objects in the visual scene are not at the high black-white contrasts employed in visual acuity testing, and for this reason an assessment of the patient's ability to detect stimuli at lower contrasts is very useful. Tests such as low-contrast test pictures in infancy and childhood provide important information about the distance at which the child can see facial features. Contrast sensitivity measurements can first be performed using the Enhancement Game, i.e., single low-contrast sym-

bols. The Enhancement Game is designed for assessment and training of vision at intermediate contrast levels that are used in visual communication. The game is called Enhancement Game because it will "enhance" examiners' understanding of the quality of vision among young children. It also offers opportunities to enhance and train visual functions at low contrast levels in an amblyopic eye. At the age of 3.5 to 4 years children are able to respond to the usual line tests. Low-contrast optotype tests are either visual acuity charts at low-contrast or tests with one symbol size (10M) at different contrast levels. With both tests the measurement of low-contrast functioning is quick and easy. The measurement of two points on the contrast sensitivity curve requires only 1 to 2 minutes. As mentioned above, it is important to remember that visual acuity as such does not define the quality of form vision. Children with equal visual acuity at high contrast may have either normal, slightly lower, or very poor function at low contrast levels.

The Hiding Heidi (HH) test and the LEA low-contrast symbols are two commercially available charts of contrast sensitivity for children. In a study by Leat and Wegmann,[20] normal age-related data for both tests are reported, and validity compared with the Pelli–Robson chart is measured. Eighty-eight normally sighted children were divided into four age groups: 1 to <2.5, 2.5 to <4, 4 to <6, and 6 to <8 years. An adult group with normal vision and one with low vision also took part. Contrast sensitivity was measured with the HH test, the LEA symbols at 1 m and 28 cm, and the Pelli–Robson chart, as the child's ability permitted. Results of the study suggested that the HH test and the LEA symbols at 28 cm and 1 m all showed a floor effect; that is, most children of all ages correctly responded to the lowest contrast. The authors concluded that the LEA and HH charts could not measure a true contrast threshold for children with normal vision because of the floor effect. According to this study, the LEA symbols at 28 cm gave the most useful information, once recalibrated for contrast, and may be useful to predict the performance of children with low vision, when contrast sensitivity is likely to be compromised.

AMBLYOPIA AND ITS MANAGEMENT

The postoperative compliant occlusion therapy of the normal eye in cases of unilateral congenital, developmental, or traumatic cataract may be needed to reverse or prevent amblyopia in visually immature children. In children <9 to 11 years of age an appropriate spectacle correction should be prescribed after refraction/retinoscopic examination. Full-time patching is recommended over the eye with better vision for 1 week per year of age (e.g., 3 weeks for a 3-year-old child).[21] This is followed by repeated eye examinations. Pirate patches and patches worn over glasses are less effective than patches placed directly over the eye and adherent to the skin. If a patch causes local irritation, use of tincture of benzoin on the skin is suggested before applying the patch and use of warm water compresses on the patch before removal may be helpful. It is advisable for parents to continue patching until vision is equalized or shows no improvement after three compliant cycles of patching. If a recurrence of ambylopia is likely, then part-time patching is used to maintain improved vision.

If occlusion amblyopia develops, it is advisable to patch the opposite eye for a short period (e.g.,1 day per year of age) and perform repeated examinations. In children >11 years of age, a patching trial may be considered if patching has never been done.

Noncompliance with occlusion therapy appears to be a major barrier in achieving a satisfactory visual outcome during the treatment of amblyopia. Pharmacological penalization may be useful in children with amblyopia secondary to unilateral aphakia. However, since the aphakic (or pseudophakic) eye has lost normal accommodation, pharmacological penalization does not give the aphakic eye any advantage unless the normal eye is hyperopic. The role of levodopa–carbidopa in supplementing occlusion therapy in older children with strabismic or anisometropic amblyopia has been evaluated in a recent clinical study[22] of 40 amblyopic children (19 strabismic and 21 anisometropic). All children received an average dose of 1.86 mg/kg/day (1.33 to 2.36 mg/kg/day) of levodopa and carbidopa (4:1 ratio) or a placebo in three divided doses over a 4-week period, combined with full-time occlusion. The occlusion was continued for the study duration of 3 months. Results of this study suggested that the visual acuity of the nonamblyopic eye did not deteriorate during the study in either group. Contrast sensitivity decreased by 22 units in the levodopa group and increased by 53 units in the placebo group in the first month. The contrast sensitivity in the levodopa group recovered later, by the third month of follow-up. The authors concluded that, clinically, levodopa supplementation does not offer any advantage over occlusion alone. Moreover, the risk of occlusion amblyopia could increase with the use of drugs like levodopa that might affect the plasticity of the visual cortex.

In summary, the accurate assessment of visual function in pediatric age group is important as the visual system is undergoing developmental changes and depend on the quality of visual input. Amblyopia management should be carried out within the first few years of life, when the visual system is sufficiently plastic to respond to modifications in visual input.

ACKNOWLEDGMENT

Part of this chapter was adapted from the author's previously published article—Suttle, CM. Visual acuity assessment in infants and young children. *Clin Exp Optom* 2001;84:337–345, with permission.

REFERENCES

1. Daw NW. Critical periods and amblyopia. *Arch Ophthalmol* 1998; 116:502–505.
2. Suttle CM. Visual acuity assessment in infants and young children. *Clin Exp Optom* 2001:84:337–345.
3. Becker RH, Hubisch SH, Graf MH, Kaufmann H. Preliminary report: examination of young children with LEA symbols. *Strabismus* 2000;8:209–213.
4. Kastenbaum SM, Kepford KL, Holmstrom ET. Comparison of the STYCAR and Lighthouse acuity tests. *Am J Optom Physiol Opt* 1977;54:458–463.
5. McGraw PV, Winn B. Glasgow Acuity Cards: a new test for the measurement of letter acuity in children. *Ophthalmic Physiol Opt* 1993;13:400–404.
6. Bailey IL, Lovie JE. New design principles for visual acuity letter charts. *Am J Optom Physiol Opt* 1976;53:740–745.
7. Flom MC, Weymouth FW, Kahneman D. Visual resolution and contour interaction. *J Opt Soc Am A* 1963;53:1026–1032.
8. Giaschi DE, Regan D, Kraft SP, Kothe AC. Crowding and contrast in amblyopia. *Optom Vis Sci* 1993;70:192–197.
9. Simmers AJ, Gray LS, McGraw PV, Winn B. Contour interaction for high and low contrast optotypes in normal and amblyopic observers. *Ophthal Physiol Opt* 1999;19:253–260.
10. Stuart JA, Burian HM. A study of separation difficulty its relationship to visual acuity in normal and amblyopic eyes. *Am J Optom Physiol Opt* 1976;53:217–223.
11. Fantz R. Visual perception from birth as shown by pattern selectivity. *Ann NY Acad Sci* 1965;118:793–814.
12. Robinson J, Mosley MJ, Fielder AR. Grating acuity cards: spurious resolution and the 'edge artefact'. *Clin Vis Sci* 1988;3:285–288.
13. Teller DY. The forced-choice preferential looking procedure: a psychophysical technique for use with human infants. *Inf Behav Dev* 1979;2:135–153.
14. Woodhouse JM, Adoh TO, Oduwaiye KA, et al. New acuity test for toddlers. *Ophthalmic Physiol Opt* 1992;12:249–251.
15. Suttle CM, Anderson SJ, Harding GFA. Diminution of chromatic visual evoked responses at 3 months post-term age in human infants. *Invest Ophthalmol Vis Sci* 1997;38(Suppl):S62.
16. Sokol S, Moskowitz A, McCormack G. Infant VEP and preferential looking acuity measured with phase alternating gratings. *Invest Ophthalmol Vis Sci* 1992;33:3156–3161.
17. Lewis TL, Maurer D, Brent HP. Development of grating acuity in children treated for unilateral and bilateral congenital cataract. *Invest Ophthalmol Vis Sci* 1995;36:2080–2095.
18. Riddell PM, Ladenheim B, Mast J, et al. Comparison of measures of visual acuity in infants: Teller acuity cards and sweep visual evoked potentials. *Optom Vis Sci* 1997;74:702–707.
19. Norcia AM, Tyler CW, Hamer RD. Development of contrast sensitivity in the human infant. *Vis Res* 1990;30:1475–1486.
20. Leat SJ, Wegmann D. Clinical testing of contrast sensitivity in children: age-related norms and validity. *Optom Vis Sci* 2004;81:245–254.
21. Ram J, Pandey SK. Management of infantile cataracts. In: Dutta LC, ed., *Modern Ophthalmology*. New Delhi: Jaypee, 2005;333–339.
22. Bhartiya P, Sharma P, Biswas NR, et al. Levodopa-carbidopa with occlusion in older children with amblyopia. *J AAPOS* 2002;6:368–372.

Refractive Surgery

Chapter 51

Phakic Intraocular Lenses in Children

Daljit Singh and Ravijit Singh

Interest in pediatric use of phakic intraocular lens (IOL) implants has arisen because of the degree of success achieved with various designs in adults and the growing awareness that anisometropic amblyopia requires effective management at an early age.[1–14] Among the refractive errors, high hyperopia has the most visually crippling effect. Myopic patients are less suitable cases, since the length of the eyeball has not stabilized. Laser refractive surgery is another modality that can serve the purpose, but the results obtained in higher degrees of hyperopia are less than certain.

Phakic IOL is an invasive procedure requiring good surgical skill, with a risk of early and late complications, some of which can damage the sight. Every design of phakic IOL presses and erodes the uveal tissue. The space that it occupies keeps shrinking due to the growth of the crystalline lens. If a cataract develops (natural or phakic lens induced), the phakic lens has to be explanted. Lifelong, meticulous, regular follow-up is essential for early detection and management of problems that may arise.

There are three basic types of lenses, depending on the site of fixation: posterior chamber ciliary body sulcus-supported, anterior chamber angle supported, and anterior chamber iris fixated. *Ciliary body sulcus–supported* lenses had a lengthy trial in aphakia that finally shifted the fixation of the lens to in-the-bag. Such a shift is not possible in phakic posterior chamber lenses. The *chamber angle-support* problems are the same as in aphakic eyes. In the case of *iris-fixated* lenses, the only important question is whether the iris will tolerate fixation of the lens haptics

for a long time. This question has been answered in the affirmative by the extensive use of iris-fixated lenses in pediatric and adult aphakic eyes for 25 years and in adult phakic eyes for 17 years. Fyodorov first used a posterior chamber lenses in 1986, and Fechner implanted an iris-fixated lens in a myopic eye in 1986. We first used a phakic iris-claw lens in a hyperopic eye in 1987. In 1988 Baikoff and Joly reported using angle-supported lens for phakic eyes.

ANATOMY AND PATHOPHYSIOLOGY

The posterior chamber is a triangular space of about 65 μL that has zero depth at the pupillary margin, precisely where a phakic posterior chamber lens is the thickest. There is no way to avoid friction and pressure between the lens and structures like the crystalline lens, ciliary body, and posterior iris pigment layer. Design modification can reduce the pressure on one tissue at the cost of increasing it on another. A low vault increases friction to the lens, while a high vault increases the pressure on uveal tissues. Growth of the crystalline lens from 150 to 240 μL with age adds to the uncertainty.

The haptics of an angle-supported lens, although said to be supported by the scleral spur (which is situated at a depth), actually rest and press against the corneoscleral trabeculae, Schlemm canal, ciliary body in the angle recess, and, sometimes, blood vessels and nerves nearby. To remain in place, the lens has to be somewhat larger than the space in which it lodges, which means that pressure is unavoidable. A short lens always rotates. The lens haptics may disturb the segmental blood supply of the iris and cause atrophy that shows itself as progressive ovalization of the pupil. Uveitis–glaucoma–hyphema (UGH) and cystoid macular edema (CME) are other serious possibilities.

Iris-fixated lenses concern only iris tolerance and no other tissue. The phakic iris-fixated lens is vaulted and has a concave posterior optic surface. It is more or less a floating lens with two-point iris fixation. The edge does not rub against the iris. The capillaries and other blood vessels are anatomically well supported to resist blood–aqueous barrier breakdown, in comparison to the vessels of the ciliary body, which are highly permeable. However, the iris tissue in the claw of the lens does get permanently compressed. Soon after implantation this may cause a uveal reaction. The iris of dark eyes reacts more than that of blue eyes. Microtrauma and sometimes macrotrauma have an effect on the long-term outcome of phakic lens implantation. Obviously lenses that stretch the tissues to get fixated (posterior chamber and angle supported) transmit more trauma to the tissues than iris-fixated lenses. Rubbing and injuring the eyes are important issues with young patients.

PATIENT SUITABILITY

The main reason for phakic lens implantation in children with high refractive errors is to help prevent amblyopia or to be part of its management. It is preferable that the cycloplegic refractive error be stationary, which is usually the case with hyperopia. For unilateral high myopes, a phakic lens may be implanted if the patient does not tolerate a contact lens and laser refractive surgery or extracapsular cataract extraction with low-power lens implant is considered unsuitable for a particularly young patient. If the anterior chamber is <2.8 mm deep, the patient is not suitable for a phakic lens implant. In our experience high-hyperopia patients are most suitable for phakic lenses. A hyperopic lens is thinnest at the optic edge, which keeps it away from the corneal endothelium, hence it is safer than a myopic lens, which is thickest at the optic edge. It is important to judge whether the patient is intelligent enough to refrain from rubbing the operated eye and to understand that the operated eye demands special, gentle care always. The parents have a great role to play in these cases. A phakic lens is not advised in the presence of diabetes or arthritis. A strong family history of diabetes is a matter of serious concern. Laser refractive surgery, wherever possible and successful, does not require the degree of lifetime attention that a phakic IOL does.

PREOPERATIVE MANAGEMENT

Examination

1. *Age of the patient*. Our youngest patient to date was 7 years old.

2. *Corneal diameter*. A diameter <11 mm is not suitable for angle-supported or posterior chamber lenses. However, a diameter of 9 mm is acceptable for a special 3-mm optic and 5.5-mm maximum width iris-fixated lens.

3. *Depth of the anterior chamber*. A depth of ≥3 mm is desirable. A 2.7-mm depth is the lowest acceptable limit, which may not be crossed, especially for anterior chamber lenses.

4. *Pupil size*. The pupil is smaller in brown and black eyes. Blue eyes have larger pupils, thus requiring larger optic lenses.

5. *Axial length*. All hyperopic eyes are smaller than normal. Yet the depth of the anterior chamber may be ample. The shortest axial length in our patients to date was 18.5 mm.

6. *Refractive error*. Lenses of up to +16 D (diopters) are available. If the cornea is small and the refractive need is higher, a lens with a small, 3.5 mm optic may be used. Smaller optics mean thinner lenses.

7. *Corrected visual acuity and degree of amblyopia*. These parameters should be noted.

8. *Glaucoma*. Glaucoma should be excluded.

9. *Fundus*. The fundus should be normal. High hyperopes often complain of night vision problems.

Presurgical Preparation

Nd:YAG peripheral iridectomy (PI), preferably in two places, may be performed 2 weeks before the main surgery. Laser PI works poorly in brown and black eyes; manual PI should be done at the time of surgery in these cases. For lens power calculation, proprietary tables are available for different designs. A conjunctival swab for culture and sensitivity is taken. The pupil is contracted for anterior chamber lenses and dilated for posterior chamber lens implantation.

Anesthesia and Surgical Preparation

General anesthesia with intubations is mandatory. The skin is painted with povidine–10% iodine and the conjunctiva and lid margin are thoroughly cleaned with a 5% solution. Superior rectus and lower lid sutures are my favorites. I do not like a plastic drape and a speculum, as they seem to put pressure on the eyeball. The important thing is that the cilia should not get in the way of the instruments and the IOL.

STEPS OF PHAKIC LENS IMPLANTATION

Posterior Chamber Lens

Before surgery the pupil is fully dilated. One 0.6-mm sideport is made. It is needed to inject viscoelastic material into the anterior chamber. For a foldable posterior chamber phakic lens, a 3.2-mm clear corneal incision is made on the steep meridian. The lens is introduced with angled-suture forceps or an injector. It is positioned behind the iris on a horizontal axis with a cyclodialysis spatula. It is then centered. The viscoelastic material from the posterior and the anterior chamber is aspirated with a syringe or washed out by irrigation. The pupil is contracted with an intraocular miotic, be it 1% acetylcholine or 0.5% pilocarpine. The incision line is hydrated for closure.

Angle-Supported Lens

Before surgery the pupil is contracted. A 4- to 6-mm corneoscleral or a pocket incision is made at the steepest meridian. The anterior chamber is filled with viscoelastic material. A silicone Sheets glide is inserted and more viscoelastic is injected over the glide. The phakic lens is held with a utility forceps and the inferior haptic is slipped over the glide. When the elements of the inferior haptics reach the destination in the angle, the glide is gently removed. The upper haptics is pushed into the anterior chamber, and with a double-tip manipulator it is positioned under the posterior lip of the incision. The lens is rotated to a horizontal position with a Sinskey hook. If needed, a PI is performed. In brown and black eyes, it should be a fair-sized iridectomy. Make sure the pupil is round. If not, the haptic is pulled away from the angle and then released. The incision line is closed. The anterior chamber is cleared of viscoelastic. Gonioscopy is performed to make sure about the relation of the haptics and the peripheral iris.

Iris-Fixated Lens

An iris-fixated lens differs from the other two lenses in two important respects. The angle-supported and posterior chamber lenses are larger than the space in which they lodge. The lens is pushed into the destined space, where the tissues catch the lens, which creates the fixation. An iris-fixated lens is smaller than the space in which it is inserted. It has to be fixed to the tissue (iris) by the surgeon. Lens fixation is therefore considerably more difficult than with the other two lenses. The steps of operation are as follows.

1. For comfortable surgery, two sideports and one main incision are needed. The width of the main incision varies from 4.25 to 6 mm, depending on the optic size chosen for the lens.

2. The anterior chamber is filled with viscoelastic material.

3. The convexoconcave lens is slipped in with the convex side facing anteriorly. The floating lens is then rotated into a horizontal position.

4. For fixation of the lens, the basic principle is to hold the lens and steady it in desired central position. A thin forceps, cannula OR some other device is introduced from the side port, to enclavate the right point on the midperiphery

of the iris into the claw of the lens. The lens is held by the optic with a special forceps designed for the convexoconcave configuration of the optic. The sideport instrument may be a thin forceps, a thin probe, or a thin irrigating cannula. My preference is the latter device, through which viscoelastic material is injected as needed while it is being used to enclavate the iris into the claw. The device is simple. It consists of an irrigating handle, which has a small, 26-gauge cannula at one end and a silicone pipe at the other. The silicone pipe is in turn attached to a syringe that holds viscoelastic material. The assistant pushes the material on command, so that the anterior chamber remains deep all the time. The iris has to be fixed on both sides. If a good central position of the optic is not achieved, the claw can be opened by pushing the iris back out of the claw, then refixation done (Fig. 51-1A–G).

5. A manual PI is done inside the eye by lifting the midperipheral iris and cutting it with a scissors.

6. The remaining surgical steps should follow basic intraocular surgery principles.

POSTOPERATIVE MANAGEMENT

In every kind of lens implantation very careful postoperative care is of paramount importance.

1. Prevention of postoperative inflammation receives the greatest attention. There is no possibility of taking a chance by managing without oral and local steroids. The highest dose of prednisolone according to body weight is given for the first 3 days, reduced by half for the next 7 days, again reduced by half for 15 days, then reduced by half for yet another 15 days. Antibiotic–steroid ointment is applied at bedtime. After this period the surgeon may put the patient on an oral nonsteroidal anti-inflammatory drug for a month. The regime might appear excessive, but it is important for the well-being of both the surgeon and the patient. Fluorometholone drops (0.2%) are instilled six times a day, reducing the amount by one drop every 2 weeks. Ketorolac tromethamine drops (0.5%), three times a day, are added 1 month after surgery and continued for 4 to 6 months.

2. The pupil is kept moving with 2% homatropine and 5% phenylepherine, once or twice a day.

3. Regarding follow-up, the pediatric phakic lens patient is examined daily for 7 days, then every 2 weeks for 3 months, every 2 months for 6 months, and, thereafter, twice a year. At every visit uncorrected and corrected visual acuity and intraocular pressure are examined. The pupil is dilated and slit-lamp examination is performed. Gonioscopy and endothelial cell count are done every year (Fig. 51-2). The patient and the parents are advised to

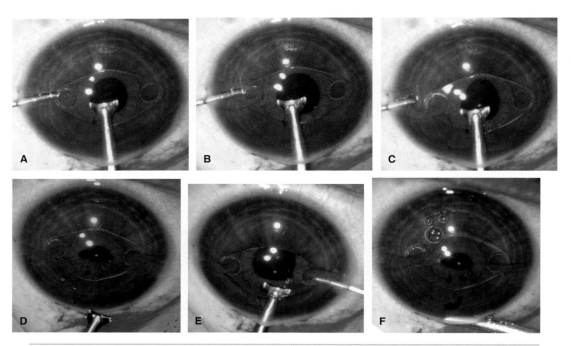

FIGURE 51-1. A. The convexoconcave optic of the phakic claw lens is held in the central position with a special dolphin tail–like holding forceps. The anterior chamber is kept full with viscoelastic pushed as needed from the sideport with a 26-gauge cannula. The same cannula is used in the fixation of the claw to the iris. **B.** The claw of the lens, which is in contact with the iris, is lifted and opened by the cannula, then released; as it snaps back, it holds the iris underneath. The iris is pushed further into the claw by a tangential-to-the-pupil movement of the cannula on the surface of the iris, which carries it through the claw. **C.** After the claw is fixed, some viscoelastic is pushed into the anterior chamber, before the lens-holding forceps is withdrawn. The convexoconcave construction of the lens optic and the viscoelastic underneath it minimize the chances of forceps–crystalline lens contact. **D.** The phakic lens (Singh version in this case, which has eccentric claws) is fixed on both sides. The fold of the iris in one of the claws seems to be excessive. **E.** The thick fold of the iris is reduced by pushing back some of the iris, out of the claw. This is a delicate step, to be performed without striking the crystalline lens under the iris. **F.** The right amount of iris is in the claws. A midperipheral iridotomy has been done by lifting and cutting the iris inside the anterior chamber. The pupil looks oval due to overcontraction with intracameral miotic. It becomes normally round in 24 hr.

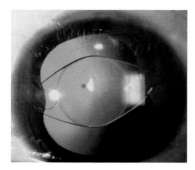

FIGURE 51-2. A phakic iris-claw lens. The pupil can be dilated for thorough examination of the eye. Every part of the lens and the iris tissue in contact with it is available for examination under the slit-lamp microscope. The lens is away from the angle of the anterior chamber, the crystalline lens, and the corneal endothelium.

make an immediate appointment if there is ever pain and redness of the eye or diminution of vision.

COMPLICATIONS

Early

1. Pupil block glaucoma can be caused by closure of the PI by inflammatory exudates, retained viscoelastic material, or closure of the PI by the lens haptic. This is a dire emergency and should be treated by a YAG-laser iridotomy or a manual iridectomy. It happens mostly in posterior chamber lens implantations.

2. Inflammatory reactions such as aqueous flare and pigment cell deposits on the implanted lens are very common. They disappear in a few weeks. A severe reaction such as synechia formation and exudates calls for intensive treatment. Explantation may be required in some patients at an early date.

3. Size mismatch when the lens is small is apparent from lens decentration and release of pigment and inflammation. A large posterior chamber lens pushes the iris anteriorly. In both cases either an explant or an exchange is required.

4. Hyphema is caused by either the PI or a torn iris root (owing to clumsy iris fixation in the claw). This condition resolves spontaneously.

5. An injury to the crystalline lens during surgery can lead to a cataract.

Late

1. Acute or subacute inflammation can occur with any kind of phakic IOL. The important signs are ciliary congestion, deposits on the IOL, and synechia and exudate formation. Most inflammations resolve with energetic treatment. If the response is poor or the condition recurs, the phakic lens should be explanted and anti-inflammatory treatment continued.

2. Cataract formation is an important issue with posterior chamber phakic lenses but not with anterior chamber lenses. Depending on the design and the version, phakic lens–crystalline lens contact is unavoidable. Adhesions may form. Cataract formation is a serious complication if it occurs at a young age.

3. A phakic posterior chamber lens can erode the iris and ciliary body by pressure and friction. Erosion is a very serious development and is manifested by an uneven shallow anterior chamber, signs of inflammation, microhyphema, and transillumination defects. Regular careful follow-up helps with early detection and suitable management, before the situation gets out of hand.

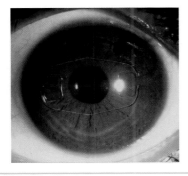

FIGURE 51-3. A worst phakic iris-claw lens in a 10-year-old child, 2 years after surgery. The claws in the Worst design are at 180°. In brown and black eyes, an optic of 4.25 mm is sufficient. Because of the vaulted construction and concave posterior surface of the optic, the iris moves freely under the lens.

4. Ovalization of the pupil is peculiar to angle-supported lenses and is not uncommon. It is caused by iris tucking with the haptics or by ischemic and fibrotic changes in the periphery of the iris. Once ovalization starts, it is progressive. It is better to explant at an early date.

5. Endothelial loss can occur due to surgical trauma, chronic inflammation, and glaucoma. Whatever lens style is used, it is good practice to keep a close watch on endothelial cell counts during follow-up (Fig. 51-3).

SURGICAL RESULTS

The first young patient we operated on was a 13-year-old girl with high hyperopia and albinism. A special iris-fixated hyperopic lens with opaque haptics was used. A +14-D lens was used. Her vision increased to 20/120 in both the eyes. Follow-up 12 years after the surgery showed quiet eyes, unchanged vision, fair tolerance to bright light, and an endothelial cell count of 2,400.

In a few albino patients, we have implanted a zero-power opaque phakic iris-claw lenses with a central aperture to mitigate photophobia. Refractive results are good with every kind of phakic IOL if the tables provided by the lens makers are used. The visual results in young patients are interesting since many of our patients are selected for surgery to overcome refractive amblyopia. In recent years we have implanted iris-fixated lenses in a number of pediatric hyperopic patients. The results are as follows for 18 patients between 7 and 16 years of age, the average being 11.9 years. The axial length varied between 18.5 and 21.88 mm, with an average of 20.8 mm. Depth of the anterior chamber varied between 2.7 and 3.8 mm, with an average of 3.1 mm. K reading varied between 37.9 and 45.5 D, the average being 42.2 D. The IOL power varied between +7 and +16 D, the average being 11.4 D. Postoperative follow-up varied from 3 to 50 months, the average being 11 months. The best corrected visual acuity (BCVA) preoperatively varied from 6/60 to 6/18, with an average of 6/39. The postoperative BCVA varied between 6/60 and 6/6, the average being 6/22. The average gain in lines was 2. The lines gained were as follows: two patients gained 5 lines, three patients gained 4 lines, four patients gained 2 lines, and six patients gained 1 line, while one patient showed no gain. No line was lost by any patient. No secondary operation was done. Endothelial cell study was done with a contact-type Bioptics specular endothelial microscope. The average endothelial cell loss was 3%.

During the past 2 years, we have studied the results of wave-guided photorefractive keratectomy (PRK) in a group of 23 young hyperopic patients. These patients had a brown or black iris. Their ages varied from 7 to 16 years, with an average of 12.7 years. The average refractive error was 5 D, the maximum being 12 D; the average cylindrical error was 1.3 D, the maximum being 6 D. Final refractive error varied from −1 to 4 D spherical and 0 to +1 D cylindrical. The follow-up varied between 6 and 24 months. Preoperative BCVA varied from 6/60 to 6/9, with an average of 6/32. Postoperative BCVA varied from 6/60 to 6/9, with an average of 6/28. Average line gain was 0.3. One patient lost 2 lines, 1 patient lost 1 line, 12 patients neither lost nor gained, 8 patients gained 1 line, and only 1 patient gained 2 lines. Three patients had a slight temporary haze. Average endothelial cell loss 4 months after PRK was 10.5%.

Comparing the phakic lens and wave-guided PRK cases, it is clear that in our patients, phakic lens implants have given far better early and stable visual results. All the cases selected for PRK had an anterior chamber depth of <2.7 mm. It is possible that future studies with PRK, LASEK, or LASIK will show results comparable to those with phakic IOLs. The only advantage of refractive surgery is that it is intraocularly noninvasive.

COMMENTS

An ideal lens should have minimal contact with the uveal tissue. A "no–uveal touch" lens is not yet available. The lens should be easy to implant and explant if need be. It should be available for examination from end to end. It should not cause cataract formation, should not cause shedding of the uveal pigment, and should not touch the corneal endothelium.

The most important issue is long-term safety, in terms of many years. All the benefits are derived from the optic and all the problems are the handiwork of the haptics. Being an invasive procedure for an otherwise healthy eye, a phakic lens implantation is not to be taken lightly. It is not a single event as an act of insertion but is the beginning of a lifelong commitment to careful service to maintain the eye in a healthy condition.

Our visual results in younger patients have been satisfying with one particular lens, the iris-fixated lens. More studies of this nature are needed to establish the long-term safety of this and other designs of phakic IOLs in children. Until laser refractive surgery is able to achieve visual results close to those with phakic IOLs, the latter will be needed for implantation in selected cases.

REFERENCES

1. Assetto V, Benedetti S, Pesando P. Collamer intraocular contact lens to correct high myopia. *J Cataract Refract Surg* 1996;22:551–556.
2. Baikoff G, Arne JL, Bokobza Y, et al. Angle-fixated anterior chamber phakic intraocular lens for myopia of −7 to −19 diopters. *J Refract Surg* 1998;14:282–293.
3. Fechner PU, Haigis W, Wichmann W. Posterior chamber myopia lenses in phakic eyes. *J Cataract Refract Surg* 1996;22:178–182.
4. Fechner PU, Singh D, Wulff K. Iris-claw lens in phakic eyes to correct hyperopia: preliminary study. *J Cataract Refract Surg* 1998;24:48–56.
5. Menezo JL, Avino JA, Cisneros A, et al. Iris claw phakic intraocular lens for high myopia. *J Refract Surg* 1997;13:545–555.
6. Perez-Santonja JJ, Iradier MT, Benitez del Castillo JM, et al. Chronic subclinical inflammation in phakic eyes with intraocular lenses to correct myopia. *J Cataract Refract Surg* 1996;22:183–187.
7. Rosen E, Gore C. Staar Collamer posterior chamber phakic intraocular lens to correct myopia and hyperopia. *J Cataract Refract Surg* 1998;24:596–606.
8. Sanders DR, Brown DC, Martin RG, et al. Implantable contact lens for moderate to high myopia: phase 1 FDA clinical study with 6 month follow-up. *J Cataract Refract Surg* 1998;24:607–611.
9. Sanders DR, Martin RG, Brown DC, et al. Posterior chamber phakic intraocular lens for hyperopia. *J Refract Surg* 1999;15:309–315.
10. Trindade F, Pereira F, Cronemberger S. Ultrasound biomicroscopic imaging of posterior chamber phakic intraocular lens. *J Refract Surg* 1998;14:497–503.
11. Verma A, Singh D. Active vision therapy for pseudophakic amblyopia. *J Cataract Refract Surg* 1997;23:1089–1094.
12. Wiechens B, Winter M, Haigis W, et al. Bilateral cataract after phakic posterior chamber top hat-style silicone intraocular lens. *J Refract Surg* 1997;13:392–397.
13. Zaldivar R, Davidorf JM, Oscherow S, et al. Combined posterior chamber phakic intraocular lens and laser in situ keratomileusis: bioptics for extreme myopia. *J Refract Surg* 1999;15:299–308.
14. Zaldivar R, Davidorf JM, Oscherow S. Posterior chamber phakic intraocular lens for myopia of −8 to −19 diopters. *J Refract Surg* 1998;14:294–305.

Pediatric Refractive Surgery

M. Edward Wilson, Jr. and Rupal H. Trivedi

Pediatric cataract surgery results in loss of the natural crystalline lens prior to completion of a complex process know as emmetropization. As part of this amazing process, marked changes in globe axial length (from 17 to 24 mm on average) are accompanied by compensatory changes in the curvature of the crystalline lens. As a result of these offsetting changes, the refractive error in most children changes very little despite marked changes in the length and size of the eye. After the crystalline lens is removed surgically, every millimeter of axial growth of the globe changes the refractive error of the eye by more than 2.5 D (diopters). Therefore, pediatric aphakia is a medical diagnosis carrying a high risk for amblyopia and disruption of visual system development. It is also an excellent indication for refractive surgery.

The most common refractive surgery performed on children is intraocular lens (IOL) implantation. Variations of this procedure are discussed throughout this book. These variations include primary implantation, secondary implantation, phakic IOLs, piggyback IOLs, multifocal IOLs, and even accommodating IOLs. Epikeratophakia is another nonlaser refractive surgical procedure introduced to treat pediatric aphakia.[1,2] In this procedure, a custom-made donor lenticule was sewn in place after the recipient's corneal epithelium was removed. The "freeze-dried" lenticule did not always regain its clarity, and even when it was clear, refractive surprises were relatively common. The procedure has been abandoned in favor of IOL implantation and contact lens wear. Despite this, we had some success stories using epikeratoplasty. A few patients, doing well, are still followed up at our clinic.

The excimer laser revolutionized refractive surgery in the 1990s. Radial keratotomy, the refractive precursor to excimer laser vision correction, had rarely been used on children. Laser vision correction, however, has been used on children with a wide range of refractive errors and diagnoses. Hutchinson[3] has reviewed reports on 234 pediatric eyes (≤18 years of age) treated with laser refractive surgery. The data are summarized in Table 52-1.[3–20]

As time passes, more and more children will be presenting for treatment with significant pseudophakic myopia. Surgical options include IOL exchange, implantation of a myopic IOL as a piggyback, and laser refractive surgery. Herein, Hutchinson's[3] review of the following three questions is summarized.

1. Does the pediatric cornea respond differently to the excimer laser than the adult cornea?
2. What is the ideal laser refractive procedure for children?
3. Are refractive outcomes predictable and stable in children?

In addition, two articles published since the Hutchinson review are summarized.

Throughout this book, we have been pointing out differences between pediatric cataract surgery and adult cataract surgery. Logically, one would conclude that the pediatric cornea is likely to respond differently to laser refractive surgery compared to the adult cornea. Also, a higher percentage of complications might be expected. However, as Hutchinson[3] points out, complications such as haze, regression, diffuse lamellar keratitis, and even corneal flap problems have not occurred in children to a greater extent than in adults. Combining the results of seven studies, Hutchinson reported no haze or trace haze in 73% (79 of 108) of eyes treated with photorefractive keratectomy (PRK) or laser in situ keratomileusis (LASIK) for myopia. No eyes had severe haze. Isolated examples of transient haze of a moderate or severe degree have been reported but these are associated with treatment of high amounts of myopia and failure to comply with postoperative steroids.

Hutchinson[3] found reports of 107 children who underwent LASIK and reported on the incidence of complications. A single case each of epithelial ingrowth, Bowman wrinkles, mild diffuse lamellar keratitis, and herpes simplex keratitis were found. Two eyes had intraoperative complications resulting in free flaps. Late corneal

▶ **TABLE 52-1**   **Summary of Pediatric Refractive Surgery, 1995 to 2003**

Study	Procedure	Eyes (n)	Mean Age (Yr)	Age Range (Yr)	Mean SEQ	SEQ Range	Attempted[a] Correction
Anisomyopia							
Leibole et al. (4)	LASEK or PRK	25	9.3	5 to 16	−11.5	−3.2 to −24.2	Match. Maximum = −15.5 D
Astle et al. (5)	PRK	18	6.3	1 to 6	−10.7	−0.75 to −25	Varies. Maximum = −17.5 D
Paysee et al. (6)	PRK	8	6.3	2 to 13	−13.6	−9 to −21	−10.0 (−7 to −11.5)
Bluestein et al. (7)	PRK	7	13	9 to 18	−9.9	ND	Match
Rybintseva & Sheludchenko (8)	LASIK	18	ND	9 to 17	−10.24	ND	Match or total
Nucci & Drack (9)	PRK	11	11.5	9 to 14	−7.2	−5.4 to −9.0	ND; Assume total
Nucci & Drack (9)	LASIK	3	13.3	13 to 14	−10.5	−9.4 to −12.9	ND; Assume total
Nassaralla & Nassaralla (10)	LASIK	9	11.5	8 to 15	−7.6	−2.5 to −13	ND; Assume total
Davis et al. (11)	LASIK	5	ND	5 to 8	ND	−5.0 to −13.6	ND; Assume match
Agarwal et al. (12)	LASIK	16	8.4	5 to 11	−14.9	−9.0 to −23.0	ND; Assume total
Autrata et al. (13)[b]	*PRK*	*13*	*11.5*	*7 to 15*	*−8.9*	*−6.5 to −11.7*	*ND; Assume total*
Rashad (14)[b]	*LASIK*	*14*	*9.4*	*7 to 12*	*−7.9*	*−4.6 to −12.5*	*Total*
Alio et al. (15)[b]	*PRK*	*6*	*6*	*5 to 7*	*−9.6*	*−4.2 to −14.5*	*Total*
Nano et al. (16)[b]	*PRK*	*5*	*12.4*	*11 to 14*	*−7.9*	*−4.0 to −11.0*	*ND; Assume total*
Singh (17)[b]	*PRK*	*6*	*10.8*	*11 to 14*	*−12.1*	*−6.2 to −17.7*	*Total*
Anisohyperopia							
Paysee et al. (6)	PRK	3	See above	See above	4.7	+ 4.2 to + 5.2	Total
Guthrie et al. (18)	PRK	2	10	9 to 11	4.2	+ 2.7 to + 5.7	+ 3 to + 5.5
Singh (17)[b]	*PRK*	*3*	*13*	*10 to 15*	*7.6*	*+ 6.5 to + 8.5*	*10 to 15 D*
Bilateral Myopia							
Astle et al. (5)	PRK	22	See above	See above	See above	See above	See above
Rybintseva & Sheludchenko (8)	LASIK	40	See above	See above	−7.47	ND	Total
Bilateral Hyperopia							
Davidorf (19)	LASIK	2	16	NA	7.25	ND	5.25

Reprinted with permission from Hutchinson AK. Pediatric refractive surgery. Curr Opin Ophthalmol 2003;14:267-275.

Note. Snellen visual acuity measurements rounded to the nearest factor of 10 unless 20/25 or better.

LASEK, laser assisted epithelial mileusis; LASIK, laser in situ keratomileusis; PRK, photorefractive keratectomy; SEQ, spherical equivalent; ND, not documented; BCVA, best corrected visual acuity; UCVA, uncorrected visual acuity.

[a]Match - attempted correction was to match the refractive error of the fellow eye; Total - attempted correction was the total refractive error.

[b]Data in italics from Primack et al. (20).

flap complications were not found but long-term follow-up is needed since children sustain more trauma on average than adults. One study reported an endothelial cell loss of 1.4% at 6 months and 3.6% after 12 months in nine children after LASIK.[10] According to Hutchinson, this is similar to the rate of cell loss after adult refractive surgery.

The ideal procedure for children would be one that is painless, requires little cooperation, has a precise refractive predictability that is stable over time, has a low risk for loss of best corrected visual acuity, and is adjustable (or can be advanced). In addition, it must withstand the rigors of the normally traumatic development of a child into an adult. This ideal procedure does not exist. Each of the currently available procedures has pluses and minuses when pediatric use is anticipated. LASIK allows faster visual rehabilitation and requires a shorter course of postoperative medications. The corneal flap, however, may be vulnerable to childhood trauma. PRK would hold up much better to trauma but heals more slowly and requires a longer course of postoperative medications. LASEK (laser-assisted subepithelial keratectomy) has been used in children as a variation in the PRK procedure but more data are needed before its role in pediatric refractive surgery can be defined. Each of these procedures could be used for the moderate degrees of myopia that will develop in most pseudophakic children and young adults. If high

▶ **TABLE 52-1** Summary of Pediatric Refractive Surgery, 1995 to 2003 (continued)

| | | | | | | | | % Losing Lines | % Gaining Lines | % Gaining Lines | Mean Follow-up |
Mean UCVA	Mean BCVA	Mean SEQ	SEQ Range	Mean UCVA	Mean BCVA	% BCVA ≥20/40	% UCVA ≥20/40	BCVA	UCVA	BCVA	(mo)
ND	ND	ND	ND	ND	ND	ND	ND	0	ND	84	ND
ND	20/70	−0.2	−4.0 to +2.9	ND	20/40	ND	ND	7.5	ND	55.9	12
ND	ND	−2.2	−6.2 to +1.25	ND	ND	ND	ND	ND	ND	57	9
20/1000	20/220	ND	ND	20/200	20/170	0	0	14.3	100	85.7	12
20/500	20/35	−2.0	ND	20/70	20/30	ND	ND	22.0	ND	ND	18
ND	20/110	−0.2	−1.0 to +0.7	20/100	ND	ND	ND	0	ND	ND	20
ND	20/170	−1	−0.2 to −1.5	20/150	ND	ND	ND	0	ND	ND	20
20/560	20/60	−0.2	−1.7 to +2.0	20/50	20/50	44	33	0	100	55	13
ND	ND	ND	−5.7 to +1.0	ND	ND	33.3	ND	0	ND	80	ND
ND	20/40	−1.4	−2.5 to 0	20/70	20/40	62.5	18.7	12.5	ND	12.5	12
20/800	20/40	−1.1	−2.0 to −0.5	20/40	20/30	76.9	30.8	0	100	69.2	24
40/200	20/50	−0.5	−1.5 to 0	20/30	20/30	100	71.4	0	100	100	12
ND	20/240	−2	−5.0 to −0.5	ND	20/50	66.6	ND	0	ND	100	33
20/800	20/400	−2.2	−3.0 to −1.5	20/100	20/70	0	0	0	100	20	12
ND	20/150	−2.9	−6.5 to −0.5	ND	20/90	66.6	ND	0	ND	100	11.8
ND	ND	0.3	−0.7 to +1.2	ND	ND	ND	ND	ND	ND	See above	9
ND	20/80	0.1	0 to 0.2	20/70	ND	0	0	ND	ND	ND	ND
20/110	20/110	0.4	+0.7 to +0.2	ND	20/70	33.3	ND	0	ND	67	8.3
See above	See above	See above	See above	ND	See above	ND	ND; See above		ND; See above	See above	
20/290	20/30	−0.67	ND	20/40	20/30	ND	ND	7.5	ND	ND	18
20/70	ND	1.7	ND	20/25	ND	100	100	ND	100	ND	ND

myopia develops, an IOL exchange would likely be chosen over laser refractive surgery.

Based on the available literature, Hutchinson concluded that refractive outcomes are less predictable and are likely to be less stable than in adults. As more data are collected, nomograms designed specifically for children, perhaps even specific to pseudophakic children, will be developed. After cataract surgery children are most likely to need laser refractive surgery at the end of their growing years. At this age, predictability and stability may approach those found in adults.

Two recent articles that have appeared in the literature since Hutchinson's review article merit mention here.

O'Keefe and Nolan[21] reported on six children (seven eyes) treated with LASIK at ages ranging from 2 to 12 years. Five of the children had myopic anisometropic amblyopia and one had bilateral myopia. All were treated under general anesthesia using the Technolas 217 excimer laser (Bausch and Lomb) with the video tracker engaged. A shield was applied continuously for the first 24 hr postoperatively and a residual corneal thickness >410 μm was ensured. The Hansatome microkeratome with a modified smaller suction ring was used to make the incision, which was hinged superiorly. No intraoperative or postoperative complications were reported and no myopic regression had occurred at the 2 year follow-up.

Autrata and Rehurek[22] reported a prospective comparative study of 27 children who underwent laser refractive surgery compared with a control group of 30 children who had conventional contact lens treatment. All of the children had myopic anisometropic amblyopia. Patching treatment was identical in the two groups. The mean age of the laser-treated children was 5.4 years. The contact lens–treated group averaged 5.1 years. Within the laser-treated group, PRK was performed on 13 eyes and LASIK on 14 eyes. No significant complications were noted. At the 2-year follow-up, the best corrected visual acuity of the amblyopic eyes was better in the laser-treated group ($P < 0.05$) than in the contact lens–treated group. Binocular vision improvement expressed as the proportion of patients who gained fusion and stereopsis was better overall in the laser-treated group (78%) than in the contact lens–treated group (33%; $P < 0.05$).

REFERENCES

1. Morgan KS, McDonald MB, Hiles DA, Aquavella JV, Durrie DS, Hunkeler JD, Kaufman HE, Keates RH, Sanders DR. The nationwide study of epikeratophakia for aphakia in older children. *Ophthalmology* 1988;95:526–532.
2. Uusitalo RJ, Uusitalo HM. Long-term follow-up of pediatric epikeratophakia. *J Refract Surg* 1997;13:45–54.
3. Hutchinson AK. Pediatric refractive surgery. *Curr Opin Ophthalmol* 2003;14:267–275.
4. Leibole MA, Berdy GJ, Packwood E, et al. Laser refractive (LASEK and PRK) surgical correction of high anisometropic myopia in ambyopic children. Presented at annual meeting of ARVO, Fort Lauderdale, FL, 2002.
5. Astle WF, Huang PT, Ells AL, Cox RG, Deschenes MC, Vibert HM. Photorefractive keratectomy in children. *J Cataract Refract Surg* 2002;28:932–941.
6. Paysee EA, Coats DK, Hamill MB, et al. Photorefractive keratectomy for anisometropia in children with amblyopia refractory to conventional treatment. Presented at 28th annual meeting of AAPOS, Seattle, WA, 2002.
7. Bluestein EC, Hutchinson AK, Saunders RA, et al. Photorefractive keratectomy for the treatment of myopic anisometropic amblyopia. Presented at annual meeting of American Academy of Ophthalmology, New Orleans, LA, 2001.
8. Rybintseva LV, Sheludchenko VM. Effectiveness of laser in situ keratomileusis with the Nidek EC-5000 excimer laser for pediatric correction of spherical anisometropia. *J Refract Surg* 2001;17(Suppl 2):S224–S228.
9. Nucci P, Drack AV. Refractive surgery for unilateral high myopia in children. *J AAPOS* 2001;5:348–351.
10. Nassaralla BR, Nassaralla JJ Jr. Laser in situ keratomileusis in children 8 to 15 years old. *J Refract Surg* 2001;17:519–524.
11. Davis JS, Dhaliwal DK, Kira DT, et al. Treatment of pediatric anisometropic myopia with laser in situ keratomileusis (LASIK): a pilot study. Presented at annual meeting of AAPOS, Orlando, FL, 2001.
12. Agarwal A, Agarwal A, Agarwal T, Siraj AA, Narang P, Narang S. Results of pediatric laser in situ keratomileusis. *J Cataract Refract Surg* 2000;26:684–689.
13. Autrata R, Rehurek J, Holousova M. Photorefractive keratectomy in high myopic anisometropia in children. *Cesk Slov Oftalmol* 1999;55:216–221.
14. Rashad KM. Laser in situ keratomileusis for myopic anisometropia in children. *J Refract Surg* 1999;5:429–435.
15. Alio JL, Artola A, Claramonte P, Ayala MJ, Chipont E. Photorefractive keratectomy for pediatric myopic anisometropia. *J Cataract Refract Surg* 1998;24:327–330.
16. Nano HD Jr, Muzzin S, Irigaray F. Excimer laser photorefractive keratectomy in pediatric patients. *J Cataract Refract Surg* 1997;23:736–739.
17. Singh D. Photorefractive keratectomy in pediatric patients. *J Cataract Refract Surg* 1995;21:630–632.
18. Guthrie EA, Salvador G, Wright KW. Pediatric PRK for hyperopic anisometropic amblyopia. Presented at annual meeting of ARVO, Fort Lauderdale, FL, 2001.
19. Davidorf JM. Pediatric refractive surgery. *J Cataract Refract Surg* 2000;26:1567–1568.
20. Primack JD, Azar NF, Azar DT. Pediatric refractive surgery. *Int Ophthalmol Clin* 2001;41:19–34.
21. O'Keefe M, Nolan L. LASIK surgery in children. *Br J Ophthalmol* 2004;88:19–21.
22. Autrata R, Rehurek J. Laser-assisted subepithelial keratectomy and photorefractive keratectomy versus conventional treatment of myopic anisometropic amblyopia in children. *J Cataract Refract Surg* 2004;30:74–84.

Miscellaneous Issues and Views

Chapter 53

Traumatic Cataracts in Children

M. Edward Wilson, Jr., Rupal H. Trivedi, and Suresh K. Pandey

Ocular trauma is a leading cause of unilateral blindness. Children are particularly vulnerable to ocular injury, especially sports-related ocular injury. Seventy-one percent of sports-related and recreational eye injuries are reported to occur in individuals <25 years of age, while about 6% occur in children <5 years of age. Prevention of eye injuries is of utmost importance and is the team responsibility of parents, teachers, coaches, ophthalmologists, pediatricians, and optometrists.[1] The American Academy of Pediatrics and the American Academy of Ophthalmology has published a joint statement recommending types of protective lenses and frames for specific sports.[1]

CLASSIFICATION OF OCULAR TRAUMA

The Ocular Trauma Classification Group has designed a standardized system for reporting mechanical injury associated with open- and closed-globe trauma. The system is based on the injury type, grade (based on visual acuity), zone, and presence or absence of an afferent papillary defect.[2,3] We provide a short summary of the reporting system below. However, interested readers are referred to the detailed description published by Kuhn and Pieramici[2,3] and to the American Society of Ocular Trauma Web site (http://www.asotonline.org).

Closed-Globe Injury

The eye wall (sclera and cornea) does not have a full-thickness wound. Mechanism of injury can be (1) contusion (blunt force), (2) superficial foreign body, (3) partial-thickness sharp force (lamellar laceration), or (4) a combination of the above.

Open-Globe Injury

The eye wall has a full-thickness wound. Mechanism of injury can be as follows.

1. *Rupture.* Full-thickness wound of the eye wall caused by a blunt object. The impact results in a momentary increase in intraocular pressure (IOP) and an inside-out injury mechanism.

2. *Laceration.* Full-thickness corneal and/or scleral wound caused by a sharp object.

3. *Penetrating injury.* Single full-thickness laceration of the eye wall usually caused by a sharp object, with no exit wound.

4. *Intraocular foreign body (IOFB).* Retained foreign object(s) causing an entrance laceration(s).

5. *Perforating injury.* Two full-thickness lacerations, with the entrance and exit wounds are caused by the same agent.

OCULAR TRAUMA AND CATARACT

The crystalline lens may be involved in any case of ocular trauma. Traumatic cataract may be an immediate, early, or late sequel of any ocular trauma. Trauma has been reported to be responsible for up to 29% of all childhood cataracts.[4] At the Storm Eye Institute, our database includes 47 eyes (10.5%) with traumatic cataract, of 450 total childhood cataract surgeries. The majority of traumatic cataract cases occur in children who are playing or involved in sport-related activities. Commonly implicated objects include knives, BB guns, firecrackers, sticks, thorns, rocks, pencils, arrows, airbags, paintballs, and toys.

Blunt trauma is responsible for coup and countercoup ocular injury.[5] *Coup* is the mechanism of direct impact. It is responsible for the Vossius ring (imprinted iris pigment) sometimes found on the anterior lens capsule following blunt injury. *Countercoup* refers to distant injury caused by shockwaves traveling along the line of concussion. When the anterior surface of the eye is struck bluntly, there is a rapid anterior–posterior shortening accompanied by *equatorial expansion*. This equatorial stretching can disrupt the lens capsule, zonules, or both. Combinations of coup, countercoup, and equatorial expansion are responsible for the formation of traumatic cataracts following blunt ocular injury. *Penetrating trauma* that directly compromises the lens capsule often leads to cortical opacification at the site of injury. If the rent is sufficiently large, the entire lens rapidly opacifies. When the capsular rent is small, however, the capsule may seal and the cortical cataract may remain localized.

Cataracts caused by blunt trauma classically form stellate– or rosette-shaped posterior axial opacities that may be stable or progressive, whereas penetrating trauma with disruption of the lens capsule forms cortical changes that may remain focal if small or may progress rapidly to total cortical opacification. Anterior and/or posterior capsule defect, intralenticular foreign body, partial/total zonular loss, dislocation, and subluxation of the lens are often found in combination with traumatic cataract. Other associated complications include glaucoma (phacolytic, phacomorphic, pupillary block, and angle recession), phacoanaphylactic uveitis, retinal detachment, choroidal rupture, hyphema, retrobulbar haemorrhage, traumatic optic neuropathy, and globe rupture. Anterior capsule rupture (with flocculent lens matter in the anterior chamber) may be associated with an increased IOP and/or possible lens-induced uveitis (e.g., phacoanaphylactic and phacotoxic endophthalmitis).

In the setting of traumatic cataract, the ophthalmologist must first "take a step back" and examine other ocular injuries in detail.[6] The cataract surgeon should be suspicious of injury to other ocular structures. Management depends on the degree and type of injury. Localized traumatic cataracts (especially if not in the visual axis) may be managed conservatively, while more significant lens opacities generally require cataract extraction. Similarly, capsular perforation may be managed with observation if small and not centrally located. Frequently, such injuries will develop only very localized opacification of the underlying cortex, without progression to generalized cataracts.

The initial patient evaluation is one of the most important critical steps in the management of any traumatic cataract. Data gathered during this examination, to a large extent, direct further investigations and establish immediate priorities. One of the most important aspects of this first examination is the description of the exact circumstances of the injury. This facilitates the development of risk estimates for occult injuries, such as IOFB, chemical exposure, and posterior rupture of the globe.

Examination

Before Dilation

1. Best corrected visual acuity (BCVA)

2. Fixation preference

3. Pupillary reflex: The presence of afferent pupillary defect may be indicative of traumatic optic neuropathy.

4. IOP (if there is no evidence of ocular rupture)

5. Iris: The clinical evaluation should also include a careful predilation examination of the iris for transillumination defects. If present, it should be documented, and following dilation, the underlying lens surface should also be inspected for an anterior capsular defect that indicates a penetrating injury or IOFB.

6. Zonule: Although detection of zonular loss is not always possible prior to pupil dilation, suggestive findings include an increase in myopic refractive error, abnormal peripheral lens curvature in one or more quadrants, an abnormal light reflex on retinoscopy, a visible lens equator, or vitreous in the anterior chamber.

After Dilation

1. *Slit-lamp examination* (after pupillary dilation) is recommended if feasible. This helps to identity and document the type of cataract, position and stability of the lens, integrity of the lens capsule, and status of the anterior segment. When slit-lamp examination is not possible in the awake state, it can be done using a portable instrument in the operating room in conjunction with the examination using the operating microscope.

2. A *posterior segment examination*, including examination of the retinal periphery, should be carried out in detail if the view through the lens allows. Otherwise B-scan ultrasonography is advisable in all eyes preoperatively.

3. *Gonioscopy* may be helpful for evaluating angle structures and for recognizing vitreous at the lens equator or areas of loss of zonular support.

4. If intraocular lens (IOL) implantation is planned, all eyes need to have keratometry and immersion A-scan ultrasound for globe axial length measurement. Even when corneal scarring is present, keratometry of the injured eye should be attempted. Changes in corneal curvature as the

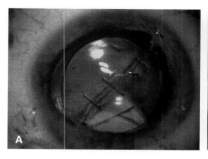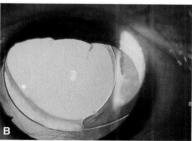

FIGURE 53-1. A. A 7-year-old boy presented with a history of trauma with knife. A heparin-surface-modified (Pharmacia 722C) IOL implanted. **B.** Two-month postoperative photo in a 14-year-old child.

result of an injury will change the IOL power needed to achieve the refractive goal. At times the keratometry readings of the fellow eye need to be used, but this will further compromise the accuracy of the postoperative refraction in relation to the postoperative goal.

A *guarded prognosis* for anatomical and functional outcome is to be thoroughly explained to the patient and the patient's relatives. The full extent of the eye injuries is not always known prior to cataract surgery. The patient and relative must understand that IOL implantation is not always possible at the initial surgery. It is also important to explain about the possible need for additional surgeries depending on the type of injury (retinal detachment, keratoplasty for dense corneal scar obstructing visual axis, etc.). The use of an IOL in traumatic cataracts is well accepted (Fig. 53-1A and B). It offers a constant, maintenance-free optical correction and, as such, helps in the prevention of amblyopia. Malplacement of the IOL is more common, in traumatic cataracts since damage to the capsular bag, zonules, and iris may predispose to decentration and pupil capture. In addition, contact lens wear may be helpful after ocular trauma to help compensate for an irregular corneal curvature caused by a healed corneal wound. However, children often have difficulty wearing these lenses due to discomfort and poor motivation to wear the lens.

With this background, we now describe some of our experience with IOL implantation in eyes with traumatic cataract at Storm Eye Institute. Then we discuss some of the relevant issues related to pediatric traumatic cataracts.[7–21] These include (a) timing of surgery for pediatric traumatic cataracts, (b) cataract surgery and IOL implantation, (c) postoperative complications, and (d) visual results.

ANALYSES OF EYES OPERATED ON FOR TRAUMATIC CATARACTS AT STORM EYE INSTITUTE

For this chapter, we analyzed 23 consecutive eyes with traumatic cataract. Peoperative characteristics and postoperative results of these 23 eyes are included in Table 53-1.

Ages at IOL implantation ranged from 3.5 to 13.8 years (mean, 6.9 ± 2.5 years). Only 5 (21.0%) of the total 23 patients were females. All 23 children had unilateral cataracts. Nine eyes (39.0%) suffered blunt injury and 14 (60.0%) had penetrating injuries with prior repair of a corneoscleral laceration. The injury preceded cataract surgery by 1 day to 7 years. Nineteen patients (82.6%) had cataract surgery within 3 months of the initial injury. Treatment prior to IOL implantation included repair of the corneoscleral laceration secondary to penetrating trauma in 13 children (56.5%) and repair of a limbal rupture after blunt injury in 1 case (4.3%). Six patients (26.0%) had undergone amblyopia therapy prior to cataract surgery. Preoperative best corrected visual acuity (BCVA) ranged from 20/40 to possible light perception.

An IOL implantation was performed at the time of cataract removal in 20 children (87.0%), while 3 eyes (13.0%) underwent secondary IOL implantation. Two of these patients (who underwent secondary IOL implantation) demonstrated amblyopia preoperatively (vision, 20/50 and 20/100 with poor fusion or strabismus). Traumatic cataracts were noted to be "dense," "white," or "total" in 14 of the patients (60.0%), "cortical" in 4 (17.3%), and posterior subcapsular in 2 patients (8.6%), who underwent a primary IOL implantation procedure. Ten patients (43.4%) had an anterior capsule rupture due to the ocular injury noted at presentation or at the time of surgery (Fig. 53-2A and B). Thirteen cases (56.5%) had a mechanical vitrector anterior capsulotomy, and in seven children (30.4%), the anterior capsulotomy was completed manually. An IOL was placed in the capsular bag in 13 (56.2%) eyes and in the ciliary sulcus in 9 eyes (39.1%), and in 1 eye (4.3%) the IOL was placed in the anterior chamber. Six foldable lens designs manufactured with hydrophobic acrylic biomaterial were used, and 14 eyes received rigid PMMA lenses. Fourteen patients (60.8%) (age range, 3.5 to 10 years) received a primary posterior capsulotomy and anterior vitrectomy. This was done in one case of traumatic posterior capsule rupture and in all patients <6 years old. Overall, the BCVA in 18 patients (78.2%) was 20/20 to 20/40 at the last follow-up visit. Three patients (13.0%) attained 20/50 to 20/80 vision, and two patients (8.6%) 20/140 or less. The mean follow-up was 113 ± 99 weeks (range, 4 to 403 weeks). The most common postoperative

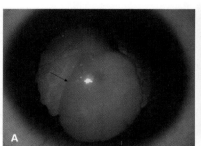 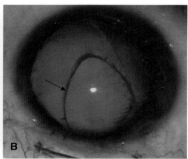

FIGURE 53-2. A. Traumatic cataract associated with ruptured anterior capsule (black arrow) and zonular loss in a 5-year-old boy **B.** After irrigation/aspiration.

complication was development of visually significant posterior capsular opacification (PCO) in five eyes (21.7%). The posterior capsule was left intact in six eyes (26%) during the cataract surgery and IOL implantation procedure. Of the six children with an intact posterior capsule, five cases (83.0%) developed PCO and required Nd:YAG laser posterior capsulotomy. In addition, two patients (8.6%) also required anterior vitrectomy and posterior capsulotomy, as Nd:YAG laser posterior capsulotomy was not successful in improving the visual acuity. One of these patients (Table 53-1, case 10) suffered a sharp penetrating injury at the age of 5 years, had undergone multiple Nd:YAG capsulotomies, and required surgical posterior membranectomy and anterior vitrectomy 14 months following IOL placement. At 7-year follow-up the patient was able to achieve a BCVA of 20/20. We have noticed IOL dislocation and pupillary capture in one (4.3%) and two (8.6%) cases, respectively. Dislocation of the IOL was seen in a 4-year-old child (Table 53-1, case 8) who had suffered zonular loss and lens subluxation at the time of injury. A polymethylmethacrylate (PMMA) IOL (Pharmacia Inc., model 815A) was implanted in the ciliary sulcus. This child did well for 19 months of follow-up but then presented with poor vision. The IOL was dislocated into the vitreous. Of two eyes with pupillary capture, the IOL was fixated in the capsular bag in one case and within the ciliary sulcus in another. Both had central corneal scars, anterior capsule rupture, and iris damage. An attempt to correct the pupillary capture was made in both cases. In the latter case (7-year-old; Table 53-1, case 9), no recurrence of the pupil capture has been seen. In the former (3.5-year-old; Table 53-1, case 12) the pupil capture was corrected 3 weeks postoperatively. However, the IOL optic recaptured when iris-to-posterior capsule adhesion was reformed. No further intervention was attempted and no persistent inflammation was noted. The BCVA in this case was 20/140 at 66-week follow-up due to a central corneal scar and poor compliance with glasses or contact lenses for corneal astigmatism and amblyopia therapy. Occurrence of amblyopia in six patients (26.0%) was also associated with poor visual outcome. Three patients (13.0%) developed strabismus postoperatively requiring strabismus surgery.

Timing of Surgery for Pediatric Traumatic Cataract

The timing of traumatic cataract surgery in children is important. Some authors have reported IOL implantation at the time of primary repair.[8] While the development of amblyopia in children necessitates prompt removal of a cataract when it develops, in our experience, cataract surgery is not necessarily required at the time of initial repair even when anterior capsular rupture is present. We prefer to defer cataract surgery and IOL implantation while the inflammatory response is treated with topical steroids. Ten of our patients (43.4%) had anterior capsule rupture and crystalline lens involvement at the time of injury and had their cataract surgery deferred for times ranging between 2 days and 6 months (average, 20 days). Cataract surgery with IOL implantation can often be safely delayed to allow a complete evaluation of damage to intraocular structures. It is important to rule out associated injury (e.g., posterior capsule rupture, vitreous hemorrhage, and retinal detachment) using ancillary methods such as B-scan ultrasonography and to allow healing after the primary repair. However, medically uncontrolled ocular hypertension may occasionally necessitate earlier cataract surgery. Cataract surgery and IOL implantation (combined during the primary repair of ocular trauma) may be considered in younger children predisposed to amblyopia.

Cataract Surgery and IOL Implantation

General principles of pediatric cataract surgery and IOL implantation described elsewhere in this book should be followed. Specific differences are described below.

- *Anesthesia.* General anesthesia is preferable even in older children who might otherwise be cooperative for local anesthesia.
- *Incision.* Although corneal tunnel incisions have become routine, we still recommend a scleral tunnel incision when operating on a traumatic cataract. The integrity of the capsular bag and the zonular support is often in question. If conversion from a planned foldable IOL insertion to a rigid PMMA IOL insertion is needed,

scleral wounds are more easily enlarged to the 6- to 7-mm length that may be required.

- *Synechiolysis*. Traumatic cataracts are often associated with posterior synechiae and it is necessary to perform synechiolysis in these eyes. Iris repositior instruments or high-viscosity viscoelastic material can be used for this purpose.

- *Anterior capsule management*. Management of the lens capsule in traumatic cataract cases may be difficult due to a ruptured lens capsule with flocculent lens matter in the anterior chamber. Creation of an intact capsulorhexis may be difficult in such a situation. A vitrectorhexis is a good alternative to manual capsulorhexis. Thirteen eyes (56.5%) had a mechanical vitrector anterior capsulotomy, and in seven eyes (30.4%) the anterior capsulotomy was completed manually. Very dense fibrous capsule can be removed with radiofrequency diathermy or Fugo plasma blade. Staining of the anterior lens capsule may be helpful to enhance visibility in these eyes with a "torn anterior capsule" or "white cataract." Anterior capsule staining can be successfully done using a nontoxic capsular dye such as 0.5% indocyanine green or 0.1% trypan blue.

- *Hydrodissection*. Avoid doing *hydrodissection* in such cases if the integrity of the posterior capsule is suspicious.

- *Posterior capsule and vitreous management*. Management of the posterior capsule depends on the age of the patient and status of the posterior capsule (intact versus torn). In our results, a primary posterior capsulotomy was performed in 14 eyes (60.8%); 9 of these patients (39.1%) underwent a pars plana posterior capsulotomy and 5 patients (21.7%) had the posterior capsulolotomy performed using an anterior approach. In young patients (too young to sit still at the Nd:YAG laser) with complex trauma, proper placement of the IOL is paramount. If this can be accomplished best by leaving the posterior capsule intact at the initial cataract surgery, plan a secondary surgery to remove the center of the posterior capsule after the IOL has become healed into the lens capsule. This staged approach may be better for surgeons unaccustomed to operating on young children. PCO occurs quickly in most cases of complex traumatic cataract surgery. Therefore, prepare the family that the best vision will likely come after this planned second surgery. Repair of iris defects or other more elective surgical maneuvers can also be done during this secondary procedure, which is often done 4 to 8 weeks after the initial cataract removal.

- *IOL Implantation*. Continued advances in IOL designs, biomaterial, and power calculations are making this decision easier in the pediatric population. BenEzra and associates[9] had reported a better visual acuity and less strabismus in children with traumatic cataract after implanting an IOL, compared to those wearing contact lenses. In-the-bag placement of the IOL haptics improves implant stability and minimizes uveitis and pupillary capture.[19] Fifteen of our 21 eyes with primary implantation had the IOL placed in the capsular bag. In-the-bag fixation is believed by most to be the best site for IOL implantation, as it sequesters the implant from uveal structures, reduces the chance of lens decentration, and delays PCO formation.[22] However, traumatic cataract cases often present unique challenges, as it is not always possible to fixate the IOL haptics in the capsular bag due to anterior and/or posterior capsule tears from trauma or the difficult surgical procedure. If the IOL must be placed in the ciliary sulcus, as with extensive traumatic posterior capsule rupture, try to capture the IOL optic through the anterior capsulotomy. If this can be done, it will eliminate the risk of pupil capture. Since the iris sphincter is often damaged in trauma, pupil capture of sulcus-fixated IOLs is higher in traumatic as opposed to nontraumatic IOL sulcus fixation.

- *Iris suture*. Occasionally iris may require suturing. Iridodialysis defects are usually repaired at the time of IOL implantation using a series of double-armed 10.0 prolene sutures on a long, straight STC-6 needle. A small paracentesis is made 180° away from the iridodialysis. Both needles of the double-armed prolene are passed through the paracentesis (one at a time) and across the anterior chamber. The needle is allowed to pick up the peripheral detached edge of the iris base and then exits the sclera as close to where that iris segment should naturally attach as possible. Each double-armed prolene is passed in a mattress fashion and is tied external to the sclera. Rather than using a scleral flap, we simply leave the suture ends long and tuck them under the conjunctiva toward the fornix. This seems to prevent suture ends from gradually eroding through the conjunctiva. Cuts and tears in the pupil margin are also often closed with the same type of suture material. This can be done at the initial surgery (Fig. 53-3 A–D) but is often easier when done as a secondary procedure in a well-healed pseudophakic eye (Fig. 53-4).

- *Removal of corneal suture*. Do not forget to remove corneal sutures from the original traumatic globe rupture repair if they are present and wound healing has been completed.

- *Postoperative medication*. Depending on the case, we may sometime increase the frequency of steroid drops. Also, a short course of systemic steroids may be indicated. If IOP control had been a problem after the original trauma, perhaps during hyphema resolution, it is likely that elevated IOP will be seen transiently after cataract surgery. Prophylactic oral Diamox is recommended during the early healing phase in such cases.

TABLE 53-1 Overview of Ocular Traumatic Cataract and Follow-up

Patient Code	Age (years)	Sex	Type of Trauma/Cause	Injury to IOL Interval (months)	Type of Cataract	Pre-op BCVA	Pre-op Complications	IOL Fixation/IOL Material	Post-op BCVA	Post-op Complications	Post-op Follow-up (weeks)
1	8.5	M	Blunt/B-B	0.5	Total	HM	Posterior lens rupture; hyphema; ↑IOP	Ciliary sulcus/PMMA	20/20	None	180
2	4.7	M	Blunt/Belt buckle	3	Cortical + anterior capsule plaque	20/100	Lid + canalicular laceration	Capsular bag/Acrylic	20/30	None	7
3	10.0	F	Penetrating/Glass	2	Total	HM	Inferior corneal scar; iris damage; lens rupture	Capsular bag/PMMA	20/30	YAG to fibrous band iris to corneal scar	103
4	4.3	M	Penetrating/Toy	0.7	Total	HM	Central corneal scar; lens rupture; iris damage	Ciliary sulcus/Acrylic	20/80	Corneal scar in visual axis; contact lens intolerance	119
5	7.4	M	Penetrating/Stick	1	PSC	CF	Superior corneal scar; lens rupture	Capsular bag/Acrylic	20/20	None	78
6	6.0	F	Penetrating/Pencil	1	Total	LP	Peripheral corneal scar; lens rupture	Ciliary sulcus/PMMA	20/20	None	127
7	10.0	F	Penetrating/Unknown object	19	Total	HM	Peripheral corneal scar	Capsular bag/PMMA	20/25	None	102
8	4.3	M	Blunt/Metal tray	24	Cortical with subluxation	20/100	Zonule loss; deprivation myopia	Ciliary sulcus/PMMA	20/80	IOL dislocation 19 months post-op	204
9	7.0	M	Penetrating/Knife	2.5	(Secondary IOL)	20/100	Posterior synechiae; aphakic	Ciliary sulcus/PMMA	20/20	Pupil capture of IOL 4 weeks post-op	90
10	4.9	M	Penetrating/Wire	0.03	Cortical	20/80	Lens rupture	Capsular bag/PMMA	20/20	YAG for PCO twice, then PPV	403

Case	Age	Sex	Mechanism/Object		Cataract	Pre-op BCVA	Injury	IOL location/type	Post-op BCVA	Complications/Other	
11	7.0	M	Blunt/B-B	1	Total	HM	Hyphema; iridodialysis; lens rupture	Capsular bag/PMMA	20/30	YAG for PCO; partial pupil capture	401
12	3.5	M	Penetrating/Box cutter	0.3	Total	LP	Lens rupture; iris damage; posterior synechiae	Capsular bag/PMMA	20/125	Recurrent pupil capture of IOL	66
13	9.5	F	Penetrating/Pocket knife	26	(Secondary IOL)	20/50	Control corneal scar; iris damage	Ciliary sulcus/Acrylic	20/40	None	267
14	6.0	M	Penetrating/Bed post	0.9	Total	LP	Rupture lens; posterior synechiae; hypopyon	Capsular bag/Acrylic	20/30	YAG for PCO	70
15	11.0	F	Penetrating/Knife	72	Cortical	20/100	Zonule loss	Capsular bag/PMMA	20/30	YAG for PCO	320
16	7.0	M	Blunt/Unknown object	84	Cortical + PSC	20/200	None	Capsular bag/PMMA	20/30	None	43
17	13.8	M	Penetrating/Glass	2	Total	CF	Lens rupture; posterior synechiae	Capsular bag/Acrylic	20/25	YAG for PCO	131
18	7.5	M	Blunt/Rock	6	Total	4/300	Iris sphincter tear	Capsular bag/PMMA	20/25	None	15
19	3.7	M	Penetrating/Toy	2.7	(Secondary IOL)	20/80	Inferior corneal tear; no capsular support	Anterior chamber/PMMA	20/25	None	164
20	5.3	M	Blunt/Car antenna	1	Total	HM	Hyphema; lens rupture; zonule loss; iridodialysis	Capsular bag/PMMA	20/40	Pupil capture of IOL	34
21	6.5	F	Penetrating/Wire	18	PSC	2/400	Retinal detachment; vitreous hemorrhage	Capsular bag/Acrylic	20/100	None	49
22	8.0	M	Penetrating/Ice	2.3	PSC; ASC	20/60	Central corneal laceration	Capsular bag/Acrylic	20/30	None	4
23	4.3	M	Penetrating/Toy	3	Total	LP	Lens rupture; corneal scar	Capsular bag/Acrylic	20/40	None	16

IOL, intraocular lens; BCVA, best corrected visual acuity; Pre-op, preoperative; Post-op, postoperative; PCO, posterior capsular opacification; PMMA, polymethylmethacrylate); HM, hand movement; CF, count fingers; LP, light perception; PSC, posterior subcapsular cataract; ASC, anterior subcapsular cataract; YAG, yttrium-aluminum-garnet laser.

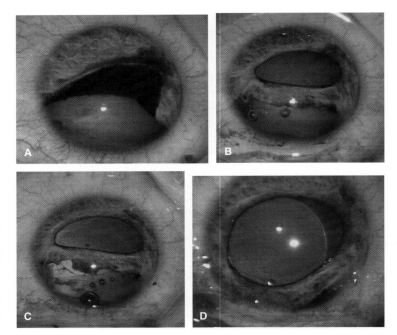

FIGURE 53-3. A 12-year-old boy presented with a history of trauma 2 months previously. **A.** Traumatic cataract was associated with iridodialysis and loss of zonules in superior 5 clock hours. Iris was folded. **B.** Reposition of folded iris. **C.** After irrigation/aspiration. **D.** Iris was sutured with 10/0 prolene as the primary procedure, and an AcrySof (SN60, Alcon laboratory) IOL implanted.

Postoperative Complications

The main postoperative complications following pediatric cataract surgery with IOL implantation include PCO and/or secondary membrane formation, pupillary capture, IOL precipitates, and decentration/dislocation of the implant. Complications in our series included visually significant PCO in five cases (21.7%), pupillary capture in two cases (8.6%) and IOL dislocation in one case (4.34%). Posterior capsule opacification developed in 5 of the 6 children when the posterior capsule was left intact. We continue to recommend planned primary posterior capsulotomy in children too young to undergo an awake Nd:YAG laser capsulotomy. Occurrence of pupillary capture can be reduced after precise fixation of the IOL within the capsular bag. The one eye that developed pupillary capture after in-the-bag IOL placement had a ruptured anterior capsule and iris damage prior to IOL implantation. Had it been possible to maintain an anterior capsular opening smaller than the IOL optic, pupillary capture could have been avoided. Iris-to-posterior capsule adhesions re-formed in this patient, causing recurrence of the pupillary capture. Decentration/dislocation of an IOL can occur because of traumatic zonular loss and/or inadequate capsular support. Capsular bag placement of the IOL combined with a capsule tension ring is a reported method that may be helpful in the presence of zonular dehiscence/loss. These capsular tension rings have now been approved by the U.S. Food and Drug Administration for use in adults. They are not recommended when the integrity of the posterior capsule has been breeched. Posterior capture of the IOL optic may be useful, at times, to obtain better centration of the implanted IOL. Asymmetric IOL fixation, with one of the haptics in the capsular bag and the other in the ciliary sulcus, can also lead to decentration and should, therefore, be avoided. Complete IOL dislocation can occur after trauma. Explantation or repositioning of the IOL may be necessary in some cases presenting with significant decentration/dislocation.

Besides PCO, pupillary capture, and implant decentration, poor visual outcome was also associated with amblyopia and retinal scar in six and one cases (26 and 4.3%, respectively). Three of our patients with significant amblyopia had marked traumatic astigmatism and were poorly compliant with glasses or contact lens wear. Poor compliance with occlusion therapy was also a factor in poor visual outcome. All of the patients with resultant vision ≤20/80 were at an age to be at risk for amblyopia. Amblyopia can develop preoperatively with cataract or aphakia, owing to corneal astigmatism, PCO, or loss of accommodation with an IOL. Compliance with amblyopia therapy is necessary

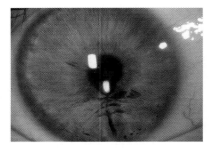

FIGURE 53-4. An 11-year-old girl with a history of traumatic cataract removal and secondary IOL implantation. Iris repaired (10/0 prolene) after 2.5 years of IOL implantation. Photo taken 2 months after iris repair.

> **TABLE 53-2** Studies of Posterior Chamber Intraocular Lens Implantation in Children with Traumatic Cataracts

Study (Ref. No.)	Number of Patients	Age Range (yr)	Mean Follow-up (yr)	BCVA (≥6/12) (%)	Complications (%)		
					Fibrous Anterior Uveitis	Pupillary Capture	PCO
Anwar et al. (8)	15	3–8	3.2	73.3	NR	NR	40
Bienfait et al. (10)	23	0.4–11	6.5	70.1	0	9	83
Eckstein et al. (14)	52	2–10	2.9	67	19	41	92
Gupta et al. (16)[a]	22	3–11	0.9	45	81.8	9	27
Koenig et al. (18)	8	4–17	0.8	87	NR	NR	37
Pandey et al. (19)	20	4–10	2.5	85	45	20	60
BenEzra & Hemo (24)	23	2–13	6.2	65.2	NR	26	100
Bustos et al. (28)	19	3–15	0.7	79	26	10.5	21

BCVA, best corrected visual acuity; PCO, posterior capsule opacification; NR, not reported.
[a] Four patients had an anterior chamber IOL.

in younger children to get maximum visual outcome, even following an excellent surgical result.

Visual Results

The prognosis for retention of good vision in pediatric eyes suffering traumatic cataracts has greatly improved over the last few decades. Binkhorst and Gobin,[23] in 1964, reviewed a case series originally published by McKimura in 1961. Twenty-six children with unilateral traumatic cataracts had been treated at McGill University Hospital and the University of California Medical Center in San Francisco. Despite treatment, most of the patient's visual acuity was in the range of counting fingers; only one child retained a visual acuity better than 20/200. Binkhorst and Gobin[23] argued that the visual prognosis for young children after treatment for a traumatic cataract need not be so poor. They recommended the use of IOLs in this situation and suggested that this treatment would improve the visual outcomes in children with lenticular opacity. BenEzra and Hemo[24] and Hiles and coworkers[25] reported the visual outcome and postoperative complications of pediatric traumatic cataract cases using contact lenses and/or IOLs in the 1990s. Several surgeons from throughout the world, often in countries with high traumatic cataract rates and conditions prohibitive of contact lens wear, have recently reported successful IOL implantation in injured children.[8–10,12,16,18,26,27] Our results (as well as the experience of several other authors) confirm that good visual outcome is frequently possible following IOL implantation in children (Table 53-2). In our patients, 78% achieved a BCVA of 20/40 or better after a mean follow-up of 2.3 years. In a comparable series, Koenig et al.[18] reported 20/40 or better visual acuity in 87% (seven of eight) of eyes undergoing IOL implantation for pediatric traumatic cataracts. The average follow-up in their series was 10 months. Gupta et al.[16] reported that 9 (50%) of 18 children with unilateral

traumatic cataracts achieved 20/40 (or better) visual acuity after IOL implantation, with an average follow-up of 12 months. In many cases corneal leukomata contributed to decreased postoperative visual acuity. Similarly, Anwar et al.,[8] Bustos et al.,[28] BenEzra et al.,[9] Eckstein et al.,[14] Pandey et al.,[19] and, recently, Brar et al.[27] reported visual acuity of 20/40 or better in 73.3, 79.0, 65.2, 67.0, 85, and 62% of cases, respectively, after traumatic cataract surgery with IOL implantation in children (Table 53-2).

CONCLUSION

To summarize, traumatic cataract can present many medical and surgical challenges to the ophthalmologist. It adds the challenges presented by childhood cataract. Comprehensive examinations, careful planning for surgical management, and close follow-up are necessary for a favorable outcome in these cases. We support the continued use of IOLs in children in eyes with traumatic cataracts. Further prospective studies are probably needed to specifically address the optimum timing of cataract–IOL surgery in cases of pediatric traumatic cataract. However, based on our experience, we suggest primary repair of the injury first and cataract–IOL surgery after 2 to 4 weeks of topical steroid and atropine treatment. This delay may be helpful in achieving the optimum surgical outcome by reducing the postoperative inflammation in these eyes and allowing healing to occur. Long delays before cataract removal must be avoided during the amblyopia-prone years, which extend to approximate the age of 8 years.

REFERENCES

1. Protective eye wear for young athletes. A joint statement of the American Academy of Pediatrics and the American Academy of Ophthalmology. *Ophthalmology* 1996;103:1325–1328.

2. Kuhn F, Morris R, Witherspoon CD, Heimann K, Jeffers JB, Treister G. A standardized classification of ocular trauma. *Ophthalmology* 1996;103:240–243.
3. Pieramici DJ, Sternberg P Jr, Aaberg TM, Bridges WZ Jr, Capone A Jr, Cardillo JA, et al. A system for classifying mechanical injuries of the eye (globe). The Ocular Trauma Classification Group. *Am J Ophthalmol* 1997;123:820–831.
4. Eckstein M, Vijayalakshmi P, Killedar M, Gilbert C, Foster A. Aetiology of childhood cataract in south India. *Br J Ophthalmol* 1996;80:628–632.
5. Datiles MB, Magno BV. Cataract: clinical types. In: *Duane's Ophthalmology.* Philadelphia: Lippincott Williams & Wilkins, 2001.
6. Harlan JB, Pieramici DJ. Evaluation of patient with ocular trauma. *Ophthalmol Clin North Am* 2002;15:153–161.
7. Kamlesh, Dadeya S. Management of paediatric traumatic cataract by epilenticular intraocular lens implantation: long-term visual results and postoperative complications. *Eye* 2004;18:126–130.
8. Anwar M, Bleik JH, von Noorden GK, el-Maghraby AA, Attia F. Posterior chamber lens implantation for primary repair of corneal lacerations and traumatic cataracts in children. *J Pediatr Ophthalmol Strabismus* 1994;31:157–161.
9. BenEzra D, Cohen E, Rose L. Traumatic cataract in children: correction of aphakia by contact lens or intraocular lens. *Am J Ophthalmol* 1997;123:773–782.
10. Bienfait MF, Pameijer JH, Wildervanck de Blecourt-Devilee M. Intraocular lens implantation in children with unilateral traumatic cataract. *Int Ophthalmol* 1990;14:271–276.
11. Blumenthal M, Yalon M, Treister G. Intraocular lens implantation in traumatic cataract in children. *J Am Intraocul Implant Soc* 1983;9:40–41.
12. Cheema RA, Lukaris AD. Visual recovery in unilateral traumatic pediatric cataracts treated with posterior chamber intraocular lens and anterior vitrectomy in Pakistan. *Int Ophthalmol* 1999;23:85–89.
13. Churchill AJ, Noble BA, Etchells DE, George NJ. Factors affecting visual outcome in children following uniocular traumatic cataract. *Eye* 1995;9:285–291.
14. Eckstein M, Vijayalakshmi P, Killedar M, Gilbert C, Foster A. Use of intraocular lenses in children with traumatic cataract in south India. *Br J Ophthalmol* 1998;82:911–915.
15. Gradin D, Yorston D. Intraocular lens implantation for trau-matic cataract in children in East Africa. *J Cataract Refract Surg* 2001;27:2017–2025.
16. Gupta AK, Grover AK, Gurha N. Traumatic cataract surgery with intraocular lens implantation in children. *J Pediatr Ophthalmol Strabismus* 1992;29:73–78.
17. Hemo Y, BenEzra D. Traumatic cataracts in young children. Correction of aphakia by intraocular lens implantation. *Ophthalmic Paediatr Genet* 1987;8:203–207.
18. Koenig SB, Ruttum MS, Lewandowski MF, Schultz RO. Pseudophakia for traumatic cataracts in children. *Ophthalmology* 1993;100:1218–1224.
19. Pandey SK, Ram J, Werner L, Brar GS, Jain AK, Gupta A, et al. Visual results and postoperative complications of capsular bag and ciliary sulcus fixation of posterior chamber intraocular lenses in children with 'traumatic cataracts. *J Cataract Refract Surg* 1999;25:1576–1584.
20. Krishnamachary M, Rathi V, Gupta S. Management of traumatic cataract in children. *J Cataract Refract Surg* 1997;23(Suppl 1):681–687.
21. Blum M, Tetz MR, Greiner C, Voelcker HE. Treatment of traumatic cataracts. *J Cataract Refract Surg* 1996;22:342–346.
22. Ram J, Pandey SK, Apple DJ, Werner L, Brar GS, Singh R, et al. Effect of in-the-bag intraocular lens fixation on the prevention of posterior capsule opacification. *J Cataract Refract Surg* 2001;27:1039–1046.
23. Binkhorst CD, Gobin MH. Injuries to the eye with lens opacity in young children. *Ophthalmologica* 1964;148:169–183.
24. BenEzra D, Hemo I. Traumatic cataract in children: visual results following correction with contact or intraocular lenses. *Eur J Implant Refract Surg* 1990;2:325–328.
25. Hiles DA, Cheng KP, Biglan AW. Aphakic optical correction with intraocular lenses for children with traumatic cataracts. *Eur J Implant Refract Surg* 1990;2:275–283.
26. Pandey SK, Werner L, Escobar-Gomez M, Roig-Melo EA, Apple DJ. Dye-enhanced cataract surgery. Part 1: Anterior capsule staining for capsulorhexis in advanced/white cataract. *J Cataract Refract Surg* 2000;26:1052–1059.
27. Brar GS, Ram J, Pandav SS, Reddy GS, Singh U, Gupta A. Postoperative complications and visual results in uniocular pediatric traumatic cataract. *Ophthalmic Surg Lasers* 2001;32:233–238.
28. Bustos FR, Zepeda LC, Cota DM. Intraocular lens implantation in children with traumatic cataract. *Ann Ophthalmol* 1996;28:153–157.

Pediatric Cataracts in Developing-World Settings

M. Edward Wilson, Jr. and Rupal H. Trivedi

Worldwide, an estimated 1.4 million children are blind, of whom approximately 190,000 (14%) are blind owing to bilateral unoperated cataract, complications of surgery, amblyopia due to delayed surgery, or the presence of other associated anomalies.[1] Pediatric cataract blindness presents an enormous problem to developing countries in terms of human morbidity, economic loss, and social burden.[2] Managing cataracts in children remains a challenge, even in the industrialized world. Treatment is often difficult and tedious and requires a dedicated team effort. Since the future of any society is in children, it is time to give childhood cataract treatment the attention that adult cataract treatment has received for many years.[2] To assure the best long-term outcome for cataract-blind children, appropriate pediatric surgical techniques need to be defined and adopted by ophthalmic surgeons of developing countries. This chapter focuses on practical guidelines and recommendations for ophthalmic surgeons and health planners dealing with childhood cataract in the developing world.

Characteristics of developing nations have *high birth and infant mortality rates* and high rates of curable and preventable blindness.[3] A child becomes bilaterally blind every minute, primarily within developing nations.[2,4] Of the 1.4 million blind children in the world, approximately 90% live in Asia and Africa, and 75% of all causes are preventable or curable.[2] The prevalence of blindness varies according to the socioeconomic development of the country and the mortality rate of those <5 years of age. In developing countries the rate of blindness can be as high as 1.5 per 1,000 population. Compared to industrialized countries, this figure is 10 times higher.[2,5–14] As reported by Foster and Gilbert,[15] about 0.5 million children become blind each year. For those who survive childhood, the burden of disability in terms of "blind-years" is huge. The child who goes blind today is likely to remain with us into 2050.[6] Restoring the sight of one child blind from cataracts may be equivalent to restoring the sight of 10 elderly adults.[6]

Irrespective of the cause, childhood blindness has far-reaching effects on the child and family throughout life. It profoundly influences educational, employment, personal, and social prospects. The control of childhood blindness has been identified as a priority of the World Health Organization's (WHO) global initiative for the elimination of avoidable blindness by the year 2020.[16,17]

An uneven distribution of ophthalmologists, pediatricians, and anesthetists creates unique challenges in developing world settings. In general, health services are concentrated in the larger cities, and people living in rural areas often live beyond the reach of the services provided by health care delivery teams. In India, a country that has an estimated backlog of 4 million patients with cataract, there is approximately 1 ophthalmologist for every 100,000 people. Great Britain has a similar ratio of 1 ophthalmologist to 100,000 people but essentially no cataract backlog! The National Program for Control of Blindness (NPCB) in India believes that the output of ophthalmologists in India is low because of underutilization and the low number of surgeons in rural regions, where the prevalence of blindness is high.

GUIDELINES AND RECOMMENDATION FOR HEALTH PLANNERS AND SURGEONS

It is very important to *improve the early identification and referral* of children with cataracts by educating and training pediatricians, rural health clinic personnel, midwives, and eye-camp workers to screen for loss of the eye's red reflex and poor visual functioning in newborn, toddlers, and school-aged children. An early surgical intervention and prompt optical rehabilitation are mandatory to prevent irreversible deprivational amblyopia. The same is true for reopacification of the visual axis.

Since the number of qualified ophthalmologists available is limited, the bulk of ophthalmic surgical screening is done by ophthalmic assistants in some areas. However, the primary health care worker can also be taught to identify cataracts. Ophthalmic assistants, working with primary health workers, can maximize the efficiency of a limited eye care system by screening and referring only patients requiring surgery or other specialized attention. It is also important to emphasize that all types of eye staff need to have the stimulus of continuing education and eye seminars to provide the necessary incentive and encouragement in what is often a difficult field and to provide updating of their knowledge and skills.

Most developing nations provide health delivery services through a tiered system, with central hospitals supporting smaller and rural hospitals and health delivery centers.[3] In Africa and Asia, for example, many countries have established a three-tiered system, consisting of primary, secondary, and tertiary levels. The primary health care worker can diagnose and treat the most prevalent disease and refer complicated cases to treatment facilities. The usual referral resource for the primary health care worker is the secondary facility. Provincial, district, and subdistrict hospitals and health centers serve as secondary medical units. Ophthalmologists are assigned to provincial and sometimes to district hospitals. The central urban hospital, usually attached to a medical school, is the tertiary resource. There may be several tertiary hospitals in larger states, provinces, or countries serving large geographic regions. This facility usually is a large general hospital and offers a wide range of specialty services. We believe that the treatment of cataract blind children should be done in *specialized, well-equipped, high-volume surgical centers*, where cataract operations on children are done on a regular basis.

There are many persons who have close contact with the community, especially at the village level. These persons, by use of appropriate knowledge, could help in the prevention of blindness. For example, the school teacher, mukhi (leader of the village), *Pujari* (person taking care of temple and religious activity), and others have great influence in villages in India.

Ocular surgical services are sometimes provided by *mobile eye units* based at the central or provincial hospital level.[18,19] These units visit villages and rural health centers. They are staffed by ophthalmic assistants or ophthalmic nurses and are supervised by ophthalmologists. Eye camps have been used for this purpose and may be cost effective. However, organizers at the Aravind Eye Hospital in Madurai, India, have found that in their setting it is more cost effective to bus patients to the hospital for surgery, after screening in the local area, than to provide local cataract camps.[3] Mobile eye units often are used where health delivery, services, roads, communications, and transport are poorly developed.

Publicity may be accomplished through a variety of mechanisms at several levels using health care personnel, radio, television, and other media. Service organizations (e.g., Lions Club, Rotary Club) are often involved in promotional activities.

In some regions, a fear of increased postoperative infection during warmer weather caused the operating season to be abbreviated. In India, generally, the "eye operating season" is a period of 2 to 3 months during cooler weather. Also, the harvest season may be a time of reduced surgery since travel to a centralized treatment facility may not be possible without loss of the family livelihood.

A significant influence in persuading parents to allow their child to undergo cataract surgery is likely to be the example of other children in the community who have had sight restored by such an operation. A reputation for good results from surgery is the major influence in the decision-making process for parents. Thus, in the initial phase, *"patient selection"* is very important. Patients with good visual potential (bilateral dense cataracts without nystagmus or microphthalmia in children who are progressing developmentally) should be operated on first to assure that parents and community leaders will trust and believe in the surgery being offered to the blind children.

In some locations the facilities are in place but are *underutilized*. Valuable resources of trained staff have often been wasted, or at best poorly used, because they have not been given even the basic equipment to carry out their work—even though the equipment is often inexpensive and simple. Basic instruments to diagnose ophthalmic disorders should be provided (visual acuity charts, torch, direct ophthalmoscope, etc.) to such a setup.

The NPCB in India published the results of the evaluation of training for ophthalmic surgeons in extracapsular cataract extraction (ECCE) and intraocular lens (IOL) placement.[30] It may have changed now, but those results showed that 14 of 66 training sites did not have operating microscopes.[20] Fourteen sites did not have an A-scan ultrasound machine for globe axial length measurements; 28 did not have a keratometer. This was the scenario in the adult cataract surgery setup. Without some help and some changes, the chances of having A-scan ultrasound and keratometry capability in the operating room for pediatric patients are low. More importantly, 42 of the 66 sites did not have a vitrectomy machine. For pediatric cataract surgery, a vitrectomy machine is needed, along with a supply of functioning cutters and tubing.

Power fluctuations and outages are additional challenges in the developing-world setting when surgical procedures, like pediatric cataract surgery, depend on automated machinery. The development of better battery-operated vitrectomy cutting instruments would be helpful in these settings.

It could be argued that all that has to be done is to transfer the well-proved methods and instrumentation from the

West to all areas of the world and all problems would be solved![21] Even if such a transfer were possible, nothing could be farther from the truth. For example, no matter how many vitrector machines were made available, this would not solve the problem. The machines would break down and the cost of a vitrector handpiece would prevent its routine use. We have witnessed a setup where a phacoemulsification machine was available and the surgeons were proficient enough to use this technology, but because the tips were not available the machine was not being used! In general, it is advisable to chose instruments that have reusable tubing sets and handpieces for use in developing-world settings. In addition, investments in biomedical maintenance and repair training will pay off almost as well as the surgical training itself.

For surgical methods applied to third-world ophthalmic problems to be appropriate, they must be cost effective, time effective, and sight effective. Surgical techniques described in other chapters in this book can be followed when treating children with pediatric cataract. However, we must remember that with the great difficulties of communication and follow-up existing in third-world situations, it is best to do a *"once and for all"* rather than a staged procedure. For this reason it may be right to do a more comprehensive procedure rather than trying a method that may need to be repeated.

SIMULTANEOUS BILATERAL PEDIATRIC CATARACT SURGERY OR IMMEDIATELY SEQUENTIAL CATARACT SURGERY

Some authors[2,22–25] have proposed simultaneous pediatric cataract surgery to manage the backlog of cataract blindness in the developing world. The fears of bilateral blinding endophthalmitis or bilateral postoperative wound rupture have made unilateral surgery the normal procedure in the industrialized world. In the amblyopic years, surgery in the second eye is usually done within a few days or weeks of the initial surgery. In the developing world, this cautious approach may not be practical. To avoid the risks and costs of a second anesthesia and to make maximal use of the vitrector tubing and cutter, simultaneous bilateral surgery on children may be given consideration.[2]

GENERAL ANESTHESIA VIA ENDOTRACHEAL INTUBATION OR LARYNGEAL MASK AIRWAY (LMA)

A detailed review of the techniques of general anesthesia at ophthalmic care centers in the developing world is beyond the scope of this chapter. Cost and effectiveness are both very important when choosing anesthetic agents in a developing-world setting. We recommend that pediatric cataract surgery be performed under general anesthesia with constant monitoring of the vital signs.

Ophthalmic surgeons in Guatemala have utilized modern inhalation agents via LMA combined with peribulbar lidocaine and marcaine in children to facilitate maintenance of anesthesia on as little inhalation agent as possible.[2] If necessary, ophthalmic surgeons should be given a special course in general anesthesia for eye surgery.

Considering the limited resources and availability of anesthetists in remote areas of the developing world, ketamine provides a safe and potent intravenously administered anesthetic of short duration for pediatric populations. Ketamine combines analgesic and sleep-producing effects without significant cardiovascular and respiratory depression. The most common side effects are the so-called "emergence phenomenon," which includes disorientation, vivid dreams, and sensory or perceptual illusion. Literature has reported the use of ketamine anesthesia in combination with peribulbar lidocaine for pediatric cataract surgery.[26,27] While an anesthetist is not always available, the anesthesia is always administered by a person trained in pediatric airway management and resuscitation. A pulse oximeter is used as part of the vital sign monitoring. This technique has the advantage of using ketamine as the dissociative anesthesia and peribulbar lidocaine (combined with ocular massage) as the local anesthetic agent to anesthetize the ocular tissues and to counter the effect of increased intraocular pressure caused by the ketamine. The authors concluded that ketamine may be useful in a simple ophthalmic setup in the developing world. Hennig, from Lahan, and Ruit, from Kathmandu (both in Nepal), have been using intravenous ketamine with good results. Hennig has added a small Pulseoxy/ECG for monitoring and an oxygen concentrator. He has also found that most of the children in Nepal older than 5 years can be operated on using local anesthesia (e-mail communication, Albrecht Hennig).

SURGICAL INSTRUMENT AND STERILIZATION

It is also much easier to ensure that a few instruments are maintained in good condition at all times rather than a large and complicated set. Simpler methods are generally used for sterilization of the instruments. Sharp instruments are simply sterilized by immersion in an efficient antiseptic solution such as 2% Savlon (a mixture of hibitane and cetrimide) together with an antirust agent such as sodium nitrite. This method is simple and inexpensive and does not depend on electricity or the integrity of a sterilizer. All other nonsharp surgical instruments can be sterilized by boiling (protecting the points with a rubber or silicone tube (2-ram sheath). When protected in this way, the use of trays and racks is unnecessary. In all cases, soft or rain water must be used for boiling to prevent damaging the instruments with deposits from hard water. Again, this method is simple and inexpensive, and almost universally applicable, even in very simple and rural situations.[21]

Due to poor compliance and the difficulty in following these pediatric patients in the developing world, we suggest a primary posterior capsulotomy followed by an anterior vitrectomy for children up to at least 8 years of age and perhaps even older, depending on the availability of a Nd:YAG laser.

USE OF IOLs FOR PEDIATRIC CATARACT SURGERY IN THE DEVELOPING WORLD

Aphakic glasses, contact lenses, and IOLs have been proposed as methods of visual rehabilitation after pediatric cataract surgery. Pros and cons of these options have been described somewhere else in this book. Implantation of an IOL during cataract surgery in the developing world seems to be a practical option, while other methods of visual rehabilitation (aphakic glasses and contact lenses) are less suitable in these settings. It is difficult to replace spectacles once broken or damaged, due to the expense and unavailability. Contact lenses are impractical for most patients in the developing world because of environmental and hygienic problems. Regular follow-up visits to eye care clinics are problematic due to the cost and distance of travel. Contact lenses are expensive and easily lost. An IOL can provide a full-time correction with optics that closely simulate those of the crystalline lens. In the industrialized world, IOL implantation at the time of cataract surgery is rapidly becoming the most common means of optical correction for children beyond infancy. In a recent study done in Africa, Yorston and coworkers[28] also recommend IOL implantation as the treatment of choice for most children with cataracts in the developing world. We agree with this assessment. In addition, Yorston has proposed that the IOL in young children be placed in the ciliary sulcus, with the optic captured through an anterior and a posterior vitrectorhexis (Fig. 54-1). We agree and recommend this technique whenever PMMA IOLs are utilized in young children in the developing world. These IOLs are well polished and inexpensive. However, they are not flexible enough to safely be placed into the capsular bag of a young child, especially when high-viscosity ophthalmic viscosurgical devices are not available. We recommend that a vitrector be used to remove the cataract and to make an identically sized anterior and posterior capsular opening. These openings should be 1 to 2 mm smaller than the IOL optic. A generous vitrectomy should also be performed if possible. The IOL is then placed into the ciliary sulcus and captured posterior to the

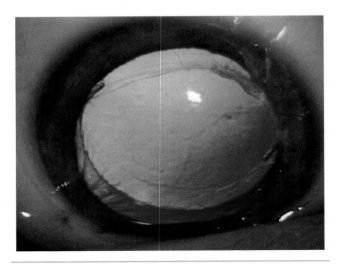

FIGURE 54-1. Optic capture through anterior and posterior capsule opening (haptics in the ciliary sulcus).

dual capsule openings. Recurrent visual axis opacification may be low using this technique (even if cortical cleanup is suboptimal) since the capsulotomy edges will seal to create a closed Sommering's ring.

Efforts to manufacture high-quality polymethylmethacrylate (PMMA) IOLs inexpensively in the developing world are ongoing.[29] Financial self-sufficiency can be attained by the physician as cataract surgery programs are able to recover costs from user fees. The IOL-producing facilities in Madurai, India (Aurolab of Aravind Eye Hospital), and in Nepal and Eritrea (Fred Hollows Foundation facilities) are successful examples. The major disadvantage of foldable IOLs is cost. Foldable lenses made from hydrophobic acrylic biomaterials (AcrySof; Alcon, Fort Worth, TX, USA) have become the most commonly implanted IOL for children in the United States, but are prohibitively expensive (more than US $100) for use in most of the developing world. As an advocate of IOL implantation, an Australian not-for-profit, nongovernmental developmental aid organization, the Fred Hollows Foundation, sought to identify and remedy these impediments. The first was the availability of good-quality, low-cost posterior chamber IOLs. In the mid-1990s, the Foundation built lens-manufacturing facilities in Eritrea and Nepal to produce lenses certified to the quality standards required in industrialized markets. The Foundation has built two internationally accredited IOL manufacturing laboratories, which produce high-quality IOLs for 3.5% of the competitor's price (www.hollows.org). In addition to their role in cataract management, the factories are examples of good manufacturing practice for other industries in the developing world. They also generate export income for these two countries, with the profit supporting blindness prevention. In collaboration with

Australian business, the Foundation has also developed a coaxial surgical microscope and YAG laser.

Selecting the best IOL power to implant in a growing child presents unique challenges even in industrial countries. The lack of instrumentation in the developing-world operating-room setting, such as the handheld keratometer and the A-scan ultrasound, increases the difficulty of selecting the appropriate IOL power to use for pediatric cataract surgery. To minimize the need to exchange IOLs later in life when a large myopic shift occurs, it has been advised to undercorrect children with IOLs so that they can grow into emmetropia or mild myopia in adult life.

CONCLUSION

To summarize, the acceptability, accessibility, and affordability of cataract surgical services must each be carefully addressed to improve efficiency. In some locations the facilities are in place but underutilized, because there is a lack of knowledge, monetary constraints, or a negative public perception of the surgery owing to poor results using inadequate or poorly time treatment. Inadequate ophthalmic and anesthesiology staff, lack of ophthalmic surgical instruments, and poor equipment maintenance are also widespread in developing countries. Other problems include the logistic complexities of identifying the children who will benefit most for surgery and arranging reliable transportation to the treatment center.

We recommend the following steps to improve the long-term visual outcome of children with cataracts, regardless of the cause of those cataracts.[2] These recommendations are in addition to the many ongoing efforts aimed at the eradication of childhood cataracts through such programs as rubella vaccination and nutritional improvements. The steps should be funded by nongovernment organizations and regional eye centers through donations and cost recovery plans. Our recommendations to facilitate the application of these surgical steps are as follows. (1) Improve the early identification and referral of children. (2) Designate regional centers for the treatment of pediatric cataracts. (3) Set up a twinning relationship between each regional developing-world pediatric cataract center and an industrialized world center that has experience with pediatric cataract surgery.

REFERENCES

1. Gilbert CE, Rahi JS, Quinn GE. Visual impairment and blindness in children. In: Johnson GJ, Weale R, Minassian DC, West SK, eds. *The Epidemiology of Eye Disease,* 2nd ed. London: Arnold, 2003.
2. Wilson ME, Pandey SK, Thakur J. Paediatric cataract blindness in the developing world: surgical techniques and intraocular lenses in the new millennium. *Br J Ophthalmol* 2003;87:14–19.
3. Schwab LT, Taylor HR, Nauze JL. Cataract and delivery of surgical services in developing nations. In: *Duane's Ophthalmology.* Baltimore: Lippincott Williams and Wilkins, 2001:chap 57.
4. WHO. Press release. Geneva: World Health Organization, 2002.
5. Gilbert C, Foster A. Childhood blindness in the context of VISION 2020—The right to sight. *Bull WHO* 2001;79:227–232.
6. Foster A, Gilbert C, Rahi J. Epidemiology of cataract in childhood: a global perspective. *J Cataract Refract Surg* 1997;23:601–604.
7. Hoyt CS, Good WV. The many challenges of childhood blindness. *Br J Ophthalmol* 2001;85:1145–1146.
8. Hoyt CS, Good WV. The many challenges of childhood blindness. *Arch Dis Child* 2001;85:452–453.
9. Cunningham ET Jr, Lietman TM, Whitcher JP. Blindness: a global priority for the twenty-first century. *Bull WHO* 2001;79:180.
10. Steinkuller PG, Du L, Gilbert C, Foster A, Collins ML, Coats DK. Childhood blindness. *J AAPOS* 1999;3:26–32.
11. Foster A. Cataract and "Vision 2020—The right to sight" initiative. *Br J Ophthalmol* 2001;85:635–637.
12. O'Sullivan J, Gilbert C, Foster A. The causes of childhood blindness in South Africa. *So Afr Med J* 1997;87:1691–1695.
13. Rahi JS, Gilbert CE, Foster A, Minassian D. Measuring the burden of childhood blindness. *Br J Ophthalmol* 1999;83:387–388.
14. Foster A. Childhood blindness in India and Sri Lanka. *Indian J Ophthalmol* 1996;44:57–60.
15. Foster A, Gilbert C. Epidemiology of childhood blindness. *Eye* 1992;6:173–176.
16. Thylefors B. Avoidable blindness. *Bull WHO* 1999;77:453.
17. Thylefors B. A mission for vision. *Lancet* 1999;354 (Suppl IV):44.
18. Venkataswamy G. Massive eye relief project in India. *Am J Ophthalmol* 1975;79:135–140.
19. Civerchia L, Ravindran RD, Apoorvananda SW, Ramakrishnan R, Balent A, Spencer MH, et al. High-volume intraocular lens surgery in a rural eye camp in India. *Ophthalmic Surg Lasers* 1996;27:200–208.
20. Thomas R. The cataract scene. *Indian J Ophthalmol* 2003;51:209–210.
21. Taylor J. Appropriate methods and resources for third world ophthalmology. In: *Duane's Ophthalmology.* Baltimore: Lippincott Williams and Wilkins, 2001:chap 58.
22. Zwaan J. Simultaneous surgery for bilateral pediatric cataracts. *Ophthalmic Surg Lasers* 1996;27:15–20.
23. Totan Y, Bayramlar H, Cekic O, Aydin E, Erten A, Daglioglu MC. Bilateral cataract surgery in adult and pediatric patients in a single session. *J Cataract Refract Surg* 2000;26:1008–1011.
24. Guo S, Nelson LB, Calhoun J, Levin A. Simultaneous surgery for bilateral congenital cataracts. *J Pediatr Ophthalmol Strabismus* 1990;27:23–25.
25. Smith GT, Liu CS. Is it time for a new attitude to "simultaneous" bilateral cataract surgery? *Br J Ophthalmol* 2001;85:1489–1496.
26. Pun MS, Thakur J, Poudyal G, Gurung R, Rana S, Tabin G, et al. Ketamine anaesthesia for paediatric ophthalmology surgery. *Br J Ophthalmol* 2003;87:535–537.
27. Thakur J, Reddy H, Wilson Jr. ME, Paudyal G, Gurung R, Thapa S, et al. Pediatric cataract surgery in Nepal. *J Cataract Refract Surg* 2004;30:1629–1635.
28. Yorston D, Wood M, Foster A. Results of cataract surgery in young children in east Africa. *Br J Ophthalmol* 2001;85:267–271.
29. Natchiar GN, Thulasiraj RD, Negrel AD, Bangdiwala S, Rahmathallah R, Prajna NV, et al. The Madurai Intraocular Lens Study. I. A randomized clinical trial comparing complications and vision outcomes of intracapsular cataract extraction and extracapsular cataract extraction with posterior chamber intraocular lens. *Am J Ophthalmol* 1998;125:1–13.
30. National Program for Control of Blindness. Evaluation of training of ophthalmic surgeons in ECCE/IOL cataract surgery: results of study done between July to October 1999. New Delhi: NPCB, Ministry of Health & Family Welfare, Government of India.

Pediatric Cataract Surgery and Intraocular Lens Implantation

Practice Styles and Preferences of the 2001 ASCRS and AAPOS Memberships

M. Edward Wilson, Jr., Luanna R. Bartholomew, and Rupal H. Trivedi

Childhood cataract is the major preventable cause of life-long visual impairment. In recent years, technical and technological advances in adult cataract surgery have helped pediatric cataract surgeons to safely operate on pediatric eyes. Increasing numbers of surgeons now accept intraocular lens (IOL) implantation pseudophakia as a mode of aphakic rehabilitation in pediatric cataract surgery. However, many other issues in the management of the pediatric cataract patient remain.

To learn more about the worldwide practice styles and ophthalmic patterns of pediatric cataract surgery, we queried adult-subspecialty and pediatric-subspecialty cataract surgeons about their pediatric cataract surgery and IOL implantation practices. Some of the 2001 results were compared with the results of the first American Society of Cataract and Refractive Surgery (ASCRS) and American Association for Pediatric Ophthalmology and Strabismus (AAPOS) surveys of IOL implantation in children that were distributed in 1993.[1]

MATERIALS AND METHODS

In October 2001, a 36-question survey of the demographics, practice patterns, surgical preferences, and preoperative and postoperative care in pediatric cataract surgery was mailed to 8,935 ASCRS members (5,980 domestic, 2,955 international) and to 980 AAPOS members (826 domestic, 154 international). The ASCRS respondents

This chapter in its entirety was first published in *J Cataract Refract Surg* 2003;29(September):1811–1820. Reprinted with permission.

were asked to mail or facsimile the completed surveys to ASCRS, which submitted the facsimiles to the Medical University of South Carolina, Storm Eye Institute (MUSC-SEI), Charleston, South Carolina, for analysis. The AAPOS respondents were asked to mail or facsimile the completed surveys to MUSC-SEI. Names of those returning questionnaires to ASCRS were placed in a drawing for a handheld electronic organizer. There were no financial rewards or incentives for returning the AAPOS questionnaires.

Questionnaire responses were compiled and analyzed at MUSC-SEI using Microsoft Excel 2000 spreadsheets and analytical tools. The number of questionnaires without a response to a question were noted as no response.

RESULTS

Demographics

The overall return rate for ASCRS was 12.6% and for AAPOS, 41.0%. The response rate by country or region is shown in Table 55-1. Respondents who were currently retired were omitted from further evaluation (Table 55-2). Seven hundred sixty-one ASCRS respondents (67.4%) and 111 AAPOS respondents (28.0%), although practicing physicians, were not doing pediatric cataract surgery (Table 55-3). The pediatric patients of these physicians were referred to other surgeons. Questionnaires from surgeons currently performing pediatric cataract surgery were available for self-evaluation of their pediatric cataract surgery techniques and procedures.

▶ **TABLE 55-1** Country or Region of Survey Respondents

Country	ASCRS Respondents (%)	AAPOS Respondents (%)
United States	905 (80.1)	343 (85.3)
Europe	74 (6.5)	3 (0.7)
Canada	39 (3.5)	14 (3.5)
Asia	30 (2.7)	7 (1.7)
Latin America	24 (2.1)	6 (1.5)
United Kingdom	13 (1.2)	8 (2.0)
Balkans	6 (0.5)	0
Australia	5 (0.4)	5 (1.2)
Middle East	5 (0.4)	10 (2.5)
Africa	3 (0.3)	0
Caribbean	3 (0.3)	0
Other, but unspecified	19 (1.7)	1 (0.2)
Unable to determine[a]	3 (0.3)	0
Retired, not applicable	1 (0.1)	5 (1.2)

[a]Front page of facsimile not received.

▶ **TABLE 55-2** Survey Questionnaire Details

Parameter	ASCRS Respondents (%)	AAPOS Respondents (%)
Domestic mailings	5,980 (66.9)	826 (84.3)
International mailings	2,955 (33.1)	154 (15.7)
Returned questionnaires	1,130 (12.6)	402 (41.0)
Retired physician[a]	1 (0.1)	5 (1.2)
Review of self-evaluation[b]	1,129 (99.9)	397 (98.8)

[a]Omitted from further evaluation.
[b]Front page of three facsimile questionnaires not received; back page included.

▶ **TABLE 55-3** Practice Patterns of Survey Respondents

Practice Pattern	ASCRS Respondents (%)	AAPOS Respondents (%)
Currently performing PCS (ASCRS, *n* = 1,129; AAPOS, *n* = 397)	368 (32.6)	286 (72.0)
If not currently performing PCS (ASCRS, *n* = 761; AAPOS, *n* = 111), PCS patients were referred to		
Pediatric ophthalmologist	612 (80.4)	63 (56.8)
Adult cataract surgeon	37 (4.9)	28 (25.2)
Either	112 (14.7)	20 (18.0)
No response	0	0

PCS, pediatric cataract surgery.

▶ **TABLE 55-4** Overall Satisfaction with Surgical Outcomes in Pediatric Cataract Patients (ASCRS, *n* = 368; AAPOS, *n* = 286)

Outcome	ASCRS Respondents (%)	AAPOS Respondents (%)
Completely satisfied	153 (41.6)	77 (26.9)
Partially satisfied	193 (52.4)	200 (69.9)
Not satisfied	8 (2.2)	3 (1.0)
Uncommitted	6 (1.6)	2 (0.7)
No response	8 (2.2)	4 (1.4)

Cataract Surgery

Table 55-4 shows physicians' satisfaction with their pediatric cataract surgical outcomes. Three hundred sixty-four ASCRS respondents (98.9%) indicated the minimum patient age at which they had performed such surgery; all AAPOS pediatric cataract surgeons responded to a similar query (Table 55-5).

Table 55-6 shows the approximate number of pediatric cataract surgeries performed annually by each respondent. More than 50.0% of respondents in the ASCRS group performed fewer than 10 pediatric cataract surgeries per year (71.5%); most AAPOS respondents (85.0%) performed fewer than 20 pediatric cataract surgeries per year.

Details of cataract surgery practice procedures are shown in Table 55-7. Routine performance of hydrodissection was performed by 256 ASCRS respondents (69.9%) and 104 AAPOS respondents (36.4%). Table 55-8 shows the reasons for omission of this step.

Table 55-9 shows how many respondents performed posterior capsulotomies, and when and how, and Table 55-10 the maximum patient age at which posterior capsulotomy was routinely performed. Table 55-11 shows the anterior capsulotomy preferences.

▶ **TABLE 55-5** Minimum Age of Patients Having Cataract Surgery by Respondents Currently Performing It (ASCRS, *n* = 364; AAPOS, *n* = 286)

Minimum Age	ASCRS Respondents (%)	AAPOS Respondents (%)
Overall mean ± SD	2.3 ± 3.7 yr	1.9 ± 8.6 mo
Overall median	0.5 yr	0.5 mo
≤2 yr	262 (72.0)	284 (99.3)
≤1 mo	114 (31.3)	256 (89.5)
≤1 wk	4 (1.1)	90 (31.5)

▶ **TABLE 55-6** Pediatric Cataract Surgery Procedures Performed per Year (ASCRS, *n* = 368; AAPOS, *n* = 286)

Annual Cases	ASCRS Respondents (%)	AAPOS Respondents (%)
<10	263 (71.5)	137 (47.9)
10–20	60 (16.3)	106 (37.1)
20–50	26 (7.1)	29 (10.1)
>50	15 (4.1)	13 (4.5)
No response	4 (1.1)	1 (0.3)

Vitrectomy preference was ascertained to determine whether it was routinely performed at the time of cataract surgery and, if so, by what technique (Table 55-12). Table 55-13 shows the maximum patient age at which vitrectomy was routinely performed.

Table 55-14 shows the use of ophthalmic viscosurgical devices.

Intraocular Lens Implantation

Three hundred forty-five ASCRS respondents (93.8%) and 256 AAPOS respondents (89.5%) were currently doing pediatric cataract surgery and implanting IOLs in children.

▶ **TABLE 55-7** Surgical Procedure Details (ASCRS, *n* = 368; AAPOS, *n* = 286)

Detail	ASCRS Respondents (%)	AAPOS Respondents (%)
Incision location		
Superior	234 (63.6)	241 (84.3)
Temporal	127 (34.5)	40 (14.0)
No response	7 (1.9)	5 (1.7)
Tunnel incision		
Scleral	217 (59.0)	198 (69.2)
Corneal	139 (37.8)	77 (26.9)
Limbal	2 (0.5)	1 (0.3)
No response	10 (2.7)	10 (3.5)
Irrigation/aspiration[a]		
Single port	218 (59.2)	179 (62.6)
Bimanual	122 (33.2)	112 (39.2)
No response	28 (7.6)	5 (1.7)
Sutured closure		
Tunnel only	186 (50.5)	160 (55.9)
Paracentesis only	6 (1.6)	3 (1.0)
Both	82 (22.3)	113 (39.5)
Neither	73 (19.8)	8 (2.8)
No response	21 (5.7)	2 (0.7)

[a] Multiple responses allowed.

▶ **TABLE 55-8** Routine Hydrodissection or Reasons Respondents Did Not Perform Hydrodissection During Pediatric Cataract Surgery

Pararameter	ASCRS Respondents (%)	AAPOS Respondents (%)
Routinely perform hydrodissection (ASCRS, *n* = 368; AAPOS, *n* = 286)	256 (69.6)	104 (36.4)
No response	16 (4.3)	5 (1.7)
If not performing hydrodissection (ASCRS, *n* = 96; AAPOS, *n* = 177), why not?		
Do not feel it is necessary	72 (75.0)	133 (75.1)
Found it was ineffective	10 (10.4)	7 (4.0)
Don't know about its use	2 (2.1)	17 (9.6)
Other (posterior capsule integrity risk)	4 (4.2)	10 (5.6)
No reason given	8 (8.3)	10 (5.6)

Three hundred fifty-four ASCRS respondents and 270 AAPOS respondents indicated the youngest patient on whom they had performed IOL implantation (Table 55-15). Table 55-16 shows the minimum patient age at which they would perform or advise unilateral and bilateral IOL implantation.

▶ **TABLE 55-9** Posterior Capsulotomy Preferences (ASCRS, *n* = 368; AAPOS, *n* = 286): Multiple Responses Were Allowed

Preference	ASCRS Respondents (%)	AAPOS Respondents (%)
Posterior capsulotomy		
Performed routinely	247 (67.1)	260 (90.9)
No response	18 (4.9)	6 (2.1)
Before IOL implantation	144 (39.1)	122 (42.7)
After IOL implantation	153 (41.6)	137 (47.9)
No response	71 (19.3)	30 (10.5)
Posterior capsulotomy technique		
Capsulorhexis	152 (41.3)	31 (10.8)
Automated vitrector cut	159 (43.2)	247 (86.4)
Radiofrequency endodiathermy	5 (1.4)	2 (0.7)
Other (laser, needle, pars plana)	8 (2.2)	10 (3.5)
No response	74 (20.1)	15 (5.2)

▶ **TABLE 55-10** Maximum Age of Patients Who Routinely Received a Posterior Capsulotomy at the Time of Cataract Surgery (ASCRS, *n* = 247; AAPOS, *n* = 260)

Patient Age (yr)	ASCRS Respondents (%)	AAPOS Respondents (%)
1	93 (37.7)	69 (26.5)
2	76 (30.8)	93 (35.8)
5	34 (13.8)	69 (26.5)
9	10 (4.0)	9 (3.5)
12	4 (1.6)	2 (0.8)
17	2 (0.8)	1 (0.4)
No age specified	28 (11.3)	17 (6.5)

▶ **TABLE 55-13** Maximum Age of Pediatric Patients Who Routinely Received a Vitrectomy at the Time of Cataract Surgery (ASCRS, *n* = 201; AAPOS, *n* = 263)

Patient Age (yr)	ASCRS Respondents (%)	AAPOS Respondents (%)
1	83 (41.3)	88 (33.5)
2	53 (26.4)	85 (32.3)
5	31 (15.4)	61 (23.2)
9	11 (5.5)	8 (3.0)
12	4 (2.0)	2 (0.8)
17	2 (1.0)	2 (0.8)
No age specified	17 (8.5)	17 (6.5)

▶ **TABLE 55-11** Anterior Capsulotomy Preferences (ASCRS, *n* = 368; AAPOS, *n* = 286): Multiple Responses Were Allowed

Preference	ASCRS Respondents (%)	AAPOS Respondents (%)
Anterior capsulotomy technique		
Can opener	26 (7.1)	69 (24.1)
Capsulorhexis	315 (85.6)	174 (60.8)
Vitrectorhexis	45 (12.2)	153 (53.5)
Radiofrequency endodiathermy	6 (1.6)	4 (1.4)
Other (laser)	1 (0.3)	2 (0.7)
No response	16 (4.3)	5 (1.7)

▶ **TABLE 55-14** Ophthalmic Viscosurgical Device Use (ASCRS, *n* = 368; AAPOS, *n* = 286)

OVD Preference	ASCRS Respondents (%)	AAPOS Respondents (%)
Single agent		
Cohesive	179 (48.6)	216 (75.5)
Superviscous cohesive	41 (22.9)	60 (27.8)
Viscoadaptive	18 (4.9)	5 (1.7)
Dispersive	95 (25.8)	28 (9.8)
Combined agents		
Cohesive + cohesive	2 (0.5)	9 (3.1)
Cohesive + viscoadaptive	4 (1.1)	2 (0.7)
Two cohesive + viscoadaptive	1 (0.3)	0
Dispersive + cohesive	46 (12.5)	15 (5.2)
Dispersive + viscoadaptive	3 (0.8)	0
No response	20 (5.4)	11 (3.8)

OVD, ophthalmic viscosurgical device.

▶ **TABLE 55-12** Vitrectomy Preferences (ASCRS, *n* = 368; AAPOS, *n* = 286)

Preference	ASCRS Respondents (%)	AAPOS Respondents (%)
Vitrectomy		
Performed routinely	201 (54.6)	263 (92.0)
No response	25 (6.8)	7 (2.4)
Optic capture prevents vitrectomy need	60 (16.3)	16 (5.6)
No response	59 (16.0)	35 (12.2)
Vitrectomy technique		
Anterior 1 port	101 (27.4)	130 (45.5)
Anterior 2 port	98 (26.6)	85 (29.7)
Pars plana	45 (12.2)	43 (15.0)
No response	124 (33.7)	28 (9.8)

▶ **TABLE 55-15** The Minimum Age of Patients in Whom Respondents Had Implanted IOL (ASCRS, *n* = 354; AAPOS, *n* = 270)

Minimum Age	ASCRS Respondents (%)	AAPOS Respondents (%)
Overall mean ± SD	4.0 ± 4.1 yr	1.8 ± 1.6 yr
Overall median	2.0 yr	1.5 yr
≤2 yr	192 (54.2)	221 (81.9)
≤1 mo	17 (4.8)	23 (8.5)
≤1 wk	0	1 (0.4)

▶ **TABLE 55-16** The Minimum Patient Age at Which Respondents Would Advise IOL Implantation (ASCRS, $n = 358$; AAPOS, $n = 285$)

Minimum Age	ASCRS Respondents (%)	AAPOS Respondents (%)
Unilateral IOL implantation		
Overall mean ± SD	2.1 ± 2.8 yr	1.4 ± 1.4 yr
Overall median	1.5 yr	1.0 yr
≤2 yr	266 (74.3)	254 (89.1)
Bilateral IOL implantation		
Overall mean ± SD	3.3 ± 3.8 yr	2.2 ± 2.2 yr
Overall median	2.0 yr	2.0 yr
≤2 yr	231 (64.5)	221 (77.5)

▶ **TABLE 55-18** Intraocular Lens Materials Routinely Implanted in Pediatric Cataract Surgery Patients (ASCRS, $n = 368$; AAPOS, $n = 286$): Multiple Responses Were Allowed

IOL Material	ASCRS Respondents (%)	AAPOS Respondents (%)
Acrylic		
Hydrophobic	246 (66.8)	205 (71.7)
Hydrophilic	9 (2.4)	3 (1.0)
Silicone	25 (6.8)	5 (1.7)
PMMA	87 (23.6)	70 (24.5)
HSM PMMA	18 (4.9)	5 (1.7)
Other, but unspecified	4 (1.1)	0
No response	13 (3.5)	22 (7.7)

PMMA, polymethylmethacrylate; HSM, heparin-surface-modified.

Of ASCRS respondents, 76.4% performed fewer than 10 IOL implantations per year, and of AAPOS respondents, 64.0% (Table 55-17). Table 55-18 shows the preferred IOL material routinely implanted.

Table 55-19 shows what postoperative refraction was aimed for after IOL implantation at various ages. Table 55-20 shows whether respondents agreed or disagreed with a series of conditions as contraindications to IOL placement in a child. Table 55-21 shows several IOL considerations with no ranking order of importance.

Drug Modalities

Table 55-22 shows which patient treatment modalities, including intracameral miotics, were used preoperatively and postoperatively.

Examination Under Anesthesia

Table 55-23 shows how frequently surgeons would advise that a child be examined under anesthesia.

▶ **TABLE 55-17** Number of Pediatric IOL Implantations per Year (ASCRS, $n = 368$; AAPOS, $n = 286$)

Cases	ASCRS Respondents (%)	AAPOS Respondents (%)
<10	281 (76.4)	183 (64.0)
10–20	54 (14.7)	69 (24.1)
20–50	21 (5.7)	20 (7.0)
>50	7 (1.9)	7 (2.4)
No response	5 (1.4)	7 (2.4)

DISCUSSION

For comparison, 1993 IOL survey data[1] were summarized in a manner similar to the presentation format of the 2001 survey data. Table 55-24 summarizes the IOL practice patterns; a comparison with the data 8 years later (Table 55-15) shows a nearly 5-fold increase in the number of ASCRS respondents and a more than 13-fold increase in the number of AAPOS respondents implanting IOLs in children 2 years old and younger. Thus, an increasing number of physicians accept IOL implantation pseudophakia as a mode of aphakic rehabilitation during or after pediatric cataract surgery in the early years of life. Comparison of the unilateral and bilateral data with those 8 years later (Table 55-16) shows the minimum mean advisement age for IOL implantation dropped by more than half for ASCRS and AAPOS respondents in both the unilateral and the bilateral categories.

Table 55-25 summarizes the 1993 survey[1] IOL styles and preferences. Over the 8-year period (Table 55-21), preference for fixation of an IOL in the ciliary sulcus of a child appears unchanged, as is disfavor of placement of an anterior chamber lens.

Manual-tear capsulorhexis remains the most commonly used method of pediatric anterior capsulotomy by both groups (Tables 55-11 and 55-25), with little interest shown in the can-opener technique. Although not part of the 1993 survey, vitrectorhexis was accepted as an alternative technique for the highly elastic pediatric anterior capsule by more than half of AAPOS respondents who use it routinely but by only one tenth of ASCRS respondents. This difference may reflect the pediatric ophthalmologists' comparatively greater experience using the vitrector for cataract surgery in infants and less experience with manual continuous curvilinear capsulorhexis (CCC). The

▶ **TABLE 55-19** The Postoperative Refraction Aimed for by Age Category After IOL Implantation (ASCRS, $n = 368$, No Response = 25; AAPOS, $n = 286$, No Response = 14)

Refraction Aim	Patient Age, Respondents (%)				
	6 mo	12 mo	2 yr	5 yr	10 yr
High hyperopia					
ASCRS	34 (9.2)	6 (1.6)	1 (0.3)	0	0
AAPOS	45 (15.7)	8 (2.8)	0	0	0
Moderate hyperopia					
ASCRS	100 (27.2)	101 (27.4)	40 (10.9)	9 (2.4)	2 (0.5)
AAPOS	98 (34.3)	103 (36.0)	44 (15.4)	3 (1.0)	0
Mild hyperopia					
ASCRS	76 (20.7)	121 (32.9)	175 (47.6)	117 (31.8)	32 (8.7)
AAPOS	42 (14.7)	85 (29.7)	178 (62.2)	125 (43.7)	21 (7.3)
Emmetropia					
ASCRS	9 (2.4)	20 (5.4)	72 (19.6)	174 (47.3)	257 (69.8)
AAPOS	1 (0.3)	6 (2.1)	37 (12.9)	133 (46.5)	227 (79.4)
Mild myopia					
ASCRS	21 (5.7)	19 (5.2)	22 (6.0)	28 (7.6)	40 (10.9)
AAPOS	1 (0.3)	1 (0.3)	4 (1.4)	7 (2.4)	17 (5.9)
No response					
ASCRS	103 (28.0)	76 (20.7)	33 (9.0)	15 (4.1)	12 (3.3)
AAPOS	85 (29.7)	69 (24.1)	9 (3.1)	4 (1.4)	7 (2.4)

Note. High hyperopia, ≥7 diopters (D); moderate hyperopia, ≥3 D but <7 D; mild hyperopia, >0 D but <3 D; mild myopia, −2 to −1 D.

vitrectorhexis technique is reported to perform better than manual CCC in laboratory and clinical settings.[2–4]

Hydrodissection is accepted as a routine approach for adult cataract surgery; however, use of this step in pediatric cataract surgery is not universally accepted (Table 55-8).

Routine posterior capsulotomy and vitrectomy in very young patients remain almost universally accepted (Table 55-9). Interest in automated vitrector-cut capsulotomy is replacing a former preference for the capsulorhexis technique in pediatric patients (Tables 55-9 and

▶ **TABLE 55-20** Contraindications to IOL Placement in a Child (ASCRS, $n = 368$, No Response = 9; AAPOS, $n = 286$, No Response = 0): Multiple Responses Were Allowed

Contraindication	Respondents (%)			
	ASCRS		AAPOS	
	Agree	Disagree	Agree	Disagree
Microphthalmia	257 (69.8)	86 (23.4)	191 (66.8)	80 (28.0)
Anterior segment dysgenesis or abnormalities	247 (67.1)	96 (26.1)	188 (65.7)	74 (25.9)
Inadequate or incomplete capsule support	224 (60.9)	111 (30.2)	188 (65.7)	80 (28.0)
Persistent fetal vasculature	185 (50.3)	142 (38.6)	99 (34.6)	156 (54.5)
Glaucoma	120 (32.6)	213 (57.9)	138 (48.3)	127 (44.4)
Aphakic fellow eye	74 (20.1)	241 (65.5)	44 (15.4)	197 (68.9)
Posterior lenticonus	24 (6.5)	291 (79.1)	8 (2.8)	238 (83.2)
Bilateral lens opacity	11 (3.0)	309 (84.0)	7 (2.4)	237 (82.9)
Other[a]	28 (7.6)	0	34 (11.9)	0
Other, unspecified	1 (0.3)	0	1 (0.3)	0
No choice indicated	17 (4.6)	42 (11.4)	14 (4.9)	41 (14.3)

[a]Ocular anomalies; only seeing eye; parental refusal; patient age; retinal detachment.

▶ **TABLE 55-21**   Intraocular Lens (IOL) Considerations (ASCRS, *n* = 368; AAPOS, *n* = 286)

Preference	ASCRS Respondents (%)	AAPOS Respondents (%)
When capsule fixation is not an option, then		
Ciliary sulcus fixation	234 (63.6)	222 (77.6)
No response	20 (5.4)	12 (4.2)
Anterior chamber IOL	40 (10.9)	36 (12.6)
No response	19 (5.2)	8 (2.8)
Iris claw IOL	50 (13.6)	14 (4.9)
No response	18 (4.9)	8 (2.8)
Multifocal alternate IOL	23 (6.3)	5 (1.7)
No response	17 (4.6)	8 (2.8)
Endocapsular ring	52 (14.1)	7 (2.4)
No response	17 (4.6)	5 (1.7)
Down-sized pediatric IOL	126 (34.2)	83 (29.0)
No response	45 (12.2)	37 (12.9)
Routine intracameral miotic	148 (40.2)	165 (57.7)
No response	19 (5.2)	7 (2.4)

▶ **TABLE 55-23**   When Ocular Examination Under Anesthesia Is Advisable (ASCRS, *n* = 368; AAPOS, *n* = 286)

Advisable	ASCRS Respondents (%)	AAPOS Respondents (%)
Never	12 (3.3)	17 (5.9)
Semiannually	121 (32.9)	83 (29.0)
Annually	44 (12.0)	34 (11.9)
Only as needed	163 (44.3)	148 (51.7)
No response	28 (7.6)	4 (1.4)

55-25). However, controversy still exists regarding at what age the posterior capsule should be left intact. More than 50% of the 1993 ASCRS[1] and 2001 ASCRS and AAPOS respondents recommended posterior capsulotomy and vitrectomy before the age of 5 years (Tables 55-9 and 55-10). In the 2001 survey, more than 60% of respondents recommended routine posterior capsulotomy and vitrectomy in all cataract patients 2 years old or younger at the time of surgery (Table 55-10).

There is no consensus in the literature on the ideal postoperative refraction after IOL implantation. Although a few surgeons indicated a preference for emmetropia or even mild myopia after surgery at all ages, the more common aim was for hyperopia until age 5 years, where the preference for emmetropia began to emerge (Table 55-19). This trend recognizes the significant myopic shift after cataract surgery in young children.[5]

Implantation of an endocapsular ring has not been approved by the U.S. Food and Drug Administration, and multifocal IOLs are not commonly implanted in children. Although not specifically addressed in our survey, we believe that multifocal IOLs are being used more often in teenage eyes in which axial growth is complete. We also believe that truly accommodating IOLs, when developed, will become popular for implantation in children.

Of surgeons currently performing cataract surgery in pediatric patients, 72.0% of ASCRS respondents and 99.3% of AAPOS respondents performed surgery in children 2 years old or younger (Table 55-5). The AAPOS respondents, however, performed surgery in patients at a much lower median minimum age (0.5 month) than ASCRS

▶ **TABLE 55-22**   Treatment Modalities Routinely Used Preoperatively and Postoperatively (ASCRS, *n* = 368, No Response = 17; AAPOS, *n* = 286, No Response = 2): Multiple Responses Were Allowed

Treatment	Respondents (%) ASCRS Preoperative	ASCRS Postoperative	AAPOS Preoperative	AAPOS Postoperative
Topical antibiotic	252 (68.5)	312 (84.8)	102 (35.7)	265 (92.7)
Systemic antibiotic	13 (3.5)	32 (8.7)	2 (0.7)	10 (3.5)
Topical steroid	86 (23.4)	331 (89.9)	23 (8.0)	276 (96.5)
Systemic steroid	7 (1.9)	39 (10.6)	5 (1.7)	53 (18.5)
Nonsteroidal antiinflammatory	93 (25.3)	115 (31.3)	27 (9.4)	24 (8.4)
Topical antiglaucoma drug	12 (3.3)	53 (14.4)	2 (0.7)	12 (4.2)
Systemic antiglaucoma drug	2 (0.5)	9 (2.4)	0	2 (0.7)
Cyclopentolate	132 (35.9)	56 (15.2)	94 (32.9)	77 (26.9)
Atropine	24 (6.5)	60 (16.3)	17 (5.9)	119 (41.6)
Other[a]	12 (3.3)	5 (1.4)	10 (3.5)	5 (1.7)
No modality indicated	57 (15.5)	9 (2.4)	127 (44.4)	3 (1.0)

[a]Tropicamide; phenylephrine; disinfectant; cycloplegic; pilocarpine.

▶ **TABLE 55-24** Overview of 1993 Survey[1] of Pediatric IOL Practice Patterns

Practice Pattern	1993 ASCRS Respondents (%)	1993 AAPOS Respondents (%)
Returned questionnaires	1039	234
Have implanted IOLs	372 (35.8)	124 (53.0)
Currently implanting IOLs	284 (27.3)	107 (45.7)
Minimum patient age ≤2 yr (ASCRS, n = 372; AAPOS, n = 124)	41 (11.0)	16 (12.9)
Minimum patient age would advise unilateral IOL implantation		
Overall mean	3.0 to 5.0 yr	4.2 yr
Overall median	NA	3.0 yr
≤ 2 yr (ASCRS, n = 284; AAPOS, n = 107)	53 (18.7)	NA
Minimum patient age would advise bilateral IOL implantation		
Overall mean	6.0 to 9.0 yr	7.0 yr
Overall median	NA	5.0 yr
≤2 yr (ASCRS, n = 284; AAPOS, n = 107)	40 (14.1)	NA

NA, not asked on questionnaire.

▶ **TABLE 55-25** Overview of 1993 Survey[1] of Pediatric IOL Styles and Preferences (ASCRS, n = 284; AAPOS, n = 107)

Style/Preference	1993 ASCRS Respondents (%)	1993 AAPOS Respondents (%)
Anterior capsulotomy technique		
Can opener	43 (15.1)	NA
Capsulorhexis	238 (83.8)	NA
Perform posterior capsulotomy routinely at the time of surgery	142 (50.0)	NA
Using capsulorhexis	108 (38.0)	NA
Maximum patient age for routine posterior capsulotomy		
5 yr	85 (30.0)	NA
12 yr	23 (8.1)	NA
17 yr	14 (4.9)	NA
When capsule fixation of the IOL is not an option, then		
Ciliary sulcus fixation	190 (66.9)	NA
Anterior chamber lens	40 (14.1)	19 (17.8)

NA, not asked on questionnaire.

respondents (0.5 year). These results show that physicians are gaining more experience with pediatric cataract surgery with or without IOL implantation, even in the early weeks of a child's life.

The current preference for superior placement and scleral (rather than corneal) tunnel incisions in the survey may reflect the increased tendency for children to rub and otherwise traumatize their eyes after surgery. Superiorly placed wounds are protected by the brow and by Bell's phenomenon.

Although the outcomes of pediatric cataract surgery have improved in recent years, most ASCRS and AAPOS respondents remained only partially satisfied with their outcomes. Growing pediatric eyes present many challenges not commonly faced in adults. Also, more than 70% of ASCRS respondents and more than 60% of AAPOS respondents performed fewer than 10 IOL implantations per year. Because the volume of childhood cataract surgery and IOL implantation is small, consideration should be given to increasing referrals to designated regional centers, where experience with these cases can be concentrated. Less than 15% of respondents were performing 20 or more pediatric cataract surgeries annually, and less than 10% were performing 20 or more IOL implantations in children per year (Table 55-17).

In conclusion, the trends and preferences in the management of pediatric cataract among ASCRS and AAPOS members have evolved since the ASCRS and AAPOS IOL survey references 8 years ago. Pseudophakia continues to be accepted and performed in younger patients. We expect practice preferences for pediatric cataract surgery and IOL implantation to continue to change over time, but not always in step with adult cataract survey trends. Because pediatric eyes differ in many ways from adult eyes, monitoring these changing trends will be important to ensure the best surgical outcomes in children.

REFERENCES

1. Wilson ME, Bluestein EC, Wang X-H. Current trends in the use of intraocular lenses in children. *J Cataract Refract Surg* 1994;20:579–583.
2. Wilson ME, Bluestein EC, Wang X-H, Apple DJ. Comparison of mechanized anterior capsulectomy and manual continuous capsulorhexis in pediatric eyes. *J Cataract Refract Surg* 1994;20:602–606.
3. Wilson ME, Saunders RA, Roberts EL, Apple DJ. Mechanized anterior capsulectomy as an alternative to manual capsulorhexis in children undergoing intraocular lens implantation. *J Pediatr Ophthalmol Strabismus* 1996;33(4):237–240.
4. Andreo LK, Wilson ME, Apple DJ. Elastic properties and scanning electron microscopic appearance of manual continuous curvilinear capsulorhexis and vitrectorhexis in an animal model of pediatric cataract. *J Cataract Refract Surg* 1999;25:534–539.
5. Plager DA, Kipfer H, Sprunger DT, et al. Refractive change in pediatric pseudophakia: 6-year follow-up. *J Cataract Refract Surg* 2002;28:810–815.

Step-by-Step Approach for Management of Pediatric Cataracts

Suresh K. Pandey, M. Edward Wilson, Jr., and Rupal H. Trivedi

The aim of pediatric cataract surgery is to provide and maintain a clear visual axis and a focused retinal image. The long-term visual outcome is often negatively affected by the development of amblyopia secondary to the cataract itself or owing to postoperative reopacification of the ocular media. Cataract surgery in children remains complex and challenging. One of the major challenges for pediatric cataract–intraocular lens (IOL) surgery has been the adaptation of techniques used for adult cataract–IOL surgery. However, pediatric cataract–IOL surgery is quite different from surgery for adult cataracts. The propensity for increased postoperative inflammation and capsular opacification, a refractive state that is constantly changing due to growth of the eye, difficulty in documenting anatomic and refractive changes due to poor compliance, and a tendency to develop amblyopia are the factors that make cataract surgery in the child different from that in the adult.

A detailed overview of pediatric cataract surgery and various surgical techniques has been published by the authors elsewhere[1–3] and also discussed in other chapters of this book. This chapter highlights the step-by-step approach for managing pediatric cataracts. It is also intended to be an overview of pediatric surgery for those who usually operate on adults. It summarizes many points made throughout this book (Fig. 56-1).

PEDIATRIC CATARACT-IOL SURGERY

The Incision

Children have thin sclera and markedly decreased scleral rigidity compared with adults. Scleral collapse results in increased vitreous upthrust (positive vitreous pressure). Collapse of the anterior chamber is much more common when operating on pediatric eyes. Pediatric cataracts can be removed through a relatively small wound, as the lens has no hard nuclei. Therefore, wounds should be con-

structed to provide a snug fit for the instruments that pass into the anterior chamber. When an IOL is not being implanted, two stab incisions are usually made at or near the limbus. These incisions should not be larger than necessary for the instruments being used. For instance, a micro vitreoretinal (MVR) blade creates a 20-gauge opening that is ideal for a 20-gauge vitrector/aspirator to enter the anterior chamber. A 20-gauge blunt-tipped irrigating cannula can also be used through a separate MVR blade stab incision. If the instrument positions need to be reversed, the snug fit is maintained. While some surgeons prefer phacoaspiration, a bimanual technique using an irrigating handpiece and a separate aspiration handpiece is preferred by pediatric ophthalmologists. Anterior chamber stability is maintained by limiting wound leak and using a high irrigation setting.

When a rigid IOL is being implanted, a scleral tunnel wound is utilized most often. A half-thickness scleral incision is made initially approximately 2 or 2.5 mm from the limbus and dissected into clear cornea. It is enlarged to the size necessary for IOL insertion. Closure is recommended using a synthetic absorbable suture such as 10-0 Biosorb or Vicryl. When a foldable IOL is being implanted, a corneal tunnel is preferred since it leaves the conjunctiva undisturbed. The corneal tunnel should begin near the limbus (so-called "near clear" incision) for maximum healing and should be sutured with a synthetic absorbable suture. Unlike adults, tunnel incisions do not self-seal in children.[4] According to a study,[5] self-sealing wounds failed to remain watertight in children <11 years of age, especially when an anterior vitrectomy was combined with cataract extraction. In older children (>11 years) the wounds remained self-sealing. The authors attributed this to low scleral rigidity resulting in fish-mouthing of the wound, leading to poor approximation of the internal corneal valve to the overlying stroma. Closure is recommended using a synthetic absorbable suture such as 10-0 Biosorb or Vicryl.

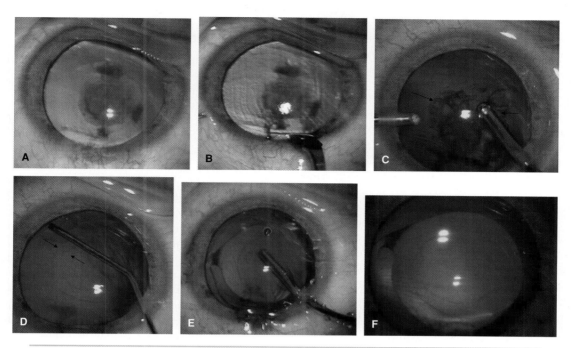

FIGURE 56-1. A 4-year-old child with bilateral cataracts. **A.** Preoperative. **B.** Corneal incision. **C.** Bimanual irrigation/aspiration after performing vitrectorhexis (arrows). **D.** Injection of viscoelastic between the anterior and the posterior capsule (arrows) facilitates in-the-bag intraocular lens implantation. **E.** Removal of viscoelastic material is essential to prevent a postoperative intraocular pressure spike. **F.** Postoperative appearance of in-the-bag fixated single-piece AcrySof IOL.

While the temporal wound presents the same advantages in children as it does in adults, the location is more easily traumatized by children. The superior approach allows the wound to be protected by the brow and Bell's phenomenon in the trauma-prone childhood years. Both scleral tunnels and corneal tunnels can be easily made from a superior approach since children rarely have deep-set orbits or overhanging brows. Positioning the patients on the operating table with a slight chin-up posture also helps made the superior approach easier. Locating the site of tunnel according to the preexisting astigmatism (e.g., temporally in against-the-rule astigmatism) has not been done as often in younger children since most of these patients will wear glasses after surgery anyway. Whether the preoperative astigmatism can be altered by the site of the tunnel incision has not been studied well in children. While wound-related astigmatism is common immediately after surgery in children, due to low scleral rigidity, these eyes tend to return to their preoperative state by 3 months after surgery.

Anterior Capsulotomy

The anterior capsule is highly elastic in the pediatric patient and poses challenges in the creation of the capsulotomy. While a manual continuous curvilinear capsulorhexis (CCC) is ideal for adults, it is more difficult to perform in young eyes. When performing a manual CCC in a child, the following technical recommendations are offered.

1. Use a highly viscous ophthalmic viscosurgical device (OVD) to fill the anterior chamber and flatten the anterior capsule. A slack anterior capsule will be easier to tear in a controlled fashion.

2. Regrasp the capsulorhexis edge frequently and begin with a smaller capsulotomy than desired. Because of the elasticity, the opening will be larger than it appears once the forceps release the capsule flap.

3. Force when tearing must often be directed toward the center of the pupil to control the turning of the CCC edge along a circular path.

4. If the capsule begins to extend peripherally, stop before the edge is out of sight under the iris. Converting to a vitrector cut capsulotomy or a radiofrequency diathermy capsulotomy is recommended when this occurs. Using a small-incision capsulorhexis forceps will allow conversion to vitrector instruments when needed without leakage around the vitrector handpiece during use.

While a CCC is a reasonable option beyond age 2, it will be very difficult for even the experienced surgeon when attempted on an infant eye. Alternative anterior capsulotomy methods as discussed below will be more consistently successful than manual CCC in infancy.

A mechanized circular anterior capsulectomy has been tested in both laboratory and clinical settings by the authors. This technique, now known as *vitrectorhexis*, has proved to be a very effective alternative to CCC for young children when the CCC may be difficult to control. Interested readers can refer to a published article (by M.E.W.) for details on the vitrectorhexis technique and management of the anterior capsule in these cases.[6]

When creating a vitrectorhexis, the following surgical caveats are offered. Use a vitrector supported by a Venturi pump. Peristaltic pump systems will not cut the anterior capsule easily. A separate infusion port is recommended. Maintain a snug fit of the instruments in the incisions through which they are placed. The anterior chamber of these soft eyes will collapse readily if leakage occurs around the instruments, making the vitrectorhexis more difficult to complete. A MVR blade can be used to enter the eye. The vitrector and the blunt-tip irrigating cannula (Nichamin cannula; Storz) or irrigation hand-piece (Alcon Greishaber 170-01) fit snugly into the MVR openings. Do not begin the capsulotomy with a bent-needle cystotome. Merely place the vitrector, with its cutting port positioned posteriorly, in contact with the center of the intact anterior capsule. Turn the cutter on and increase the suction using the foot pedal until the capsule is engaged and opened. A cutting rate of 150 to 300 cuts/min and an aspiration maximum of 150 to 250 (these settings are for the Alcon Accurus and the Stortz Premier—adjustments may be needed for other machines) are recommended. With the cutting port facing down against the capsule, engage the capsule and enlarge the round capsular opening in a spiral fashion to the desired shape and size. Any lens cortex that escapes into the anterior chamber during the vitrectorhexis is aspirated easily without interrupting the capsulotomy technique. Care should be taken to avoid leaving any right-angle edges, which could predispose to radial tear formation. The completed vitrectorhexis should be slightly smaller than the size of the IOL optic being implanted. The vitrector creates a slightly scalloped edge but inspection by both the dissecting microscope and the scanning electron microscope has revealed that the scallops roll outward to leave a smooth edge. Any capsular tags or points created at the apex of a scalloped cut from the vitrector are located in an area of low biomechanical stress much like an irregular outside-in completion of a CCC. These tags do not predispose to radial tear formation as demonstrated by finite element method computer modeling.

A third option for creating an anterior capsulotomy in a child is available with the use of high-frequency endodiathermy (Kloti radiofrequency endodiathermy). The Fugo plasma blade has also been introduced recently for use in making an anterior capsulotomy. The Fugo Blade is discussed elsewhere in this book.

Lens Substance Aspiration (Phacoaspiration)

Pediatric cataracts are soft. Phacoemulsification is not needed. Lens cortex and nucleus can be aspirated with an irrigation/aspiration or vitrectomy handpiece. When using the vitrector, bursts of cutting can be used intermittently to facilitate the aspiration of the more "gummy" cortex of young children. The phacoemulsification handpiece can also be used when aspirating pediatric lens material if the surgeon is more comfortable with this instrument. Hydrodissection has been thought to be less useful in children than in adults. However, a recent study[7] has shown the intraoperative benefits of performing multiquadrant hydrodissection: an overall reduction in the operative time and the amount of irrigating solution used and facilitation of lens substance removal. A fluid wave can sometimes be generated in older children but not reliably in infants and toddlers. Cortical material strips easily from the pediatric capsule even in the absence of hydrodissection. Attempts at hydrodelineation should be discouraged in children since it does not aid in lens removal and may lead to capsular rupture. Posterior polar cataracts in children are contraindicated for hydrodissection because of fragility in the posterior capsule.

Primary IOL Implantation

General consensus exists that IOL implantation is appropriate for most children undergoing cataract surgery beyond their second birthday.[8] In contrast, the advisability of IOL implantation in infancy is still being questioned. It is well known that the majority of the eye's axial growth occurs during the first 2 years of life. This rapid eye growth makes selection of an IOL power for an infant difficult.

When placing an IOL in a child's eye, in-the-bag implantation is strongly recommended. Care should be taken to avoid asymmetrical fixation, with one haptic in the capsular bag and the other in the ciliary sulcus. This can lead to decentration of the IOL. In contrast to adults, dialing of an IOL into the capsular bag can be difficult in children. Often the IOL will dial out of the capsular bag rather than into it. This tendency can be blunted somewhat by the use of highly viscous OVDs. Foldable hydrophobic acrylic IOLs are used increasingly in children. The AcrySof hydrophobic acrylic IOL (Alcon Laboratories, Ft. Worth, TX, USA) has been shown to be very biocompatible for the child's eye, as per author's experience.[9] The newer one-piece AcrySof is especially suited for small soft eyes and can be inserted into the capsular bag with ease. The short-term data suggest that implantation of the AcrySof single-piece hydrophobic acrylic IOL is safe in the pediatric eye.[10] While silicone IOLs are infrequently utilized in children, the second-generation silicone material appears to be an acceptable alternative for older children. When capsular fixation is not possible, sulcus placement of an IOL in a child is acceptable. To avoid decentration, rigid polymethylmethacrylate (PMMA) IOLs are recommended instead of foldable IOLs when sulcus fixation is anticipated.

Secondary IOL Implantation

The vast majority of children undergoing secondary IOL implantation have had a primary posterior capsulectomy and anterior vitrectomy. If adequate peripheral capsular support is present, the IOL is placed into the ciliary sulcus or in the reopened capsular bag. Viscodissection and meticulous clearing of all posterior synechiae between the iris and the residual capsule are mandatory. An all-PMMA heparin-surface-modified IOL rather than a foldable acrylic lens is recommended for sulcus placement. Prolapsing the IOL optic through the fused anterior and posterior capsule remnants is useful in preventing pupillary capture and ensuring lens centration. When inadequate capsular support is present for sulcus fixation in a child, implantation of an IOL is not recommended unless every contact lens and spectacle option has been explored fully.

IOL Power Selection

Selecting the best IOL power to implant in a growing child presents unique challenges. While Gordon and Donzis[11] have documented the axial growth pattern of normal eyes in children, controversy still exists about whether the pseudophakic eye grows predictably along that same curve. In the normal phakic child, there is little change in refraction (0.9 D [diopter] from birth through adulthood on average) because the power of the natural lens decreases dramatically as the eye grows axially. However, an IOL placed in a child's eye cannot change in power to match the growth of the eye. An IOL chosen for emmetropia in early childhood is likely to leave the patient highly myopic as he grows older. For children beyond age 2, studies are available to help the surgeon predict the growth of the eye on average.[12] When operating on children between 2 and 8 years of age, many surgeons have advised selecting an IOL power that will leave mild to moderate hyperopia, milder with increasing age. Other authors have advocated aiming for emmetropia regardless of age when operating beyond age 2. This approach avoids potentially amblyogenic residual hyperopia but is likely to lead to the development of significant myopia later.

Management of the Posterior Capsule

The advent of vitreous suction cutting devices for removing the center of the posterior capsule and a portion of the anterior vitreous during the initial surgery in young children undergoing cataract surgery dramatically decreased the need for secondary surgery. A primary posterior capsu-

lotomy and anterior vitrectomy during IOL implantation in the pediatric cataract gives the best chance for maintaining a long-term clear visual axis. Neodymium–yttrium aluminum garnet (Nd:YAG) laser posterior capsulotomies are usually necessary in children when the posterior capsule is left intact. Larger amounts of laser energy are often needed compared to adults, and the posterior capsule opening may close, requiring repeated laser treatments or a secondary pars plana membranectomy.

POSTOPERATIVE MANAGEMENT

Medications

When pediatric cataract surgery is performed under general anesthesia, a patch and shield are usually placed over the eye for the first postoperative night. Immediately at the end of surgery, a drop of dilute (5%) Povidone iodine is placed on the operative eye. An antibiotic steroid ointment and atropine ointment are placed on the eye prior to the patch and shield. The eye is examined on the first postoperative day. Topical atropine (0.5% in children <1 year of age and 1% thereafter) is utilized once per day for 2 to 4 weeks. Prednisolone acetate is used topically six times per day for 2 weeks and then three or four times per day for an additional 2 weeks. An antibiotic drop is used for 1 week only. Any residual refractive error is corrected after the wound stabilizes and the synthetic absorbable sutures dissolve. Oral steroids are rarely used by the authors.

Follow-up

The eye patch and shield are removed on the first postoperative day. The use of glasses or the shield during the day and the shield at night is recommended for at least 1 week postoperatively. Postoperative examinations are scheduled at 2 weeks, 4 weeks, 3 months, and 6 months postoperatively. Yearly examinations under anesthesia should be considered in children undergoing cataract surgery to measure intraocular pressure, examine the peripheral retina, monitor eye growth using A-scan ultrasound, and examine the position of the IOL and detect any secondary membrane or aftercataract formation. Once children become old enough and cooperative enough to undergo these examinations awake, the serial examination under anesthesia becomes unnecessary.

MANAGEMENT OF PEDIATRIC TRAUMATIC CATARACTS

Trauma is a common cause of unilateral cataract in children. At the time of presentation after the trauma to the eye, primary repair of a corneal or scleral wound may be needed along with a complete evaluation of damage to the intraocular structures (e.g., posterior capsule rupture, vitreous hemorrhage, and retinal detachment). The authors prefer to defer cataract surgery and IOL implantation in traumatic cataract patients, even when anterior lens capsule has been ruptured. A delay of 1 to 4 weeks may be helpful to allow corneal healing and to reduce the inflammatory response.[13] Longer delays are avoided in children within the amblyopic ages of 0 to 8 years. Implantation of IOL is preferred in the cases of traumatic cataracts with corneal injuries, because contact lenses may be difficult to fit. Placement of the IOL in the capsular bag is preferred when capsular support is available. Ciliary sulcus fixation of the IOL can also be done in the absence of adequate capsule support for in-the-bag placement, but with a greater incidence of uveitis, pupillary capture, etc., as reported in a recent study.[14]

CONCLUSION

In summary, surgical management of cataracts in children is markedly different from that in adults due to numerous reasons. Not only are the eyes smaller because of age but also many are microphthalmic. Decreased scleral rigidity and increased vitreous up-thrust make surgical manipulations within these eyes more difficult. The anterior chamber is often unstable; the capsule management requires special considerations and the propensity for postoperative inflammation is increased. Ocular growth makes selection of an IOL power difficult. Children do not always comply with postoperative instructions. Examinations of the eye after surgery are also often incomplete. The long expected lifespan after surgery for children also deserves consideration when surgical decisions are made. These special patients are uniquely challenging. The best surgical techniques for children will evolve most efficiently with optimal cooperation and collaboration between pediatric ophthalmologists and adult cataract surgeons. Our rec-

ommendations for a step-by-step approach to pediatric cataract–IOL surgery summarized in this chapter may be useful for surgeons and help to fine-tune pediatric cataract–IOL surgery.

REFERENCES

1. Wilson ME. Pediatric cataract surgery. In: Chang DF, ed. *Ophthalmic Hyperguides*. Thorofare, NJ: Slack, 2002 (www.ophthalmic.hyperguides.com).
2. Wilson ME, Pandey SK, Werner L, et al. Pediatric cataract surgery: current techniques, complications and management. In: Agarwal S, Agarwal A, Sachdev MS, Mehta KR, Fine IH, Agarwal A, eds., *Phacoemulsification, Laser Cataract Surgery and Foldable IOLs*. New Delhi: Jaypee Brothers, 2000:369–388.
3. Pandey SK, Wilson ME, Trivedi RH, et al. Pediatric cataract surgery and intraocular lens implantation: current techniques, complications and management. *Int Ophthalmol Clin* 2001;41:175–196.
4. Gimbel HV, Sun R, DeBrouff BM. Recognition and management of internal wound gape. *J Cataract Refract Surg* 1995;21:121–124.
5. Basti S, Krishnamachary M, Gupta S. Results of sutureless wound construction in children undergoing cataract extraction. *J Pediatr Ophthalmol Strabismus* 1996;l33:52–54.
6. Wilson ME. Anterior capsule management for pediatric intraocular lens implantation. *J Pediatr Ophthalmol Strabismus* 1999;36:1–6.
7. Vasavada AR, Trivedi RH, Apple DJ, et al. Randomized, clinical trial of multiquadrant hydrodissection in pediatric cataract surgery. *Am J Ophthalmol* 2003;135:84–88.
8. Wilson ME. Intraocular lens implantation: Has it become the standard of care for children? (Editorial). *Ophthalmology* 1996;103:1719–1720.
9. Wilson ME, Elliott L, Johnson B, et al. AcrySof™ acrylic intraocular lens implantation in children: Clinical indications of biocompatibility. *J AAPOS* 2001;5:377–380.
10. Trivedi RH, Wilson ME Jr. Single-piece acrylic intraocular lens implantation in children. *J Cataract Refract Surg* 2003;29:1738–1743.
11. Gordon RA, Donzis PB. Refractive development of the human eye. *Arch Ophthalmol* 1985;103:785–789.
12. McClatchey SK, Dahan E, Maselli E, et al. A comparison of the rate of refractive growth in pediatric aphakic and pseudophakic eyes. *Ophthalmology* 2000;107:118–122.
13. Peterseim MM, Pandey SK, Wilson ME, et al. Outcome of traumatic cataract surgery and intraocular lens implantation in children. Presented at the AAPOS Meeting, Orlando FL, March 2001.
14. Pandey SK, Ram J, Werner L, et al. Visual results and postoperative complications of capsular bag versus sulcus fixation of posterior chamber intraocular lenses for traumatic cataract in children. *J Cataract Refract Surg* 1999;25:1576–1584.

Chapter 57

My Preferred Approach

M. Edward Wilson, Jr. and Rupal H. Trivedi

For this chapter, we have invited 11 of the world's most experienced pediatric cataract surgeons to share with us their individual "preferred approach" to surgery on children. Four of the surgeons are pediatric ophthalmologists from the United States (Dr. Al Biglan from Pittsburgh, Pennsylvania; Dr. Earl Crouch from Norfolk, Virginia; Dr. Scott Lambert from Atlanta, Georgia; and Dr. David Plager from Indianapolis, Indiana). One surgeon, Dr. Sam Masket, is an adult cataract surgeon from Los Angeles, California. Our international surgeons represent a wide and diverse geography: Dr. David BenEzra is from Israel; Dr. Elie Dahan is from South Africa; Dr. Michael O'Keefe is from Ireland; Dr. Abhay Vasavada is from India; Dr. David Yorston is from Kenya; and Dr. Charlota Zetterstom is from Sweden.

We asked each of our surgeons to fill in the appropriate information regarding the following 10 aspects of pediatric cataract surgery.

1. What is your preoperative routine?
2. What incision do you use? Is it closed with sutures?
3. How do you make the anterior capsulotomy?
4. What viscosurgical device do you prefer?
5. How do you remove the lens contents? Include machine settings if applicable.
6. What IOL size, material, brand do you prefer?
7. Do you implant all children? Or only children above a certain age? Any contraindication to IOL?
8. How do you handle the posterior capsule?
9. When do you perform anterior vitrectomy?
10. Describe your postoperative medication and follow-up schedule.

The responses were edited slightly for formatting, but the content was left as submitted. At the end of the chapter, we provide some summary comments to point out areas of agreement among and areas of disagreement between our guest experts. You will find pearls throughout the surgeons' responses that will help you to develop your own preferred approach.

*Dr. BenEzra

Preoperative routine: Tropicamide 0.5% and Cyclogyl 1% (two drops), three times before surgery.

Incision: Two ports initially (1.2 mm each). One for the anterior chamber maintainer, the other for the ocutome device. The wound is enlarged to 3.2 mm if soft lens IOL is inserted (no sutures). The wound is enlarged to 5.5 mm if PMMA IOL lens is inserted (two or three 10-0 sutures).

Anterior capsulotomy: I use the ocutome, a round capsulectomy.

Viscosurgical device: I use only viscoelastic for insertion of the IOL. I use Healon or Biolon.

Lens removal: I use a linear cutting and aspiration device set according to evolving needs and the lens constitution. Prefer either the Storz Premiere or the Alcon Accurus.

IOL preference: PMMA (Hanita or AOL), Acrylic (Alcon).

Implantation inclusions and exclusions: I implant all children, provided they are 6 weeks of age or older. The only contraindication is a child younger than 6 weeks or the parents (after thorough explanation) are against the use of IOL and willing to use contact lenses.

Posterior capsule management: I perform a round posterior capsulectomy using the same instrument (ocutome-type vitrector) as for the anterior capsulectomy and aspiration of the lens material.

Anterior vitrectomy: After the posterior capsulectomy and before the IOL insertion.

Post operative medication:
1. Tropicamide 0.5% × 2/d for 3 weeks;
2. Gentamycin 0.3% × 4/d for 2 weeks;
3. Dexamycin drops × 6/d for one week decreasing the dosage by one drop/day each following week. Total use for 6 weeks post operation;
4. Dexamycin ointment × 1/d for 3 weeks.

Routine Follow-up:
1. The day following surgery;
2. One week after surgery, perform refraction and prescribe correction as needed;
3. One month after surgery;
4. Three months after surgery; refraction and adaptation of the correction.
5. Six months after surgery. Bifocals are prescribed if needed
6. Twelve months after surgery.

*Dr. Biglan

Preoperative routine: My preoperative routine includes a history of the pregnancy and birth followed by a careful assessment of the morphology, density, and location of the lens opacity. Care is taken to identify lens subluxation or any dehiscence in the posterior lens capsule. Children with monocular cataracts are not evaluated with ancillary testing. Children with bilateral cataracts or cataracts that are progressive without a positive family history will receive evaluation with a urine test for reducing substances and amino acids. If there is dysmorphology, genetic evaluation will be obtained. During the office visit, other children and, if available, relatives will have their lenses evaluated when indicated. The horizontal diameters of both corneas are measured. Keratometry is also performed on both eyes. The extent of the cataract and the effect that the opacity has on visual acuity is estimated based on the size and density of the cataract. If the child is old enough to cooperate, age-appropriate recognition acuities will be obtained. I sketch a diagram in the clinical record to document the location, morphology, and density of the opacity. The intraocular pressure is measured and an attempt is made to visualize the optic nerve, fovea, and retinal structures. If age and cooperation permit, obtain contact A scan biometry (without immersion). I use both the Holladay and the SRK II formulae to calculate the power of the IOL. For children unable to cooperate, these tests are performed in the operating room, just prior to the procedure. Since I have an interest in the growth of the eye and related structures during early childhood, measurements are routinely obtained for both eyes. A date for surgery will be selected and if an intraocular lens is going to be used, appropriate consent is obtained. Outpatient surgery is performed on all patients older than one month. Those children who are younger than one month of age are observed overnight by our anesthesia department. The child is brought to a "holding area" outside of the operating room where the child is allowed to be with the parents until the room is ready to accept the child. When the room is prepared, the child is brought to the operating room and placed under general anesthesia. As soon as the child is anesthetized, I instill a drop each of 1% or 2% Cyclogyl and 2.5%

phenylephrine into each eye. This is repeated five minutes later. Following endotracheal intubation, keratometry is performed using a Nidek handheld keratometer to measure the central corneal curvature. Intraocular pressures are then measured using a Perkins applanation tonometer, a Tonopen, and a Schiotz tonometer. Following this, an A-scan is performed. If the posterior segment is not able to be visualized, a B-scan will also be performed. If a rigid gas-permeable contact lens is going to be used, it is fit with a trial set of single-cut aphakic lenses with varying posterior curvatures. The lenses are fit with fluorescein and a cobalt blue light to assess the lens fit. Prior to commencing, a "time out" is taken to review the procedure and site of surgery with the entire operative team. The eye is prepped with 5% Betadine solution and a drop of Betadine is instilled into the cul-de-sac. The lashes are sequestered with an adhesive barrier drape, and an open-bladed Barraquer lid speculum is inserted.

Incision: I make a two-plane incision in the anterior limbal area using a keratome. The incision site is made at 12 o'clock and the site is prepared with a peritomy of the limbal conjunctivae using a Vannas scissors. Bleeding is controlled with an eraser tip bipolar cautery. The initial incision is approximately 2.0 mm; large enough to insert a bent-tip 25-gauge needle to perform a capsulorrhexis. When a foldable IOL is used, the incision is later opened with the keratome to 3.2 mm. The incision is always sutured closed with a figure-8, 9-0 polygalactin suture (Vicryl).

Anterior capsulotomy: The capsulotomy is performed under Healon or Healon GV using either a bent 25-gauge needle or a fine-tipped capsulorrhexis forceps. If the capsule begins to tear radially, I abandon the capsulorrhexis and proceed with a vitrectorhexis using a coaxial irrigating guillotine-cutting instrument. I avoid hydrodissection. This step has not been found to be useful and can be dangerous if there is a dehiscence in the posterior lens capsule.

Viscosurgical device: Healon, Healon GV.

Lens removal: I prefer to use a single incision and a coaxial irrigation guillotine-cutting instrument to remove the cataract. This tip is a modification of the Ocutome tip. Irrigation fluid is balanced salt, BSS plus with 1 ampule of epinephrine added to the bottle. The bottle height is set at 60 cm. The aspiration pressure is set as a maximum of 240 mm and the cutting speed is set at 300 cuts per minute. The aspiration pressure and irrigation are controlled by the Millennium unit designed by Storz, but upgraded by Bausch & Lomb. Following the capsulotomy, I use the aspiration–irrigation mode to aspirate the central portion of the lens. I try to leave some cortex in front of the posterior lens capsule to prevent inadvertent opening of the posterior lens capsule. During the lensectomy, the cutting mode is used only if lens material occludes the tip or if there is a membrane or the lens has a consistency that does not aspirate well. Once the central portion, or nucleus, has been removed, I use the same tip to begin aspiration of the cortical material. The lens cortex aspirates well and usually delaminates from the capsule. The cortex is engaged by the aspiration port and is drawn to the center of the lens. I am obsessive in removing all lens cortex from the peripheral lens capsule. I use a combination of 45- and 90-degree 0.3 mm aspiration–irrigation tips to achieve complete removal of the lens cortex.

IOL preference: Our group has been using an AcrySof lens manufactured by Alcon. Rather than jumping on the latest lens design or new material or coating, we have tried to standardize the lens we use for consistency in calculations and assessing the results of our surgery. We change the style and material of the IOL as infrequently as possible. We currently use the MA-60 lens, which has a 6 mm optic and is a hydrophobic acrylic product. We are currently evaluating a change to a single-piece, clear acrylic lens inserted using an injector.

Implantation inclusions and exclusions: I remain uncomfortable implanting children with monocular cataracts under 9 to 12 months of age. For children who have bilateral cataracts, I will usually not use an implant until 12 to 14 months of age. In my experience, bilateral cataracts are most common at birth. I am uncomfortable in using bilateral implants in these children. Cataracts that are acquired will usually occur later, usually after 4 or 5 years of age. Most infants with congenital bilateral cataracts still receive a lensectomy and contact lens rehabilitation. The lensectomy is performed in such a manner as to preserve sufficient capsule for a secondary implant if the child becomes contact lens intolerant or when the growth of the eye has stabilized. If prepared well, it is sometimes possible to reopen the capsular bag and insert the secondary implant. Many of these children are now receiving secondary implants in their early teens. The infants that we are currently treating will have the benefits of evolution of products and the possibility of implanting a lens that has the capability to provide improved optical quality or even accommodation. Contraindications for implants are a corneal diameter of less than 9 mm, preexisting glaucoma, and dislocation of the lens.

Posterior capsule management: Following implantation of the lens, I have been using a 20-gauge high-speed vitrectomy instrument slid beneath the displaced lens optic and the anterior leaflet of the lens capsule. I perform a posterior capsulectomy and anterior vitrectomy. If the capsule has a tear or threatens to tear radially, I close the corneal–scleral incision. I then insert a chamber-maintaining port in the peripheral cornea, and then make a separate incision at the pars plana and insert a 20-gauge, high-speed cutting tip to perform a posterior capsulectomy and anterior vitrectomy through the pars plana. If I have difficulty removing the entire lens cortex, or if the pupil does not dilate or a lens is placed in the ciliary sulcus, I will perform an iridotomy.

Anterior vitrectomy: See above

Postoperative medication and follow-up: At the completion of the procedure, I inject 50 mg of cefazolin into the subconjunctival space. At a separate location, I inject Dexamethasone, 0.4 mm/cc. Tobradex solution is applied to the eye and is continued four times a day for 2 weeks. The patient is given a bottle of atropine 1% to bring to the office for possible use. I am using less atropine in the immediate postoperative period than I have in the past.

Patients are seen within 48 hours following the procedure. The eye is shielded for the first 3 days. If there are no complications, children are seen 7 days after the surgery and then every 2 weeks. Refractions are started at 3 weeks following the procedure and once stable (usually within 4 to 5 weeks), a prescription for glasses is provided to the patient. If the child is 2 years of age or older, a bifocal segment is added to the spectacle overcorrection. If a contact lens is used in an infant, the child is refracted within a week of the procedure and a lens is ordered and is delivered following a discussion with the parents on care of the lens and demonstration of appropriate insertion and removal techniques.

*Dr. Crouch

Preoperative routine: My preoperative routine consists of a complete eye exam, including manifest, cycloplegic, and auto refraction; A-scan ultrasound; B-scan ultrasound in the case of dense cataracts; keratometry; and detailed informed consent. Povidine iodide is given at the time of preparation for surgery.

Incision: Preferred incision is posterior scleral beveled or small frown incision with endocapsular fixation. Clear corneal incision is sometimes utilized as well. In active children, the incision is closed with 10-0 nylon sutures.

Anterior capsulotomy: Since 1996, automated mechanical anterior capsulorhexis has been preferred.

Viscosurgical device: I prefer Healon GV viscoelastic.

Lens removal: The lens nucleus and cortex is aspirated with the Alcon mechanical supravitrectomy unit with cutting rate at 200 cycles per minute and aspiration at 400 mm Hg.

IOL preference: The intraocular lens preferred is the foldable acrylic IOL (Acrysof, Alcon Labs, Irvine CA, MA60BM or MA30BA).

Implantation inclusions and exclusions: I do not implant all children. In children older than 12 months, I will implant IOLs in unilateral and bilateral cataracts. In children younger than 12 months, I will have a lengthy informed consent discussion with the parents and obtain written consent on an IRB–approved consent form. Contraindications to IOL: uncontrolled uveitis, uncontrolled glaucoma, PHPV, microphthalmia with corneal diameter less than 10 mm.

Posterior capsule management: The posterior capsule is left intact in patients older than 8 years of age. A YAG capsulotomy can generally be performed in this older age group when indicated. For patients younger than 8 years of age, pars plana posterior capsulotomy and anterior vitrectomy are performed.

Anterior vitrectomy: Anterior vitrectomy is performed with cutting rate at 600 cycles per minute and aspiration at 200 mm Hg.

Postoperative medication and follow-up: Patients are treated postoperatively with topical 1% prednisolone acetate every 4 hours for 4 weeks, topical 1% cyclopentolate hydrochloride once daily for 4 weeks, and Ocuflox ophthalmic every 4 hours for 2 weeks. No systemic steroids are prescribed. Postoperative cycloplegic refractions are performed at 4 weeks and 8 weeks. Any residual refractive error is corrected with glasses or contact lens. If fixation preference or two lines visual acuity difference is observed, amblyopia therapy is instituted.

*Dr. Dahan

Preoperative routine: The preoperative routine includes: pregnancy history (illnesses, use of drugs), family history (to determine if the cause is a genetic condition or the case is sporadic), complete check up by a pediatrician (bloods according to pediatrician request), full ophthalmic examination (if necessary under general anaesthetic), B-mode and A-mode ultrasound of both eyes (to detect relative microphthalmia), and biometry of both parents (to predict an approximate value of the future adult IOL power).

Incision: I prefer a limbal incision and for that purpose I disinsert the conjunctiva to uncover the surgical limbus. The incision starts at the surgical limbus as a 3 mm tunnel into clear cornea, long enough to accommodate a 5.7 mm PMMA optic. I close my incision tightly with a minimum of 3 separate 10-0 nylon sutures with buried knots. Children's wounds tend to dehisce easily, especially if the patient rubs his operated eye. Unsutured clear corneal incisions are contraindicated in pediatric cases. Postoperative astigmatism due to tight sutures is not an issue in pediatric cases because the operated eye first needs amblyopia treatment in the majority of the cases.

Anterior capsulotomy: The anterior capsulotomy can easily be done with a vitrectomy apparatus and a chamber maintainer. It provides a practical controlled manner to achieve the exact size opening. Capsulorrhexis under high viscosity viscoelastic is an alternative, but it is probably an unnecessary surgical procedure. Often the capsulorrhexis size cannot be controlled and it results in anterior capsule phimosis.

Viscosurgical device: I prefer to use the purest type viscoelastic from nonanimal origin (bacterial fermentation, genetic engineering) because of the increased immune reaction in children.

Lens removal: It is relatively easy to use a lens cortex aspiration cannula (Visitec, Katena) on a 2 cc syringe with an anterior chamber maintainer (ACM). The aspiration of the lens cortex is done manually because it provides more control than machine aspiration. Irrigation/aspiration cannula causes A/C collapse and iris prolapse when it is retrieved from the eye. Maintaining a deep A/C with constant irrigation (ACM) throughout the procedure reduces the iatrogenic trauma of the operation.

IOL preference: The overall diameter of a pediatric IOL should be between 10.5 mm and 12 mm. PMMA is still the best material because of its long-proven safety and chemical stability (over 50 years of use with excellent results). Hydrophilic acrylics are second choice. Silicone material should be avoided because of its short history and its lower biocompatibility.

Implantation inclusions and exclusions: In unilateral congenital cataract I implant an IOL from age of 6 weeks as long as the infant weighs more than 3 kg. The power of the IOL should be 80% of the calculation for emmetropia to allow the child to grow into emmetropia later on in adult life and to prevent high myopization. In bilateral equal congenital cataracts, I prefer to implant when the child has reached the age of 2 years as a secondary procedure (PC IOL in the sulcus). The IOL power should be 90% of the calculation for emmetropia. In bilateral congenital cataracts, the primary procedure consists of cataracts aspiration with elective posterior capsulotomy and anterior vitrectomy. Aphakic correction during the first 2 years of life can be done with contact lenses or glasses. This approach is preferred because there is no danger of rivalry amblyopia in bilateral congenital cataract, whereas in unilateral congenital cataract the risk for deep amblyopia is very high. When IOLs are implanted in both eyes in an infant, the risk of uneven surgical results is very high and amblyopia occurs in the less successful eye. Furthermore, a secondary implantation is easily done in a 2-year-old child when the eye is closer to its adult size. In developmental cataracts, I implant when visual acuity is lower than 20/60 in one of the eyes.

Posterior capsulotomy: I do an elective posterior capsulotomy with a vitrectomy apparatus and an ACM in all children younger than 8 years of age. Amblyopia can develop until 8 years of age when capsule opacification occurs and when adequate follow-up fails.

Anterior vitrectomy: I do an elective posterior capsulotomy and elective anterior vitrectomy in all children younger than 8 years of age. Amblyopia can develop until 8 years of age when capsule opacification occurs and when adequate follow-up fails. Posterior capsulotomy alone in children younger than 8 years is not sufficient to prevent visual axis opacification because the anterior vitreous serves as a scaffold for lens fibers to grow on.

Postoperative medication and follow-up: When an ACM is used during pediatric cataract surgery, there is no need for systemic steroids because all the prostaglandins have been washed away and the eye is as quiet as in adult modern cataract surgery. Topical antibiotic/steroids combination every 2 hours for the first 3 days and every 4 hours for the next 2 weeks are sufficient. The patient is seen on day 1, 3, 7, 14, and at 1 month, 2 months, 3 months, and thereafter every 3 months. Temporary corrective glasses are prescribed at day 7 or as soon as the media has cleared. Aggressive amblyopia treatment is initiated as soon as the media is cleared. In unilateral congenital cataracts, half-day occlusion is continued until 5 years of age and gradually reduced to zero at 12 years of age.

*Dr. Lambert

Preoperative routine: I dilate the patients with 1% cyclopentolate and 2.5% neosynephrine.

Incision: I make a 3 mm scleral tunnel superiorly and a paracentesis site. I close the wound with 9-0 vicryl sutures.

Anterior capsulotomy: I make the anterior capsulotomy with Katena forceps, except in infants or children with abnormalities of the anterior capsulotomy—in these children I use the vitreous cutting instrument to make the capsulotomy.

Viscosurgical device: I prefer Healon GV in infants and Healon in older children.

Lens removal: I remove the lens contents with the vitreous cutting instrument (cutting 100, suction either 150 or 200).

IOL preference: I use the Alcon AcrySof SA-60 in children when I implant the lens in the capsular bag. For sulcus fixation I use a Chiron all PMMA lens.

Implantation inclusions and exclusions: I implant all children with normal capsular bags. I do not implant children with ectopia lentis, uveitis, or severe microphthalmos.

Posterior capsulotomy: In children under 5 years of age or children with a posterior capsule opacity I perform a primary posterior capsulotomy with the vitreous cutting instrument. In older children I leave the posterior capsule intact and perform a YAG capsulotomy either in the operating room with a LASIG YAG laser or in the clinic.

Anterior vitrectomy: I perform an anterior vitrectomy in children under 5 years of age.

Postoperative medication and follow-up: I prescribe prednisolone acetate and an antibiotic qid and atropine qd. I usually use the prednisolone for 1 month and the antibiotic for 1 week. I examine patients on postoperative day 1, 7, and 30 and then at 3 months and 6 months. My schedule then varies based on the age of the patient. I continue to see young children every 3 months, whereas I usually see older children annually.

*Dr. O'Keefe

Preoperative routine: There are 3 main considerations in the preoperative assessment of any child for cataract surgery: timing of the operation, simultaneous bilateral surgery, and timing of implant insertion. Timing of surgery is determined by the age of the child; for children 1 year of age and younger, surgery should be done as soon as possible; in infants it should certainly be performed in the first 12 weeks and preferably in the first 4 weeks. In older children, timing is not critical. The second issue in cases of bilateral cataracts is the question of unilateral versus bilateral simultaneous surgery. My preferred option is to do each eye separately, and I perform surgery on the second eye within 1 week of the first. I rarely do bilateral surgery unless there is a serious anaesthetic or medical consideration. The third main consideration is the question of implant insertion. This remains a controversial area in children younger than 1 year of age and sporadically in children younger than 2 years. I do implant the eyes of children who are younger than 1 year of age. Clearly if one decides on this policy, the implant power becomes an important issue. My policy is to make children younger than 1 year about 6 diopters hyperopic, children between 1 and 2 years 3 to 4 diopters hyperopic, children 2 to 5 years 2 diopters hyperopic, and children 6 to 8 years of age about 1 diopters hyperopic. Beyond the age of 8 years old, I try and make them emmetropic. Another major consideration is the assessment of parents and proper counselling. In children left aphakic, parents are instructed on contact lens insertion and its management, and the need for regular follow-up appointments is made clear.

Incision: I make a clear corneal incision at the 12 o'clock position using a keratome knife. At the end of surgery I suture this wound tightly, using 10-0 vicryl sutures.

Anterior capsulotomy: I use the kloti diathermy system to do an anterior capsulotomy, and I make this 5 mm in diameter. In younger children, I rarely do a manual capsulotomy because of the great difficulty and the possibility of a radial tear; in older children this is not a major issue, and it is easier to do a manual capsulotomy.

Viscosurgical device: I use viscoelastic in all patients and at surgery, and I favor Healon GV.

Lens removal: I remove the lens material using a side port incision and bimanual technique using the phaco machine. With this technique I can remove all of the soft lens matter, which I think is a particularly important consideration in younger children. I use heparin 5000 units to 500 mL infusion bottle—yields a concentration of ten IU/mL for intracameral use. I believe this helps to reduce postoperative inflammation.

IOL preference: I have changed from Pharmacia one-piece heparin-coated implant to the AcrySof foldable implant. This has improved my technique because the incision is smaller and I can more easily insert the implant into the capsular bag with the new folding devise for this implant. I believe that the ability to put the implant into the capsular bag does improve the postoperative outcome both in terms of reaction and visual acuity.

Implantation inclusions and exclusions: For 10 years I have used implants in all children irrespective of age. My contraindications to implant insertion include microphthalmic eyes, eyes with other anatomical disorders, and parents who I believe will be poorly compliant with follow-up.

Posterior capsulotomy: Presently I adopt two main approaches to the posterior capsule: in some children I remove the posterior capsule using the kloti diathermy system through the clear corneal incision and then do an anterior vitrectomy. Following this I insert the implant into the capsular bag. Alternatively, I do a clear corneal incision and through this I insert the implant into the capsular bag. I close the wound and through a pars plicata approach I use the vitrector to remove the posterior capsule and do a core vitrectomy. I do an anterior vitrectomy in all children up to the age of 6 years. In children older than 6 years of age I leave the posterior capsule intact because it is less likely to immediately thicken and is easier to open the capsule in an awake child using a YAG laser.

Anterior vitrectomy: See above

Postoperative medication and follow-up: Postoperative management is a very important issue in younger children, particularly in infants up to the age of 1 year and even up to the age of 2. Children up to the age of 1 year all receive intracameral steroids at the end of surgery at a dosage of 250 micrograms into the anterior chamber. Postsurgery, they receive intensive topical steroids in the form of Pred Forte every 2 hours and topical antibiotic about 4 times a day. I administer IV hydrocortisone about 1 mg per kg for 3 days and reduce orally over about 1 week. I dilate all pupils postsurgery. In older children this regime is not necessary. I manage them with a topical steroid drop and the frequency depends on the age of the child. These are continued for the period of 1 month and then reduced to zero. They all receive topical dilating drops for about 2 weeks to mobilize the pupil. All children receive the appropriate glasses to correct the residual refractive change, and I begin patching as soon as possible after surgery. The patching regime is 40% of the waking day for children younger than 1 year old and about 80% of the waking day for children older than 1 year. This is monitored frequently. I perform an annual examination under anaesthesia of all patients up to the age of 5 years of age. This helps to monitor their refractive change, the axial length, their corneal curvature, and intraocular pressure. Capsular opacification is still a significant issue, even in children who have had vitrectomy performed. Although the posterior capsulectomy and vitrectomy has significantly reduced this problem, it is still an issue in younger children. Therefore, one has to be prepared to reopen the capsule using the horizontally mounted YAG laser or by means of a repeat surgical technique through the pars plicata.

Phacoemulsification has transformed our approach to pediatric cataract surgery: it has resulted in small incisions and more complete aspiration of the soft lens material and IOL insertion has become a more acceptable alternative option. As we gain more experience, profound eye growth, choice of implant power, and approach and management of the posterior capsule vitrectomy and of postoperative inflammation are still real issues. Further advances in adjustable implants, refractive techniques, intracameral agents to reduce inflammation and capsular reopacification should result in less morbidity and better visual outcome.

*Dr. Masket

Preoperative routine: Preoperative eye drops are started 2 hours before surgery. Each of the following drops are given four times at $1/2$ hour intervals: Atopine 0.5% (except in Down's syndrome), Cyclogyl 1.0%, phenlyephrine 2.5%, antibiotic (currently Vigamox).

Incision: Incision was originally a superior sclerocorneal tunnel, then sclerocorneal temporal, now back to superior sclerocorneal tunnel 3 mm long by 2.5 mm wide. This placement is based on my unpublished data that indicate a very strong tendency for little induced astigmatism in superior incisions and marked increased WTR astigmatism with temporal incisions. In addition, two paracenteses are created for bimanual removal of cataract. The main incision is used for the capsulorhexis and lens implantation. The incision is closed with 9-0 nylon sutures with knots buried. Smaller sutures often cheese-wire the tissue. Typically I use three sutures and perform an intraoperative Siedel test. Conjunctival closure is accomplished with buried 10-0 vicryl sutures.

Anterior capsulotomy: Anterior capsulotomy is generated with a sharp cystitome for the initial central puncture followed by use of a forceps (Masket) with a centripetal vector. Copious use of Healon 5 allows a very high success rate.

Viscosurgical device: Healon 5 for capsulorhexis and Healon or Healon GV for implantation.

Lens removal: Lens contents are removed in bimanual I/A manner with default settings.

IOL preference: I prefer three-piece hydrophobic acrylic IOLs with square edge design to help retard PCO; I have used primarily Alcon MA60 lenses and more recently the AMO Sensar E.

Implantation inclusions and exclusions: I implant all cases if possible, but my surgery has been limited to patients older than 1 year.

Posterior capsulotomy: The posterior capsule will require a capsulectomy in almost all patients younger than the age of 4 or 5. However, I have a strong preference to leave the capsule intact at the initial surgery, unless the child cannot return for EUA and capsulectomy/vitrectomy at 6 to 12 weeks postoperatively. I have a concern that a primary capsulectomy could tear peripherally and jeopardize the long term success of in the bag implantation. When performed secondarily, I have never encountered a problem, as the capsule has thickened and will not tear. At secondary surgery I enter the pars plana 2.5 mm posterior to the limbus and use the MVR blade to engage the central aspect of the posterior capsule. Next, the vitrectomy hand-piece is used to create a central 4.5 mm capsulectomy with a slow cutting rate and vacuum at 200 mmHg. Infusion is carried out through the limbus with a separate cannula. Next, the vitrector is turned posteriorly and an anterior vitrectomy carried out with a high cutting rate and vacuum at 100 mmHg. Both incisions are closed with absorbable material. Above age 5 to 6 I leave the capsule intact, particularly if the child is amenable to laser capsulotomy.

Anterior vitrectomy: Vitrectomy is always performed if a surgical capsulotomy is required.

Postoperative medication and follow-up: Atropine and steroid/antibiotic ointments are applied along with a patch and shield. One day after surgery, topical steroids (1% prednisolone) and antibiotics are given 6 times daily by drops (if possible). A steroid antibiotic ointment may be used if the parents cannot manage the drops. The antibiotic is discontinued after 1 week, while the steroids are tapered over 6 weeks. I prefer that the child wear the shield nightly for a week or two, varying with age and social setting. Under many circumstances (such as when siblings are also present) I prefer that the shield be worn during the day for a week. The child is followed at 1 day, 1 week, 3 weeks, and 6 weeks to observe healing. Amblyopia is managed as appropriate.

*Dr. Plager

Preoperative routine: Measurements for IOL are taken in the OR at beginning of each case with portable keratometer and A-scan. No preoperative antibiotics or other medications are typically used except for a povidone–iodine prep in the OR.

Incision: I use one of two techniques depending on whether I am planning to do a primary posterior capsulectomy. For children younger than approximately 4 years or in patients with opaque posterior capsules, a vitrectomy instrument is used for the entire procedure—anterior capsulotomy, cortex removal, posterior capsulectomy, and anterior vitrectomy. In this case, the incision is done with a 20 G MVR blade in clear cornea superiorly. A second peripheral cornea incision is made for the infusion cannula. In older children with clear posterior capsules, the incision is a single 2.5 mm superior clear cornea incision that facilitates a manual CCC with forceps and fits the one-piece I/A handpiece. In either case, the incision is enlarged to 3 mm for IOL insertion and closed with one x-shaped 10-0 vicryl suture. I think placement of a suture in these incisions is important in children because their activity level in the immediate post op period may place a self-sealing incision in jeopardy.

Anterior capsulotomy: In children destined for primary posterior capsulectomy/anterior vitrectomy, the anterior capsulotomy is done with the vitrectomy instrument. In older children, the anterior capsulotomy is a CCC with forceps.

Viscosurgical device: I do not have strong preference.

Lens removal: When using the vitrectomy instrument in young children, suction is used variably up to 250 with cutting rate of 250 (used intermittently as needed to clear the port). When using the I/A technique, the aspiration is controlled with the foot pedal as needed. In all cases except for the cutting required of some dense membranes in PHPV eyes or for tough capsules after long standing trauma, aspiration alone is adequate for pediatric lenses. Phacoemulsification is never required.

IOL preference: For most cases, I prefer the Acrysof family of lenses. For in-the-bag placement, the Acrysof SA60AT is very nice—easy to inject securely and reliably in the capsular bag. In the rare case where sulcus fixation is necessary, such as for some secondary IOL placements or in some trauma cases, the Acrysof MA series of lenses with PMMA haptics works well. In cases where the stability of a single-piece IOL is desired, the Pharmacia 722-C is preferred.

Implantation inclusions and exclusions: I tend not to implant IOLs in babies with bilateral cataracts except in special circumstances such as when an unusually informed family specifically requests it or in cases where the follow up is expected to be inadequate for successful contact lenses or glasses (rare). Babies with unilateral cataracts receive an IOL only in cases in which the family is well versed in the relative and potential benefits and disadvantages of this option. Other relative contraindications include eyes that are too small, uveitis (especially due to JRA), or insufficient capsular support.

Posterior capsulotomy: In my experience, the posterior capsule tends to opacify to a visually significant degree in 18 to 24 months on average. Therefore, if I feel the child will not be able to cooperate sufficiently for a YAG capsulotomy within 18 months post operatively, I will do a primary posterior capsulotomy/anterior vitrectomy. In most cases, the capsulectomy/vitrectomy is done through the pars plana after the IOL has been placed in the capsular bag and the anterior incision closed. On occasion, I will do the posterior capsulectomy/vitrectomy through the anterior incision prior to placement of the IOL, but my general preference is not to run the risk of getting vitreous in the anterior chamber.

Anterior vitrectomy: Any time I do a primary posterior capsulotomy, I also do an anterior vitrectomy.

Postoperative medication and follow-up: Subconjunctival steroids are injected only in infants and when there is more than the usual inflammation, such as with some traumatic cataracts. Typical post-op drop regimen includes a topical antibiotic/steroid combination—for example, Tobradex and a topical 1% prednisolone drop, each three times daily for the first week. The drops are then weaned over 1 month or more depending on the inflammatory response. Atropine drops are used PRN—often in infants to keep synechiae from forming and rarely in older children.

*Dr. Vasavada

Preoperative routine: To begin, we cannot overstress the importance of counseling and examination under anesthesia before surgical management. Thorough counseling of parents is extremely helpful. Examination under anesthesia [EUA] with fully dilated pupils is mandatory in both the eyes. It includes examination under operating microscope, tonometry, binocular indirect ophthalmoscopy, keratometry, and axial length measurement. Intraocular lens power is calculated using modified SRK II formula. Topical and systemic antibiotic is started a day prior to surgery. One percent atropine sulfate eyedrops are instilled the night before surgery and in the morning of surgery. Cyclopentolate 1% and phenylephrine 10% eyedrops are instilled three times every hour prior to surgery.

Incision: I make an incision on the steeper meridian based on keratometric readings. I prefer a 3.0 mm in width limbal incision with 2 mm in length internal entry into clear cornea creating a self-sealing valvular incision. In view of the expected low rigidity, I suture the main incision and side-port incisions with 10-0 nylon.

Anterior capsulotomy: I aim for a small anterior capsulorhexis because the elasticity of the pediatric capsule creates an opening that is larger than expected. I use a combination of cystitome and forceps through the main incision to accomplish the capsulorhexis. Initial puncture is made with the cystitome [26-gauge needle] in the center, and a small flap is raised. The flap is grasped by the Utrata forceps, and the rhexis is completed with the forceps. Frequent grasping and regrasping of the flap is essential to control the size of the rhexis. If the capsulorhexis is judged to be small, a definitive larger rhexis is performed.

Viscosurgical device: High viscosity 1.4% sodium hyaluronate (HealonGV or Hyvisc plus) proves indispensable in pediatric cataract surgery. In very intumescent total cataracts, I use Healon 5.

Lens removal: Except in a white mature cataract or a suspected preexisting posterior capsule defect, I perform multiquadrant hydrodissection because it eases the lens aspiration procedure. Lens contents are removed with a bimanual irrigation and aspiration. Separate irrigation and aspiration minimizes the anterior chamber fluctuations and aids in thorough removal of cortex, which is especially crucial in small eyes. Usual machine settings are vacuum 400 mmHg and aspiration flow rate 25 cc per minute (Alcon Legacy 20000) or vacuum 500+ mmHg and aspiration flow rate 25 cc per minute both in linear mode (Alcon Infiniti).

IOL preference: I prefer Acrysof IOL implantation (Alcon). I use single-piece Acrysof with 5.5 mm optic diameter and 12.5 mm overall diameter because the short-size IOLs are not generally available. I believe that adult-size IOLs can cause excessive pressure on uveal structures and produce low-grade uveitis even when they are placed in bag in infants and small children. I feel downsizing of the adult-size IOLs would be of great help in reducing the incidence of uveal inflammation, particularly in children younger than 1 year of age. I had an opportunity of evaluating three-piece short-size Acrysof IOL 10.5 mm overall size/5.5 mm optic, and they worked well.

Implantation inclusions and exclusions: I implant IOL in all age groups—the youngest patient has been 16 days old. It is mandatory to fixate IOL in the bag younger than 1 year of age. Ciliary fixation is a contraindication in the children younger than 1 year. Other contraindications to IOL implantation are microcornea (corneal diameter less than 9.5 mm), microphthalmos (axial length less than 17 mm), preexisting glaucoma, and aniridia.

Posterior capsulotomy: I perform posterior continuous curvilinear capsulorhexis (PCCC) in children up to 8 years old at the time of surgery. The capsule bag and the anterior chamber are filled with high-viscosity sodium hyaluronate. The initial puncture is made with a 26-gauge cystitome. The cystitome engages the central capsule, lifts it toward the surgeon, and at the same time initiates the puncture. A flap is created by grasping the inferior margin of the puncture with Utrata forceps. The flap is then grasped and regrasped with forceps to accomplish a PCCC of about 3.0 mm.

Anterior vitrectomy: I perform anterior vitrectomy in children younger than 2 years of age at the time of surgery. My machine settings are cut rate 400 cuts per minute, AFR 40 cc per minute and vacuum 400 mmHg (Advanced Technology irrigation ocutome probe, Alcon Legacy 20,000) or cut rate 800 cuts per minute, AFR 40 cc per minute and vacuum 400 mmHg (Alcon Infiniti). The vitrectomy probe is kept steady with the port directed posteriorly within the area of PCCC. A central anterior vitrectomy with a depth of about 2 mm is adequate. With Acrysof implantation, I do not perform anterior vitrectomy along with PCCC in children older than 2 years of age. However, these children need to be followed-up carefully. The rate of visual axis obscuration without vitrectomy is about 25%.

Postoperative medication and follow-up: Postoperative treatment comprises prednisolone acetate 1% eyedrops and ciprofloxacin 0.3% eyedrops six times a day tapered over 3 months, Timolol maleate 0.25% eyedrops twice a day for 1 month, Ketorolac tromethamine 0.3% eyedrops three times a day for 1 month, and cyclopentolate 1% eyedrops twice a day for 2 weeks—once at night for 2 weeks and alternate days for 2 weeks. The patients are followed up on the first postoperative day and at 1 month, 6 months, and every 6 months thereafter. We have appointed a secretarial person to look after the follow-up schedule and ensure that the patient is followed up at the scheduled period. This has given a very satisfactory follow-up rate.

*Dr. Yorston

Preamble: Some of our standard practice differs from the experience of surgeons in Europe and North America, so I will give a brief description of our working environment. Kikuyu Eye Unit is the largest eye clinic in East Africa. It is very well equipped by the standards of most African eye clinics. However, compared to tertiary care centers in wealthy countries, our resources are very limited. For example, the only available IOL is a single-piece PMMA lens, with an overall diameter of 12.5 mm. We have no specialist pediatric anesthetist. Our only viscoelastic is hydroxypropyl methylcellulose (HPMC). Spectacle frames suitable for infants and young children are difficult to obtain. Many of our patients travel long distances to obtain treatment but are unable to afford regular return journeys for follow-up. The average annual income in Kenya is $340 per person. Because of the poverty and the lack of specialist eye clinics, many patients present late. It is not unusual to see a 3-year-old child who has had dense cataracts since birth, but who has never previously seen an ophthalmologist. A typical presentation would be a 6-month-old infant with bilateral dense cataracts since birth. Unless otherwise stated, this is the patient being treated in the following paragraphs.

Preoperative routine: The most important element is to counsel the family so that they realize the necessity of follow-up and understand that surgery is the beginning of treatment and not the end of it. The child is admitted with the mother, and they share a bed—as is customary in East Africa. In older children, biometry is performed. In infants, biometry is carried out after the child is anesthetized. Topical steroids (Predsol 1%) and antibiotics (gentamicin 0.3%) are started the day before surgery.

Incision: The main incision is a scleral tunnel; however, two 20 G corneal incisions are made for the AC-maintainer and the vitrectomy probe. Because of the elasticity of the infant sclera, and the risk of trauma, all wounds, including the 20 G corneal incisions, are closed with interrupted 10-0 nylon sutures. The corneal sutures are usually removed at 1 week.

Anterior capsulotomy: In older children with a lamellar cataract, I attempt a continuous curvilinear capsulorhexis, using a bent 25-gauge needle under HPMC. In an infant with a mature cataract, I would perform the anterior capsulectomy with a vitrector, as described by Dr. Wilson.

Viscosurgical device: We only have HPMC.

Lens removal: I insert an AC maintainer through a 20 G stab incision in the superonasal cornea. I then insert the vitrector through an inferotemporal 20 G corneal stab incision. After removing the anterior capsule with a high suction and low cutting speed, I use suction alone to extract the lens matter. There is usually some lens matter remaining behind the inferotemporal incision. This can be reached via the main superior scleral tunnel.

IOL preference: We import low-cost ($3) single-piece PMMA IOLs from India. These are manufactured to a high quality and have been tested at the Storm Eye Institute. The same design of IOL is used for all our patients. The optic diameter is 6 mm, and the overall diameter is 12.5 mm. The IOL is available in 0.5 D steps from 10 D to 30 D. We have had some experience of using acrylic IOLs, and these appear to carry a lower risk of postoperative fibrin formation. However, they are currently too expensive for widespread use in Africa. We have also used single-piece HEMA lenses ("Iogel"). However, we found late dislocation was a problem with these IOLs, and they are no longer manufactured.

Implantation inclusions and exclusions: We do not operate on children younger than 3 months old, as we do not have adequate anesthetic facilities to guarantee their safety. We would consider an IOL in all children older than 3 months. The major contraindication is microphthalmos. If the corneal diameter is less than 9 mm, I would not implant an IOL. If it is less than 10 mm, I would be cautious about IOL insertion. Other contraindications include absence of adequate capsular support or chronic uveitis. I would use an IOL in a traumatic cataract, providing there was sufficient capsule remaining. Because we do not have highly viscous viscoelastics, such as Healon GV, and because we are using a rigid 12.5 mm IOL, we have found that attempts to place the IOL in the capsular bag usually lead to asymmetric fixation in infantile cataract. We place the haptic in the sulcus, and then push the optic backwards through the posterior capsulectomy. This keeps the IOL central and prevents pupil capture of the implant. In older children we would place the IOL in the capsular bag.

Posterior capsulotomy: In children younger than 5 years of age, or in any child in whom follow-up is likely to be impossible, we would perform a primary posterior capsulectomy. We usually do this with a vitrector prior to inserting the IOL. In older children, in whom it may be possible to insert the IOL in the capsular bag, the posterior capsulectomy is performed through the pars plana, 3 mm posterior to the limbus, after the IOL has been inserted. We have found that needle capsulotomies are often inadequate in the long term and seriously compromise the view of the posterior segment.

Anterior vitrectomy: As a routine when a primary posterior capsulectomy is performed. If we wish to leave the posterior capsule intact, I try to avoid disturbing the vitreous as well.

Postoperative medication and follow-up: Over 30% of our patients develop fibrinous uveitis. African children are at particularly high risk of uveitis following cataract surgery and lens implantation. We keep them on topical prednisolone sodium phosphate 1% every 2 hours for 1 week and daily cyclopentolate 0.5% or 1%. At 1 week after surgery we carry out an examination under anesthesia and remove any corneal sutures. The second eye is usually operated on at the same time. Because we have found amblyopia to be much more common in the second eye, we now routinely occlude the first eye following surgery until the second eye is operated. The frequency of review depends on the child's age. Up to 1 year of age, we prefer to see the child, and refract them, every 3 months. From 1 to 2 years of age, they are seen every 4 months. From 2 to 5 they are seen every 6 months. Over 5 years of age, an annual follow-up is sufficient. If they develop amblyopia, then the better eye is occluded according to a schedule based on the child's age. During the occlusion treatment, they are likely to require more frequent review. Family members are taught to provide visual stimulation, and to encourage the child to use their sight as much as possible. If there is a residual visual impairment (which is common in view of the late presentation) additional support is provided to ensure that the children receive the best possible education for their level of visual

function. The outcomes of these techniques have been published:

Yorston, D., Foster A., and Wood, M. Results of cataract surgery in young children in East Africa. *Br J Ophthalmol.* 2001;85:267–271.
Gradin D, Yorston D. Results of IOL implantation in traumatic cataract in children. *J Cat Ref Surg.* 2001;27:2017–2025.

*Dr. Zetterström

Preoperative routine: Combination drops of cyclopentolate and phenylephrine.
Incision: Corneal closed with a 10-0 nylon suture.
Anterior capsulotomy: Bent needle and capsulorhexis forceps.
Viscosurgical device: Healon GV.
Lens removal: With aspiration–irrigation.
IOL preference: One-piece Acrysof from Alcon, the new yellow one to protect the maculae in the future.
Implantation inclusions and exclusions: I implant all children but newborns with bilateral cataract operated on during their first days of life.
Posterior capsulotomy: Posterior rhexis same as the anterior.
Anterior vitrectomy: In all cases under the age of 6 to 7 years old and cases with cataract because of uveitis.
Postoperative medication and follow-up: Depending on age, more drops and more extensive follow-up in younger patients.

SUMMARY

Pediatric cataract surgery continues to change and evolve. Our expert surgeons have given us their preferences as of 2004, when they answered the questions posed. This is as up-to-date as possible. With that said, however, these progressive surgeons are always looking for ways to improve their technique. The reader is urged to contact the authors of this book or any of the surgeons listed in this chapter when questions arise about whether to incorporate a new technique or a new device into the pediatric protocol.

We will now summarize the opinions of the surgeons and give our perspective on their answers. For the preoperative routine, most surgeons use dilating drops before surgery and apply povidone iodine during the preoperative prep. Dr. Yorston uses preoperative gentamicin. Dr. Masket uses preoperative Vigamox (Alcon). A comprehensive eye examination of the child, either in the clinic or in the operating room, is needed to help categorize the cataract type, which is related to the cataract etiology, and to detect other eye abnormalities that may be associated with the cataract. Dr. Biglan recommends also examining the other children in the family and any relatives who are available. Likewise, Dr. O'Keefe emphasized examining the parents of any child with a cataract. Dr. Dahan goes one step further by recommending biometry (globe axial length and keratometry) on the parents to help predict the growth of the eye in the child. This can aid the selection of an IOL power.

The surgeons are split between clear corneal tunnels and limbal/scleral tunnels for incision preference. Most operate from a superior approach, although Dr. Vasavada states that he prefers an incision on the steeper "K" reading obtained during keratometry. All reported using sutures to close the incisions. Dr. BenEzra sutures a 5.5 mm incision used to insert a PMMA IOL but does not suture a 3 mm incision used to insert a foldable IOL. For all the others, each incision is closed with either 10-0 (nine surgeons) or 9-0 (two surgeons) sutures of vicryl or nylon.

The most commonly used anterior capsulotomy technique for younger children, among our experts, was the vitrectorhexis (six surgeons). Drs. Masket, Vasavada, and Biglan use the manual capsulorhexis at all ages, although Dr. Biglan specifically stated that he converts to a vitrectorhexis if he has problems with the manual capsulorhexis. Dr. O'Keefe prefers the Kloti diathermy capsulotomy at all ages. Most of the other surgeons use a manual anterior capsulorhexis in older children and a vitrectorhexis in younger children.

Various viscosurgical devices were listed by our surgeons. Healon GV seems to be the most commonly used, followed by "regular" Healon. Dr. Masket has now started using Healon 5 for the IOL insertion step, and Dr. Vasavada stated that he uses Healon 5 when faced with a total cataract in a child.

The vitrector handpiece or bimanual irrigation–aspiration hand-pieces are used most often for removing the substance of the cataract in a child. Dr. Dahan, however, prefers a manual cannula for this step. Drs. Dahan and Yorston use PMMA IOLs for children preferentially.

Dr. BenEzra uses either a PMMA or an acrylic IOL. The others use the hydrophobic acrylic AcrySof (Alcon) IOL. In the AcrySof family of lenses the single-piece SA series and the single-piece "blue-blocker" SN series are very popular for in-the-bag placement in children. Several surgeons mentioned switching to a PMMA IOL if the sulcus, rather than the capsular bag, was being utilized for fixation.

IOLs are implanted by all of our expert surgeons when a child is operated at age 12 months or older. Drs. Benezra, Dahan, Lambert, O'Keefe, Vasavada, and Yorston also recommend IOLs in very young infants. Dr. Plager implants very young infants if their cataract is unilateral but prefers to manage bilateral neonatal cataracts by leaving the eyes aphakic initially. Dr. Biglan will implant an IOL unilaterally at 9 months of age but reserves bilateral IOL implantation for children 12 months of age and older. Dr. Crouch preserves to implant IOLs only at age 12 months or older whether the cataracts are unilateral or bilateral. Interestingly, Dr. Vasavada states that IOLs should never be placed in the ciliary sulcus in infancy. Yet, Dr. Yorston reports that he always places IOLs in the ciliary sulcus when implanting infants.

The majority of our expert surgeons perform a posterior capsulotomy and an anterior vitrectomy when cataracts are removed from patients younger than 5 years of age. Drs. Crouch and Vasavada extend the posterior capsulotomy up to age 8 years. Dr. Dahan performs a YAG laser posterior capsulotomy in the operating room. Dr. Masket prefers a staged procedure in which the posterior capsulotomy is performed through the pars plana 6 to 12 weeks after the primary cataract surgery. Topical steroids are given by most of our surgeons for 4 weeks after surgery. Dr. Vasavada continues postoperative medications for 3 months. Dr. Dahan prefers only 2 weeks with 3 days of postoperative topical steroids.

Articles Relevant to Pediatric Cataracts Published by the Editors in Peer-Reviewed Journals

1. **Wilson ME Jr,** Bluestein EC, Wang XH. Current trends in the use of intraocular lenses in children. *J Cataract Refract Surg* 1994;20:579–583.

2. **Wilson ME Jr,** Apple DJ, Bluestein EC, Wang XH. Intraocular lenses for pediatric implantation: biomaterials, designs, and sizing. *J Cataract Refract Surg* 1994;20:584–591.

3. **Wilson ME Jr,** Bluestein EC, Wang XH, Apple DJ. Comparison of mechanized anterior capsulectomy and manual continuous capsulorhexis in pediatric eyes. *J Cataract Refract Surg* 1994;20:602–606.

4. Wang XH, **Wilson ME Jr,** Bluestein EC, Auffarth G, Apple DJ. Pediatric cataract surgery and intraocular lens implantation techniques: a laboratory study. *J Cataract Refract Surg* 1994;20:607–609.

5. Bluestein EC, **Wilson ME Jr,** Wang XH, Rust PF, Apple DJ. Dimensions of the pediatric crystalline lens: implications for intraocular lenses in children. *J Pediatr Ophthalmol Strabismus* 1996;33:18–20.

6. **Wilson ME Jr,** Saunders RA, Roberts EL, Apple DJ. Mechanized anterior capsulectomy as an alternative to manual capsulorhexis in children undergoing intraocular lens implantation. *J Pediatr Ophthalmol Strabismus* 1996;33:237–240.

7. **Wilson ME Jr.** Intraocular lens implantation: Has it become the standard of care for children? *Ophthalmology* 1996;103:1719–1720.

8. Andreo LK, **Wilson ME Jr,** Saunders RA. Predictive value of regression and theoretical IOL formulas in pediatric intraocular lens implantation. *J Pediatr Ophthalmol Strabismus* 1997;34:240–243.

9. Hutchinson AK, **Wilson ME Jr,** Saunders RA. Outcomes and ocular growth rates after intraocular lens implantation in the first 2 years of life. *J Cataract Refract Surg* 1998;24:846–852.

10. Andreo LK, **Wilson ME Jr,** Apple DJ. Elastic properties and scanning electron microscopic appearance of manual continuous curvilinear capsulorhexis and vitrectorhexis in an animal model of pediatric cataract. *J Cataract Refract Surg* 1999;25:534–539.

11. Buckley E, Lambert SR, **Wilson ME Jr.** IOLs in the first year of life. *J Pediatr Ophthalmol Strabismus* 1999;36:281–286.

12. O'Neil JW, Hutchinson AK, Saunders RA, **Wilson ME Jr.** Acquired cataracts after argon laser photocoagulation for retinopathy of prematurity. *J AAPOS* 1998;2:48–51.

13. **Pandey SK,** Ram J, Werner L, Brar GS, Jain AK, Gupta A, Apple DJ. Visual results and postoperative complications of capsular bag and ciliary sulcus fixation of posterior chamber intraocular lenses in children with traumatic cataracts. *J Cataract Refract Surg* 1999;25:1576–1584.

14. Lambert SR, Buckley EG, Plager DA, Medow NB, **Wilson ME Jr.** Unilateral intraocular lens implantation during the first six months of life. *J AAPOS* 1999;3:344–349.

15. Olitsky SE, Waz WR, **Wilson ME Jr.** Rupture of the anterior lens capsule in Alport syndrome. *J AAPOS* 1999;3:381–382.

16. **Wilson ME Jr,** Englert JA, Greenwald MJ. In-the-bag secondary intraocular lens implantation in children. *J AAPOS* 1999;3:350–355.

17. **Wilson ME Jr,** Anterior capsule management for pediatric intraocular lens implantation. *J Pediatr Ophthalmol Strabismus* 1999;36:314–319.

18. McClatchey SK, Dahan E, Maselli E, Gimbel HV, **Wilson ME Jr,** Lambert SR, Buckley EG, Freedman SF, Plager DA, Parks MM. A comparison of the rate of refractive growth in pediatric aphakic and pseudophakic eyes. *Ophthalmology* 2000;107:118–122.

19. Englert JA, **Wilson ME Jr.** Postoperative intraocular pressure elevation after the use of Healon GV in pediatric cataract surgery. *J AAPOS* 2000;4:60–61.

20. Apple DJ, Ram J, Foster A, Pang Q (**Pandey SK, Trivedi RH, Wilson ME Jr,** documented major contributor). Elimination of cataract blindness: a global perspective entering the new millennium. *Surv Ophthalmol* 2000;45(Suppl 1):S1–S196.

21. Peterseim MW, **Wilson ME Jr.** Bilateral intraocular lens implantation in the pediatric population. *Ophthalmology* 2000;107:1261–1266.

22. Vasavada AR, **Trivedi RH.** Role of optic capture in congenital cataract and intraocular lens surgery in children. *J Cataract Refract Surg* 2000;26:824–831.

23. **Pandey SK,** Werner L, Escobar-Gomez M, Roig-Melo EA, Apple DJ. Dye-enhanced cataract surgery. Part 1. Anterior capsule staining for capsulorhexis in advanced/white cataract. *J Cataract Refract Surg* 2000;26:1052–1059.

24. **Pandey SK,** Werner L, Escobar-Gomez M, Werner LP, Apple DJ. Dye-enhanced cataract surgery. Part 3. Posterior capsule staining to learn posterior continuous curvilinear capsulorhexis. *J Cataract Refract Surg* 2000;26:1066–1071.

25. **Wilson ME Jr.** Intraocular lenses for children in the year 2000: When is oversight by the institutional review board or food and drug administration required? *J AAPOS* 2000;4:325.

26. Donahue SP, Byrne D, **Wilson ME Jr,** Sinha D. Aphakic glaucoma in children. *J AAPOS* 2000;4:389–390.

27. **Wilson ME Jr.** Anterior capsule management for pediatric intraocular lens implantation. *J Pediatr Ophthalmol Strabismus* 1999;36:314–319.

28. Lambert SR, Lynn M, Drews-Botsch C, Loupe D, Plager DA, Medow NB, **Wilson ME Jr,** Buckley EG, Drack AV, Fawcett SL. A comparison of grating visual acuity, strabismus, and reoperation outcomes among children with aphakia and pseudophakia after unilateral cataract surgery during the first six months of life. *J AAPOS* 2001;5:70–75.

29. **Pandey SK,** Werner L, Apple DJ. Staining the anterior capsule. *J Cataract Refract Surg* 2001;27:647–648.

30. **Trivedi RH,** Izak AM, Werner L, Macky TA, **Pandey SK,** Apple DJ. Interlenticular opacification of piggyback intraocular lenses. *Int Ophthalmol Clin* 2001;41:47–62.

31. **Pandey SK, Wilson ME Jr, Trivedi RH,** Izak AM, Macky TA, Werner L, Apple DJ. Pediatric cataract surgery and intraocular lens

implantation: current techniques, complications, and management. *Int Ophthalmol Clin* 2001;41:175–196.

32. **Wilson ME Jr,** Peterseim MW, Englert JA, Lall-Trail JK, Elliott LA. Pseudophakia and polypseudophakia in the first year of life. *J AAPOS* 2001;5:238–245.

33. **Wilson ME, Jr.** The challenge of pediatric cataract surgery *J AAPOS* 2001;5:265–266.

34. Vasavada AR, **Trivedi RH,** Singh R. Necessity of vitrectomy when optic capture is performed in children older than 5 years. *J Cataract Refract Surg* 2001;27:1185–1193.

35. **Wilson ME Jr,** Elliott L, Johnson B, Peterseim MM, Rah S, Werner L, **Pandey SK.** AcrySof acrylic intraocular lens implantation in children: clinical indications of biocompatibility. *J AAPOS* 2001;5: 377–380.

36. Alexandrakis G, Peterseim MM, **Wilson ME Jr.** Clinical outcomes of pars plana capsulotomy with anterior vitrectomy in pediatric cataract surgery. *J AAPOS* 2002;6:163–167.

37. **Pandey SK,** Werner L, **Wilson ME Jr,** Izak AM, Apple DJ. Anterior capsule staining. Techniques, recommendations and guidelines for surgeons. *Indian J Ophthalmol* 2002;50:157–159.

38. **Wilson ME Jr, Pandey SK,** Thakur J. Paediatric cataract blindness in the developing world: surgical techniques and intraocular lenses in the new millennium. *Br J Ophthalmol* 2003;87:14–19.

39. Vasavada AR, **Trivedi RH,** Apple DJ, Ram J, Werner L. Randomized, clinical trial of multiquadrant hydrodissection in pediatric cataract surgery. *Am J Ophthalmol* 2003;135:84–88.

40. Kruger SJ, **Wilson ME Jr,** Hutchinson AK, Peterseim MM, Bartholomew LR, Saunders RA. Cataracts and glaucoma in patients with oculocerebrorenal syndrome. *Arch Ophthalmol* 2003;121: 1234–1237.

41. **Trivedi RH, Wilson ME.** Single-piece acrylic intraocular lens implantation in children. *J Cataract Refract Surg* 2003;29:1738–1743.

42. **Wilson ME Jr,** Bartholomew LR, **Trivedi RH.** Pediatric cataract surgery and intraocular lens implantation: practice styles and preferences of the 2001 ASCRS and AAPOS memberships. *J Cataract Refract Surg* 2003;29:1811–1820.

43. **Wilson ME Jr, Trivedi RH,** Hoxie JP, Bartholomew LR. Treatment outcomes of congenital monocular cataracts: the effects of surgical timing and patching compliance. *J Pediatr Ophthalmol Strabismus* 2003;40:323–329; quiz 353–354.

44. Vasavada AR, Nath VC, **Trivedi RH.** Anterior vitreous face behavior with AcrySof in pediatric cataract surgery. *J AAPOS* 2003;7: 384–388.

45. Lambert SR, Lynn M, Drews-Botsch C, DuBois L, **Wilson ME Jr,** Plager DA, Wheeler DT, Christiansen SP, Crouch ER, Buckley EG, Stager D Jr, Donahue SP. Intraocular lens implantation during infancy: perceptions of parents and the American Association for Pediatric Ophthalmology and Strabismus members. *J AAPOS* 2003;7: 400–405.

46. **Trivedi RH, Wilson ME Jr,** Bartholomew LR, Lal G, Peterseim MM. Opacification of the visual axis after cataract surgery and single acrylic intraocular lens implantation in the first year of life. *J AAPOS* 2004;8:156–164.

47. Vasavada AR, **Trivedi RH,** Nath VC. Visual axis opacification after AcrySof intraocular lens implantation in children. *J Cataract Refract Surg* 2004;30:1073–1081.